Clinical Scenarios in Surgical Oncology

Clinical Scenarios in Surgical Oncology

Editor

Vijay P. Khatri, MD, FACS

Associate Professor of Surgery
University of California, Davis School of Medicine
Davis, California

Division of Surgical Oncology
University of California
Davis Cancer Center
Sacramento, California

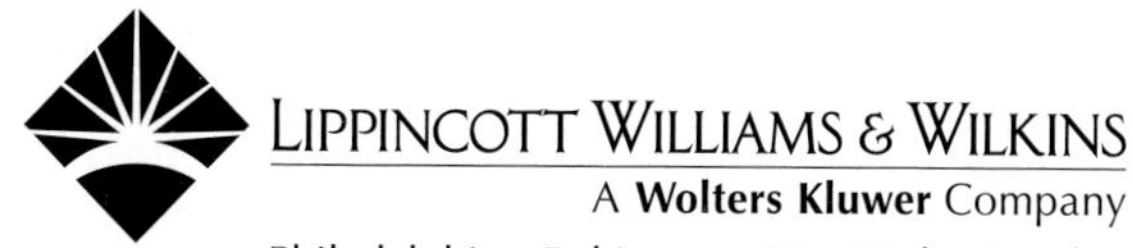

Acquisitions Editor: Brian Brown
Managing Editor: Julia Seto
Project Manager: Fran Gunning
Marketing Manager: Adam Glazer
Manufacturing Manager: Ben Rivera
Design Coordinator: Doug Smock
Production Services: Nesbitt Graphics, Inc.
Printer: Edwards Brothers

Library of Congress Cataloging-in-Publication Data

Clinical scenarios in surgical oncology / editor, Vijay P. Khatri.
    p. ; cm. — (Clinical scenarios in surgery series)
  Includes bibliographical references and index.
  ISBN 0-7817-5466-6 (alk. paper)
  1. Cancer—Surgery—Case studies. I. Khatri, Vijay P. II. Series. [DNLM: 1. Neoplasms—surgery—Case Reports. 2. Diagnostic Techniques, Surgical—Case Reports. 3. Neoplasms—diagnosis—Case Reports. QZ 268 C641 2006]
  RD651.C56 2006
  616.99'4059—dc22
                              2005007328

Clinical Scenarios in Surgery
Clinical Scenarios in Thoracic Surgery
Edited by Robert Kalimi, MD

Clinical Scenarios in Vascular Surgery
Edited by Gilbert R. Upchurch Jr, MD

contents

Contributing Authors xiii

Foreword by Charles M. Balch xx

Foreword by Umberto Veronesi xxiii

Preface xxv

Case 1. Squamous Cell Cancer of the Oral Cavity 1
M. Abraham Kuriakose and Subramanya Iyer

Case 2. Squamous Cell Cancer of the Oropharynx 5
M. Abraham Kuriakose and Subramanya Iyer

Case 3. Squamous Cell Cancer of the Nasopharynx 8
Brigette B.Y. Ma and Anthony T. C. Chan

Case 4. Squamous Cell Cancer of the Larynx 12
Jean-Louis Lefebvre and David Pasquier

Case 5. Squamous Cell Cancer of the Hypopharynx 15
Jean-Louis Lefebvre and David Pasquier

Case 6. Cervical Lymph Node Metastases With Unknown Primary 18
Kerwin F. Shannon and Christopher J. O'Brien

Case 7. Parotid Gland Tumor 23
Kerwin F. Shannon and Christopher J. O'Brien

Case 8. Non-Small Cell Cancer of the Lung (Early and Advanced Stage) 29
Thomas W. Stamp and Alex G. Little

Case 9. Small Cell Cancer of the Lung 32
Frank Detterbeck

Case 10. Pancoast Tumor 36
Alden M. Parsons and Frank Detterbeck

Case 11. Mediastinal Tumors 41
Larry R. Kaiser

Case 12. Solitary Pulmonary Nodule 44
Larry R. Kaiser

Case 13. Pulmonary Metastases 47
Harvey I. Pass

Case 14. Mesothelioma 51
Harvey I. Pass

Case 15. Chest Wall Tumors 59
Antonio Briccoli and Michele Rocca

Case 16. Cervical Esophageal Cancer 63
Simon Law and John Wong

Case 17. Squamous Cell Cancer of the Mid-esophagus 68
Simon Law and John Wong

Case 18. Adenocarcinoma at the Gastroesophageal Junction With
Barrett's Esophagus 74
Andreas Sendler and J. Rüdiger Siewert

Case 19. Gastric Adenocarcinoma 78
Andreas Sendler and J. Rüdiger Siewert

Case 20. Linitis Plastica 83
Andreas Sendler and J. Rüdiger Siewert

Case 21. Gastric Lymphoma 87
Vinod Narra and Stephen R. T. Evans

Case 22. Gastrointestinal Stromal Tumor of the Stomach 90
Toshirou Nishida

Case 23. Duodenal Adenocarcinoma 95
Keith D. Lillemoe and Alyssa D. Wait

Case 24. Small Bowel Adenocarcinoma 98
Hiromichi Ito and Edward E. Whang

Case 25. Distal Ileal Carcinoid Tumor 101
Eric Benoit and Edward E. Whang

Case 26. Gastrointestinal Stromal Tumor of the Small Bowel 106
Vijay P. Khatri

Case 27. Appendiceal Carcinoid 111
Arnold C. Goede and Marc C. Winslet

Case 28. Pseudomyxoma Peritonei 114
Paul H. Sugarbaker

Case 29. Malignant Colon Polyp 119
Paris P. Tekkis and John M. A. Northover

Case 30. Early Colon Carcinoma 123
Shingo Tsujinaka and Steven D. Wexner

Case 31. Locally Advanced Colon Carcinoma 126
Susan M. Cera and Steven D. Wexner

Case 32. Colon Carcinoma With Synchronous Hepatic Metastases 131
Vijay P. Khatri

Case 33. Proximal Rectal Adenocarcinoma 136
Christoph A. Maurer and Emanuel Burri

Case 34. Distal Rectal Adenocarcinoma 140
Christoph A. Maurer and Emanuel Burri

Case 35. Rectal Adenocarcinoma With Pelvic Sidewall/Bladder Invasion 146
Kimberly A. Varker and Harold J. Wanebo

Case 36. Recurrent Rectal Cancer 150
Kimberly A. Varker and Harold J. Wanebo

Case 37. Rectal Carcinoid 155
Arnold C. Goede and Marc C. Winslet

Case 38. Rectal/Pelvic Gastrointestinal Stromal Tumor 159
Toshirou Nishida

Case 39. Squamous Cell Cancer of the Anal Canal 165
Vivek Chaudhry and Herand Abcarian

Case 40. Anal Margin Squamous Cell Cancer 170
Vivek Chaudhry and Herand Abcarian

Case 41. Anal Melanoma 173
Merrick I. Ross and Matthew T. Ballo

Case 42. Hepatoma With Cirrhosis 178
Norihiro Kokudo and Masatoshi Makuuchi

Case 43. Management of Solitary Liver Lesions 183
Vijay P. Khatri and Henri Bismuth

Case 44. Colorectal Liver Metastases 188
Brendan C. Visser and Robert S. Warren

Case 45. Neuroendocrine Liver Metastases 194
Bernard Meunier and Bernard Launois

Case 46. Gallbladder Carcinoma 199
Yoshio Shirai and Katsuyoshi Hatakeyama

Case 47. Hilar Cholangiocarcinoma 203
Vijay P. Khatri and Henri Bismuth

Case 48. Intrahepatic Cholangiocarcinoma 209
Bernard Meunier and Bernard Launois

x Contents

Case 49. Periampullary/Pancreatic Head Carcinoma 214
Keith D. Lillemoe and Alyssa D. Wait

Case 50. Cystic Neoplasm of the Pancreas 217
James M. Kiely and Henry A. Pitt

Case 51. Early Invasive Breast Cancer 223
Susan S. Chang and Armando E. Giuliano

Case 52. Locally Advanced Breast Cancer 228
Robyn M. Moncrief and Monica Morrow

Case 53. Inflammatory Breast Cancer 232
Robyn M. Moncrief and Monica Morrow

Case 54. Locally Recurrent Breast Cancer 236
Lloyd A. Mack and Walley J. Temple

Case 55. Breast Cancer During Pregnancy 241
John T. Vetto

Case 56. High-Risk Patient With Lobular Carcinoma in Situ 245
Helen Krontiras and Kirby I. Bland

Case 57. Ductal Carcinoma in Situ 249
Samuel W. Beenken and Kirby I. Bland

Case 58. Paget's Disease of the Breast 253
Emiel J. Rutgers

Case 59. Axillary Metastases With Unknown Breast Primary 257
Maureen A. Chung and Blake Cady

Case 60. Male Breast Cancer 261
Stefano Zurrida and Giovanna Gatti

Case 61. Extremity Soft Tissue Sarcoma 265
Vijay P. Khatri

Case 62. Retroperitoneal Sarcoma 273
Vijay P. Khatri

Case 63. Chondrosarcoma of the Pelvis 279
Martin M. Malawer and Kristen Kellar Graney

Case 64. Osteosarcoma of the Humerus 286
Martin M. Malawer and Kristen Kellar Graney

Case 65. Ewing's Sarcoma of the Femur 293
Robert W. Rödl

Case 66. Chordoma 299
Alessandro Gronchi and Marco Fiore

Case 67. Cutaneous Melanoma 303
Julie R. Lange and Charles M. Balch

Case 68. Recurrent In-Transit Melanoma 307
Douglas L. Fraker

Case 69. Melanoma Presenting With Regional Lymph Node Metastases 311
Michael S. Sabel and Vernon K. Sondak

Case 70. Merkel Cell Carcinoma 316
Michael S. Sabel and Vernon K. Sondak

Case 71. Squamous Cell Cancer of the Skin 321
Marlyanne M. Pol-Rodriguez and Désirée Ratner

Case 72. Basal Cell Cancer of the Skin 330
Adam Ian Rubin and Désirée Ratner

Case 73. Kaposi Sarcoma in Acquired Immunodeficiency Syndrome 335
A. Marini and Ulrich Hengge

Case 74. Pheochromocytoma 339
Bertil Hamberger and Anna-Lena Hjelm-Skog

Case 75. Management of Incidental Adrenal Lesion .343
Jeffrey A. Norton

Case 76. Gastrinoma 347
Jeffrey A. Norton

Case 77. Insulinoma 350
Jeffrey A. Norton

Case 78. Well-Differentiated Thyroid Carcinoma (Papillary and
Follicular Carcinoma) 354
Ashok R. Shaha and Vijay P. Khatri

Case 79. Medullary Carcinoma of the Thyroid 362
Jeffrey F. Moley

Case 80. Parathyroid Adenoma 365
Julie Ann Sosa and Robert Udelsman

Case 81. Parathyroid Carcinoma 369
Sanziana A. Roman and Robert Udelsman

Case 82. Adrenal Adenocarcinoma 372
William C. Huang and John A. Libertino

Case 83. Seminomatous Testicular Carcinoma 377
Richard S. Foster

Case 84. Nonseminomatous Testicular Carcinoma 379
Richard S. Foster

Case 85. Renal Tumor 382
Marcus L. Quek and Donald G. Skinner

Case 86. Bladder Cancer Presenting as Hematuria 386
Marcus L. Quek and Donald G. Skinner

Case 87. Prostate Cancer 389
Martin I. Resnick

Case 88. Ovarian Cancer 393
Ron E. Swensen and Benjamin E. Greer

Case 89. Incidental Ovarian Mass at Laparotomy 397
Ron E. Swensen and Benjamin E. Greer

Case 90. Symptomatic Splenomegaly 402
Jeff Kolff and Jeffrey Brodsky

Case 91. Cancer of Unknown Origin 409
David R. Spigel and F. Anthony Greco

Index 413

contributing authors

Herand Abcarian, MD
Turi Josefsen Professor and Head
Department of Surgery
University of Illinois-Chicago
and
Chief of Service
Department of Surgery
University of Illinois Medical Center
Chicago, Illinois

Charles M. Balch, MD, FACS
Executive Vice President and CEO
American Society of Clinical Oncology
Alexandria, Virginia
and
Professor of Surgery and Oncology
Department of Surgery
Johns Hopkins Medical Institutions
Baltimore, Maryland

Matthew T. Ballo, MD, FACS
Associate Professor
Department of Radiation Oncology
M.D. Anderson Cancer Center
Houston, Texas

Samuel W. Beenken, MD
Section of Surgical Oncology
University of Alabama at Birmingham
Birmingham, Alabama

Eric Benoit, MD
Clinical Fellow
Department of Surgery
Harvard Medical School
and
Department of Surgery
Brigham & Women's Hospital
Boston, Massachusetts

Henri Bismuth
Centre Hepato-Biliaire
Departement de Chirurgie Hepato-Biliaire
Hopital Paul Brousse
Villejuif, France

Kirby I. Bland, MD
University of Alabama at Birmingham
Chairman, Department of Surgery
Birmingham, Alabama

Antonio Briccoli, MD
Associate Professor
Department of Surgery
University of Bologna
and
Chief
Department of Surgery
Instituto Ortopedico Rizzoli
Bologna, Italy

Jeffrey Brodsky, MD
Department of Surgery
Hahnemann University Hospital
Philadelphia, Pennsylvania

Emanuel Burri, MD
Fellow
Hospital of Liestal
Liestal, Switzerland

Blake Cady, MD
Professor of Surgery
Department of Surgery
Brown Medical School
and
Interim Director
Comprehensive Breast Center
Rhode Island Hospital
Providence, Rhode Island

Susan M. Cera, MD
Colorectal Surgeon
Department of Colon and Rectal Surgery
Cleveland Clinic Florida
Naples, Florida

Anthony T. C. Chan, MD, FRCP
Professor and Chief of Service
Department of Clinical Oncology
Prince of Wales Hospital,
Chinese University of Hong Kong
Hong Kong

Susan S. Chang, MD
Surgical Oncology Fellow
John Wayne Cancer Institute
Santa Monica, California

Vivek Chaudhry, MD
Assistant Professor
University of Illinois at Chicago
and
Division Head of General Surgery
Department of Surgery
Provident Hospital of Cook County
Chicago, Illinois

Maureen A. Chung, MD, PhD
Assistant Professor of Surgery
Department of Surgery
Brown Medical School
and
Surgical Oncologist
Department of Surgery
Rhode Island Hospital
Providence, Rhode Island

Frank Detterbeck, MD
Professor of Surgery, Chief of Thoracic Surgery
Yale Cancer Center
Associate Director, Department of Surgery
Yale University
and
Yale New Haven Hospital
New Haven, Connecticut

Stephen R.T. Evans, MD
Robert Coffey Professor and Chair
Department of Surgery
Georgetown University Hospital
Washington, DC

Marco Fiore, MD
Fellow in Surgical Oncology
Department of Surgery
Istituto Nazioinale per lo studio e la cura dei Tumori
Milan, Italy

Richard S. Foster, MD
Department of Urology
Indiana University School of Medicine
Indianapolis, Indiana

Douglas L. Fraker, MD, FACS
Jonathon Rhoads Professor of Surgery
Division of Surgical Oncology
University of Pennsylvania
Philadelphia, Pennsylvania

Giovanna Gatti, MD
Assistant Professor, Division of Breast Surgery
European Institute of Oncology
Milan, Italy

Armando E. Giuliano, MD
Clinical Professor of Surgery
University of California-Los Angeles
Los Angeles, California
and
Chief of Surgical Oncology
John Wayne Cancer Institute
Santa Monica, California

Arnold C. Goede, MBChB, MRCS
Surgical Research Fellow
Department of Surgery
Royal Free University College Medical School
and
Honorary Surgical Fellow
Academic Department of Surgery
Royal Free Hampstead NHS Trust
London, United Kingdom

F. Anthony Greco, MD
Medical Director
Department of Medical Oncology
Sarah Cannon Research Institute
and
Director, Sarah Cannon Medical Center
Nashville, Tennessee

Benjamin E. Greer, MD
Professor and Director
Division of Gynecologic Oncology
Department of Obstetrics and Gynecology
University of Washington School of Medicine
Seattle, Washington

Alessandro Gronchi, MD
Consultant Surgical Oncologist
Melanoma and Sarcoma Unit
Department of Surgery
National Cancer Institute
Milan, Italy

Bertil Hamberger, MD, PhD, FRCS
Professor of Surgery
Department of Surgical Sciences
Section of Surgery
Karolinska Hospital
Stockholm, Sweden

Katsuyoshi Hatakeyama, MD, FACS
The First Department of Surgery
Niigata University School of Medicine
Niigata, Japan

Ulrich Hengge, MD
Department of Dermatology
Heinrich-Heine University
Düsseldorf, Germany

Anna-Lena Hjelm-Skog
Assistant Professor
Department of Oncology
Karolinska Hospital
Stockholm, Sweden

William C. Huang, MD
Department of Urology
Tufts University School of Medicine
Burlington, Massachusetts

Hiromichi Ito, MD
Senior Resident in Surgery
Brigham & Women's Hospital
Boston, Massachusetts

Subramanya Iyer, MS, MCh, FRCS
Professor
Departments of Head and Neck Surgery
and Plastic Reconstructive Surgery
Amrita Institute of Medical Sciences and Research Centre
Kerala, India

Larry R. Kaiser, MD
The John Rhea Barton Professor and Chairman
Department of Surgery
University of Pennsylvania
and
Chief, Department of Surgery
Hospital of the University of Pennsylvania
Philadelphia, Pennsylvania

Kristen Kellar Graney, BS
Master's Degree Candidate
Interdisciplinary Program in Tumor Biology
Georgetown University
and
Clinical Researcher
Orthopedic Oncology Department
Washington Cancer Institute at Washington Hospital
  Center
Washington, DC

Vijay P. Khatri, MD, FACS
Associate Professor of Surgery
University of California, Davis School of Medicine
Davis, California
and
Division of Surgical Oncology
University of California, Davis Cancer Center
Sacramento, California

James M. Kiely, MD
Research Resident
Department of Surgery
Medical College of Wisconsin
Milwaukee, Wisconsin

Norihiro Kokudo, MD
Associate Professor
Department of Surgery,
Hepato-Biliary-Pancreatic Surgery Division
University of Tokyo, Faculty of Medicine
and
Deputy Chief
Department of Surgery,
Hepato-Biliary-Pancreatic Surgery Division
University of Tokyo Hospital
Tokyo, Japan

Jeff Kolff, MD
Department of Surgery
University of Pennsylvania
Philadelphia, Pennsylvania

Helen Krontiras, MD
Assistant Professor
Department of Surgery, Section of
  Surgical Oncology
University of Alabama at Birmingham
Birmingham, Alabama

M. Abraham Kuriakose, MD, DDS, FRCS
Professor and Chairman
Head and Neck Institute
Amrita Institute of Medical Sciences
and Research Centre
Kerala, India
and
Associate Professor, New York University
New York, New York

Julie R. Lange, MD, ScM
Assistant Professor
Department of Surgery
Johns Hopkins School of Medicine
and
Department of Surgery
John Hopkins Hospital
Baltimore, Maryland

Bernard Launois, MD, FACS
Emeritus Professor of Surgery
School of Medicine
Au-Bz Leon Bernard
and
Hopital Pontchaillou
Rennes, France

Simon Law, MS, MA (Cantab),
MBBChir, FRCSEd, FACS
Professor of Surgery
Department of Surgery
University of Hong Kong Medical Centre
Queen Mary Hospital
Hong Kong

Jean-Louis Lefebvre, MD
Professor, ENT Head and Neck Surgery
Lille University Medical School
and
Chief, Department of Head and Neck Cancer
Centre Oscar Lambret
Lille, France

John A. Libertino, MD
Chairman and Professor
Institute of Urology
Department of Urology
Tufts University School of Medicine
and
Lahey Clinic Medical Center
Burlington, Massachusetts

Keith D. Lillemoe, MD
Jay L. Grosfeld Professor and Chairman
Department of Surgery
Indiana University School of Medicine
and
Surgeon-in-Chief
Indiana University Hospital
Indianapolis, Indiana

Alex G. Little, MD
Professor and Elizabeth Berry Gray Chair of Surgery
Department of Surgery
Wright State University School of Medicine
and
Miami Valley Hospital
Dayton, Ohio

Brigette B.Y. Ma, FRACP
Assistant Professor
Department of Clinical Oncology
Prince of Wales Hospital
Chinese University of Hong Kong
Hong Kong

Lloyd A. Mack, MD, FRCSC
Research Associate
Department of Oncology and Surgery
University of Calgary
and
Surgical Oncologist
Department of Oncology and Surgery
Tom Baker Cancer Centre
University of Calgary
Calgary, Alberta, Canada

Masatoshi Makuuchi, MD
Department of Surgery
Hepato-Biliary-Pancreatic Surgery Division
Artificial Organ and Transplantation Division
University of Tokyo
Tokyo, Japan

Martin M. Malawer, MD, FACS
Professor of Orthopedics
and Director of Orthopedic Oncology
and Professor of Pediatrics
Georgetown University School of Medicine
Professor, Orthopaedic Surgery
George Washington University School of Medicine
  and Health Sciences
Washington, DC

A. Marini
Department of Dermatology
Heinrich-Heine University
Düsseldorf, Germany

Christoph A. Maurer, MD, FACS, FRCS
Associate Professor
Department of Surgery
Basel University
Basel, Switzerland
and
Chief, Department of Surgery
Kantonsspital Liestal
Liestal, Switzerland

Bernard Meunier
Department of Oncological Surgery
School of Medicine
Au-Bz Leon Bernard
and
Hopital Pontchaillou
Rennes, France

Jeffrey F. Moley, MD
Professor of Surgery
Washington University in St. Louis
St. Louis, Missouri

Robyn M. Moncrief, MD
Department of Surgery
Northwestern University School of Medicine
Chicago, Illinois

Monica Morrow, MD
G. Willing Pepper Chair in Cancer Research and
Chairperson
Department of Surgery
Fox Chase Cancer Center
and
Professor of Surgery
Temple University School of Medicine
Philadelphia, Pennsylvania

Vinod Narra, MD
Department of Surgery
Henry Ford Hospital
Detroit, Michigan

Toshirou Nishida, MD, PhD
Associate Professor
Department of Surgery
Osaka University School of Graduate Medicine
and
Chief, Department of Surgery
Osaka University Hospital
Osaka, Japan

John M. A. Northover, MD, FRCS
Professor of Intestinal and Colorectal Disorders
Imperial College, London
Colorectal Cancer Unit
Cancer Research UK
St Mark's Hospital for Intestinal
and Colorectal Disorders
London, United Kingdom

Jeffrey A. Norton, MD
Professor of Surgery
Department of Surgery
Stanford University
and
Chief, Surgical Oncology
Department of Surgery
Stanford University Medical Center
Stanford, California

Christopher J. O'Brien, MD, FRACS
Professor
Department of Surgery
University of Sydney
and
Director, Sydney Cancer Centre
Royal Prince Alfred Hospital
Sydney, Australia

Alden M. Parsons, MD
Department of Surgery
The University of North Carolina at Chapel Hill
and
Cardiothoracic Surgery Resident
Division of Cardiothoracic Surgery
University of North Carolina Memorial Hospital
Chapel Hill, North Carolina

David Pasquier, MD, MSc
Radiation Oncology Department
Universtiy Lille II
and
Centre O. Lambret
Lille, France

Harvey I. Pass, MD
Thoracic Oncology Program
Karmanos Cancer Institute and
John D. Dingell VA Medical Center
Wayne State University
Detroit, Michigan

Henry A. Pitt, MD
Professor of Surgery
Department of Surgery
Medical College of Wisconsin
Milwaukee, Wisconsin

Marlyanne M. Pol-Rodriguez, MD
Postdoctoral Residency Fellow
Department of Dermatology
Columbia University Medical Center
New York, New York

Marcus L. Quek, MD
Clinical Instructor
Department of Urology
Keck School of Medicine at the University of
Southern California
and
USC/Norris Comprehensive Cancer Center
Los Angeles, California

Désirée Ratner, MD
George Henry Fox Associate Clinical
Professor of Dermatology
Department of Dermatology
College of Physicians and Surgeons of Columbia
University
and
Director of Dematologic Surgery
Department of Dermatology
Columbia University Medical Center of the New York
Presbyterian Hospital
New York, New York

Martin I. Resnick, MD
Lester Persky Professor and Chairman
Department of Urology
Case Western Reserve University
School of Medicine
and
Director, Department of Urology
University Hospital of Cleveland
Cleveland, Ohio

Michele Rocca
General Surgery Unit
Instituto Ortopedico Rizzoli
Bologna, Italy

Robert W. Rödl, MD
Department of Orthopaedics
University Hospital of Muenster
Münster, Germany

Sanziana A. Roman, MD
Assistant Professor
Department of Surgery
Yale University
and
Chief of Endocrine Surgery
Department of Surgery
Yale New Haven Hospital
New Haven, Connecticut

Merrick I. Ross, MD, FACS
Professor of Surgery
Chief, Melanoma Section
Department of Surgical Oncology
M.D. Anderson Cancer Center
Houston, Texas

Adam Ian Rubin, MD
Postdoctoral Residency Fellow
Department of Dermatology
Columbia University College of Physicians and Surgeons
and
Resident in Dermatology
Department of Dermatology
Columbia University Medical Center
New York Presbyterian Hospital
New York, New York

Emiel J. Rutgers, MD, PhD
Chairman of Breast Cancer Group
Department of Surgery
Netherlands Cancer Institute
Amsterdam, Netherlands

Michael S. Sabel, MD, FACS
Assistant Professor of Surgery
Department of Surgery
University of Michigan
Ann Arbor, Michigan

Andreas Sendler, MD
Technische Universität München
and
Department of Surgery
Klinikum rechts der Isar
München, Germany

Ashok R. Shaha, MD, FACS
Professor of Surgery
Department of Surgery
Cornell University Medical College
Attending Surgeon
Department of Surgery
Memorial Sloan-Kettering Cancer Center
New York, New York

Kerwin F. Shannon, MBBS, FRACS
Consultant Surgeon
Sydney Head & Neck Cancer Institute
Royal Prince Alfred Hospital
Camperdown, Australia

Yoshio Shirai, MD, PhD
Associate Professor
Division of Digestive and General Surgery
Niigata University Graduate School of Medical
  and Dental Sciences
Niigata City, Japan

J. Rüdiger Siewert, MD
Chirurgische Klinik und Poliklinik
Klinikum rechts der Isar der Technischen
Universität München
München, Germany

Donald G. Skinner, MD
Professor and Chairman
Department of Urology
Keck School of Medicine at University
  of Southern California
USC/Norris Comprehensive Cancer Center
Los Angeles, California

Vernon K. Sondak, MD, FACS
H. Lee Moffitt Cancer Center
University of South Florida College of Medicine
Tampa, Florida

Julie Ann Sosa, MA, MD
Assistant Professor of Surgery and Clinical Epidemiology
Department of Surgery
Yale University School of Medicine
and
Attending Physician
Department of Surgery
Yale-New Haven Hospital
New Haven, Connecticut

David R. Spigel, MD
Associate Director of Clinical Research
Sarah Cannon Research Institute
Nashville, Tennessee

Thomas W. Stamp, MD
Resident Instructor
Department of Surgery
Wright State University School of Medicine
Dayton, Ohio

Paul H. Sugarbaker, MD, FACS, FRCS
Director, Peritoneal Surface Malignancy Program
Department of Surgical Oncology
Washington Hospital Center
Washington, DC

Ron E. Swensen, MD
Assistant Professor, Division of Gynecologic Oncology
Department of Obstetrics and Gynecology
University of Washington School of Medicine
Seattle, Washington

Paris P. Tekkis, MD, FRCS
Senior Lecturer
Department of Surgical Oncology and Technology
Imperial College London
and
Consultant Colorectal Surgeon
Department of Surgical Oncology and Technology
St. Mary's Hospital
London, United Kingdom

Walley J. Temple, MD, FRCSC, FACS
Professor, Department of Oncology and Surgery
University of Calgary
and
Chief, Division of Surgical Oncology
Department of Surgery
Foothills Medical Center
Calgary, Alberta, Canada

Shingo Tsujinaka, MD
Department of Colorectal Surgery
Cleveland Clinic Florida
Weston, Florida

Robert Udelsman, MD, MBA

Lampman Professor of Surgery and Oncology, Chairman
Department of Surgery
Yale University School of Medicine
and
Surgeon-in-Chief
Department of Surgery
Yale-New Haven Hospital
New Haven, Connecticut

Kimberly A. Varker, MD

Postdoctoral Research Fellow
Arthur C. James Comprehensive Cancer Center
The Ohio State University
Columbus, Ohio

John T. Vetto, MD, FACS

Associate Professor
Department of Surgery
Division of Surgical Oncology
Oregon Health & Science University
Portland, Oregon

Brendan C. Visser, MD

Department of Surgery
University of California at San Francisco
San Francisco, California

Alyssa D. Wait, MD

Surgical Resident
Department of Surgery
Indiana University School of Medicine
Indianapolis, Indiana

Harold J. Wanebo, MD, FACS

Chairman Emeritus, Department of Surgery
Director, Surgical Oncology Fellowship
Roger Williams Medical Center
Providence, Rhode Island

Robert S. Warren, MD

Professor of Surgery
and
Chief, Surgical Oncology Program
Department of Surgery
University of California
San Francisco, California

Steven D. Wexner, MD, FACS, FRCS(Ed)

Professor, Department of Surgery
Ohio State University
Columbus, Ohio
and
Clinical Professor of Surgery
University of South Florida College of Medicine
Tampa, Florida
and
Chairman, Department of Colorectal Surgery
Cleveland Clinic Florida
Weston, Florida

Edward E. Whang, MD

Assistant Professor
Department of Surgery
Harvard Medical School
and
Associate Surgeon
Department of Surgery
Brigham & Women's Hospital
Boston, Massachusetts

Marc C. Winslet, MS, FRCS

Division Head
Division of Surgery and Interventional Sciences
Royal Free and University College Medical School
University College London
and
Department Head
Department of Surgery
Royal Free Hospital NHS Trust
London, United Kingdom

John Wong, PhD, FRACS, FACS

Chairman, Department of Surgery
The University of Hong Kong
Queen Mary Hospital
Hong Kong

Stefano Zurrida, MD

Scientific Director's Office
European Institute of Oncology
Milan, Italy

by Charles M. Balch, MD, FACS

Clinical Scenarios in Surgical Oncology has a distinctive and valuable approach to education, especially for the busy clinical surgeon. Instead of the traditional didactic approach used in most textbooks, *Clinical Scenarios in Surgical Oncology* uses a comprehensive series of clinical presentations and case studies that cover the entire gamut of disease sites and clinical presentations. The editor has captured the rich experience of experts across many surgical disciplines to provide an invaluable, practical, and efficient resource that will be helpful to every surgeon.

The variable presentation of cancer requires more clinical judgment and individual treatment planning than almost any other surgical specialty. Some surgical oncology textbooks serve as an important reference source when we need to review a cancer subject in depth, such as preparing for a tumor board or giving a teaching conference. There are other circumstances in which the busy clinical surgeon needs a handy reference guide readily available in the office, the clinic, or on the surgical unit of their hospital. This is one of those books.

Imagine yourself on a busy day in the hospital or office. You are about to provide a surgical oncology consult for a patient with a very unusual or uncommon presentation. There are very few reference sources from which you can rapidly obtain practical clinical information in this circumstance. *Clinical Scenarios in Surgical Oncology*, edited by Dr. Vijay Khatri, is the source you can go to for information about the clinical presentation, including diagnostic work-up, surgical options to be considered, intraoperative decision making, and postoperative management. A few examples of the chapters in this book of uncommon or unusual clinical presentations for which you, the reader of this foreword, might be consulted, include male breast cancer, breast cancer during pregnancy, Merkel cell carcinoma, rectal carcinoid, pseudomyxoma peritonei, linitis plastica of the stomach, anal melanoma, chordoma, insulinoma, pancoast tumor of the lung, oral cavity cell carcinoma, and cervical nodal metastasis from an unknown primary. However, among its 91 clinical scenarios, this book also contains practical clinical and surgical recommendations about more common presentations from a distinguished group of experts in the field. These include parotid gland tumors, solitary pulmonary nodules, cervical esophageal cancer, gastric adenocarcinoma, colon cancer with synchronous hepatic metastasis, recurrent rectal cancer, solitary liver metastasis, gall bladder carcinoma, locally advanced breast cancer, Paget disease of the breast, axillary metastasis from unknown breast primary, extremity soft-tissue sarcoma, retroperitoneal sarcoma, in-transit melanoma, pheochromocytoma, parathyroid adenoma, renal tumors, prostate cancer, and incidental ovarian mass at laparotomy. All these chapters are written by renown experts in surgical oncology in a format that is very useful for clinical surgeons.

Clinical Scenarios in Surgical Oncology is well written and well illustrated. The target audience is the busy clinical surgeon who needs a resource when consulting patients with difficult or complex circumstances, especially those with uncommon or unusual clinical presentations of their cancer. The 91 clinical scenarios address virtually every clinical presentation for all anatomic sites that would be referred to general surgeons, general surgical oncologists, thoracic surgeons, head/neck surgeons, gynecologic surgeons, abdominal surgeons, plastic surgeons, and dermatologic surgeons. Surgical residents, surgical oncology fellows, and nurse oncologists would also find this an extremely valuable educational resource.

I would heartily recommend this book as an all-encompassing resource to all surgical specialities who treat cancer patients. It is not a book one necessarily reads from cover to cover. Instead, it is a resource that the surgeon would use almost daily as they encounter patients with difficult clinical presentations or for consultations for which the busy surgeon needs a single reference to guide the treatment planning for their oncology patient.

Charles M. Balch, MD, FACS
Executive Vice President and CEO
American Society of Clinical Oncology
Alexandria, VA
Professor of Surgery and Oncology
Johns Hopkins Medical Institutions
Baltimore, Maryland

Surgical management of malignant diseases represents an exemplary model of multidisciplinary therapeutics. The combined modality approach to the treatment of cancer patients that includes primary surgical treatment, radiation therapy, chemotherapy, and immunotherapy requires careful integration. *Clinical Scenarios in Surgical Oncology* provides such a practical "case-based" approach to the successful management of solid neoplasms. For this endeavor, Dr. Khatri has assembled leaders in the field of surgical oncology from around the globe to provide a truly international flavor for the reader. The content of this textbook is therefore relevant to clinicians around the world.

There are more than 90 chapters with major sections on cancers in all sites, ranging from head and neck cancer, thoracic malignancies, intra-abdominal organ cancers, breast, soft tissue and bone sarcoma, skin cancers, endocrine tumors, and gynecological and urologic cancers. Each chapter begins with a case presentation which engages the reader in a real-patient scenario and thus facilitates the learning process. The case then naturally progresses with the differential diagnosis, appropriate examinations, and a definitive diagnosis through a logical pathway of investigations. This is followed by a comprehensive "therapeutic and operative approach," a concise discussion of the disease, and finally a closure of the case. The select bibliography of articles provides the reader with alternative viewpoints for selection of diagnostic and treatment approaches. Finally, an abundance of relevant clinical photographs augments the textbook.

This textbook is an excellent, user-friendly guidebook for anyone who cares for or manages patients with solid neoplasms—particularly residents, fellows, and practitioners of general surgical oncology. For this reason, it would be a worthy addition to most surgical and oncological libraries.

Umberto Veronesi, MD
Director, European Institute of Oncology
Via Ripamonti 435
Milan 20141, Italy

<h1 style="text-align:right">preface</h1>

To study the phenomenon of disease without books
is to sail an uncharted sea, while to study books
without patients is not to go to sea at all.
SIR WILLIAM OSLER

The secret of health for both mind and body is not to mourn
for the past, worry about the future, or anticipate troubles,
but to live in the present moment wisely and earnestly.
SIDDHARTHA GAUTAMA BUDDHA

Management of cancer involves complex decision making and can be challenging for residents, fellows in medical and surgical oncology, as well as physicians in practice. This is primarily because treatment of malignancy has evolved into a multidisciplinary approach with appropriate integration of surgery, chemotherapy, and radiation therapy. The specialty also requires tactical incorporation of imaging studies in the diagnosis and follow-up of patients. Sequencing of the various therapeutic modalities is influenced not only by the stage of presentation but also the overall goals (cure vs. palliation) established for the individual patient. Even though physicians may be familiar with the general treatment concepts for individual cancers, management has to be tailored to the individual patient to achieve optimal outcome.

Contemporary oncology textbooks provide comprehensive review of site-specific cancers, but application of this information to patient management can still be formidable. The objective of this textbook, which is part of an exciting "Clinical Scenarios" series, was to have prominent leaders provide current multidisciplinary management of common malignancies in the format of a clinical case review. Such a teaching format is uniquely suited to surgical oncology as it provides the fund of knowledge in a practical fashion and reviews the critical decision making involved in interdisciplinary management of patients with malignancy.

In the editor's own experience, mere reading of standard textbooks is often not adequate in preparing trainees for optimal cancer patient care. A case management–oriented teaching style is exceptionally conducive in promoting improved understanding of the principles of oncology. These illustrative cases should also be useful to other ancillary care providers such as nurses, nurse practitioners, and physician assistants. The additional advantage of such an educational approach is that even though individual cancer clinical scenarios are presented in this textbook, the management principles can be easily translated to similar cases encountered in the physicians practice.

The textbook has 91 chapters grouped into 20 major anatomic cancer sites that encompass the spectrum and breadth of everyday surgical oncology. In keeping with the established format of "Clinical Scenarios," each chapter begins with a case presentation that logically guides the reader through the real-life clinical process of differential diagnosis, relevant investigations, and a comprehensive treatment plan. Ample clinical photographs compliment the succinct text.

Compiling this textbook has been a challenging and rewarding project. I hope it serves the goal of communicating the principles of cancer management and provides insight into multidisciplinary practice.

ACKNOWLEDGMENTS

> *Great discoveries and improvements invariably involve the*
> *cooperation of many minds. I may be given credit for*
> *having blazed the trail, but when I look at the*
> *subsequent developments I feel the credit is*
> *due to others rather than myself.*
> *ALEXANDER GRAHAM BELL*

The editor is deeply indebted to each of the contributors and above all the senior authors who represent leading authorities in the field of surgical oncology. Special gratitude is extended to Drs. Charles Balch and Umberto Veronesi, two "megastars" of surgical oncology, for providing the Forewords. Their lifelong pursuit of improving management of malignancies through elegant clinical trials has been a model for many young surgical oncologists. Appreciation is extended to Brian Brown, Acquisitions Editor at Lippincott Williams & Wilkins, for his assistance with the conceptual plan and for stewarding this endeavor through the various phases of publication. Molly Connors' tireless pursuit to achieve timely completion of the textbook was admirable, and I am grateful for her efforts. Thanks also go to Maria McColligan of Nesbitt Graphics for the efficient production phase. I am ever grateful to the tremendous administrative support provided by both Shannon Stanley and Sandra Moura and the academic insight of Lynn Kossack.

Finally, special recognition is extended to Drs. Nicholas J. Petrelli and Michael A. Caligiuri, who have been, and continue to be, extraordinary mentors and are embodiments of true academic oncologists.

DEDICATION

This book is dedicated to my wife Anjana, who has provided unrelenting support; my children Amit and Shevani for their unconditional, unfettered love; and finally to my parents Pranjivan and Dhanuben Khatri, whose dreams are being fulfilled.

Presentation

A 56-year-old man presents to your office with a progressive painful ulcer of the tongue of 3 months' duration. The lesion started as a painless ulcer, which gradually increased in size and became painful during the past week. He reports no history of similar ulcers or of trauma. He reports smoking cigarettes for the past 20 years; however, there is no history of alcohol abuse. Examination reveals a 4.5 × 3.5-cm indurated ulceroproliferative lesion of the left lateral border of the tongue. Tongue movement is normal. There is no extension of the induration to the base of the tongue or to the floor of the mouth. The rest of the oral mucosa appears healthy. There is no palpable cervical lymphadenopathy. A direct flexible laryngoscopy performed in the office reveals normal larynx and hypopharynx.

Clinical Photograph

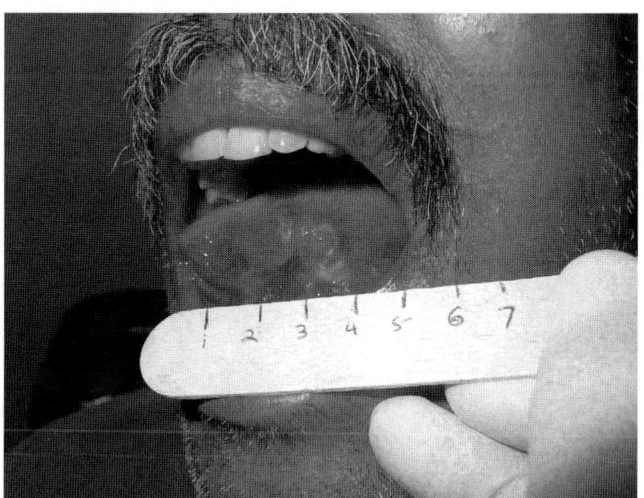

Figure 1.1

Physician Examination Report

Ulceroproliferative lesion of the left lateral border of the tongue.

Differential Diagnosis

Any oral ulcer that persists for more than 3 weeks should be considered malignant unless proved otherwise by biopsy. The painless nature of the lesion at onset and its increase in size further favor the diagnosis of a malignant lesion. The presence of induration on clinical examination is diagnostic of malignant lesions. However, because the patient complains of pain, it is necessary to exclude other reactive and inflammatory lesions. These include recurrent major aphthous ulcers and bullous lesions, such as pemphigus and pemphigoid, and the others listed later. The nonrecurrent nature of the lesion and presence of induration of the surrounding tissue make the diagnosis of reactive and inflammatory lesions less likely. Necrotizing sialometaplasia and keratoacanthoma, however, can mimic malignant ulcers. Other benign lesions likely to be considered are tuberculous ulcer and peripheral giant cell granuloma.

More than 90% of oral malignant lesions are squamous cell carcinomas. Other diagnoses to be considered are nonepidermoid malignancies (e.g., minor salivary gland tumors). These lesions usually have an intact overlying mucosa. In view of the relative rarity of other entities, the characteristic physical examination findings, and the risk factor of smoking, a provisional diagnosis of oral squamous cell carcinoma of the lateral tongue is considered for this patient.

Discussion

The oral tongue accounts for 20% to 50% of all squamous cell carcinomas of the oral cavity. Given their painless nature, they may grow considerably before a patient seeks medical help. On average, there is about 6 months' delay in the diagnosis of oral squamous cell carcinoma by primary care physicians and dentists. Many of these patients are subjected to treatment by antibiotics prior to referral for definitive treatment. In this respect, considering biopsy of any oral lesions of more than 3 weeks' duration is an important rule. Cervical nodal metastasis occurs

Differential Diagnosis Algorithm

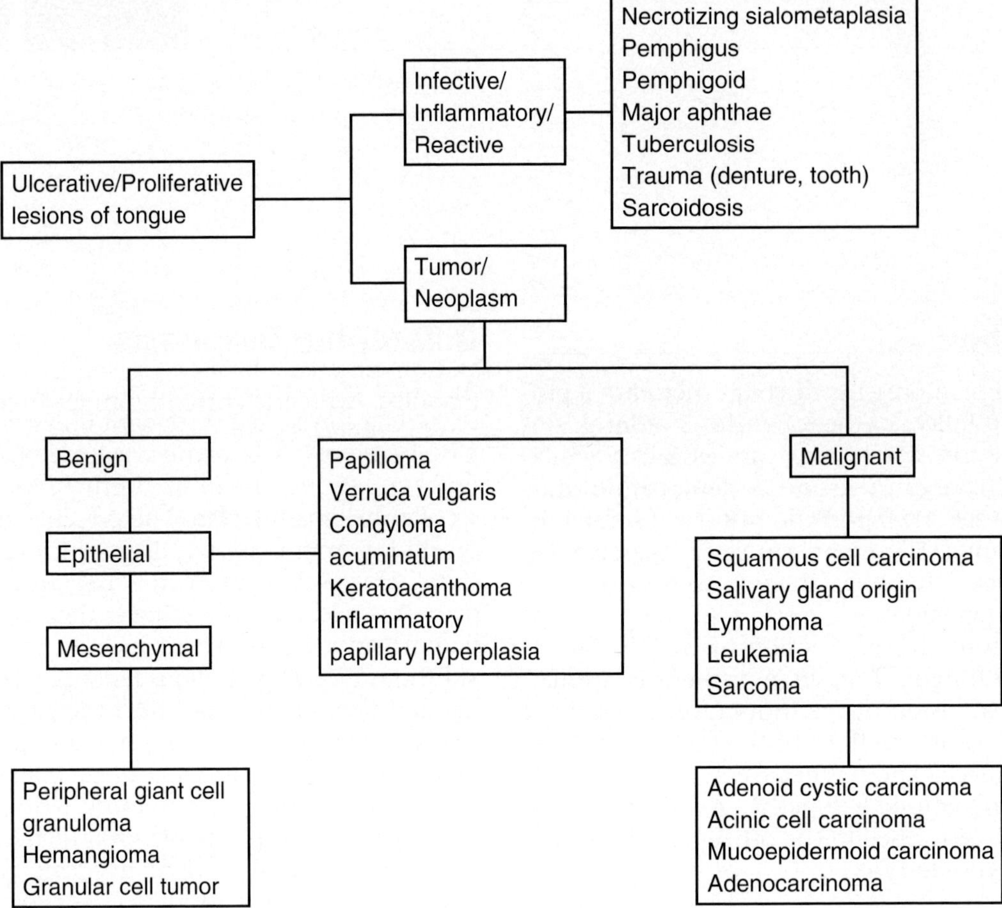

Figure 1.2

more frequently from cancer of the tongue than any other site within the oral cavity. More than 50% of patients present with a locally advanced lesion and lymph node metastasis. Even in patients without clinically obvious metastasis, there is over 30% risk of occult nodal metastasis. Biopsy of cervical lymph nodes is mandatory in establishing the diagnosis. Examination of other head and neck sites is mandatory to rule out synchronous tumors. Palpation of the tongue helps to delineate the submucosal extent of tumor and extension to the floor of the mouth and mandibular alveolus, which should be taken into consideration when planning surgical excision.

Recommendation

Computed tomography (CT) scan with contrast required to determine the extent of primary lesion and to evaluate the neck. Biopsy to confirm diagnosis.

CT Scans

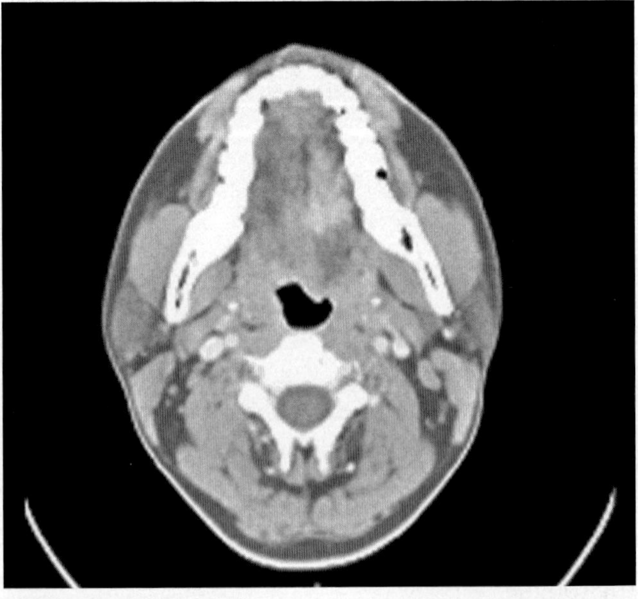

Figure 1.3A

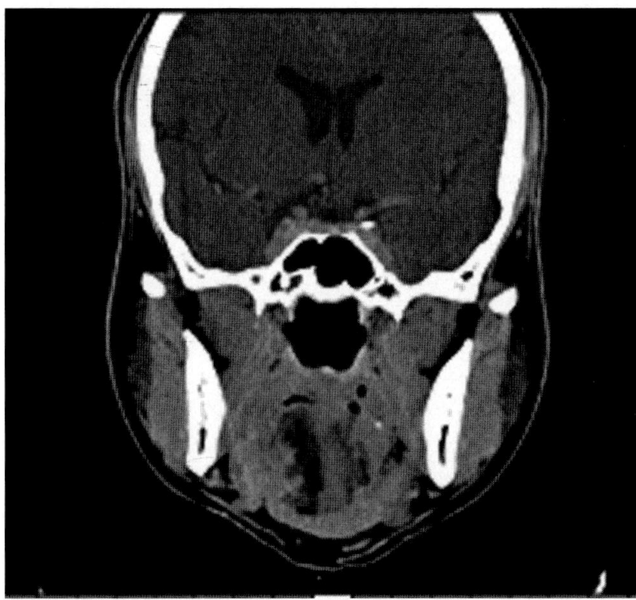

Figure 1.3B

CT Scan Report

CT scan shows tumor confined to the anterior tongue with no bone involvement. The tumor, however, was found to extend to the midline raphe. The neck showed only subcentimeter lymph nodes in the level I and level II regions. The diagnostic criteria of pathological nodes include size greater than 1.5 cm, central necrosis, round nodes, and perinodal enhancement. The diagnostic accuracy of CT scan is only 70%.

Case Continued

The patient undergoes a wedge biopsy from the edge of the lesion, which is reported as squamous cell carcinoma with moderate differentiation. There is no evidence of lymphovascular or perineural invasion.

Diagnosis

Squamous cell carcinoma of the oral tongue, T3 N0 M0; patient assigned stage III carcinoma.

◼ Approach

Curative-intent single-modality treatment by surgery is recommended. This involves paramedian mandibulotomy, wide local excision with at least a 1-cm margin, selective neck dissection of levels I through IV, and reconstruction by sensate radial forearm free flap. The decision for the need for adjuvant radiation therapy is determined based on the histopathological findings.

Discussion

A neck dissection is indicated because the possibility of occult neck metastasis with a T3 cancer of the tongue is about 50% to 70%. Other parameters that predict nodal metastasis are depth of invasion greater than 0.4 mm, tumor volume greater than 13 cm^3, and lymphovascular invasion. These parameters can serve as adjuncts to the clinical treatment decision because each has significant false-positive and false-negative rates. The necessity of neck dissection may be obviated by sentinel lymph node mapping, which is currently under investigation in head and neck cancer.

◼ Surgical Approach

For the ablative surgery, a modified radical neck dissection of levels I to IV is carried out through an upper neck incision. A wide local excision was carried out by mandibulotomy approach. The osteotomy of the mandibulotomy approach is made between the lateral incisor and canine teeth after inserting a preadapted bone plate. Frozen section of the excised tumor showed margins free of tumor.

Reconstruction was performed using a radial forearm free flap, which was harvested from the nondominant left arm after confirming the vascularity of the hand using the Allen test. The antebrachial cutaneous nerve from the flap was anastomosed to the lingual nerve, the radial artery to the facial, and the cephalic vein to the external jugular vein, and one of the venae-comitantes to an internal jugular vein tributary.

Discussion

It was conventional to perform a supraomohyoid neck dissection for tongue tumors with no lymph node metastasis to the neck, but recent evidence suggests that 10% of patients undergoing supraomohyoid neck dissection have metastasis in level IV, which would normally be missed, as level IV was not included in the surgery. It is therefore prudent to include level IV as an extended supraomohyoid neck dissection. The decision to perform mandibulotomy was made because of the infiltrative nature of the lesion. A paramedian mandibulotomy, between the incisor teeth and canine teeth, avoids muscle insertion and damage to the mental nerve. The roots of the teeth also diverge at this region, preventing loss of bone support to the teeth. Preadapted bone plates will ensure maintenance of occlusion. The insertion of two miniplates using the Champey principles offers the best bone stability. This involves placement of monocortical screws at the upper border and bicortical screws at the lower border. Frozen section analysis ascertains the margin of resection; if found inadequate, repeat resection is needed. This is true if the final pathology examination shows a positive margin and the oncological outcome is inferior even after using adjuvant radiation therapy. Of all the reconstructive modalities available for the oral cavity, the radial forearm stands out as the best donor site. The flap is pliable and therefore does not impede function. Donor site morbidity is acceptable, and the presence of a sensory nerve facilitates reinnervation. Alternate flaps for tongue defect reconstruction include the lateral arm free flap. However, if the floor of the mouth also needs reconstruction, the radial forearm free flap is a better choice as it prevents restriction of tongue mobility. Pedicled pectoralis major or nasolabial flaps have been used historically to reconstruct tongue defects. However, the functional results are far inferior to the free flaps.

Case Continued

The patient makes an uneventful recovery. Oral feeding is started on the fifth postoperative day. Definitive histopathology report confirms adequacy of margins. However, there is one metastatic node with extracapsular invasion (pT3 N1 M0). Therefore, the decision is made to offer adjuvant radiotherapy. This is started 3 weeks after the surgery. The patient receives 170 cGy per fraction in 6 weeks for a total dose of 6000 cGy. The radiation port included the tongue and ipsilateral neck; however, the contralateral parotid was spared using 3D conformal treatment planning.

Discussion

Definitive pathological examination suggests the need for adjuvant radiotherapy. Adjuvant radiotherapy is indicated in patients with multiple metastatic nodes, extracapsular extension, or unfavorable primary tumor histology (lymphovascular invasion, perineural invasion, and close surgical margin). The depth of tumor is also seen to adversely affect the prognosis.

Case Continued

Patient is discharged on the 10th postoperative day. Patient is advised to schedule regular follow-up after the radiation therapy.

Postoperative Image

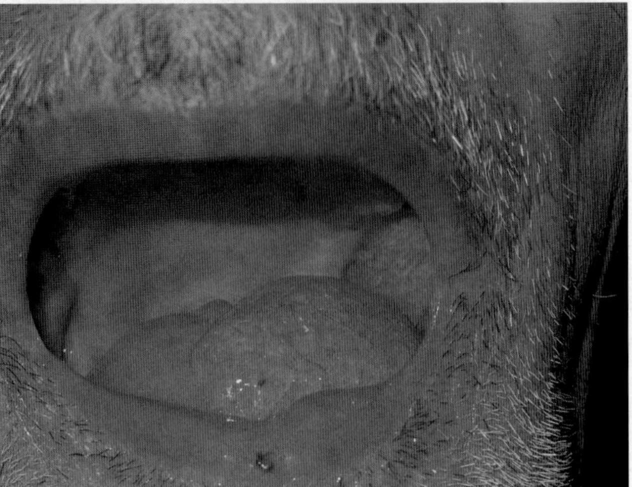

Figure 1.4

Postoperative Report

The radial forearm flap in position.

Discussion

The 5-year disease-free survival of advanced stage oral cavity tumors has improved recently with aggressive multimodality treatment and is reported to be about 60%. During follow-up examination, attention is directed toward diagnosis of recurrence in the neck or primary site, or in the lungs. Head and neck tumor patients have about a 15% lifetime risk of developing second primary tumors in the aero digestive tract. Annual chest radiography is therefore desirable.

Suggested Readings

Byers RM, Clayman GL, McGill D, et al. Selective neck dissection for squamous cell carcinoma of upper aerodigestive tract: patterns of regional failure. *Head Neck* 1999;21:499–505.

Byers RM, El-Naggar AK, YaYen L, et al. Can we detect or predict the presence of occult metastasis in patients with squamous cell carcinoma of the oral tongue. *Head Neck* 1998;20:138–144.

Clayman GL, Frank DK. Selective neck dissection of anatomically appropriate levels is as efficacious as modified radical neck dissection for elective treatment of the clinically negative neck in patients with squamous cell carcinoma of the upper respiratory and digestive tracts. *Arch Otolaryngol Head and Neck Surg* 1998;124:348–352.

Kuriakose MA, Loree TR, Spies A, et al. Sensate radial forearm flaps in tongue reconstruction. *Arch Otolaryngol Head and Neck Surg* 2001;127:1463–1466.

O'Brien CJ, Lauer CS, Fredricks S, et al. Tumor thickness influences prognosis of T1 and T2 oral cavity cancer—but what thickness? *Head Neck* 2003;25:937–945.

Vokes EE, Weichselbaum RR, Lippman SM, et al. Head and neck cancer. *N Engl J Med* 1993;328:184–194.

Presentation

A 59-year-old man presents to your office with complaints of swelling over the right side of the neck of 3 months' duration and otalgia for 1 month. He has been a chronic smoker for the last 30 years. Examination of the neck reveals enlarged lymph nodes at levels II and III on both sides. The largest node at the right level II measures about 4.5 × 4.5 cm and appears to be fixed to the underlying structures. Remaining nodes are less than 3 cm in diameter.

Clinical Photograph

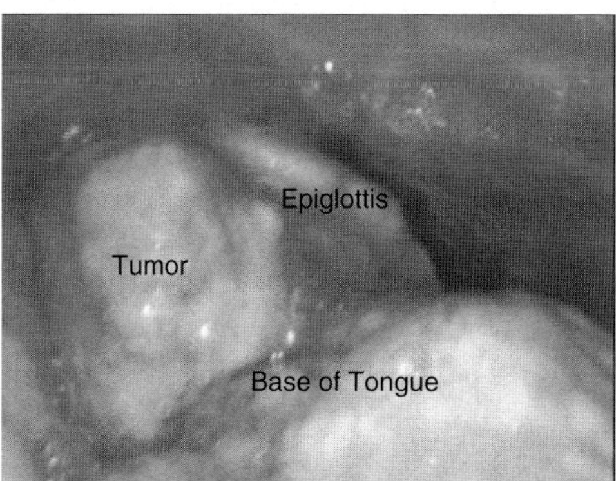

Figure 2.1

Physical Examination Report

Examination of the oral cavity reveals a proliferative growth over the base of the tongue on the right side involving the right vallecula and just reaching the midline, measuring about 4 × 4 cm. There is no extension to the larynx, and tongue movements are normal. On digital examination, induration is felt just around the lesion and reaching midline.

Differential Diagnosis

A provisional diagnosis is made of malignant tumor of the base of the tongue with secondary metastasis to the neck lymph nodes. The patient is advised to undergo biopsy from the base of the tongue and fine-needle aspiration cytology (FNAC) of the right cervical lymph node. A computed tomography (CT) scan of the neck and radiography of the chest is also advised.

Discussion

Squamous cell carcinoma of the base of the tongue usually presents as neck swelling, though some patients present with complaints of change in voice, foreign body sensation in throat, referred otalgia, odynophagia, and dysphagia. With involvement of the larynx, the patients can develop stridor. The differential diagnosis for the exophytic lesions over the base of the tongue includes benign lesions like lymphoid hyperplasia, lingual thyroid, papillomas, benign tumors of the minor salivary glands, peripheral giant cell granulomas, and migratory glossitis. Most common malignant tumors of the base of the tongue are squamous cell carcinomas, which account for about 70% of cases. About 20% are lymphomas, and the remainder are minor salivary gland tumors. Other less common malignant tumors are sarcomas, adenocarcinomas from the lingual thyroid, and metastatic tumors.

Case Continued

The patient undergoes a punch biopsy from the base of the tongue lesion and FNAC from the right level II node. The biopsy is reported as squamous cell carcinoma with moderate differentiation. The FNAC is reported as metastatic deposits of squamous cell carcinoma.

CT Scans

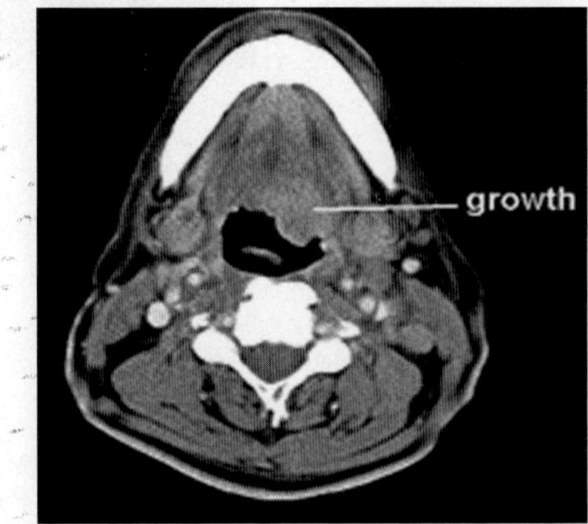

Figure 2.1A

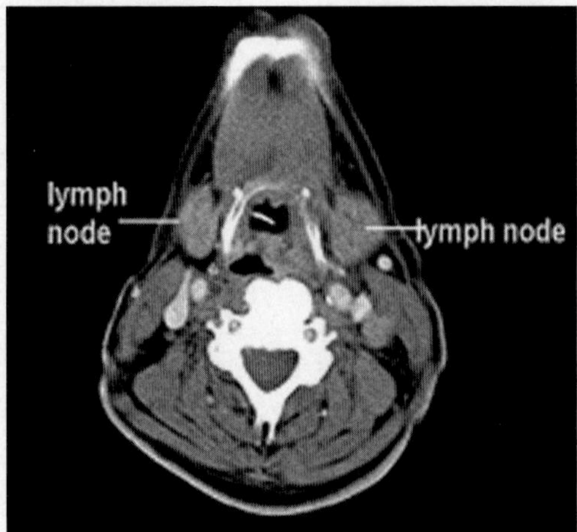

Figure 2.1B

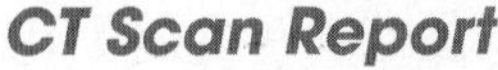

CT Scan Report

The CT scan shows an infiltrative lesion at the base of the tongue on the right side involving the vallecula. The extrinsic muscles of the tongue, pterygoid muscles, and larynx are free of disease. Level II and III nodes are present bilaterally. The largest node is about 4 cm in diameter and is present at right level II. Chest radiography is unremarkable.

Diagnosis

Moderately differentiated squamous cell carcinoma of the base of the tongue, T2 N2c M0; patient assigned stage IVa carcinoma.

Recommendation

Patient is advised to undergo external beam radiation to the primary lesion as well as the neck, followed by a bilateral neck dissection.

Discussion

Most patients with oropharynx carcinoma present with locally advanced tumors with cervical nodal metastasis. Treatment of carcinoma of the base of the tongue is controversial; most patients need to undergo a combined modality of treatment. Treatment options available are radiation therapy of the primary lesion with planned neck dissection depending on nodal status. The second option is surgery followed by radiation therapy. Emerging data suggest that concurrent chemotherapy and radiation therapy offers better loco regional control and an improvement in survival.

Generally, radiation therapy of the primary lesion is recommended, as the functional result of radiation therapy is superior to surgery. Surgery is reserved as a salvage treatment for patients with residual or recurrent disease after radiation therapy. Planned neck dissection after radiation therapy is recommended in patients with advanced neck disease (N2 or N3). There is a high incidence of bilateral metastasis in lesions of the base of the tongue; hence, treatment to the neck should address both sides.

Case Continued

The patient is referred to the radiation oncology department for radiation therapy, and external beam therapy is planned for the primary lesion and the neck bilaterally. The tumor bed receives a total dose of 72 Gy in 6 weeks, with 65 Gy in wide field by opposing lateral portals and a 7-Gy boost to the tumor bed by a submental, mandible-sparing portal. The upper neck receives 65 Gy in wide field, while the lower neck receives 50 Gy.

Discussion

Various modifications to the radiation therapy protocol are recommended to increase locoregional control without added morbidity. The recommended schedules are as follows. (a) Concomitant boost accelerated radiation therapy consisting of 72 Gy delivered over 6 weeks using 1.8 Gy/fraction to large volume with 1.5 Gy/fraction to the tumor bed in the last 12 treatments. (b) Hyperfractionation of the total dose of 81 Gy given over 7 weeks in 1.2-Gy doses twice a day. (c) Brachytherapy boost using interstitial implant as the boost dose. Improvement in disease control rate has been reported with brachytherapy boost. However, the procedure often requires a tracheostomy.

Attempts have been made to use concurrent chemotherapy and radiation therapy, a technique found to have improved the loco regional control rate in larynx and hypopharynx tumors, in the oropharynx. The technique is often associated with increased short-term and long-term complications, and its superiority over radiation therapy alone is not well established at the oropharynx.

Case Continued

The patient is reviewed 2 weeks after initiation of radiation therapy to assess response to therapy. He is found to have good response at the primary lesion and the neck. The patient is evaluated again 2 weeks after completion of radiation therapy; there is complete response at the primary and the neck. Radiation mucositis changes are seen in the oral cavity and minimal edema over the base of the tongue. A bilateral comprehensive neck dissection is planned for the patient after 4 weeks.

Surgical Approach

In view of the presence of bilateral multiple nodes initially at presentation, a bilateral planned neck dissection is done. Bilateral Schobinger's incision is placed, and skin flaps are elevated in the subplatysmal plane. Bilateral clearance of tissue from level I to V is done. Accessory nerve, internal jugular vein, and sternomastoid muscle are preserved on both sides. The wound is closed in layers. The base of the tongue is evaluated intra operatively and is found to be disease free.

Case Continued

The patient has an uneventful postoperative period; the skin sutures are removed after the 10th postoperative day. The postoperative histopathology report shows neck nodes that are free of disease. The patient is discharged after suture removal and is advised to schedule regular follow-up visits.

Discussion

The dissection is generally carried out 4 to 6 weeks after the completion of radiation therapy. By this time, the acute radiation reaction would have re-

solved and pathological interpretation is more reliable. Neck dissections are classified as follows. (a) Radical neck dissection, in which all ipsilateral lymph node groups from level I to V are removed along with the sternocleidomastoid muscle, internal jugular vein, and accessory nerve. (b) Modified radical neck dissection, in which all lymphatic structures are removed, as in radical neck dissection, along with preservation of one or more nonlymphatic structures (i.e., the sternocleidomastoid muscle, internal jugular vein, and accessory nerve). (c) Selective neck dissection, in which selected groups of lymph nodes are removed depending on the site of the primary lesion and pattern of spread. (d) Extended radical neck dissection, which includes removal of one or more lymphatic or nonlymphatic structures that are not included in radical neck dissection.

In the literature, 5-year survival for stage IV disease of the base of the tongue is reported to be in the range of about 30% to 50% of patients. About 10% to 15% of patients develop distant metastasis. Among patients who have recurrence, most experience it within 2 years; therefore, a regular monthly follow-up is recommended in the first year, with follow-ups every 2 to 3 months during the second year, and every 6 months thereafter. Chest radiography is performed annually to rule out lung metastasis.

Suggested Readings

Barrett WL, Gleich L, Wilson K, et al. Organ preservation with interstitial radiation for base of tongue cancer. *Am J Clin Oncol* 2002;25(5):485–488.

Bolner A, Mussari S, Fellin G, et al. The role of brachytherapy in the management of oropharyngeal carcinomas: the Trento experience. *Tumori* 2002;88:137–141.

Catherine KS, Bhattacharya J, Wang CC. Role of neck surgery in conjunction with radiation in regional control of node-positive cancer of the oropharynx. *Am J Clin Oncol* 2002; 25(2):109–116.

Fien MA, Lee WR, Warren RA, et al. Oropharyngeal carcinoma treated with radiation therapy: a 30 years experience. *Int J Radiat Biol Phys* 1996;32(2):289–296.

Machlay MM, Perch S, Markiewiez D, et al. Combined surgery and postoperative radiation for carcinoma of the base of tongue. Analysis of treatment outcome and prognostic valve of margin status. *Head Neck* 1997;19(6):494–499.

Malone JP, Stephens JA, Grecula JC, et al. Disease control, survival, and functional outcome after multimodal treatment for advanced-stage tongue base cancer. *Head Neck* 2004;26(7): 561–572.

Mendenhall WM, Stringer SP, Amdur RJ, et al. Is radiation therapy a preferred alternative to surgery for squamous cell carcinoma of the base of tongue? *J Clin Oncol* 2000;18(1):35–42.

Parsons JT, Mendenhall WM, Stringer SP, et al. Squamous cell carcinoma of the oropharynx: surgery, radiation therapy, or both. *Cancer* 2002;94(11):2967–2980.

Robbins KT, Clayman G, Levine PA, et al. Neck dissection classification update. *Arch Otolaryngol Head Neck Surg* 2002; 128(7): 751–758.

case 3

Presentation

A 38-year-old man of Southern Chinese ancestry presents to your office with a 3-month history of a progressively enlarging left neck mass associated with intermittent right nasal obstruction. He is otherwise well with no other symptoms. He has no significant past medical or family history and is a non-smoker.

On physical examination, the only significant finding is an enlarged, firm left upper cervical lymph node measuring 4 × 3 cm in diameter. Cranial nerve examination is normal and no abnormalities are found in other systems.

You perform a flexible nasal endoscopic examination of the nasopharynx.

Endoscopic Image

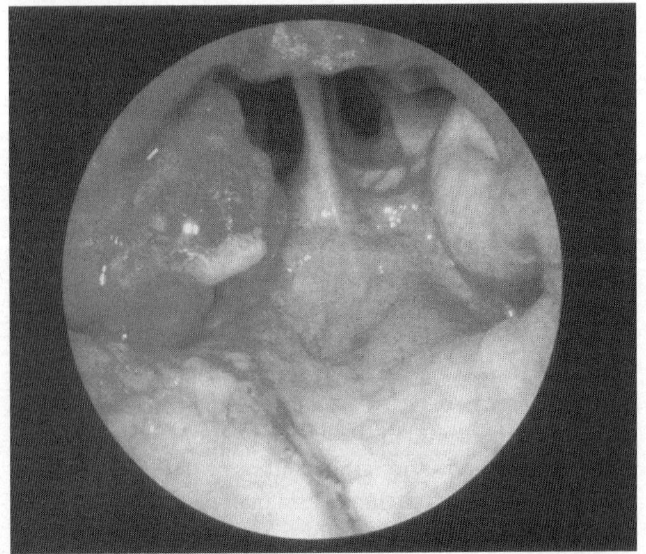

Figure 3.1

Endoscopy Report

There is a soft-tissue mass involving the left lateral and posterior walls of the nasopharynx.

Differential Diagnosis

The differential diagnosis for nasopharyngeal masses in the adult includes primary nasopharyngeal carcinoma (NPC), non-Hodgkin's lymphoma (e.g., natural killer–cell lymphoma), rhabdomyosarcoma, plasmacytoma, and adenocarcinomas of minor salivary glands. The undifferentiated and nonkeratinizing histological subtypes of NPC (World Health Organization [WHO] classification, 1991 edition, WHO types II and III) are most commonly found in Southeast Asian patients (e.g., Southern China, Hong Kong, Taiwan), whereas the keratinizing subtype (WHO type I) is more commonly found in North American or white populations. In this patient of Chinese ancestry with nasal obstruction, undifferentiated NPC is the most likely diagnosis.

Case Continued

Histopathological examination of an endoscopic biopsy of the nasopharyngeal tumor shows an undifferentiated nasopharyngeal carcinoma with strong nuclear staining for Epstein-Barr virus (EBV)-encoded RNA (EBER).

EBER is an important histological marker for NPC because it can be found in most NPC cells, with a preponderance for tumors of the undifferentiated subtype.

Discussion

NPC is endemic in Southern China, North Africa, parts of the Mediterranean basin, and the far Northern Hemisphere (e.g., Alaska, Greenland), where the disease is linked to genetic and dietary factors and is etiologically associated with EBV. The prevalence is highest in Southern China, where as many as 80 (range 10 to 150) cases per 100,000 population are reported each year. The prevalence is lowest in North America, western Europe, and Japan (one case per 100,000 population per year), where the disease is linked to tobacco and alcohol use.

The most common presenting symptom is painless cervical lymphadenopathy. Tumors limited to the nasopharynx may result in nasal symptoms such as epistaxis or obstruction. As the tumor invades the nearby soft tissues, symptoms such as tinnitus, deafness, and recurrent otitis media resulting from eustachian tube obstruction may occur. Advanced tumors invading the base of the skull or the infratemporal fossa may lead to headaches or multiple cranial nerve palsies. Histological confirmation is made primarily via biopsy of the nasopharynx with a fiberoptic nasopharyngoscope. The primary tumor should be evaluated via both computed tomography (CT) and magnetic resonance imaging (MRI) of the nasopharynx and the skull base. These scans are preferably performed before tumor biopsy, because biopsy may cause soft-tissue swelling or a hematoma, rendering radiological interpretation difficult. MRI is more sensitive than CT in evaluating the extent of soft-tissue and neurovascular invasion by the primary tumor, as well as the presence of regional nodal metastasis (especially in the retropharyngeal group of lymph nodes). However, CT is a better tool for defining bone erosion. Nonetheless, both CT and MRI are not sensitive tools for distinguishing locally recurrent or residual disease following radical radiotherapy. There is emerging evidence that positron emission tomography (PET) has a sensitivity of 100% and a specificity of 93% to 96% for detecting recurrent or residual disease at the nasopharynx, compared to 72% and 88% for CT.

MRI

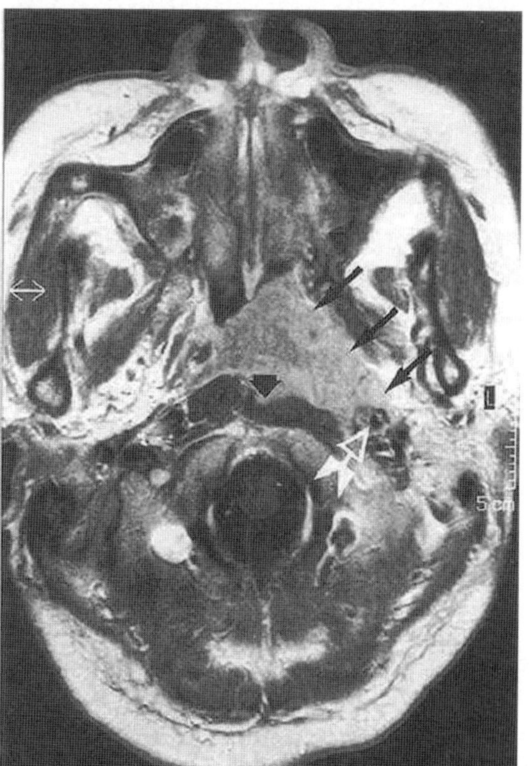

Figure 3.2

MRI Report

A T1-weighted, contrast-enhanced image of the nasopharynx reveals a nasopharyngeal soft-tissue mass involving the left lateral wall, the posterior wall, and the roof of the left nasopharynx. The tumor extends into the parapharyngeal space, partially encasing the carotid artery. There is inferior extension of the tumor into the oropharynx along the left lateral wall. The anterior nasal space is not involved. There is no involvement of the skull base. Enlargement of the left deep cervical chain is noted (5 × 4 cm maximum diameter). Retropharyngeal and supraclavicular nodes are not enlarged. *Black arrows* indicate the location of the primary tumor.

Case Continued

As part of the disease staging, MRI and CT scans of the nasopharynx and neck are obtained.

Case Continued

A bone scan, abdominal ultrasound, and CT scan of the chest are normal, with no evidence of metastases.

Diagnosis and Recommendation

According to the American Joint Committee on Cancer (AJCC) staging classification (2002, 6th edition), this patient has T2b N1 M0 (stage IIb) undifferentiated NPC. Staging of nasopharyngeal carcinoma is based on tumor invasion of the soft tissue (e.g., the oropharynx, nasal sinuses, or parapharyngeal space), bony structures, and cranial nerves and organs (e.g., brain, orbit). Distant metastases tend to involve the lungs, mediastinal nodes, liver, and bony skeleton.

Approach

The patient completed a course of radiation therapy with concurrent cisplatin followed by an additional radiation therapy boost to the left parapharyngeal area.

Discussion

Unlike other head and neck squamous cell carcinomas, radiation therapy (RT) is the primary curative treatment for NPC, while surgery is reserved for selected cases of locoregional disease recurrence (in discussion section). Conventionally, RT involves delivering external radiotherapy (either 2-dimensional or 3-dimensional planning) to the primary tumor and the involved regional lymph nodes at a total dose of 60 to 70 Gy, divided as a daily dose of 2.0 to 2.5 Gy per fraction given over 6 to 7 weeks. In the absence of distant metastasis, more than 80% of patients with AJCC stage I and II NPC will be cured with RT alone. However, 30% to 40% of patients with stage III to IV disease will develop locoregional or distant recurrence with RT alone. For patients with stage III to IV disease, the current standard of treatment is concurrent cisplatin-based chemotherapy and RT, with or without adjuvant cisplatin-based chemotherapy. This bimodality approach is supported by the results of several randomized clinical trials, demonstrating that patients with AJCC stage T3 or 4 disease, or stage N2 or 3 disease, who were treated with concurrent cisplatin and RT had better overall and disease-free survival than those treated with RT alone.

Case Continued

CT, MRI, and endoscopic assessments 3 and 6 months after RT show complete response to therapy. Around 25 months after RT, the patient develops symptoms of increasing lethargy and loss of libido. On examination, apart from a delayed relaxation phase of his ankle reflexes, there are no other abnormalities, and in particular no cranial nerve or visual field defects. The following blood tests were performed:

Thyroid-stimulating hormone (0.4–5.0 mU/L): 0.15 mU/L ↓
Thyroxine (64–154 nmol/L): 40 nmol/L ↓
Testosterone (10–35 nmol/L): 18 nmol/L
8 a.m. cortisol (140–690 nmol/L): 208 nmol/L
Complete blood cell count and renal and liver function tests were normal.

Discussion

This patient developed hypothyroidism 25 months following RT to the neck. Late toxicities of RT may include progressive neck fibrosis and therefore delayed wound healing, xerostomia from irradiation of the parotid and other salivary glands, radionecrosis of the mandible, hearing impairment, trismus, and endocrine abnormalities such as hypothyroidism and hypopituitarism. Hypothyroidism secondary to RT is common following treatment with concurrent chemotherapy and RT for head and neck cancers, with one study reporting an incidence of 27% 1 year after treatment. Progressive impairment in hypothalamic–pituitary function leading to endocrine dysfunction that requires treatment can occur in 50% of patients 5 years after cranial irradiation.

Case Continued

At 35 months, the patient complains of some asymmetry and "fullness" over the left side of the neck. He is otherwise well. On examination, the only abnormality is a probable neck swelling at the left upper cervical area. Because of radiation-induced fibrosis of the adjacent skin, it is difficult to ascertain whether the swelling is an enlarged node. Endoscopic examination of the nasopharynx reveals an atrophic mucosa, and random biopsies of the nasopharynx do not show malignant cells. An MRI of the neck performed as part of this evaluation is equivocal, showing a left-sided lymph node, measuring 1 cm, of uncertain significance. A blood sample shows an increased plasma EBV DNA level of 580 copies/mL. A repeat MRI of the neck performed 2 months later shows a 2-cm left-sided cervical lymph node at the left carotid space and C3–4 level, suggestive of regional nodal recurrence. This is confirmed cytologically via a percutaneous fine-needle aspiration of the node. The plasma EBV DNA level repeated at this time has elevated to 1,530 copies/mL. A whole-body PET scan does not show any distant metastases.

Discussion

Several circulating tumor markers are specific to NPC. Precipitating antibodies against EBV-infected cells such as IgG and IgA directed against particular components of the EB virus (e.g., antibodies against EBV capsid antigen and neutralizing antibodies against EBV-specific DNase), are commonly elevated at the time of diagnosis. However, these markers are of little value in posttreatment surveillance, unlike tumor-derived plasma EBV DNA, which is an important prognostic and diagnostic marker for newly diagnosed or recurrent NPC. Using the technique of quantitative real-time polymerase chain reaction, plasma EBV DNA has a sensitivity of 96% and specificity of 93% in the primary diagnosis of NPC. A persistently elevated EBV DNA level greater than 500 copies/mL taken 4 to 6 weeks following primary RT is associated with the presence of residual cancer and a higher risk of subsequent disease recurrence. Rising levels of EBV DNA during the follow-up period may also indicate the presence of local or distant relapse. This increase in plasma EBV DNA level can also predate clinical manifestation of relapse by several months, as with this patient. Nevertheless, plasma EBV DNA measurement remains an experimental investigation and does not replace the confirmatory role of MRI, CT, or histopathological evaluation in the diagnosis of disease recurrence.

Locoregional recurrence is potentially curable via salvage surgery or brachytherapy. Reirradiation of a recurrent tumor at the nasopharynx using conventional 2-dimensional RT is not recommended because of the significant late neurological toxicity to the adjacent, previously irradiated, normal tissue (e.g., causing trismus and damaging cranial nerves, brainstem, and temporal lobes). For small (<5 cm) and suitably located recurrent tumors at the nasopharynx that spare the eustachian tubes and nasal septum, salvage options may include interstitial brachytherapy using ^{198}Au or nasopharyngectomy. Several surgical approaches are available, including the transcervical, transoral, transpalatal, transmaxillary, posterolateral, and mid-face degloving approach. There is no single ideal surgical approach, and surgery should be individually tailored. Regional neck node recurrence is most often managed with radical neck dissection. New 3-dimensional RT planning and delivery techniques, such as intensity-modulated radiation therapy (IMRT) and stereotactic RT, can also be considered for selected patients with local recurrence, depending on the tumor extent and tolerance of adjacent tissues to reirradiation. For patients with distant metastases, or patients whose recurrent disease is not amenable to local therapy, systemic chemotherapy would be an option. Among selected patients with isolated mediastinal nodal or pulmonary metastases, complete responses to platinum-based chemotherapy and long-term survivors have been reported.

Suggested Readings

Al-Sarraf M, LeBlanc M, Giri PG, et al. Chemoradiotherapy versus radiotherapy in patients with advanced nasopharyngeal cancer: phase III randomized intergroup study 0099. *J Clin Oncol* 1998;16:1310–1317.

Chan AT, Teo PM, Johnson PJ. Nasopharyngeal carcinoma. *Ann Oncol* 2002;13:1007–1015.

Chan AT, Teo PM, Ngan RK, et al. Concurrent chemotherapy-radiotherapy compared with radiotherapy alone in locoregionally advanced nasopharyngeal carcinoma: progression-free survival analysis of a phase III randomized trial. *J Clin Oncol* 2002;20:2038–2044.

Chan KC, Lo YM. Circulating EBV DNA as a tumor marker for nasopharyngeal carcinoma. *Semin Cancer Biol* 2002;12:489–496.

Chien YC, Chen JY, Liu MY, et al. Serologic markers of Epstein-Barr virus infection and nasopharyngeal carcinoma in Taiwanese men. *N Engl J Med* 2001;345:1877–1882.

Colevas AD, Thornhill J, Adak S, et al. Hypothyroidism incidence after multimodality treatment for stage III and IV squamous cell carcinomas of the head and neck. *Int J Radiat Oncol Biol Phys* 2001;51:599–604.

Kao CH, Chieng PU, Yen RF, et al. Detection of recurrent or persistent nasopharyngeal carcinomas after radiotherapy with 18-fluoro-2-deoxyglucose positron emission tomography and comparison with computed tomography. *J Clin Oncol* 1998;16:3550–3555.

Lam KS, Wang C, Yeung RT, et al. Effects of cranial irradiation on hypothalamic-pituitary function—a 5-year longitudinal study in patients with nasopharyngeal carcinoma. *Q J Med* 1991;78:165–176.

Lee AW, Poon YF, Foo W, et al. Retrospective analysis of 5037 patients with nasopharyngeal carcinoma treated during 1976–1985: overall survival and patterns of failure. *Int J Radiat Oncol Biol Phys* 1992;23:261–270.

Shanmugaratnam KSL. The World Health Organization histological classification of tumors of the upper respiratory tract and ear. A commentary on the second edition. *Cancer* 1993;71:2689–2697.

Teo P, Yu P, Lee WY, et al. Significant prognosticators after primary radiotherapy in 903 nondisseminated nasopharyngeal carcinoma evaluated by computer tomography. *Int J Radiat Oncol Biol Phys* 1996;36:291–304.

Tsai ST, Jin YT, Mann RB, et al. Epstein-Barr virus detection in nasopharyngeal tissues of patients with suspected nasopharyngeal carcinoma. *Cancer Epidemiol Biomarkers Prev* 1998;82:1449–1453.

case 4

Presentation

A 55-year-old teacher presents with hoarseness that has worsened over the past month and now interferes with his occupation. He has a history of smoking 10 cigarettes per day for around 20 years. Using the indirect laryngeal mirror and flexible laryngoscope, you detect an irregular 1-cm lesion at the junction of the anterior and middle thirds of the left vocal fold, but mobility is not impaired. The rest of the head and neck examination is normal.

Differential Diagnosis

Because the patient is a smoker, and because dysphonia has persisted for more than 1 month and is worsening, laryngeal carcinoma is the most likely diagnosis, and needs to be confirmed with tissue biopsy. Laryngopharyngeal reflux (LPR) is the most common cause of laryngitis in adults and can present as persistent dysphonia. Features on clinical examination include erythema of the posterior third of the vocal folds and arytenoids, diffuse edema, and granuloma of the vocal process of the arytenoids. Examination of the larynx can reveal a variety of findings: erythema of the posterior third of the vocal folds and arytenoids with interarytenoid mucosal hypertrophy, subglottic edema, or mucosal thickening without significant erythema. Vocal process granulomas, with or without associated laryngeal edema, can be present.

Vocal fold nodules usually result from vocal abuse. They are often bilateral and occur at the junction of the anterior and middle thirds of the true vocal folds.

Laryngeal papillomatosis is caused by human papilloma virus and can present with hoarseness and airway obstruction if the disease is advanced. Characteristically, the laryngeal mucosa is erythematous and edematous, especially over the true vocal folds.

Tuberculous laryngitis is a common granulomatous disease of the larynx. Dysphonia, odynophagia, dyspnea, and odynophonia may occur. It is usually associated with active pulmonary tuberculosis. Laryngeal examination may reveal edematous and hyperemic mucosa involving the posterior third of the larynx or granular exophytic lesions that may mimic carcinoma.

Recommendation

A biopsy is mandatory for confirming the diagnosis. It can be obtained during the panendoscopy, which is necessary to evaluate for synchronous cancer. Computed tomography (CT) scan with contrast enhancement is the method of choice for studying the larynx. CT scan should be performed before biopsy so that abnormalities that may be caused by biopsy are not confused with tumor.

Case Continued

Biopsy reveals a well-differentiated invasive squamous cell carcinoma.

CT Scan

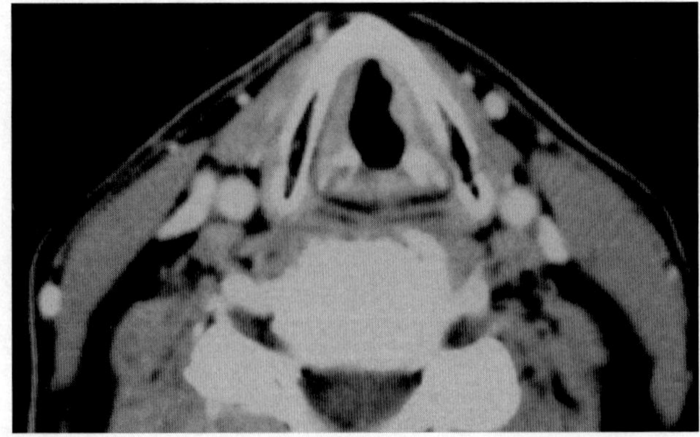

Figure 4.1

CT Scan Report

There is tissue thickening with contrast enhancement at the junction of the anterior and middle thirds of the left true vocal fold; there is no infiltration of the paraglottic space or the anterior commissure. The subglottis is not involved. There is no evidence of cartilage invasion or pathologically enlarged cervical lymph nodes.

Discussion

This case represents a T1a N0 glottic carcinoma. The tumor is limited to one vocal fold; there is neither mobility impairment nor infiltration of the supra- or subglottis. Clinical examination and endoscopy represent the most important pretreatment assessments of early glottic cancer. However, CT scan can provide useful information. For example, involvement of the paraglottic space, the anterior commissure, or the subglottis correlates with a higher local recurrence rate in glottic carcinoma treated with radiotherapy. Even in T1 glottic carcinoma treated with radiotherapy, tumor volume is correlated with local control.

Approach

Because of his occupation, the patient attached great importance to functional results; therefore, radiotherapy would be the preferred modality.

Discussion

The goal of the treatment is to cure with the best achievable functional result and with no serious complications, so the technique must be adapted to each patient.

Early laryngeal cancer is a highly curable disease and can be treated with equal success with open partial laryngectomy, transoral laser excision, or radiotherapy. Open partial laryngectomy produces cure rates ranging from 90% to 95% for T1 glottic carcinoma and 70% to 90% for T2 glottic carcinoma. Transoral laser excision is a safe and effective method. Local control rates range from 80% to 90% for T1 lesions and 70% to 85% for T2 lesions.

The major advantage of radiotherapy over partial laryngectomy or laser excision is the better quality of voice. As for radiotherapy, T1 and T2 lesions with anterior commissure involvement have low rates of local control. After radiotherapy, local control is around 90% for T1 lesions and 80% for T2 lesions. Several factors correlate with lower local control: T stage, prolonged overall treatment time, anterior commissure involvement, poor histologic differentiation, and verrucous lesions. In the series by Reddy and colleagues, local control was 88%

when anterior commissure was not involved and only 67% when anterior commissure was involved. Similarly, the degree of paraglottic space invasion is significantly associated with local control.

In the series by Rosier and colleagues, there was a trend toward less hoarseness after external radiotherapy than after laser microsurgery or partial laryngectomy, but the difference was significant only between radiotherapy and partial laryngectomy. In T1 and T2 lesions, when the functional result is important, radiotherapy treatment is preferred. If voice quality is not important, and the patient has a T1 or T2 lesion that does not involve the anterior commissure, transoral laser excision is a good option. However, voice quality after transoral laser excision is directly related to the extent of resection, and for very limited tumors, radiotherapy and laser transoral excision functional results are similar. Open partial laryngectomy has slightly poorer functional results than either laser excision or radiotherapy.

Long-term follow-up is necessary to detect recurrences at an early stage. Indeed, surgical salvage was considered to be possible only with total laryngectomy, but partial laryngectomy as salvage surgery for radiation failures is possible, essentially in T1 lesions. In the Mendenhall series, 19 of the 291 patients treated for a T1 lesion experienced local recurrence; seven patients underwent salvage hemilaryngectomy and 11 patients underwent total laryngectomy. One patient refused treatment. In the Rodriguez-Cuevas series, recurrences were salvaged with partial laryngectomy in half of the patients with acceptable functional results. The selection of a salvage surgical procedure after radiotherapy (total or partial laryngectomy) is based on the tumor extension. Arytenoid fixation, subglottic infiltration, interarytenoid invasion, pre-epiglottic space invasion, or extralaryngeal spread remain contraindications to partial laryngectomy; patients must have limited comorbidities and good pulmonary function. Cordectomy or frontolateral laryngectomy can be done with minimal morbidity and a short hospital stay, whereas more extended procedures, such as horizontal supraglottic laryngectomy or subtotal laryngectomy, induce a higher rate of complications.

Case Continued

The patient tolerates radiation well except for complaining of dry mouth and hoarseness of voice initially. Repeat endoscopy at 3 months shows no evidence of disease. He remains on strict surveillance for local recurrence and for a new upper aerodigestive tract primary cancer.

Discussion

The risk of new primary cancer related to tobacco is an important problem, especially in patients with small tumors, where the risk of a new primary exceeds the risk of recurrence. This risk is around 35% in patients who continue smoking, compared with 16% in patients who never smoked or stopped smoking after diagnosis. A high importance must be attached to smoking cessation.

Suggested Readings

Beitler JJ, Johnson JT. Transoral laser excision for early glottic cancer. *Int J Radiat Oncol Biol Phys* 2003;56:1063–1066.

Franchin G, Minatel E, Gobitti C. Radiotherapy for patients with early stage glottic carcinoma. Univariate and multivariate analyses in a group of consecutive, unselected patients. *Cancer* 2003;98:765–772.

Hermans R, Van den Bogaert W, Rijnders A, et al. Predicting the local outcome of glottic cell carcinoma after definitive radiation therapy: value of computed tomography determined tumor parameters. *Radiother Oncol* 1999;50:39–46.

Mendenhall WM, Amdur RJ, Morris CG, et al. T1-T2 squamous cell carcinoma of the glottic larynx treated with radiation therapy. *J Clin Oncol* 2001;19:4029–4036.

Mendenhall WM, Werning JW, Hinerman RW, et al. Management of T1-T2 glottic carcinomas. *Cancer* 2004;100:1786–1792.

Reddy SP, Mohideen N, Marra S, et al. Effect of tumor bulk on local control and survival of patients with T1 glottic cancer. *Radiother Oncol* 1997;47:161–166.

Rodriguez-Cuevas S, Labastida S, Gonzalez D. Partial laryngectomy as salvage surgery for radiation failures in T1-T2 laryngeal cancer. *Head Neck* 1998;20:630–633.

Rosier JF, Gregoire V, Counoy H, et al. Comparison of external radiotherapy, laser microsurgery and partial laryngectomy for the treatment of T1 N0 M0 glottic carcinomas: a retrospective evaluation. *Radiother Oncol* 1998;48:175–183.

Simpson Jones A, Fish B, Fenton JE, et al. The treatment of early laryngeal cancers (T1-T2 N0): surgery or irradiation? *Head Neck* 2004;26:127–135.

Presentation

A 58-year-old man who is a TV reporter presents to your office with a 2-month history of pharyngeal foreign body sensation. He reports a long history of tobacco consumption (around 30 cigarettes a day) and alcohol abuse (one bottle of wine a day and occasional spirits), without any evidence of other co-morbidity. Examination reveals good denture status, and flexible nasopharyngoscopic examination demonstrates an ulcerative and infiltrative lesion about 1.5 cm in diameter in the upper pyriform sinus arising within the aryepiglottic and the pharyngoepiglottic folds. The apex of the pyriform sinus as well as the posterior part of the aryepiglottic fold are free of tumor. Larynx mobility is normal. There is no other obvious abnormality of the upper aerodigestive tract. There are no palpable cervical lymph nodes.

Recommendation

Computed tomography (CT) scan of the head and neck and panendoscopy are required.

▓ CT Scans

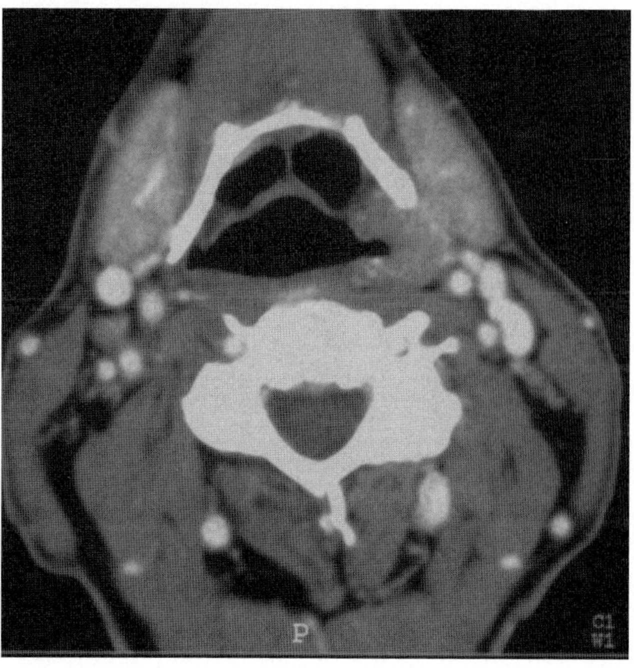

Figure 5.1A

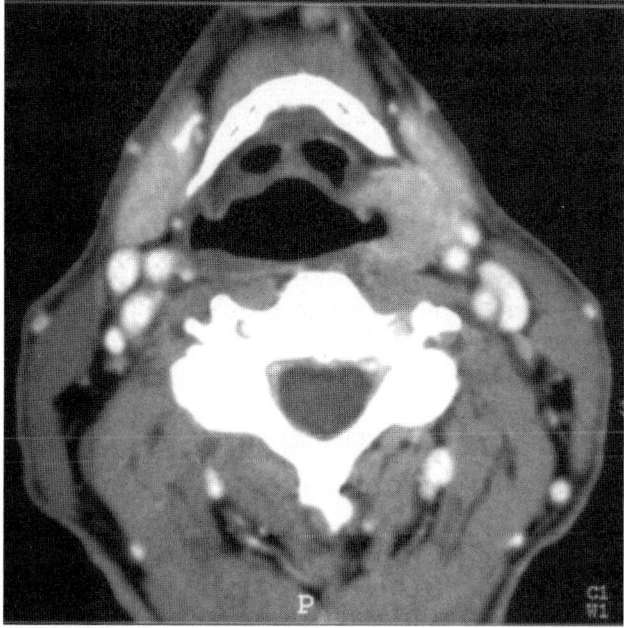

Figure 5.1B

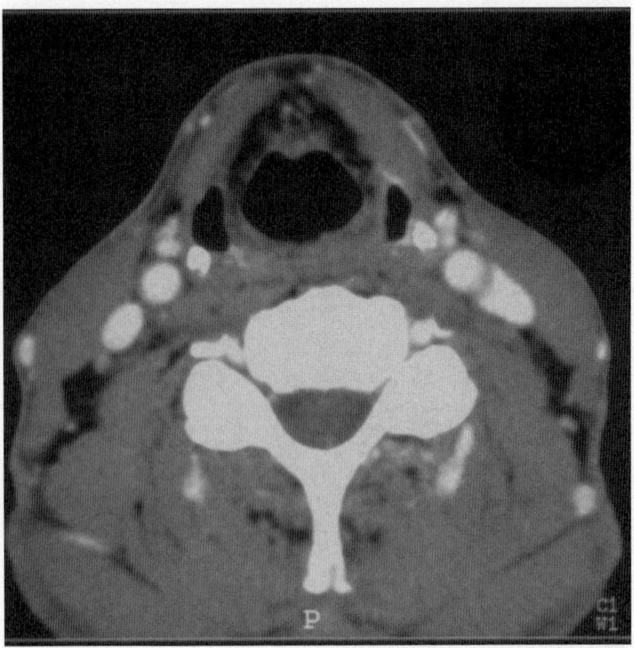

Figure 5.1C

CT Scan Report

The CT scan reveals an infiltrative lesion of the upper part of the lateral wall of the pyriform sinus extending to the anterior part of the aryepiglottic fold and reaching the thyrohyoid membrane without extending through it. The greatest diameters are 20.9×21.7 cm. The inferior part of the pyriform sinus is free and the larynx is mobile. There are no suspicious enlarged cervical lymph nodes.

Differential Diagnosis

Actually, there are very few differential diagnoses in such a situation. Such a lesion could correspond to a tuberculosis ulcer, but these lesions are most often localized on the posterior part of the pharyngolarynx. Nevertheless, tissue biopsy is mandatory.

Case Continued

The panendoscopy begins with a complete exploration of the esophagus and of the trachea and main bronchi. The oropharynx and oral cavity are carefully explored. There is no disease. The pharyngolarynx is explored directly and with rigid 30 degree and 70 degree endiscope. This confirms the presence of an ulcerative and slightly infiltrative lesion, 2 cm in diameter, of the upper part of the pyriform sinus growing down, but without extension to, the apex. Biopsy is performed.

Diagnosis

Disease is staged as T2 N0 M0, and the pathology report indicates moderately differentiated squamous cell carcinoma.

◼ Approach

There are two possible options: either partial surgery or irradiation. Because the apex is free, partial laryngopharyngectomy is feasible; in addition, only the very upper part of the medial wall of the pyriform sinus is involved, allowing a supraglottic resection sparing the arytenoid. The postoperative functional results are satisfactory in such a case. In the absence of enlarged suspicious cervical lymph nodes on the CT scan, postoperative irradiation most probably will not be necessary.

Discussion

There is no randomized comparison of the two approaches. There is a consensus that functional results are slightly better with irradiation but surgery offers better local control, particularly for endophytic lesions. Partial salvage surgery is less frequently feasible for hypopharyngeal than for laryngeal tumors that recur after irradiation. In the situation of irradiation failure (infiltrative and ulcerative tumor), due to the inferior extension of the tumor and its close contact with the thyrohyoid membrane, partial salvage surgery most probably would not be feasible, leaving only total laryngectomy as the surgical salvage option. For this patient, the chances of locoregional cure are high, and the main risk is the appearance of a second primary tumor that often occurs in the head and neck region. An exclusive surgical treatment would keep open any other option for the treatment of a second head and neck tumor. Laser endoscopic surgery is another surgical option, though in this case the endoscopic accessibility of the tumor was not sufficiently satisfactory to facilitate such an approach.

◼ Surgical Approach

A tracheotomy is performed, and a feeding tube is placed through the nasal cavity. Then, a modified neck dissection removing levels II to V is performed. A supraglottic hemipharyngolaryngectomy is performed, removing half the hyoid bone, the superior two thirds of the left thyroid ala, the superior half of the lateral wall, and the anterior half of the medial wall of the pyriform sinus in continuity with the left false vocal cord and the left half of the epiglottis. Macroscopic evaluation of the specimen reveals satisfactory margins and no metastases to the lymph nodes, to be confirmed by the pathology examination before deciding on an adjuvant treatment.

Case Continued

At the conclusion of the procedure, the patient is transferred to the recovery room, and 2 hours later, to his room in the surgery ward. The tracheotomy is removed on day 3 and speech therapy is initiated on the same day. Oral feeding is initiated on day 8, and the feeding tube is removed on day 9. The pathology report indicates that the neck dissection specimen contained 23 lymph nodes, all free of metastases, and the tumor had negative surgical margins.

Recommendation

No postoperative irradiation or chemotherapy is necessary. Psychological support for quitting tobacco and alcohol consumption should be provided. Bimonthly examinations should be performed as part of the surveillance program.

Suggested Readings

Chevalier D, Watelet JB, Darras JA, et al. Supraglottic hemilaryngopharyngectomy plus radiation for the treatment of early lateral margin and pyriform sinus carcinoma. *Head Neck* 1997;19:1–5.

Dubois JB, Guerrier B, Di Ruggiero JM, et al. Cancer of the piriform sinus: treatment with radiation alone and with surgery. *Radiology* 1986;160:831–836.

Gehanno P, Barry B, Guedon C, et al. Lateral supraglottic pharyngolaryngectomy with arytenoidectomy. *Head Neck* 1996;18:494–500.

Lefebvre JL, Chevalier D, Eschwege F. Pharyngeal walls, hypopharynx and larynx. In: Souhami RL, Tannock I, Hohenberger P, et al., eds. *Oxford textbook of oncology.* 2nd ed. Oxford: Oxford University Press; 2002:1429–1444.

case 6

Presentation

A 69-year-old woman became aware of a right upper neck swelling during an upper respiratory tract infection. Although the acute symptoms resolved, the mass persisted. She has a history of essential hypertension but is otherwise in very good health. She has smoked 20 cigarettes per day for more than 20 years, but had ceased in the 3 months prior to her presentation. She rarely drinks alcohol. She denies any throat pain, dysphagia, bleeding, or weight loss and has noticed no recent voice change. No skin tumors were removed in the past. Physical examination reveals a mass at least 3 cm in diameter, deep to the anterior border of the sternomastoid muscle with no additional evidence of adenopathy. Inspection of the oral cavity and oropharynx and flexible nasopharyngoscopy reveal no obvious abnormality.

Differential Diagnosis

A lateral neck mass presenting in an older patient, particularly one who smokes, should be considered metastatic carcinoma in a cervical lymph node until proven otherwise. The most likely diagnosis is metastatic squamous cell carcinoma (SCC), either from a mucosal or cutaneous site. Other metastatic tumors would include poorly differentiated or undifferentiated carcinomas, adenocarcinoma from head and neck or infraclavicular primaries, thyroid carcinoma, and melanoma or other cutaneous malignancies. Less commonly, a lateral neck mass may be a primary tumor of the salivary gland or thyroid, or a primary lymphoid tumor. A pulsatile mass may suggest a vascular tumor, such as a carotid body tumor. Rarely, this may be the presentation of a primary or metastatic bone or soft tissue sarcoma.

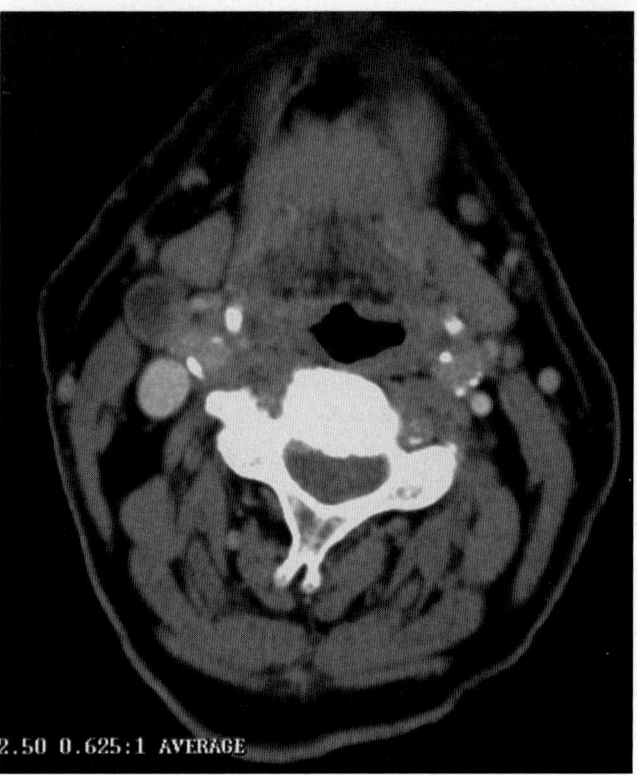

Figure 6.1

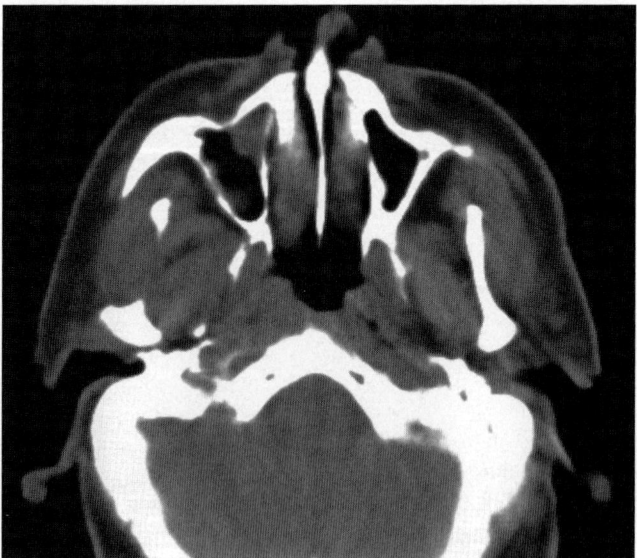

Figure 6.2

CT Scan Report

Computed tomography (CT) demonstrates a heterogeneous mass in the upper jugular chain consistent with malignant adenopathy. Figure 6.1 shows a partially cystic lymph node in the upper right neck, and Figure 6.2 reveals subtle asymmetry in the nasopharynx, suggesting a possible primary site.

Case Continued

Ultrasound results confirm the CT findings. Chest radiography reveals no pulmonary lesion. Fine-needle aspiration (FNA) biopsy shows large degenerate or necrotic cells with features consistent with SCC.

Recommendation

The patient is advised to have examination under anesthesia (EUA) and positron emission tomography (PET) scanning as part of an investigational protocol.

Approach

The entire upper aerodigestive tract should be systematically examined with the assistance of rigid endoscopes and, where possible, palpated. In the absence of a suspicious ulcer or tumor mass in the office examination, mucosal asymmetry, induration, or friability may offer the only clues to the presence of a primary tumor. In view of the CT findings, close attention should be paid to the right nasopharynx in this patient. The base of tongue, tonsils, pyriform sinuses, and postcricoid regions frequently harbor small primaries and should be carefully assessed. Biopsies should be taken from any suspicious areas. In the absence of any other abnormality, tonsillectomy should be performed.

Discussion

FNA biopsy is the most appropriate investigation of the neck mass, providing there is no specific contraindication. A diagnosis can be obtained in more than 90% of patients; therefore, open lymph–node biopsy is usually not necessary and is not recommended. If, however, FNA does not provide a diagnosis, current opinion is that an open biopsy can be performed without compromising the long-term outcome.

A thorough history and physical examination, combined with imaging and examination under anesthesia, will uncover a primary site in approximately 50% of patients presenting with a putative unknown primary. A diagnosis of metastatic SCC is easily made, but for diagnoses other than SCC, special stains of the fine-needle aspirate, or additional blood tests such as thyroglobulin, calcitonin, or prostate-specific antigen levels may provide some clue. A finding of adenocarcinoma would prompt further imaging of the thyroid, breast, and gastrointestinal tract. Poorly differentiated or undifferentiated tumors may also have primary sites above or below the clavicles. For 5% to 8% of patients presenting with a malignant neck mass, no primary site will be found.

Some have advocated "random" mucosal biopsies of the nasopharynx, tongue base, tonsils, and hypopharynx at EUA, but the diagnostic yield is small in the absence of mucosal abnormality. Biopsies should be directed by clinical and imaging findings and by the nature and location of the metastasis in the neck. Tonsillectomy is advocated because 15% to 40% of tonsils resected in this setting will contain a primary tumor. In at least one series, 10% of these tonsil tumors were found in the tonsil contralateral to the presenting neck mass; therefore, bilateral tonsillectomy has been recommended. Cystic metastases in the upper neck should raise suspicion of a tonsil or tongue base primary; for metastases lower in the neck, a primary in the cervical esophagus should be considered.

There is now considerable experience in using PET in the assessment of patients with unknown primaries, but its role is still debated. The sensitivity and specificity of PET for identifying known tumors are high and are better than CT or magnetic resonance imaging, but few additional primaries are found after careful clinical assessment, EUA, and directed biopsies as outlined earlier. Moreover, a significant false-positive rate leads to unnecessary additional investigations in some patients. Additional PET findings, other than locating the primary, lead to significant changes in management in up to 25% of patients. This investigation has been more useful in the assessment of nonsquamous tumors and in the detection of infraclavicular or metastatic disease. It may prove more cost-effective if done prior to any anatomical imaging and before biopsy.

Case Continued

At EUA, no significant mucosal abnormality is seen in the oral cavity, oropharynx, hypopharynx, or larynx. Cervical esophagoscopy is also normal. Biopsies are taken from the right nasopharynx and from the right tongue base. The patient has under-gone tonsillectomy in the distant past, and the right tonsillar fossa appears normal. No malignancy is identified in any of the biopsies.

PET Scan

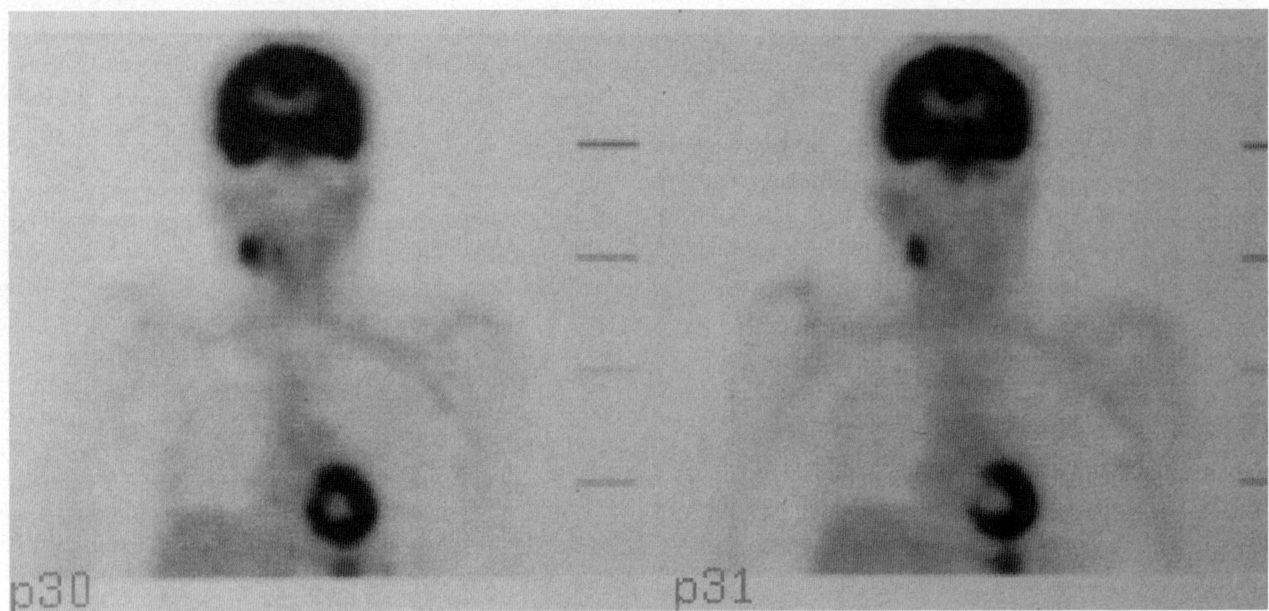

Figure 6.3

PET Scan Report

The PET scan demonstrated the presenting neck metastasis clearly. No primary site was identified, no hot spot was seen in the nasopharynx, and there was no evidence of any systemic disease.

Diagnosis

The diagnosis is metastatic SCC from an unknown primary site, with the tumor staged as Tx N2a M0 (stage III).

Recommendation

The patient is seen and assessed in a multidiscipli-nary clinic, and is offered surgical treatment in the form of a comprehensive right neck dissection, to be followed by adjuvant radiotherapy to the neck. Surgical complications discussed include wound infection, hemorrhage, seroma formation, neck stiffness and contractures, and the potential for shoulder droop and weakness should the spinal accessory nerve be injured or sacrificed. Early radia-tion effects include radiation dermatitis and mucosi-tis, with the potential for long-term xerostomia and neck fibrosis and pigmentation.

Surgical Approach

With the primary site not known, the entire nodal basin of the neck is considered at risk of harboring additional metastatic deposits, so comprehensive dissection of all five neck levels is advised. For a large, infiltrative mass in the upper neck, radical neck dissection may be necessary, but one or more of the internal jugular vein, spinal accessory nerve, or sternomastoid muscle may be preserved in an attempt to reduce the morbidity of the procedure, as long as complete excision of the tumor mass is not compromised in doing so.

Intraoperative Image

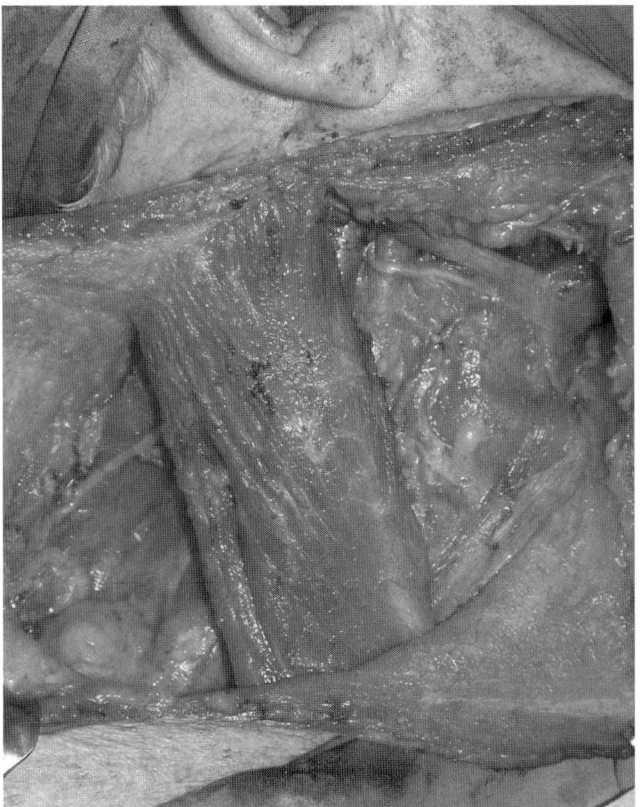

Figure 6.4

Intraoperative Report

On modified radical neck dissection, the single nodal mass proves to be quite mobile, and uninvolved fascial planes over the sternomastoid muscle and above the plane of the accessory nerve permit complete resection of the tumor with a modified dissection preserving all three major nonlymphatic structures (type III modified radical neck dissection).

Case Continued

The patient's postoperative course is uneventful. The pathology examination confirms a partially cystic SCC metastasis up to 4 cm in maximal diameter. No additional involved nodes are found. Postoperative radiotherapy is delivered to the right neck, with the patient receiving 50 Gy of the planned 54 Gy before finishing treatment early because of severe skin reaction. She is seen regularly in follow-up and remains well and free of disease 3 years following her surgery, with the primary tumor never having been found.

Discussion

As is the case for management of the neck in cases of head and neck cancer with known primaries, treatment options generally include surgery, radiotherapy, or a combination of the two. For limited neck disease with no extracapsular tumor extension, a single modality of treatment (either a neck dissection or neck irradiation alone) may be all that is necessary. Most patients, however, will present with advanced neck disease, and combination therapy is appropriate. Chemotherapy has not previously had a role in the management of this condition, but very recent studies have suggested a role for adjuvant concomitant chemoradiation following surgery for advanced neck disease from mucosal SCC.

Controversy exists regarding whether irradiation should be given only to the neck, or to all potential primary sites. There is doubt whether radiotherapy to the nasopharynx, hypopharynx, supraglottic larynx, and oropharynx is associated with a reduction in the ultimate appearance of primary tumors; however, radiotherapy is associated with significantly higher morbidity, and uses a potential treatment modality in the event of new tumors or recurrence. More extensive radiotherapy also does not appear to confer any additional survival advantage.

Primary tumors will become apparent in up to 20% of patients, and are usually associated with a worse outcome because only a minority will be salvaged. The appearance of the primary may be associated with the development of contralateral neck disease, so the appearance of a contralateral neck mass should lead to a full assessment with further EUA and biopsies. Up to 25% of patients overall may develop recurrence in the neck, with half or more of these in the contralateral neck. Ongoing surveillance is mandatory if these patients are to achieve optimal outcomes.

Although presentation with metastases implies advanced disease from the outset, aggressive treatment is warranted, because ultimate rates of disease control in the ipsilateral neck are more than 90%, and disease-specific survival at 4 years is more than 60%, with advancing neck stage adversely influencing the outcome.

Suggested Readings

Colletier PJ, Garden AS, Morrison WH, et al. Postoperative radiation for squamous cell carcinoma metastatic to cervical lymph nodes from an unknown primary site: outcomes and patterns of failure. *Head Neck* 1998;20:674–681.

Cooper JS, Forastiere AA, Jacobs J, et al. Postoperative concurrent radiotherapy and chemotherapy for high-risk squamous cell carcinoma of the head and neck. *N Engl J Med* 2004;350:1937–1944.

Fogarty GB, Peters LJ, Stewart J, et al. The usefulness of fluorine 18-labelled deoxyglucose positron emission tomography in the investigation of patients with cervical lymphadenopathy from an unknown primary tumor. *Head Neck* 2003;25:138–145.

Jereczek-Fossa BA, Jassem J, Orecchia R. Cervical lymph node metastases of squamous cell carcinoma from an unknown primary. *Cancer Treat Rev* 2004;30:153–164.

Koch WM, Bhatti N, Williams MF, et al. Oncologic rationale for bilateral tonsillectomy in head and neck squamous cell carcinoma of unknown primary source. *Otolaryngol Head Neck Surg* 2001;124:331–333.

McMahon J, Hruby G, O'Brien CJ, et al. Neck dissection and ipsilateral radiotherapy in the management of cervical metastatic carcinoma from an unknown primary. *Aust N Z J Surg* 2000;70:263–268.

Randall DA, Johnstone PA, Foss RD, et al. Tonsillectomy in the diagnosis of the unknown primary tumor of the head and neck. *Otolaryngol Head Neck Surg* 2000;122:52–55.

Presentation

A 55-year-old, previously well man presents with a history of a painless, gradually enlarging mass in the region of the right parotid for about 7 months. He presents after noticing difficulty depressing the right angle of his mouth, and being unable to close his right eye fully for the previous week. He gives a 90-pack-year history of cigarette use and has chewed tobacco for 40 years. He previously had a heavy alcohol intake, but has drunk none in the past decade. There were, however, no symptoms related to the upper aerodigestive tract. Examination reveals facial asymmetry with weakness in the distribution of upper and lower divisions of the facial nerve. There is a firm, nontender mass overlying the right angle of the mandible, somewhat mobile but with a suggestion of fixity to the overlying skin. No adenopathy is palpable elsewhere in the neck. No mucosal lesions or cutaneous tumors are present.

Clinical Photograph

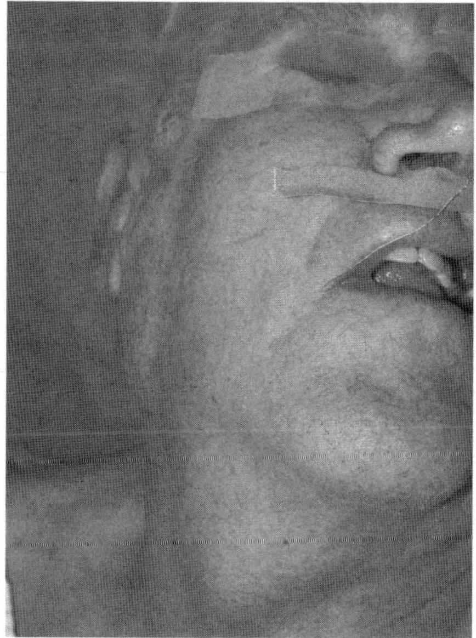

Figure 7.1

Physical Examination Report

A right parotid mass is clearly visible.

Differential Diagnosis

This man has significant risk factors for mucosal carcinoma of the upper aerodigestive tract, and careful assessment is needed to exclude a mucosal tumor. However, the presence of a mass partially overlying the angle of the mandible, in association with facial nerve weakness, strongly suggests a malignancy arising in, or metastatic to, the parotid salivary gland. In some adult populations, metastatic cutaneous malignancy is the most common cause of a parotid mass, so evidence of a current or previous squamous cell carcinoma or cutaneous melanoma should be sought. A variety of primary parotid malignancies may be the cause; mucoepidermoid carcinoma and adenoid cystic carcinoma are the most common, and both are frequently associated with perineural tumor involvement. Nonepithelial primary malignancies such as sarcoma and lymphoma are less likely, but should be considered. Most parotid tumors are benign, but these are rarely associated with facial nerve weakness. A primary neurogenic tumor or an inflammatory lesion involving the nerve is possible, as is a synchronous benign tumor and unrelated neuropathy; however, active steps should be taken to exclude malignancy even if these diagnoses are suggested. No pulmonary lesion is seen on a chest radiograph.

▦ Histopathology Slides

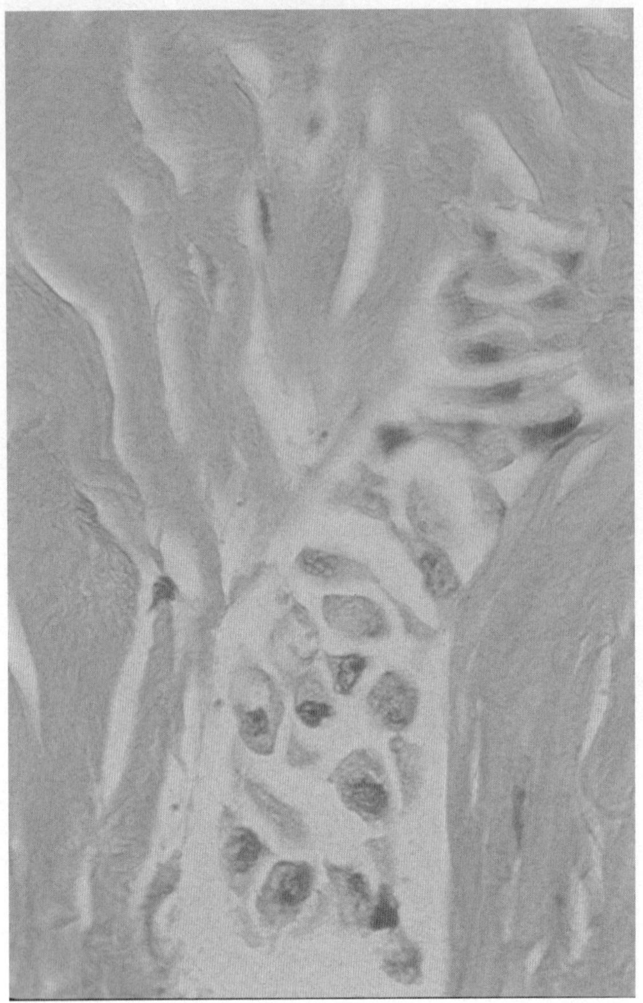

Figure 7.2A

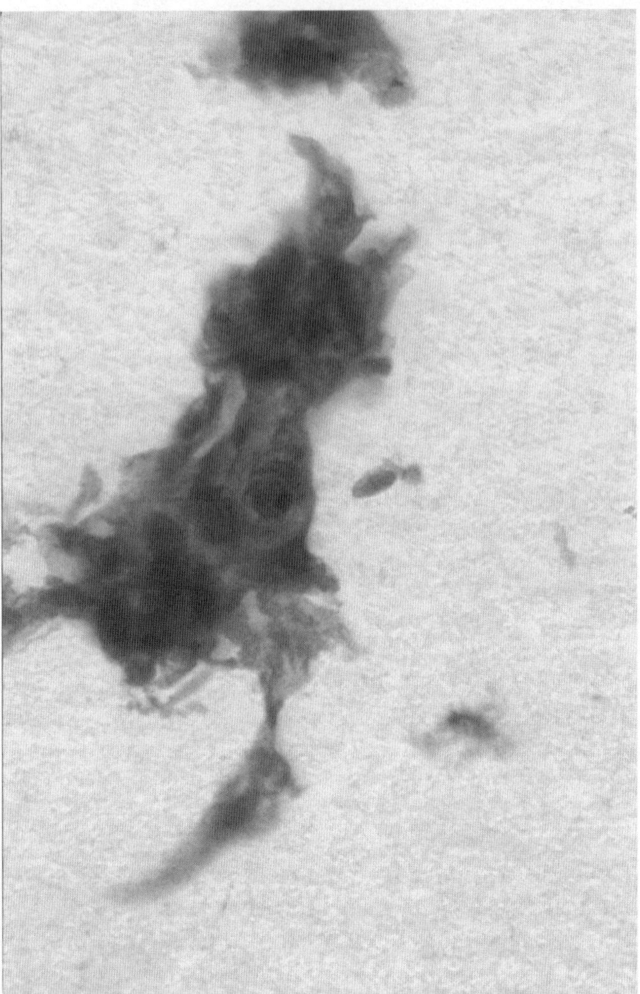

Figure 7.2B

Histopathology Report

Fine-needle aspiration (FNA) biopsy reveals large, malignant pleomorphic cells with features thought likely to be associated with mucoepidermoid carcinoma. Cell block **(A)** and Papanicolaou stain **(B)** show malignant cells with dense cytoplasms and high nuclear grades.

▦ CT Scan

CT Scan Report

Computed tomography (CT) scan of the parotid region of the head and neck shows a 4-cm enhancing mass involving the right parotid gland.

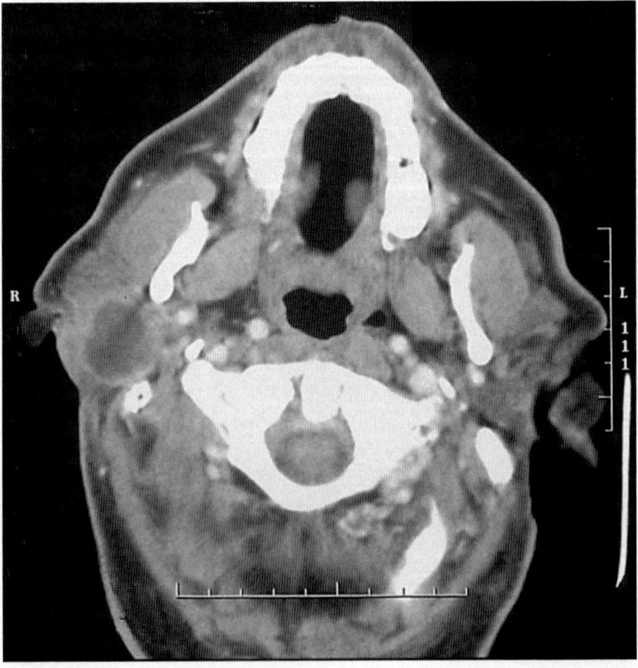

Figure 7.3

Discussion

FNA biopsy of salivary tumors has been established as an accurate and safe procedure, with a sensitivity and specificity well over 90% with experienced cytopathologists. FNA has been found to alter management of salivary masses in 35% of patients biopsied. In this case, the distinction needs to be made between a primary and a metastatic lesion that will effect management of the neck. Confirming the presence of malignancy allows appropriate counseling about the management of the facial nerve.

Imaging the parotid probably adds little to the assessment of benign lesions in the superficial lobe of the gland, but is necessary in an assessment of malignancy to accurately define the site and extent of the tumor and its relationship to neural and vascular structures and the base of the skull. Both CT scan and magnetic resonance imaging (MRI) can accurately define the relationship of the tumor to the gland and the extent of disease in the neck. CT offers better assessment of bony invasion. MRI would have provided far greater assessment of the extent of perineural spread.

Diagnosis

The history and investigations suggest a primary high-grade mucoepidermoid carcinoma arising in the right parotid gland and involving the facial nerve, with the tumor staged clinically as T4a N0 M0 (stage IVa).

Recommendation

After assessment at a multidisciplinary clinic, the patient is offered surgical treatment in the form of radical total parotidectomy with sacrifice of the facial nerve, and dissection of the lymph nodes of the upper neck. Primary reconstruction of the nerve with a nerve graft is recommended. Adjuvant radiotherapy to the parotid bed will be required, and will likely also be necessary for the neck. The patient is informed that nerve reconstruction will not result in the immediate return of facial function, and the importance of eye care postoperatively to avoid exposure keratosis and blindness is stressed. Additional procedures about the eye may prove necessary for corneal protection. Complications of the neck surgery discussed include wound collections due to hemorrhage or seroma, neck stiffness and contractures, and the potential for shoulder droop and weakness should the spinal accessory nerve be injured or sacrificed in the upper neck. There is the potential for damage to organs of hearing and balance during access to the facial nerve in the temporal bone. Harvest of the sural nerve for grafting will cause permanent sensory loss on the lateral border of the foot. Early radiation effects include radiation dermatitis and mucositis, with the potential for long-term xerostomia and neck fibrosis and pigmentation.

Surgical Approach

The parotid is approached via a right preauricular incision that is extended into an upper neck skin crease, raising a skin flap above the plane of the parotid fascia in the cheek and deep to the platysma in the neck. If skin infiltration is suspected, skin over the tumor mass is excised in continuity. The suspicion of facial nerve involvement requires radical total parotidectomy, an en bloc resection of the parotid and the tumor it contains, and sacrifice of the facial nerve. Ideally, the involvement of the nerve by tumor should be confirmed intraoperatively before the irreversible step of nerve transaction, but adequate resection of the mass should not be compromised. The presence or absence of tumor at the surgical resection margins has a significant impact on the prognosis of these carcinomas. If there is gross infiltration of the facial nerve (see Fig. 7.4A) or encasement of the nerve by the tumor, facial nerve sacrifice cannot be avoided. The facial nerve is transected as it leaves the stylomastoid foramen. After completion of the parotidectomy and neck dissection, a cortical mastoidectomy is performed to expose the proximal facial nerve and the temporal bone is drilled to expose the nerve as far as is necessary to obtain an uninvolved margin. Frozen sections should be taken from the proximal and distal nerve margins because perineural tumor may be present at sites distant from macroscopic disease.

The need for neck dissection for the clinically negative neck in major salivary gland cancers is debatable. The suspicion of a high-grade lesion in this case implies a risk of nearly 50% that occult nodal disease is present, so treatment of the neck needs to be addressed. Indications already exist for postoperative radiotherapy, and experience suggests that, as in mucosal squamous cell carcinoma, subclinical disease may be adequately treated with radiotherapy. However, because the upper neck will be entered to achieve an adequate margin on the tumor mass, little additional morbidity will be incurred to remove the upper neck nodes. Levels II and III are dissected in this patient in continuity with the parotid resection, which, if negative, may help minimize the morbidity of subsequent radiotherapy.

▨ Intraoperative Images

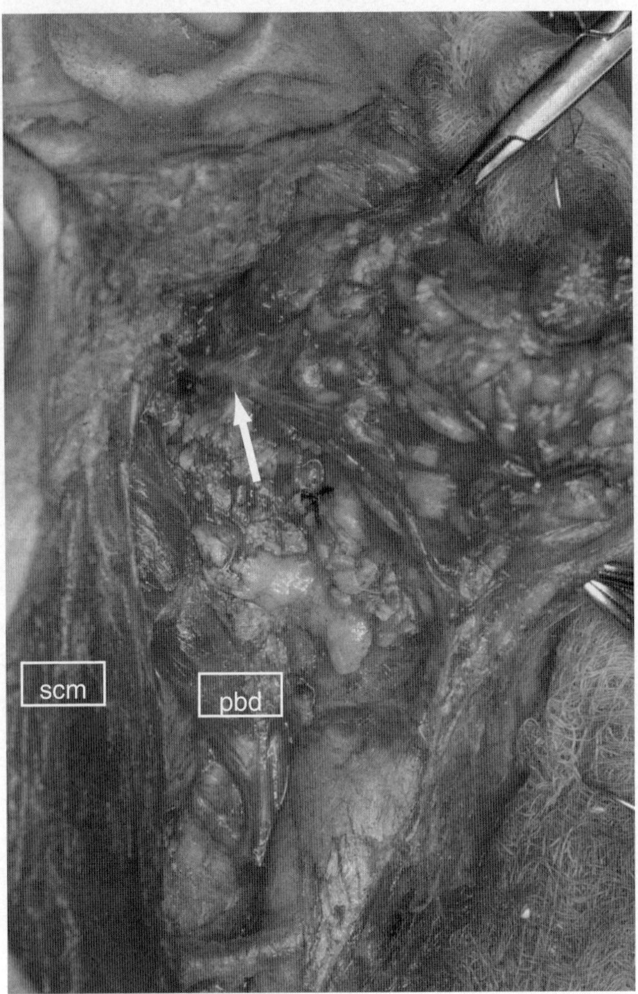

Figure 7.4A

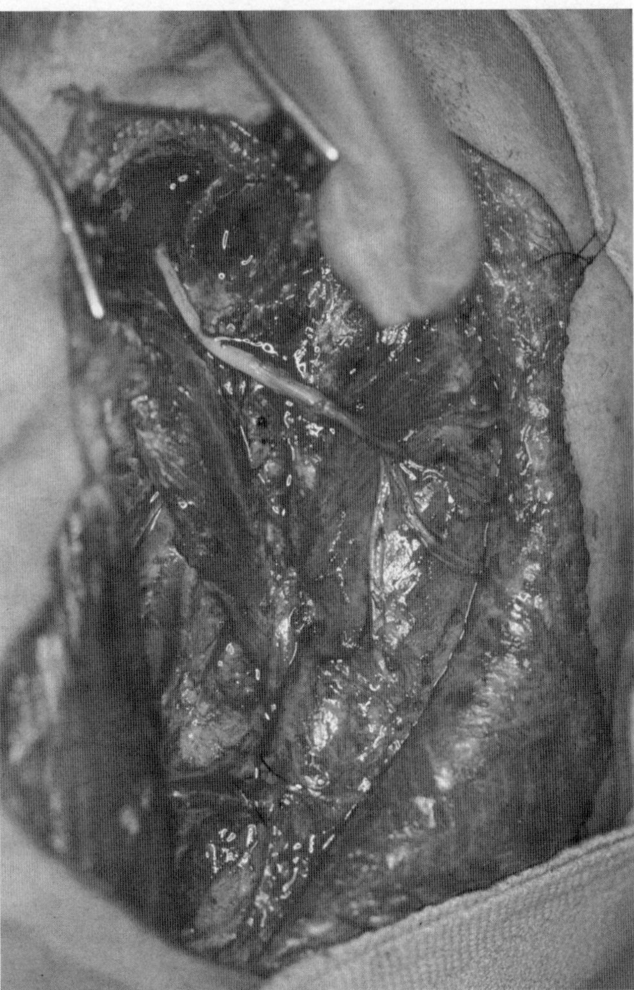

Figure 7.4B

Intraoperative Report

The facial nerve trunk is infiltrated with tumor (A, *arrow*). The sural nerve is chosen for grafting because it is a branched sensory nerve easily harvested from the distal lateral leg, the loss of which causes little morbidity. As many branches as possible are grafted, with priority given to branches to the periorbital muscles.

Case Continued

The patient has an uneventful postoperative course. The facial nerve weakness is more pronounced, but there is adequate corneal cover initially. Tarsorrhaphy is ultimately required to improve ectropion, but the patient declines insertion of a gold weight to the upper lid and suffers no complication as a result. There is obvious perivascular invasion, with gross tumor within the external jugular vein. One lymph node in level IIA is found to contain metastatic disease.

▨ Histopathology Slides

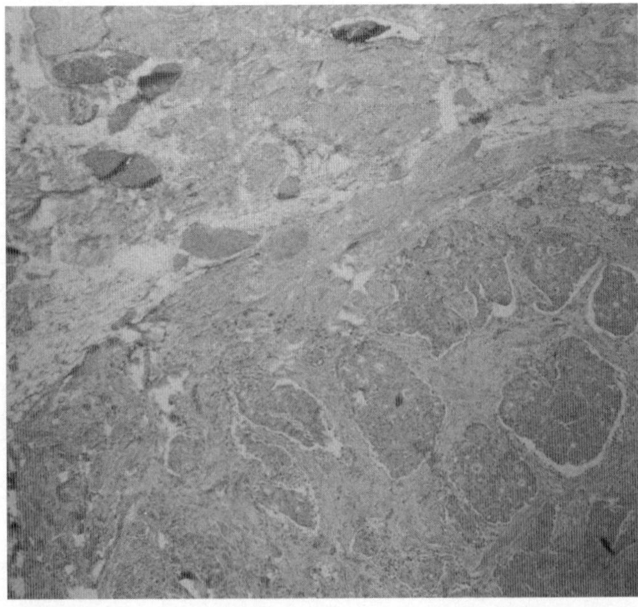

Figure 7.5A

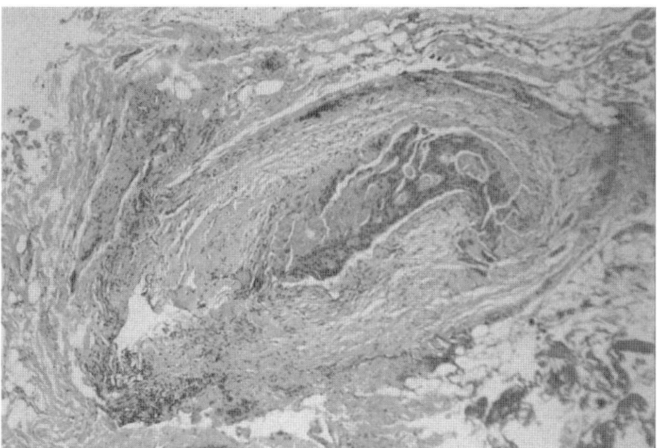

Figure 7.5B

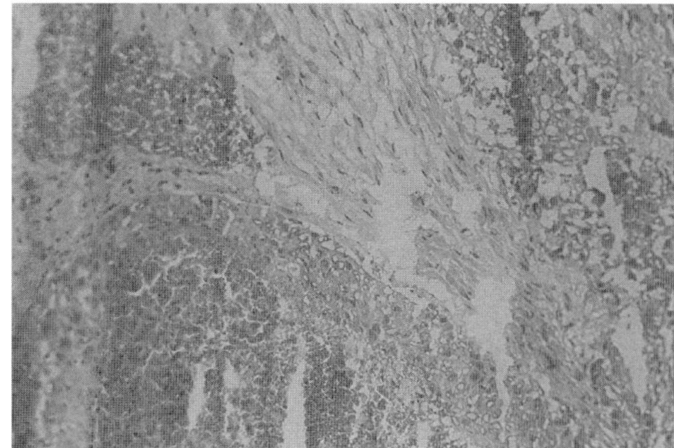

Figure 7.5C

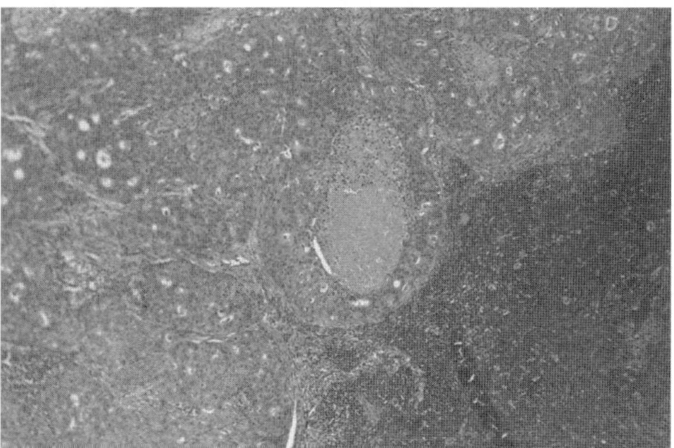

Figure 7.5D

Histopathology Report

The pathology examination confirmed a high-grade mucoepidermoid carcinoma infiltrating the main trunk of the facial nerve and further perineural tumor involving more peripheral branches, with a close margin reported on the buccal branch. Histology examination shows aggressive pathological features of (a) tumor infiltrating close to skin, (b) tumor in buccal nerve, (c) invasion of the external jugular vein, and (d) level IIA node metastasis.

Case Continued

Postoperative radiotherapy is delivered to the parotid bed and right neck, and is well tolerated. There is no evidence of recurrence 1 year following treatment, with some recovery of the resting facial tone.

Discussion

Despite the good early outcome in this patient, the prognosis for this tumor is poor. Approximately one in eight patients with primary parotid malignancies will present with facial nerve palsy, with 5-year survival in this group ranging from 0% to 27%, with a mean survival of less than 3 years from the onset of paralysis. Even without obvious nerve dysfunction, the findings of perineural invasion will double the chance of local failure. The presence of facial nerve weakness also indicated the likelihood of the presence of occult nodal metastasis. At least one in four patients with high-grade mucoepidermoid carcinoma will have occult nodal disease. As with head and neck squamous carcinomas, the presence of nodal disease reduces the chance of survival by half or more. There is general agreement that tumor grade significantly affects the outcome in mucoepidermoid carcinoma, but there is still controversy about what constitutes the most useful system for grading. Marked cellular pleomorphism, tumor necrosis, and neural and vascular invasion all indicate the aggressive nature of this tumor. High tumor grade is associated with a higher incidence of local, regional, and systemic failure, and a nearly 80% chance of dying from the disease.

Postoperative radiotherapy is recommended for patients with adverse prognostic features, including large primary tumors, high-grade tumors, perineural invasion, lymph-node metastases, and close or positive margins. When major nerves are involved, the course of the nerves is usually irradiated to their ganglion. Adding radiotherapy does not, however, replace the need to obtain adequate surgical margins where possible. Many of these adverse features are risk factors for the development of systemic disease, so no definite survival advantage has been demonstrated, but the rates of local and regional failure can be significantly reduced. Salivary gland malignancies do respond to various chemotherapeutic agents, but responses are neither complete nor durable and have not improved survival, so chemotherapy does not yet have a defined role in this disease.

Suggested Readings

Bron LP, Traynor SJ, NcNeil EB, et al. Primary and metastatic cancer of the parotid: Comparison of clinical behavior in 232 cases. *Laryngoscope* 2003;113:1070–1075.

Heller KS, Dubner S, Chess Q, et al. Value of fine needle aspiration biopsy of salivary gland masses in clinical decision-making. *Am J Surg* 1992;164:667–670.

Hicks MJ, el-Naggar AK, Flaitz CM, et al. Histocytological grading of mucoepidermoid carcinoma of major salivary glands in prognosis and survival: a clinicopathological and flow cytometric investigation. *Head Neck* 1995;17:89–95.

Hocwald E, Korkmaz H, Yoo GH, et al. Prognostic factors in major salivary gland cancer. *Laryngoscope* 2001;111:1434–1439.

Medina JE. Neck dissection in the treatment of cancer of the major salivary glands. *Otol Clin North Am* 1998;31:815–822.

Seifert G, Sobin LH. The World Health Organization's histological classification of salivary gland tumors. *Cancer* 1992;70:379–385.

Spiro RH, Armstrong JG, Harrison LB, et al. Carcinoma of major salivary glands. Recent trends. *Arch Otolaryngol Head Neck Surg* 1989;115:316–321.

Presentation

The patient is a 61-year-old man who is having knee-replacement surgery. His medical history includes osteoarthritis, mild hypertension, chronic obstructive pulmonary disease, and gastroesophageal reflux disease. He has no surgical history. His medications are a beta-blocker, some inhaled bronchodilators, a proton-pump inhibitor, and a COX-2 inhibitor. He has a 90-pack-year smoking history, and drinks alcohol occasionally. He reports an intermittent chronic cough. He has had no hemoptysis, hoarseness, chest pain, dyspnea, or facial swelling. On physical examination, pertinent findings include globally decreased breath sounds and mild expiratory wheezes. There is no dullness to chest percussion. The remainder of his physical exam is unremarkable. He brought his chest radiograph with him.

■ Chest X-Ray

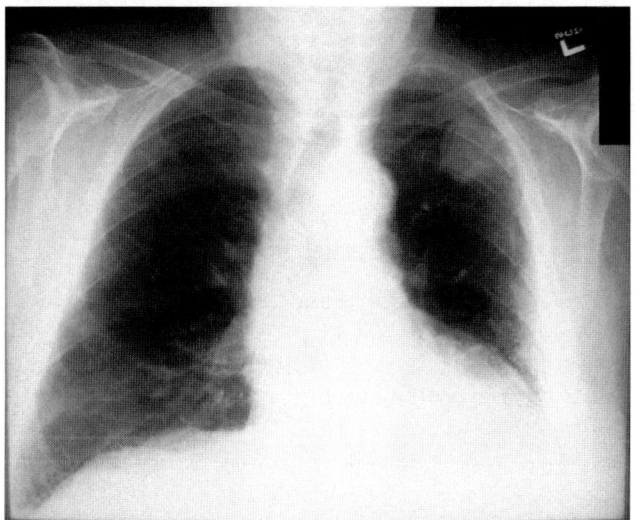

Figure 8.1

Chest X-Ray Report

There is a suspicious nodule in the left upper lobe, but otherwise lung fields are clear.

Differential Diagnosis

The most likely diagnosis of a newly identified lung mass in a 61-year-old smoker is non-small cell lung cancer (NSCLC). This is the working diagnosis until definitively excluded. When definitively excluded, alternative diagnoses can be considered, including infection, benign tumors, and metastatic disease.

Discussion

A primary lung cancer can be definitively diagnosed using four methods: sputum cytology, flexible bronchoscopy, transthoracic needle aspiration (TTNA), and at operation. Sputum cytology carries a sensitivity of 66% and specificity of 99% when done at an institution with a well-established sputum cytology program, but is rarely performed now. Reports of flexible bronchoscopy vary by tumor location. The sensitivity for central tumors is reported to be about 88%, but falls to 69% or less for peripheral tumors. Thus, nondiagnostic results of bronchoscopy for a peripheral lesion that is suspicious for cancer do not obviate the need for further evaluation. The sensitivity of TTNA is reported to be as high as 90%, but the false-negative rate is generally found to be between 20% and 30%. Thus, a nondiagnostic TTNA also does not exclude cancer. Its role in the workup of suspicious lesions is debatable because the results will not affect therapy if the patient is an acceptable candidate for lung resection. Either outcome—identifying cancer or leaving it not disproved—will lead to surgical resection. Exhaustive efforts to obtain definitive tissue diagnosis should be used in cases where neoadjuvant (preoperative) therapy is planned or surgery is not feasible. Patients with suspicious tumors, clinically early-stage disease, and those who are candidates for surgery should have appropriate surgical therapy, despite a nondiagnostic TTNA or bronchoscopy.

Recommendation

Flexible bronchoscopy.

Case Continued

Based on the likelihood of NSCLC, a flexible bronchoscopy is performed, but no abnormalities are seen. Results of bronchial brushings and washings are also negative. A TTNA is considered, but is not performed for the reasons outlined perviously; the results, diagnostic or not, would not alter the plan of treatment for this patient.

Diagnosis and Recommendation

Highly likely NSCLC. A thorough history and physical examination complemented with appropriate staging (computed tomography [CT] scan, positron emission tomography [PET] scan, mediastinoscopy) of the tumor is important in the treatment of lung cancer.

Discussion

The majority of lung cancer patients are not candidates for resection at the time of presentation because of the extent of their disease. Signs and symptoms associated with intrathoracic spread include recurrent laryngeal nerve palsy, phrenic nerve paralysis, Horner's syndrome, chest wall pain, pleuritic pain, and superior vena cava syndrome.

Staging for lung cancer can be accomplished using a variety of noninvasive and invasive modalities. Mediastinoscopy is the most accurate method for staging the mediastinum. Transbronchial needle aspiration (TBNA) and endoscopic ultrasound with needle aspiration (EUS-NA) are alternative methods to sample mediastinal lymph nodes, presently performed only in a few medical centers.

CT scan and PET scan are the primary noninvasive staging modalities. Although initially heralded as a great advance in staging the mediastinum, CT scan is not sensitive enough to be used alone. When based only on CT scanning, 5% to 15% of patients with clinical stage T1 N0 NSCLC will have mediastinal lymph node metastases. There is also a 40% false-positive rate with CT for mediastinal lymph nodes. However, when used to evaluate mediastinal lymph-node involvement, PET scan has a reported sensitivity as high as 85% and specificity as high as 88%. Studies are currently underway to evaluate the utility of combined CT and PET scanning for staging.

Mediastinoscopy remains the mainstay of mediastinal staging. Its specificity is essentially 100% and its sensitivity 90% to 95%. As mentioned earlier, CT has appreciable false-positive and false-negative rates, and PET scans also are not sufficiently sensitive.

Currently, mediastinoscopy is the procedure of choice to confirm mediastinal lymph-node status in patients after noninvasive staging. However, future experience with combined CT and PET scanning may eventually demonstrate sufficient sensitivity that mediastinoscopy can be omitted.

Case Continued

The patient has a CT scan of the chest to evaluate the possibility of involvement of other structures and the status of regional lymph nodes. A PET scan is also completed. The PET scan shows neither distant metastases (for which its accuracy is high) nor mediastinal lymph-node involvement.

◼ Chest CT Scan

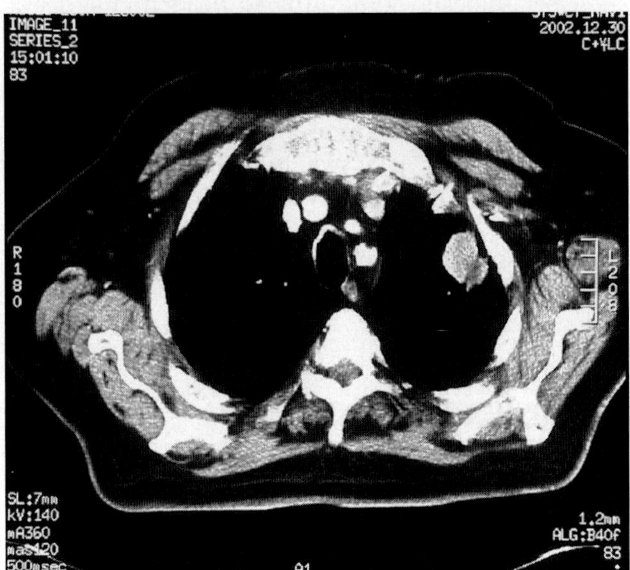

Figure 8.2

Chest CT Scan Report

There is a spiculated mass in the left upper lobe, compatible with NSCLC, contained within the visceral pleura. There is an identifiable left paratracheal lymph node, which is approximately 1 cm in diameter.

◼ Approach

Prior to undergoing a thoracotomy, the patient's physiologic condition must be considered. All patients should have a preoperative cardiac evaluation, as smoking is a significant risk factor for coronary artery disease as well as lung cancer. The patient's lung function must be carefully assessed. Pulmonary function tests (PFTs) will determine if the patient has sufficient lung function to tolerate a lung resection. In general, a forced expiratory volume in 1 second (FEV_1) greater than 2.0 L (or 80% of predicted) is acceptable for a patient requiring pneumonectomy. An FEV_1 greater than 1.5 L is sufficient for a lobectomy. Stair-climbing and arterial blood gas testing have also been used to stratify patient risk based on pulmonary function. Finally, smoking cessation preoperatively will significantly decrease the patient's morbidity and mortality, and should be encouraged in every lung cancer patient.

Surgical Approach

Mediastinoscopy allows for biopsy of mediastinal lymph nodes. Through a suprasternal incision, the pretracheal plane is developed and a mediastinoscope is used to sample the paratracheal lymph nodes. If these nodes are involved, the patient has stage III disease and should have chemotherapy, with or without radiotherapy, as neoadjuvant therapy before being considered for resection. If the mediastinoscopy shows no lymph-node involvement, the patient has stage I or II disease and is a candidate for immediate surgical resection.

After a thorough exploration of the thoracic cavity is performed, the mediastinal pleura is opened. After identification of the phrenic, vagal, and recurrent laryngeal nerves, the superior pulmonary artery and the superior and inferior pulmonary veins are individually dissected and vessels loops placed. To perform an upper lobectomy, the pulmonary artery is followed distally, which leads to the major fissure. The individual segmental branch to the upper lobe is carefully dissected, and can be transected with a linear endovascular stapler. The appropriate draining pulmonary vein is dissected and then transected. With the vessels controlled, the underlying bronchus is exposed and then transected. After the lung resection is completed, the lung is inflated and any leaks are controlled with absorbable sutures. Two chest tubes are inserted and connected to wall suction, and the incision is closed.

Case Continued

Our patient has no metastatic disease on his PET scan, and the mediastinoscopy is normal. This made his final staging T2 N0 M0. His physiologic status was judged to be sufficient for a lobectomy. Through a left thoracotomy, a left upper lobectomy was completed. Paratracheal and subcarinal lymph nodes were excised en bloc and were found not to harbor metastatic disease. Postoperatively, the patient does well. His chest tubes are removed in 3 days, and he is discharged home on postoperative day 5.

Discussion

If the patient had evidence of nodal involvement on PET scan, confirmed by mediastinoscopy, he would have stage III disease. In that event, the appropriate therapeutic approach is to begin with neoadjuvant therapy consisting of chemotherapy with or without radiotherapy prior to restaging. Patients who respond to this therapy with tumor reduction have been shown to have considerably better survival than nonresponders. For this patient, the appropriate operative procedure would still be a left upper lobectomy with excision of mediastinal lymph nodes. Postoperative morbidity and mortality are usually not increased by the neoadjuvant regimen.

Suggested Readings

Beckles MA, Spiro SG, Colice GL, et al. Initial evaluation of the patient with lung cancer: symptoms, signs, laboratory tests, and paraneoplastic syndromes. *Chest* 2003;123:97S–104S.

Beckles MA, Spiro SG, Colice GL, et al. The physiologic evaluation of patients with lung cancer being considered for resectional therapy. *Chest* 2003;123:105S–114S.

Detterbeck FC, DeCamp MM, Kohlman LJ, et al. Invasive staging: the guidelines. *Chest* 2003;123:167S–175S.

Gonzalez-Stawinski GV, Lemaire A, Merchant F, et al. A comparative analysis of positron emission tomography and mediastinoscopy in staging non-small cell lung cancer. *J Thorac Cardiovasc Surg* 2003;126:1900–1905.

Rivera MP, Detterbeck F, Mehta AC. Diagnosis of lung cancer: the guidelines. *Chest* 2003;123:29S–136S.

Silvestri GA, Tanoue LT, Margolis ML, et al. The noninvasive staging of non-small cell lung cancer: the guidelines. *Chest* 2003;123:147S–156S.

case 9

Presentation

A 66-year-old woman is referred by her primary care physician for further workup of a left lung mass. She is a former smoker, having quit in 1994. She has noted increasing shortness of breath and cough for 6 weeks, but no hemoptysis. She quit work 3 weeks ago because of increasing fatigue, and she has lost 8 pounds over the last month.

Differential Diagnosis

There is little doubt that this patient has a malignancy, although sometimes a smoldering infection such as tuberculosis (TB) or an empyema can cause similar fatigue and weight loss. The symptoms of cough and shortness of breath suggest airway compression, and thus suggest lung cancer as opposed to a primary mediastinal tumor or a pleural process. The rapidity of progression of her symptoms suggests this is a rapidly growing tumor, such as small cell lung cancer (SCLC). In addition to detailed evaluation of the clinical presentation, a computed tomography (CT) scan of the chest is helpful. The clinical findings and the radiographic characteristics generally allow a presumptive diagnosis to be made, and furthermore, usually define which tests are needed for further workup with regard to diagnosis and staging.

Recommendation

The patient should have a complete history and physical examination, and a chest CT scan.

Case Continued

A careful history discloses no other symptoms. Specifically, she denies any neurological symptoms such as headaches or focal weakness, and has no new bone or joint pains. Past medical history, family history, social history, and review of systems are unremarkable except for smoking and that her father died of lung cancer. Her physical examination is entirely normal. Notably, there are no palpable supraclavicular lymph nodes.

■ Chest CT Scans

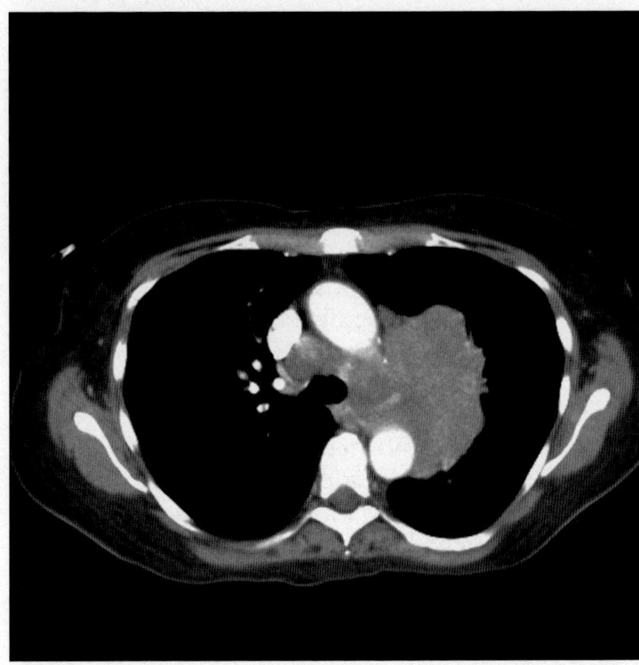

Figure 9.1A

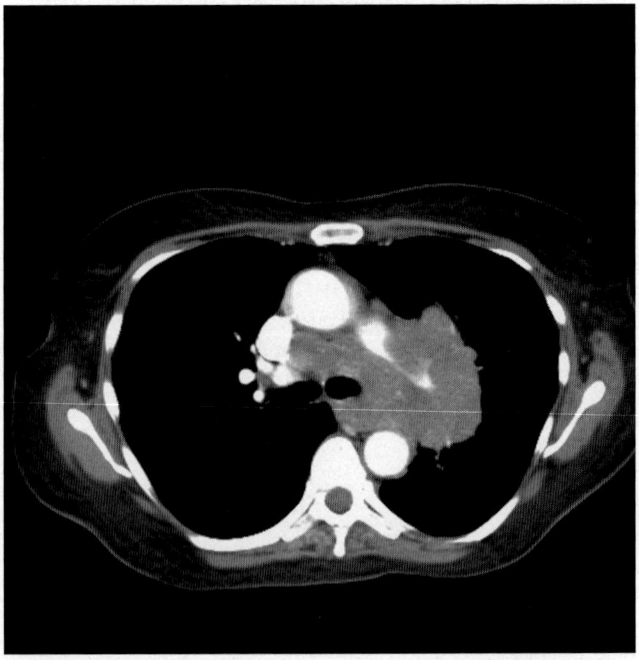

Figure 9.1B

Chest CT Scan Report

There is a large central left lung mass extending into the mediastinum. The left pulmonary artery is compressed, as is the left upper lobe bronchus. The heart, liver, and adrenal glands appear normal.

Differential Diagnosis Continued

The combination of risk factors and the radiographic appearance leave no real doubt that this is a lung cancer. The epicenter of this tumor is in the left lung, although it extends dramatically into the middle mediastinum. The rapid progression of symptoms, the central nature of the tumor, and the bulky mediastinal involvement makes SCLC very likely.

Other possible diagnoses include a non-small cell lung cancer (NSCLC), a lymphoma, or a mediastinal germ cell tumor. This tumor could be a NSCLC, although these typically have a less central epicenter and less dramatic mediastinal involvement. Although mediastinal germ cell tumors are more common in younger patients, they do occur in this age group and may be rapidly growing. However, they are typically centered in the anterior mediastinum, and the radiographic appearance of this case would be highly unusual. Lymphoma may also exhibit rapid growth, but that presentation is more common in the pediatric population and young adults. Furthermore, patients with lymphoma usually have palpable nodes in extrathoracic sites and additional areas of nodal enlargement on CT (in the anterior mediastinum, lower mediastinum, opposite hilum, neck, axilla, or upper abdomen).

This patient has nonspecific symptoms of distant metastases (fatigue and weight loss), although she does not have organ-specific symptoms (neurologic or skeletal). The physical exam does not suggest an obvious site of distant metastases that would be easy to biopsy and thereby confirm both the diagnosis and the stage.

Discussion

Approximately 15% to 20% of lung cancers are classified as SCLC. Approximately 2% to 3% of these cases have a mixed SCLC and NSCLC histologic pattern. SCLC is characterized by rapid growth and early involvement of mediastinal nodes and distant metastatic sites. The primary risk factor for SCLC is tobacco consumption. In fact, the occurrence of SCLC in a nonsmoker is so rare (0% to 3%) that one must question the diagnosis of SCLC in a patient who is a lifelong nonsmoker.

Signs and symptoms of SCLC relate to the bulk of disease and anatomic location of the tumor. In a population-based retrospective review of presenting symptoms, cough, weight loss, dyspnea, and chest pain were each present in approximately one third of patients with SCLC. Hemoptysis and hoarseness also occur frequently. Regional and mediastinal lymphadenopathy are present in the vast majority of patients. Various paraneoplastic syndromes have been reported with SCLC. These include the syndrome of inappropriate antidiuretic hormone (SIADH), hyponatremia, ectopic adrenocorticotropic hormone (ACTH) production, and Eaton-Lambert syndrome.

Case Continued

The patient undergoes bronchoscopy, which reveals abnormal endobronchial tissue in the left upper lobe bronchus.

Diagnosis

Biopsies reveal SCLC.

Discussion

In SCLC, the diagnosis is obtained by whatever method is easiest, and staging is generally based on radiographic imaging without tissue confirmation of metastatic involvement. In the absence of palpable supraclavicular nodes, bronchoscopy is a reasonable choice. Although sputum cytology and transthoracic needle aspiration are alternatives, the sensitivity of these approaches is approximately 40% to 60%, whereas it is more than 90% for bronchoscopy in cases of SCLC (and in central tumors with airway symptoms in general). Mediastinoscopy, thoracoscopy, and thoracotomy are reserved for those patients in whom other techniques have failed to yield a diagnosis.

A cytologic diagnosis of SCLC is reliable when the clinical presentation is consistent with this diagnosis. A peripheral lung mass is an extremely unusual presentation of SCLC, especially in the absence of bulky mediastinal node involvement. When a cytologic diagnosis suggests SCLC in such cases, the chances are far greater that this is an error, and that the tumor is an NSCLC or a carcinoid tumor (which also has neuroendocrine granules like SCLC). Further diagnostic tests, including resection of the mass, are indicated when the presentation is highly unusual for SCLC.

SCLC is divided into limited-stage (LS) and extensive-stage (ES) disease. LS denotes disease confined to the chest, although occasionally patients may be classified as ES if the intrathoracic disease is very extensive (a mass larger than 50% of the width of the thorax, ipsilateral pleural effusion, contralateral hilar involvement, supraclavicular involvement). Because extrathoracic metastases are present in approximately 60% of patients with SCLC, all patients with SCLC should undergo a search for distant metastases with scans, as necessary, of the brain, bones, and abdomen, and bone marrow biopsy.

Case Continued

The patient is found to have no evidence of extrathoracic disease.

Approach

The patient has limited-stage SCLC. She is treated with a combination of chemotherapy and radiation. She undergoes two cycles of etoposide and cisplatin (EP), followed by concurrent EP and radiation therapy (RT) for a total of six cycles of EP and 45 Gy of RT. She has a complete radiographic response. She then undergoes prophylactic cranial irradiation (PCI).

CT Scans

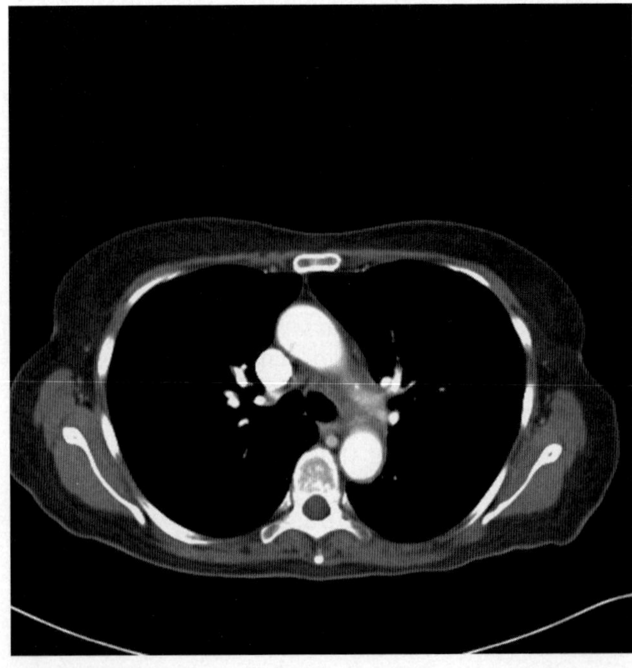

Figure 9.2A

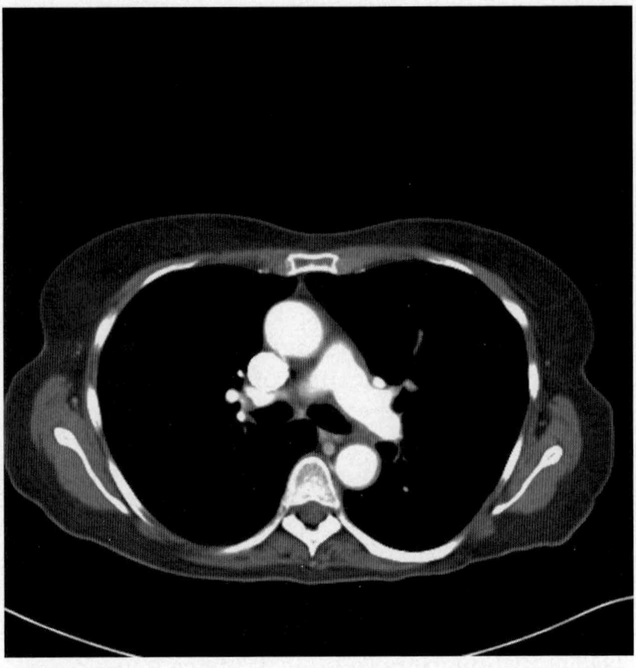

Figure 9.2B

CT Scan Report

There is complete resolution of the left hilar mass.

Discussion

Extensive-stage SCLC is treated with chemotherapy. Although the chance of cure for these patients is slim (2% to 3%), treatment is of tremendous palliative benefit. The median survival time without treatment is approximately 6 weeks, whereas with treatment it is 8 to 12 months. An objective response (more than 50% reduction in radiographic tumor dimensions) is achieved in the vast majority (80%) of patients, and a complete radiographic response is seen in approximately 25%. Consistent with this, patients generally experience a marked relief of symptoms and improvement in quality of life with chemotherapy. Patients may be candidates for second-line therapy when they relapse.

Limited-stage SCLC (LS-SCLC) is treated with a combination of chemotherapy and RT. The combination results in an improvement in 5-year survival to approximately 15% from about 10% with chemotherapy alone. The addition of RT also results in significantly improved local (intrathoracic) control, although most patients with LS-SCLC nevertheless eventually experience local recurrence. There appears to be better survival when RT is delivered early and concurrently with chemotherapy. In patients who achieve complete responses, PCI is indicated because it improves the 5-year survival rate (to 20% from 15%) and reduces the incidence of subsequent brain metastases.

Surgical Approach

The patient does not undergo surgical resection.

Discussion

In general, surgery plays an extremely limited role in patients with SCLC. The role of surgery in SCLC is restricted to patients in whom the diagnosis is either unknown or in doubt, to occasional patients who have failed nonsurgical treatment but remain resectable, and to patients enrolled in a clinical trial involving surgery.

If the accuracy of the diagnosis of SCLC is in doubt because of an atypical presentation, there should be no hesitation to proceed with a resection. Usually the tumor will be found to be an NSCLC, and resection is not detrimental if the patient really has an SCLC without mediastinal node involvement. If SCLC is found, most experts in this field believe strongly that adjuvant chemotherapy should be given, although little direct data are available on which to base this.

Occasionally patients fail to respond to chemoradiation, or experience a relapse, but have resectable tumors. These select patients should undergo surgery. There is a high probability that these patients have an NSCLC component to their tumors, and often the SCLC component of the tumor has been effectively treated by the chemoradiotherapy. There are compelling, albeit limited, data suggesting that a substantial number of these select patients can be cured by resection. In one study of surgery as a *salvage* treatment after unsuccessful chemoradiotherapy, the median survival was 31 months, with a 5-year survival rate of 32%. Most (82%) of the 28 patients were able to be completely resected, and 36% were found to have either a pure NSCLC or a tumor of mixed histology.

The high local failure rate and the low cure rate of combined chemotherapy and RT have led to a re-evaluation of the role of surgery as part of a multimodality approach. Although the reported survival rates of patients with SCLC treated with chemotherapy and surgery are better than the rates reported for chemoradiation alone, such a comparison is not valid because the series involving chemotherapy and adjuvant surgery represent a subgroup of patients with less advanced disease. Similarly, although only about 15% of all resected patients have experienced a local recurrence, it is inappropriate to compare the local failure rate of these selected patients with studies of LS-SCLC treated with chemoradiotherapy. One randomized study found no difference in survival or local control in 146 patients treated with chemotherapy, with or without surgery, followed by RT and PCI. Thus, when selection is taken into account, a multimodality approach including surgery does not appear to result in a survival benefit over chemoradiotherapy alone, although further clinical trials to define selected subsets of patients are reasonable.

Suggested Readings

Aupérin A, Arriagada R, Pignon JP, et al. Prophylactic cranial irradiation for patients with small-cell lung cancer in complete remission. *N Engl J Med* 1999;341:476–484.

Fried DB, Morris DE, Poole C, et al. Systematic review evaluating the timing of thoracic radiation therapy in combined modality therapy for limited-stage small-cell lung cancer. *J Clin Oncol* 2004;22:4837–4845.

Gillenwater HH, Socinski MA. Extensive stage small cell lung cancer. In: Detterbeck FC, Rivera MP, Socinski MA, et al., eds. *Diagnosis and treatment of lung cancer: an evidence-based guide for the practicing clinician.* Philadelphia, PA: WB Saunders; 2001:360–375.

Lad T, Piantadosi S, Thomas P, et al. A prospective randomized trial to determine the benefit of surgical resection of residual disease following response of small cell lung cancer to combination chemotherapy. *Chest* 1994;106(suppl):320S–323S.

Morris DE, Socinski MA, Detterbeck FC. Limited stage small cell lung cancer. In: Detterbeck FC, Rivera MP, Socinski MA, et al., eds. *Diagnosis and treatment of lung cancer: an evidence-based guide for the practicing clinician.* Philadelphia, PA: WB Saunders; 2001:341–359.

Shepherd FA, Ginsberg R, Patterson GA, et al. Is there ever a role for salvage operations in limited small-cell lung cancer? *J Thorac Cardiovasc Surg* 1991;101:196–200.

Simon GR, Wagner H. Small cell lung cancer. *Chest* 2003; 123:259S–271S.

case 10

Presentation

A 56-year-old woman is referred to you with left shoulder pain, which is radiating down her arm, that she has had for the last 6 months. She has been treated by an orthopaedist and a chiropractor without improvement. She works in an office and smoked one to two packs of cigarettes per day until 5 years ago. There is a family history of diabetes, lung cancer, and breast cancer. She has no other symptoms. Physical examination is unremarkable, including range of motion of her left shoulder and chest auscultation. She brings cervical spine films and shoulder radiographs from 5 months ago; they are normal. She also brings chest radiographs from 3 weeks ago.

Chest X-Rays

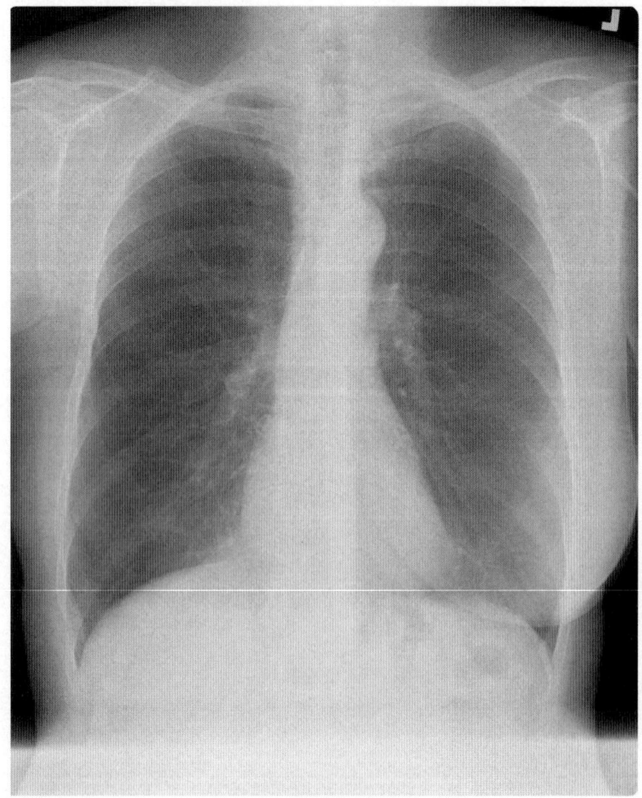

Figure 10.1A

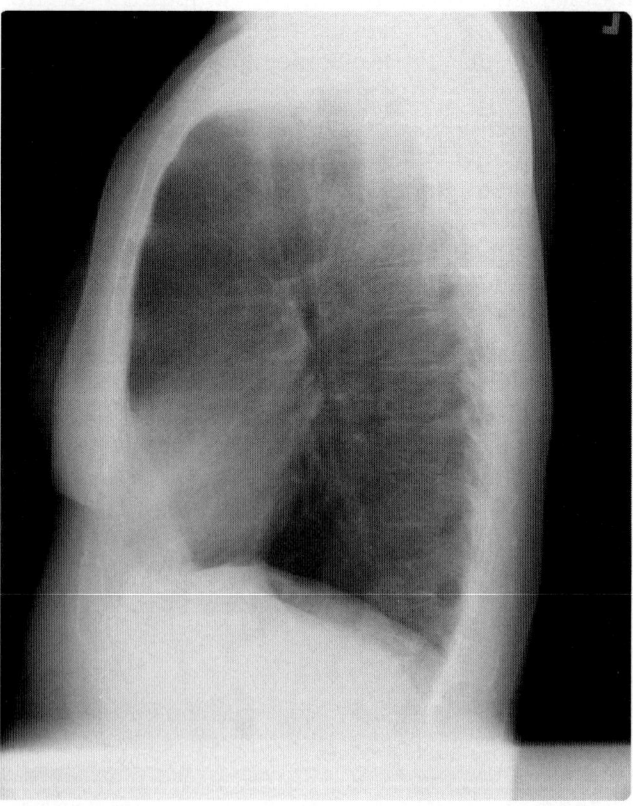

Figure 10.1B

Chest X-Ray Report

On posteroanterior (PA) and lateral chest radiographs, the heart size is normal, and the lung fields are clear, with the exception of a small opacity in the left apex.

Differential Diagnosis

This patient has a classic presentation of a Pancoast tumor, with pain radiating down the arm and a subtle, easily missed, abnormality on a chest radiograph. Often, numerous physicians treat patients with such presentations for many months before the possibility of a process arising from the chest is entertained. A Pancoast tumor is a lung cancer arising in the apex of the lung and involving structures of the apical chest wall. Patients may or may not have the classic Pancoast syndrome of pain, weakness, or numbness radiating down the arm as a result of brachial plexus involvement. Horner's syndrome occurs in approximately 20% of patients with Pancoast tumors (also known as superior sulcus tumors). More than 95% of patients with Pancoast syndrome have non-small cell lung cancer (NSCLC). Less than 5% have small cell lung cancer (SCLC), or even more rarely, another malignancy or an infectious process. Adenocarcinomas account for approximately two thirds of reported cases of Pancoast tumors, and the remaining third are squamous cell with less than 10% large cell carcinomas.

As with all lung cancers, a computed tomography (CT) scan of the chest should be obtained to further characterize the primary lesion, as well as to assess the mediastinum for lymph-node enlargement and the liver and adrenal glands for possible asymptomatic distant metastases. If patient characteristics (risk factors for lung cancer such as smoking and family history), presentation (lack of symptoms suggestive of an infection, hematologic malignancy), and radiographic features (spiculated mass) are all consistent with lung cancer, then there is little question about the diagnosis in patients with a lesion suggestive of a Pancoast tumor. Cytologic confirmation of the diagnosis can be obtained by fine-needle aspiration (FNA) of the mass, which has a diagnostic success rate greater than 90%. Bronchoscopy and sputum cytology are low-yield tests.

Recommendation

CT scan, and FNA of the left apical mass.

Case Continued

A CT scan was normal except for a spiculated left apical mass, confirmed to be an adenocarcinoma by FNA.

Diagnosis

Non-small cell Pancoast tumor with Pancoast syndrome.

Discussion

As with all lung cancers, patients with a Pancoast tumor should first undergo a careful history and physical examination to look for signs of distant metastases. Imaging tests for distant metastases (brain CT, magnetic resonance imaging [MRI], bone scan, or whole-body positron-emission tomography [PET] scan) are not necessary in the presence of a negative clinical evaluation. However, patients should undergo further evaluation of possible mediastinal-node involvement by either mediastinoscopy or PET, even if the CT scan does not demonstrate nodal enlargement. N2 lymph-node involvement is present in approximately 20% of patients with Pancoast tumors, and is a poor prognostic factor. Tumor involvement in enlarged mediastinal or supraclavicular nodes must also be confirmed by cytology or biopsy because of a high false-positive rate.

In patients without mediastinal or distant metastatic disease, MRI should evaluate tumor resectability. This is the best imaging modality to evaluate the extent of tumor involvement of the brachial plexus and bony structures because of the ability to obtain high-quality coronal and sagittal MRI images.

Recommendation

In the absence of distant disease with a normal mediastinum on CT scan of the chest, the patient should undergo mediastinoscopy and an MRI of the left brachial plexus.

Case Continued

Mediastinoscopy is negative. MRI scan is obtained.

MRI Scan

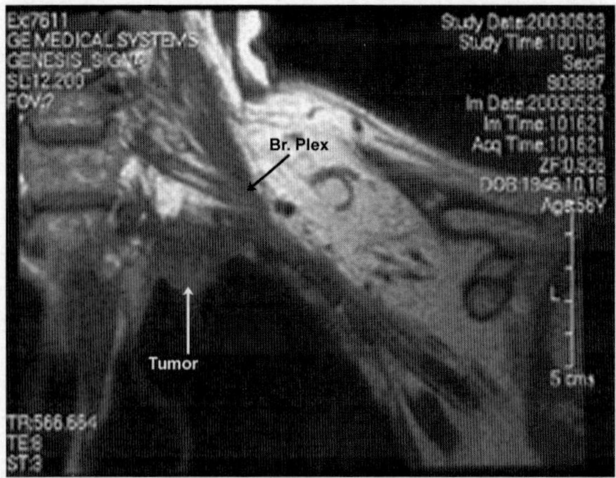

Figure 10.2A

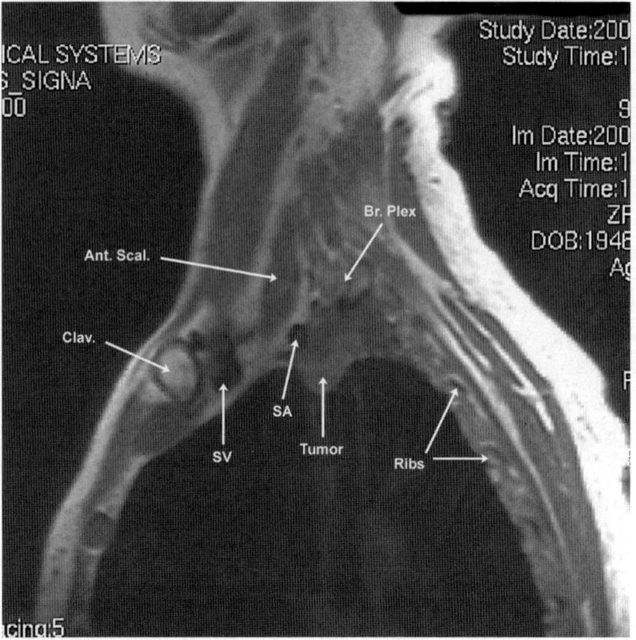

Figure 10.2B

MRI Scan Report

MRI coronal and sagittal images show a left apical tumor and its relationship to the neurovascular structures of the thoracic inlet. There is suspected involvement of the first and second ribs and the lower nerve roots of the brachial plexus. The left subclavian artery and vein are not involved.

Approach

The patient has a localized, resectable tumor with no evidence of mediastinal or distant metastases. A strategy of preoperative therapy followed by resection is chosen. Concurrent chemotherapy (two cycles of cisplatin and etoposide) and radiotherapy (RT, 50 Gy) is used for the preoperative therapy.

Discussion

Because of the peripheral location in the lung and chest wall involvement, Pancoast tumors usually present before distant metastases have occurred. As a result, surgery is usually the mainstay of a curative treatment approach. However, the location of these tumors is difficult to approach surgically, and makes resection with a wide margin problematic. Therefore, the strategy of preoperative therapy has appeal, with the rationale that resection with a limited margin may be more likely to be curative after preoperative therapy. Traditionally, 30 to 45 Gy RT is given, but the newer approach involves concurrent chemotherapy and RT. Although chemotherapy may have an effect on systemic occult micrometastases, the primary role is as a radiation sensitizer, making the preoperative local therapy more effective. The results of preoperative RT demonstrated that one third of patients underwent incomplete resection and that two thirds of patients experienced local recurrence postoperatively. Preoperative chemotherapy and RT results in an incomplete resection in less than 10% of patients, and a markedly decreased rate of local recurrence.

Appropriate selection of patients for resection depends on multiple factors. N2 node involvement has been a poor prognostic factor, making these patients unsuitable for resection unless, perhaps, the mediastinum is downstaged by preoperative therapy. Traditionally, involvement of the subclavian vessels, or invasion of a vertebral body or the neural foramina, has been viewed as a contraindication to resection. However, newer surgical approaches have been developed that allow complete resection of Pancoast tumors involving these structures. Therefore, involvement of these structures should only be a contraindication to resection in institutions that do not have experience to perform such complex resections. It must be emphasized that an incomplete resection is of no demonstrable benefit. Referral to a center with specialized expertise should be strongly considered before either labeling a patient as unresectable or attempting a resection without confidence that a complete resection can be achieved.

Patients with localized tumors that are not resectable should be treated with definitive chemoradiotherapy as a potentially curative treatment, or with radiotherapy alone as a palliative treatment. The natural history of untreated patients with Pancoast tumors is an average survival of 10 to 14 months after diagnosis, with symptoms of severe pain.

Surgical Approach

After preoperative chemoradiotherapy, a sternotomy was performed with an incision over the left clavicle toward the left deltopectoral groove. The left internal jugular vein and the left internal mammary artery were both divided to facilitate retraction of the clavicle and anterior chest wall away from the tumor. The tumor involved the upper ribs and T1 and T2 nerve roots, but not the subclavian vessels, the carotid artery, or the brachial plexus. The first and second ribs were disarticulated from the vertebral bodies and transverse processes and divided in the deltopectoral groove. The involved nerve roots were divided at the neural foramina as well as distal to the tumor. Structures including the left carotid, subclavian, and vertebral arteries, the subclavian and innominate veins, the vagus and phrenic nerves, and the thoracic duct were identified and isolated with careful dissection. A left upper lobectomy was performed, resulting in a complete en bloc resection.

the pulmonary hilum and posterior chest wall and nerve roots. However, exposure of more anterior or cephalad structures is poor until the tumor is mobilized, making it difficult to achieve negative margins along the brachial plexus beyond the nerve roots or along the subclavian vessels. Several anterior approaches have been developed, and are useful for tumors involving the middle or anterior compartments of the thoracic inlet, and perhaps for most tumors involving the posterior compartment as well. The anterior approaches include the anterior transcervical-thoracic approach and the cervicothoracic transmanubrial incision, popularized by Dartevelle (Fig. 10.4). A transsternal approach, involving an incision above the clavicle and either a median sternotomy or partial sternotomy with extension into the fourth intercostal space, allows excellent exposure of the brachial plexus, the subclavian vessels, and the vertebral bodies, as do the other anterior approaches. Exposure of the pulmonary hilum can be difficult with the transcervical-thoracic approach.

Intraoperative Image

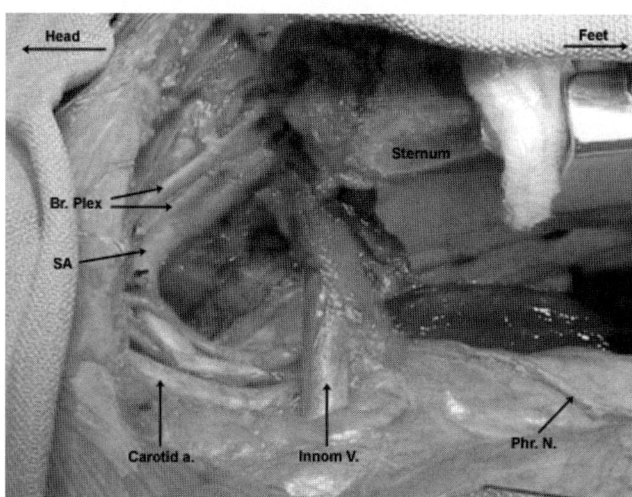

Figure 10.3

Intraoperative Report

Pancoast tumor resection through sternotomy with a transclavicular incision. Anatomy visualized postresection is detailed.

Discussion

The traditional surgical approach to a Pancoast tumor is a high posterior thoracotomy, with an incision extending around the scapula up to the base of the neck. This approach provides good exposure of

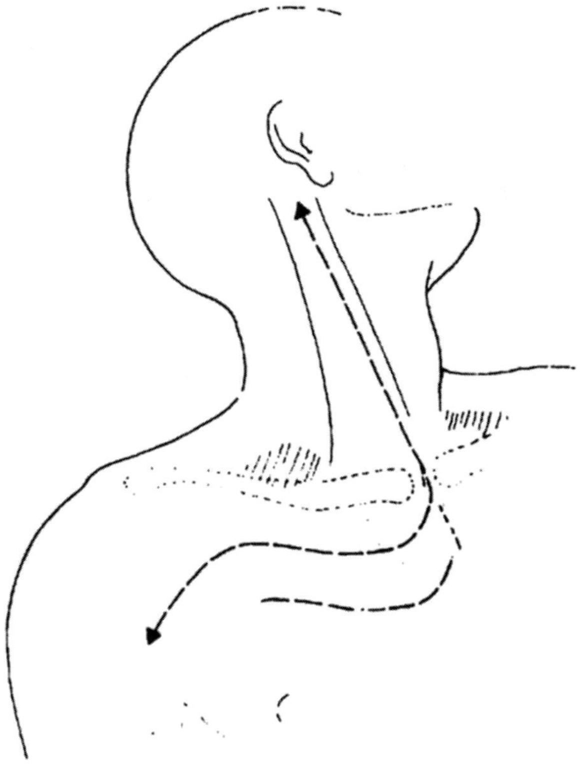

Figure 10.4 Dartevelle anterior approaches include the anterior transcervical-thoracic approach and the cervicothoracic transmanubrial incision. (From Dartevelle P, Macchiarini P. Resection of superior sulcus tumors. In: Kaiser LR, Kron IL, Spray TL, eds. *Mastery of cardiothoracic surgery.* Philadelphia, PA: Lippincott-Raven; 1998:261.)

Lobectomy has been shown to result in better survival than wedge resection of the lung; therefore, a formal lobectomy should be performed unless the patient has a projected postoperative forced expiratory volume at 1 second (FEV_1) of less than 40% of normal. Because an incomplete resection is of minimal, if any, benefit, the surgeon must be sure that the approach and techniques used allow a complete resection to be achieved.

Case Continued

At the conclusion of the procedure, the patient is extubated and transferred to the recovery room, then to the intensive care unit for monitoring. On the first postoperative day, the patient was noted to be tachypneic with decreased oxygen saturation and left lower lobe collapse on chest radiograph.

Approach

A likely etiology of this patient's early postoperative respiratory distress is poor mobilization of secretions and atelectasis secondary to uncontrolled postoperative pain. Other less likely but possible factors include diaphragmatic dysfunction from left phrenic nerve injury or chest tube malposition.

Case Continued

Due to persistent respiratory decline, the patient underwent flexible bronchoscopy, which disclosed retained secretions. With improved pain control, the patient was subsequently able to clear her own secretions successfully; she recovered uneventfully. She has returned to work and has had no evidence of recurrence to date.

Discussion

With the more traditional approach of preoperative RT and resection, 5-year survival rates of approximately 30% were achieved for Pancoast tumors. Major negative prognostic factors included an incomplete resection, N2 nodal involvement, and the presence of Horner's syndrome, subclavian artery involvement, and vertebral body invasion. Recurrence occurred in about two thirds of patients, and two thirds of recurrences were local. The brain was the most common site of distant recurrence. The addition of postoperative RT was not beneficial in either completely (R0) or incompletely (R1 or R2) resected patients.

With the advent of preoperative chemoradiotherapy and the development of surgical techniques that provide better exposure to structures at the thoracic inlet and more complete resection, the outlook is improved. It appears that involvement of adjacent structures such as the subclavian vessels or vertebral column does not confer a prohibitively poor prognosis. Even mediastinal nodal involvement may not contradict a curative approach with either definitive chemoradiotherapy alone or with resection if the mediastinum has been downstaged by induction therapy. Overall, the 2-year survival rate after chemoradiotherapy and resection is 55%, and a 5-year survival rate of 40% to 45% is anticipated.

Suggested Readings

Dartevelle PG, Chapelier AR, Macchiarini P, et al. Anterior transcervical-thoracic approach for radical resection of lung tumors invading the thoracic inlet. *J Thorac Cardiovasc Surg* 1993;105:1025–1034.

Detterbeck FC, Jones DR, Kernstine KH, et al. Special treatment issues. *Chest* 2003;123:244S–258S.

Detterbeck FC, Jones DR, Rosenman JG. Pancoast tumors. In: Detterbeck FC, Rivera MP, Socinski MA, et al., eds. *Diagnosis and treatment of lung cancer: an evidence-based guide for the practicing clinician*. Philadelphia, PA: WB Saunders; 2001: 233–243.

Detterbeck FC. Changes in the treatment of Pancoast tumors. *Ann Thorac Surg* 2003;74:1990–1997.

Rusch VW, Giroux DJ, Kraut MJ, et al. Induction chemoradiation and surgical resection for non-small cell lung carcinomas of the superior sulcus: initial results of Southwest Oncology Group Trial 9416 (Intergroup Trial 0160). *J Thorac Cardiovasc Surg* 2001;121:472–483.

Presentation

A 51-year-old man with no significant past medical history presents to his primary care physician with a 3-week history of facial swelling, lightheadedness, dizziness, and cough. The symptoms are worse when he is supine. He has only a 5-pack-year smoking history, having quit 15 years prior to presentation. The primary physician orders a computed tomography (CT) scan of the chest, and 1 week later, late on a Friday afternoon, the patient presents for evaluation.

On examination there is significant facial swelling (confirmed by the spouse), supraclavicular fullness, and dilated superficial veins on his anterior chest wall. He relates that he has noted blurring of his vision over the last 3 days and increasing shortness of breath. He can no longer tolerate lying flat. There is no palpable adenopathy and his lungs are clear. He specifically denies fevers, chills, night sweats, and weight loss.

■ CT Scan

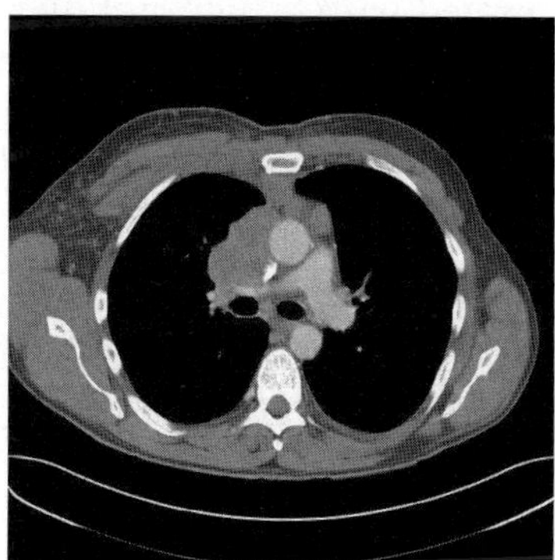

Figure 11.1

CT Scan Report

The CT scan of the chest demonstrates an invasive anterior mediastinal mass encasing the aorta and obliterating the superior vena cava.

Differential Diagnosis

The differential diagnosis of an anterior mediastinal mass depends somewhat on the age of the patient. In the adult, one must consider thymoma, lymphoma, teratoma, substernal goiter, malignant germ cell tumor, thymic carcinoma, and metastatic disease from a distant primary lesion, such as testicular cancer in men. Metastatic disease from a primary lung cancer does not commonly occur in the anterior mediastinum, but may be seen with small cell lung cancer. In this patient, either invasive thymoma or lymphoma would be the most likely diagnosis with lymphoma occurring more commonly.

Diagnosis

The patient has acute superior vena caval (SVC) syndrome and requires immediate tissue diagnosis followed by the initiation of treatment. Our suspicion is lymphoma, most likely of the non-Hodgkin's type.

■ Approach

This patient had not had anything by mouth in the preceding 8 hours, so he was immediately taken to the operating room for an incisional biopsy. With this presentation, and especially with the invasive nature of this lesion, we did not consider an excisional procedure. Because of the SVC syndrome, it is most advantageous to proceed with the diagnostic procedure in an urgent fashion so that definitive treatment may be initiated promptly. With the high likelihood of lymphoma, we felt it was not prudent to attempt needle biopsy because it is critically important to obtain enough tissue to adequately phenotype the lymphoma, which includes flow cytometry.

■ Surgical Approach

Our intent was to obtain enough material for a definitive diagnosis. This requires the cooperation of the pathologist, ideally the hematopathologist, who should be present to ascertain whether adequate diagnostic material has been obtained. Even with a large mass, this may sometimes be difficult, especially in the more fibrous lesions where there is very little cellularity. Entering the anterior mediastinum via a parasternal approach allows us to stay extrapleural, that is, out of the pleural space. This is particularly important if the lesion proves to be a thymoma, where pleural spread is known to occur, and thus we avoid violating the pleural space. The bulk of this lesion occurred to the right of the sternum, and therefore we selected a right parasternal approach. Noting the position of the lesion relative to the sternomanubrial joint on the CT scan, we elected to approach the lesion via the third interspace, a procedure known as anterior mediastinotomy (as distinct from median sternotomy).

We made a transverse parasternal incision just over the third costal cartilage. The perichondrium overlying the cartilage was incised, and the medial portion of the third costal cartilage was removed in a subperichondrial fashion. The lateral aspect of the cartilage was incised with the scalpel after the Matson periosteal elevator was placed posterior to it, and then the medial aspect was disarticulated from the sternum, allowing removal of the piece of cartilage. Removing the costal cartilage facilitates our ability to stay extrapleural. The right pleural reflection was swept laterally, taking care not to enter into it while the internal mammary vessels were identified and preserved.

The posterior perichondrium was incised and the lesion could be easily palpated. A needle may be inserted to ascertain bleeding potential, but most commonly, as we did in this case, we make a small incision directly into the mass to allow for the insertion of a standard biopsy forceps, as usually used for mediastinoscopy. We do not use electrocautery on the lesion because this may hinder the interpretation if additional material is needed. A piece of hemostatic material, such as Surgicel, may be applied, and this usually suffices to take care of the bleeding from the lesion. Multiple samples were taken and brought fresh to the waiting pathologist, who performed a touch preparation and frozen section and assessed the adequacy of the material obtained. If it is believed that more material is needed, we return to the operating room and obtain additional fresh material.

The specimens should not be placed in formalin. The touch preparations and frozen sections suggested a malignant neoplasm consistent with large cell lymphoma, but the definitive diagnosis was deferred until the permanent sections could be studied. Additional fresh tissue was obtained for permanent section, immunohistochemistry, and special studies. The incision was closed.

Case Continued

The frozen section diagnosis of large cell lymphoma was confirmed 48 hours later by immunohistochemistry.

Discussion

There is never an indication to treat a patient who presents in this fashion without first establishing a tissue diagnosis. In the past, many of these patients received urgent radiation therapy to the mediastinum without first obtaining tissue. We now know that radiation may not be the initial treatment of choice for many of these lesions, and thus the importance of obtaining the appropriate tissue. The key to initiating the appropriate treatment is the acquisition of adequate diagnostic material. Often there is a temptation to operate and attempt to resect the mass when faced with an anterior mediastinal lesion. This may be appropriate in the situation where the CT scan appears to demonstrate a mass that is well encapsulated. Yet even in these situations, one may occasionally find that one has resected a lymphoma. Usually it is not possible on frozen section for the pathologist to distinguish a thymoma from a lymphoma. The diagnosis and treatment require close coordination among the surgeon, pathologist, and oncologist. Obtaining a reliable definitive tissue diagnosis is of utmost importance. Some have advocated CT-guided fine-needle aspiration with cytologic examination. This technique is associated with a high nondiagnostic rate, and if suggestive of a lymphoma does not provide enough tissue for phenotyping or flow cytometry. It also often results in further delay in diagnosis and treatment, and we do not utilize this technique, especially in patients with acute SVC syndrome. A similar comment can be made regarding the use of a transthoracic core needle biopsy. Although histologic evaluation is possible with this technique, differentiation between a lymphocyte-rich invasive thymoma and frank lymphoma can be difficult. In a patient with an anterior mass, with or (as more commonly seen) without SVC syndrome, we prefer an incisional biopsy for diagnosis.

Anterior mediastinal masses cannot be approached via mediastinoscopy, a technique useful for lesions, or more commonly adenopathy, in the superior mediastinum, a region distinct and posterior to the anterior mediastinum. The mediastinoscope is placed just anterior to the trachea far from the location of an anterior mediastinal lesion. The most direct approach to diagnosis of an anterior mediastinal mass is the anterior mediastinotomy (Chamberlain procedure) or a modification of this procedure as described earlier for this patient. Classically, the Chamberlain procedure was described as a left parasternal mediastinotomy with removal of the second costal cartilage specifically for use in staging the aortopulmonary window in primary lung cancer. In this patient we performed a right-sided procedure via the third costal cartilage.

Anterior mediastinal masses in patients presenting with SVC syndrome usually are malignant (greater than 90% of cases). Unless there is clear evidence of cerebral edema or laryngeal edema, it usually is not necessary to treat the SVC syndrome. The administration of corticosteroids, even just for several days prior to obtaining tissue for diagnosis, may obscure the pathologic interpretation, especially if the lesion proves to be a lymphoma. An anterior mediastinal mass presenting with SVC syndrome requires immediate diagnosis and prompt treatment. SVC syndromes due to lymphoma often improve rapidly with the institution of treatment.

Case Continued

The patient was transferred to the oncology service to begin definitive treatment. Before definitive therapy can begin, the patient's disease is staged with CT scan of the abdomen/pelvis, positron-emission tomography scan, and a bone marrow biopsy. The interventional radiologist inserts a port for long-term venous access, and the patient is commenced on chemotherapy. After one cycle of therapy, some improvement was noted in the patient's symptoms.

Suggested Readings

Petersdorf SH, Wood DE. Lymphoproliferative disorders presenting as mediastinal neoplasms. *Semin Thorac Cardiovasc Surg* 2000;12:290–300.

Roberts JR, Bueno R, Sugarbaker DJ. Multimodality treatment of malignant superior vena caval syndrome. *Chest* 1999;116:835–837.

Wright CD, Mathisen DJ. Mediastinal tumors: diagnosis and treatment. *World J Surg* 2001;25:204–209.

Yoneda KY, Louie S, Shelton DK. Mediastinal tumors. *Curr Opin Pulm Med* 2001;4:226–233.

case 12

Presentation

An asymptomatic 65-year-old woman with a 40-pack-year smoking history recently relocated and presents to the office of her new primary care physician. She undergoes an initial physical examination that includes a routine chest radiograph. The chest x-ray raises the question of a faint nodular density in the right lung. The primary physician orders a computed tomographic (CT) scan of the chest and a positron emission tomographic (PET) scan, and sends the patient to a pulmonologist who performs pulmonary function testing and a bronchoscopy.

CT Scan

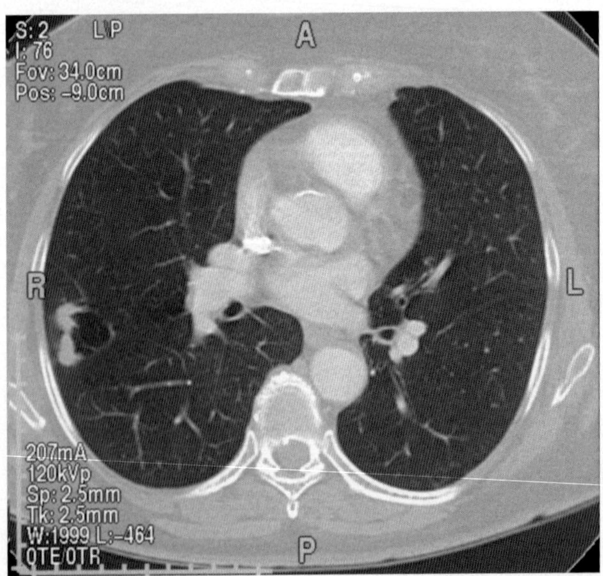

Figure 12.1

CT Scan Report

A 2.5-cm solitary pulmonary nodule is present in the posterolateral aspect of the right upper lobe.

There is no mediastinal or hilar adenopathy seen. The CT scan includes cuts through the upper abdomen; both adrenal glands are visualized and appear normal, as does the liver.

PET Scan

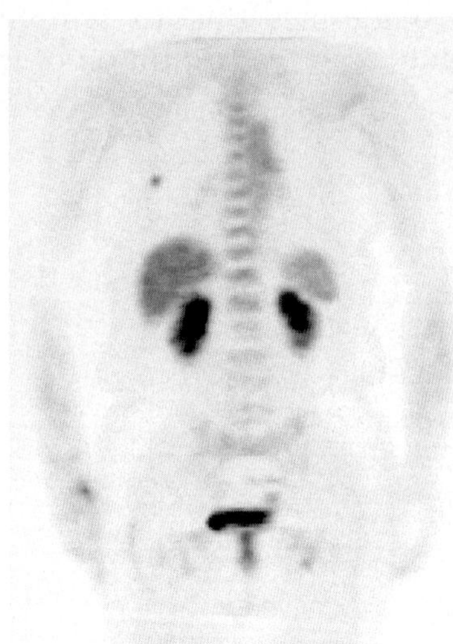

Figure 12.2

PET Scan Report

There is one area of moderate 5-fluorodeoxyglucose (FDG) accumulation within the right upper lobe nodule corresponding to the abnormality seen on the chest CT scan. The measured maximum standard uptake value (SUV) for the nodule is 2.5; this SUV value would be considered borderline with respect to malignancy.

Case Continued

The pulmonary function testing shows a forced expiratory volume at 1 second (FEV$_1$) of 1.55 L or

69% of predicted. The diffusion capacity is 71% of predicted.

The bronchoscopic examination is unremarkable, with no evidence of any mucosal abnormality or discrete endobronchial lesion. The cytology studies from the bronchial brushings and bronchoalveolar lavage show no evidence of malignancy.

Case Continued

The pulmonologist refers the patient for evaluation. On further review you find the patient to be quite healthy and very active. Her past surgical history is significant for 2 cesarean sections and a hysterectomy 24 years ago. She has no history of malignant disease but admits to a 40-pack-year smoking history, as mentioned previously. She has no palpable supraclavicular, cervical, or axillary adenopathy on examination. Her lungs are clear in all fields bilaterally and there is good air entry with no crackles or wheezes. She has no clubbing or cyanosis.

Differential Diagnosis

The differential diagnosis of a solitary pulmonary nodule is quite broad and can include both benign and malignant processes. Patient-specific factors, especially a smoking history, increase the probability that a solitary pulmonary nodule is malignant. Our patient, with her significant smoking history, has a high likelihood of harboring a primary carcinoma of the lung. In appropriate clinical settings, other possibilities include metastatic nodules from commonly encountered cancers, including breast, colon, thyroid, or renal cell carcinomas. Benign neoplasms of the lung, such as a hamartoma, can also be entertained but these lesions usually are evident on CT scan because of their characteristic "popcorn-like" calcification pattern. Other possibilities include inflammatory or infectious nodules, the most common lesion being a granuloma. Several fungal diseases, including coccidioidomycosis and histoplasmosis, may present with a solitary pulmonary nodule, as may actinomycosis. The elusive rounded atelectasis, seen as a pleural-based lesion, may also appear to be a solitary pulmonary nodule.

Diagnosis and Recommendation

A solitary pulmonary nodule is defined as a lesion less than 3 cm in size, surrounded by lung and without associated mediastinal adenopathy. Compare the film to a previous chest radiograph to determine if this is a new or an existing stable nodule.

Case Continued

The patient reports that she had a chest radiograph done 5 years ago, which was "normal;" however, the film is no longer available for review.

Approach

A solitary pulmonary nodule larger than 1 cm in a person who smokes requires a definitive tissue diagnosis. If the preoperative workup suggests localized disease and further evaluation determines that the patient can tolerate a pulmonary resection, proceed to the operating room for both definitive diagnosis and treatment. A positive PET scan is further confirmation that the lesion is malignant. A small solitary nodule may be followed with serial CT scans performed at intervals of 3 months to assess change in size. A nodule noted to be increasing in size mandates excision. A 2-year period of serial scans is required before assuming that a lesion is benign and does not need further surveillance.

Surgical Approach

The patient was taken to the operating room. General anesthesia was induced, and she was intubated with a double-lumen, left-sided, endobronchial tube. Flexible bronchoscopy was performed, and no abnormalities were seen down to the subsegmental level bilaterally. The tube was bronchoscopically positioned for isolated lung ventilation and secured in place. The patient was repositioned and underwent right video-assisted thoracic surgery (VATS) through three 2.5-cm incisions. A peripherally located right upper lobe lesion was localized and removed with a surrounding wedge of normal lung parenchyma using multiple firings of an endoscopic stapling device. Intraoperative frozen section revealed a non-small cell carcinoma of the lung. The thoracoscopic port sites were converted to a thoracotomy and a right upper lobectomy with mediastinal lymph node dissection was performed.

Discussion

In approaching a person who smokes, and who has a new solitary pulmonary nodule suspected of being a primary lung cancer, the following three questions should be addressed: (a) what is the extent of disease? (b) can the patient tolerate a definitive pulmonary resection for treatment? and (c) what is the most expedient method to obtain a tissue diagnosis and initiate treatment? If possible, a previous chest radiograph should be obtained for comparison because the presence of a nodule that has not changed in size and that, in retrospect, is present on a film taken 2 years earlier makes a benign diagnosis much more likely.

The extent of disease is surmised by a combination of history, physical examination, and radiographic studies. Subtle neurologic signs, such as blurred vision or new headaches, require a brain magnetic resonance imaging study to rule out metastatic disease. Long bone or rib pain may indicate bony metastatic disease and should be excluded with bone scan or PET imaging. Mediastinal views of the CT scan should be reviewed and mediastinoscopy performed if mediastinal adenopathy (lymph nodes larger than 1.0 cm) is present, or is suspected.

If the clinical information suggests limited disease, the surgeon needs to determine if the patient can tolerate a pulmonary resection. Activity levels usually are the best indicator of a patient's ability to tolerate a pulmonary resection, but unfortunately, these are difficult to quantify during an office visit. Pulmonary function testing, including spirometry, should be obtained in all patients who are potentially candidates for resection. Although traditionally a postoperative FEV_1 of 800 cc was suggested as a minimum, advances in operative technique, postoperative care, and a better understanding of emphysema have allowed for curative resections even in patients with advanced-staged emphysema and very poor lung function. However, these patients probably are best treated in specialized centers that have pulmonary surgeons experienced in operating on high-risk patients.

Finally, the surgeon should select the approach that allows for establishment of a diagnosis and efficient initiation of treatment. In this case of a patient with a small peripheral nodule, bronchoscopy would be expected to have a very low diagnostic yield and would better be performed at the time of surgery solely to rule out any additional, unsuspected endobronchial pathology. As

a preoperative study, it did not influence the decision making regarding this patient's care. A transthoracic needle biopsy performed either under fluoroscopy or by CT guidance is possible, but it is unlikely to change the management in this patient with apparent localized disease and acceptable pulmonary function. If the transthoracic needle biopsy is positive for carcinoma of the lung, the patient requires a pulmonary resection for treatment. If the needle biopsy is nondiagnostic, as is typical if a diagnosis of malignancy cannot be made, the patient requires an operation for diagnosis and lobectomy for treatment if the diagnosis of carcinoma is confirmed. The likelihood of obtaining a specific benign pathologic diagnosis, which would preclude surgery, is less than 15%. The chance of small cell lung cancer, a disease usually treated nonoperatively, presenting as a solitary pulmonary nodule is quite small; in such a circumstance, the initial treatment of choice would still be resection.

Case Continued

The final pathology studies revealed a stage IA (T1 N0 M0) adenocarcinoma of the lung. No further treatment is required unless the patient is eligible for any specific clinical trials evaluating adjuvant therapy. The patient is placed on routine surveillance consisting of clinical examination and chest x-ray.

Suggested Readings

Libby DM, Smith JP, Altorki NK, et al. Managing the small pulmonary nodule discovered by CT. *Chest* 2004;125:1522–1529.

Ost D, Fein A. Evaluation and management of the solitary pulmonary nodule. *Am J Respir Crit Care Med* 2000;162: 782–787.

Swanson SJ, Jaklitsch MT, Mentzer SJ, et al. Management of the solitary pulmonary nodule: role of thoracoscopy in diagnosis and therapy. *Chest* 1999;116(6 suppl):523S–524S.

Swensen SJ, Silverstein MD, Ilstrup DM, et al. The probability of malignancy in solitary pulmonary nodules: application to small radiologically indeterminate nodules. *Arch Intern Med* 1997;157:849–855.

Presentation

A 45-year-old businessman, who is otherwise healthy, and who is a nonsmoker, presents to his local physician with the complaint of a new mass in his upper thigh. Over the last 6 months, the patient had noted that there was a dull pain in his right medial thigh, and noted a mass that was nontender. Physical examination reveals a 4.5 × 6.0-cm mass in the medial aspect of his right thigh, which moved with the underlying muscle. There was no inguinal adenopathy.

Magnetic resonance imaging (MRI) of the thigh revealed a well-circumscribed mass within the musculature, which is bright on the T2-weighted gadolinium image. The patient is referred to a surgical oncologist who performs a percutaneous core biopsy of the mass. The biopsy reveals a high-grade synovial sarcoma with 2+ necrosis. A computed tomography (CT) scan of the chest is performed, which reveals no nodules. A limb-sparing resection of the mass is performed after preoperative chemotherapy and radiation therapy. The pathology examination reveals 99% necrosis of the mass, and the margins of the resection are free of tumor. The patient had a 3-month period of rehabilitation and then returned to work.

The patient is seen in follow-up by his surgeon and medical oncology team every 3 months after the resection. At each follow-up visit, a CT scan of the chest is performed as well as examination of the primary site. All chest CT scans were free of disease until 18 months after surgery.

CT Scan

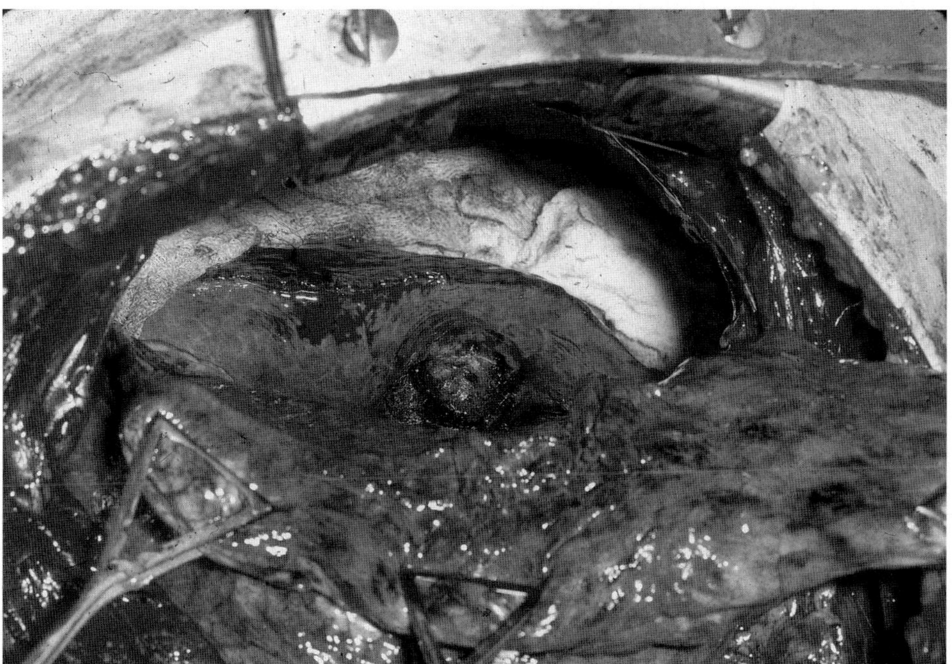

Figure 13.1

CT Scan Report

CT scan of the chest reveals a new solitary nodule in the left lower lobe, which was not present on the previous study

Differential Diagnosis

Given the prior history of a stage III high-grade sarcoma, which has an approximately 50% incidence of developing metastases over the next 18 months, the presence of a solitary pulmonary nodule most likely represents metastatic sarcoma. Nevertheless, despite the absence of a history of smoking, the possibility of a new primary lung cancer, such as bronchoalveolar carcinoma, should also be considered. The presence of a benign granuloma is also a possibility, though unlikely, because the previous CT scans were normal.

Discussion

The development of a new pulmonary nodule in a patient with a previous history of a high-grade extremity sarcoma is an ominous sign, and pulmonary metastases must be considered. This patient had never been a smoker, so the possibility of a new lung cancer is remote. Moreover, the appearance of the nodule with smooth edges, nonspiculated, is more compatible with a pulmonary metastasis than a bronchogenic lung cancer. The chance of this new nodule being a metastasis in a sarcoma patient approaches 90%. The time course for the development of pulmonary metastases after successful sarcoma resection is usually within the first 2 years after the management of the primary lesion. Sequential CT scanning at intervals of 3 months for a period of 2 to 3 years is the recommended surveillance for such patients, because it has been shown that CT is much more sensitive in detecting pulmonary metastases than plain chest radiograph. With newer generation CT scanners with multiple detectors, it is possible to detect nodules as small as 2 mm, and performing CT scanning with 5-mm cuts can be a useful test to quantitate the number of nodules bilaterally. It is unnecessary to perform further radiologic workup, except for an evaluation of the primary site, because the natural history of extremity sarcomas is usually metastasis to the lung, as opposed to bone, liver, or brain metastases. The most efficacious manner to evaluate the primary site is with an MRI of the resected bed. This is an important study because the management of the pulmonary metastasis may involve a metastasectomy, and this would be contraindicated if the primary site demonstrated a local recurrence.

Patients with sarcomas are frequently treated with chemotherapies containing doxorubicin, and it has been demonstrated that doses above 400 mg/m^2 can be associated with cardiac events, most notably impaired responses to exercise with decreases in ejection fraction. Patients treated with this chemotherapy as part of the regimen should have a stress multiple-gated acquisition (MUGA) scan or equivalent exercise scan to define whether there is any contraindication to thoracotomy.

For patients who are smokers, or who have had a history of pulmonary disease including chronic obstructive pulmonary disease, pulmonary function testing is recommended to define pulmonary risk for possible multiple wedge resections.

Diagnosis and Recommendation

Pulmonary metastases from a soft tissue sarcoma. Because the patient has been previously treated with doxorubicin (Adriamycin) chemotherapy for soft tissue sarcoma, he should have a stress MUGA or equivalent exercise scan to define whether there is any contraindication to thoracotomy. For this patient without pulmonary symptoms who has never smoked, and who is having initial metastasectomy, pulmonary function testing is optional.

Case Continued

MRI of the thigh revealed no evidence of recurrent tumor. A stress MUGA examination revealed an ejection fraction of 60% without evidence of decompensation with stress. Thin-cut CT scan revealed only the aforementioned nodule.

Approach

The most likely diagnosis is metastatic sarcoma without evidence of disease outside the lung. The indications for such a resection include the ability to resect all nodules, absence of other effective therapy, control of the primary site, and adequate pulmonary reserve, all of which are satisfied in this case. Because the patient has already received the best possible chemotherapy, it is reasonable to consider resection. The recommendation for such a situation would be exploration with complete resection of all nodules. Efficacy of the procedure will depend on whether a complete resection can be performed, and this will depend on the number of nodules and whether the resection of all the nodules can be accomplished in a way that preserves adequate pulmonary tissue/function. Moreover, the prognosis is also influenced by the disease-free interval from the time of the original primary resection. It has been shown that a disease-free interval of greater than 1 year is a good prognostic sign for efficacy of metastasectomy.

The choice of surgical approach is mildly controversial. The use of thoracoscopy is not encouraged because the ability to palpate the rest of the lung is limited unless one uses an anterior access thoracotomy. The ability to palpate the parenchyma for small nodules is crucial, and in the majority of cases, the surgeon can expect that the number of nodules found will be 2 to 3 times the number seen on the preoperative radiographic studies. These nodules can be as small as 1 to 2 mm and appear as grains of sand, which require careful palpation, marking with a suture, and assessment of whether the number is beyond that obtainable for a complete resection. The number of nodules to resect to accomplish complete resection is also controversial, and there is no set number with regard to an upper limit; however, patients with solitary nodules have a better prognosis than those with multiple nodules. Although there are no evidence-based data to choose one approach over another, many surgeons who have performed a substantial number of metastasectomies prefer the use of the median sternotomy to perform a complete exploration of both sides with bilateral simultaneous resection of nodules in each lung. Whether staged thoracotomies or median sternotomy is used, it is an absolute requirement to have one-lung anesthesia, using either a bronchial blocker or a double-lumen endotracheal tube. This greatly increases the chance of finding nodules and performing a complete resection. Nodule removal is accomplished using the automatic staplers for peripheral nodules. For deep-seated central nodules, "core-out" cautery resection has been used, as well as segmental resections. For large central nodules, lobectomy is a reasonable choice, but may influence the patient's suitability for future metastasectomies. It is safe to say the pneumonectomy is discouraged as metastasis management.

Recommendation

Median sternotomy with resection of the pulmonary metastases.

Surgical Approach

General anesthesia is induced with double-lumen technique. After performing a median sternotomy, the left lung is deflated and carefully palpated. There is a 2-cm nodule in the basilar segment of the left lower lobe.

Intraoperative Images

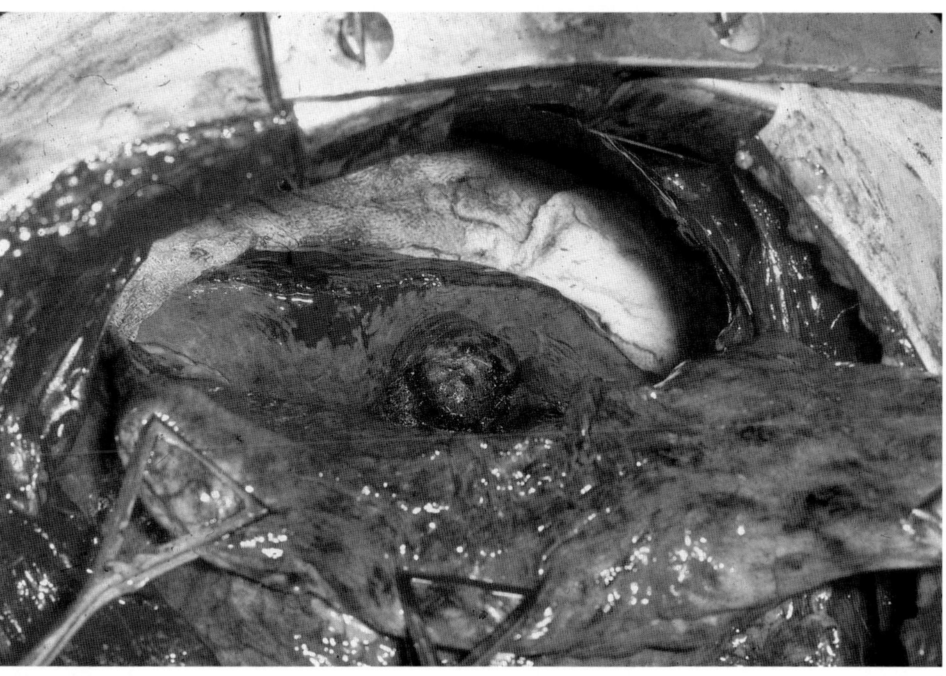

Figure 13.2

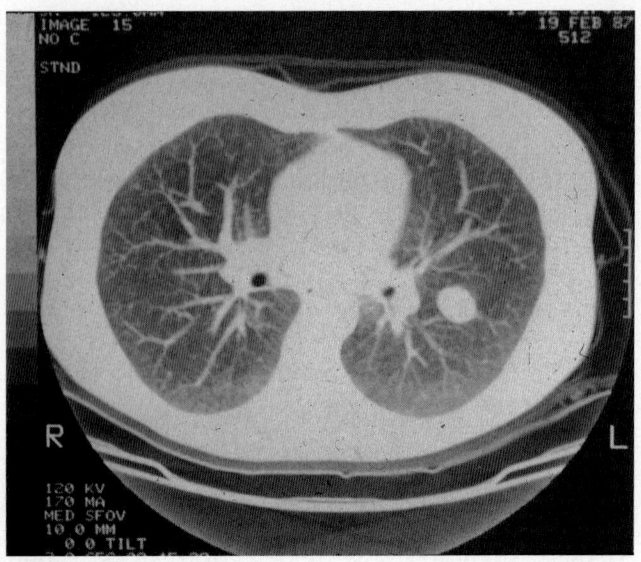

Figure 13.3

Intraoperative Report

The nodule in the left lung is located and marked with a suture. A Duval lung clamp is placed on the lung and surrounding the nodule, and the lung is pulled into the wound. Packs are placed behind the left lower lobe to elevate it into the wound.

Surgical Approach

Using a stapling device, the nodule is removed with a wedge resection with a good margin of lung parenchyma. Palpation of the rest of the left lung reveals no other nodules, and there is no disease on the parietal pleura or diaphragm. The opposite lung is also carefully palpated. A 4-mm nodule in the right upper lobe is noted on the visceral pleura, but no other nodules were palpated. At completion, the lungs are inflated and the staple line is checked for hemostasis and air leaks. Chest tubes are placed for drainage and connected to underwater seal suction. The median sternotomy is closed in the standard fashion.

Case Continued

The patient is extubated in the operating room and taken to the recovery room. His total hospital stay of 4 days is uneventful, with the chest tube removal on the third postoperative day.

Pulmonary nodules, left lower lobe 2.2 cm and right upper lobe 4 mm, were both compatible with metastatic synovial cell sarcoma.

Suggested Readings

Ambiru S, Miyazaki M, Ito H, et al. Resection of hepatic and pulmonary metastases in patients with colorectal carcinoma. *Cancer* 1998;82:274–278.

Belli L, Scholl S, Livartowski A, et al. Resection of pulmonary metastases in osteosarcoma. A retrospective analysis of 44 patients. *Cancer* 1989;63:2546–2550.

Ferson PF, Keenan RJ, Luketich JD. The role of video-assisted thoracic surgery in pulmonary metastases. *Chest Surg Clin N Am* 1998;8:59–76.

Koong HN, Pastorino U, Ginsberg RJ. Is there a role for pneumonectomy in pulmonary metastases? International Registry of Lung Metastases. *Ann Thorac Surg* 1999;68:2039–2043.

McCormack PM, Burt ME, Bains MS, et al. Lung resection for colorectal metastases. 10-year results. *Arch Surg* 1992;127:1403–1406.

Pass HI. Surgical management of pulmonary metastases. *Curr Opin Oncol* 1998;10:146–150.

Pastorino U, McCormack PM, Ginsberg RJ. A new staging proposal for pulmonary metastases. The results of analysis of 5206 cases of resected pulmonary metastases. *Chest Surg Clin N Am* 1998;8:197–202.

Pastorino U. History of the surgical management of pulmonary metastases and development of the International Registry. *Semin Thorac Cardiovasc Surg* 2002;14:18–28.

Rusch VW. Pulmonary metastasectomy. Current indications. *Chest* 1995;107:322S–331S.

Presentation

A 67-year-old man who is a retired shipyard worker with a 30-year asbestos exposure is seen in the emergency department with a history of progressive shortness of breath and cough for 6 months. Prior to this 6-month history of progressive dyspnea, he was performance status 0, with a past medical history of hypertension, and he relates a loss of appetite as well as a cough over this period. Physical examination of this former 16-pack-year smoker reveals dullness to percussion and distant breath sounds on the right side. Fortunately, the hospital had an old chest radiograph taken after an automobile accident 1 year ago, for comparison. A complete blood cell (CBC) count reveals a platelet count of 450,000/mL.

Chest X-Rays

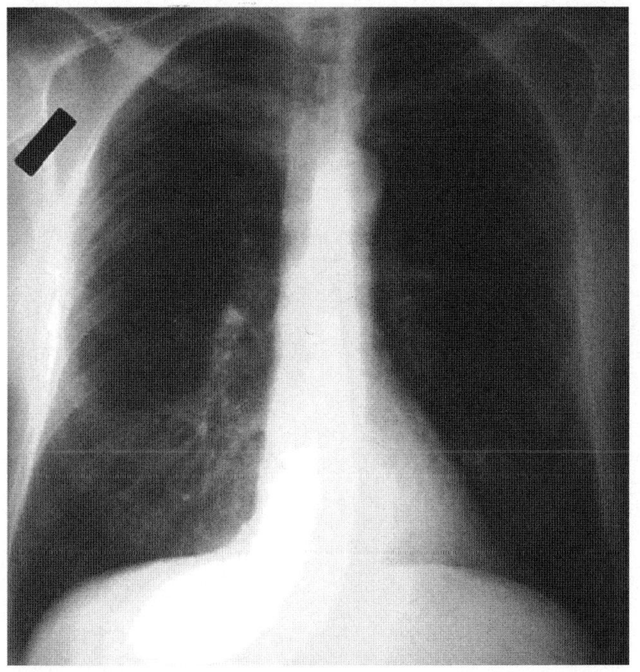

Figure 14.1

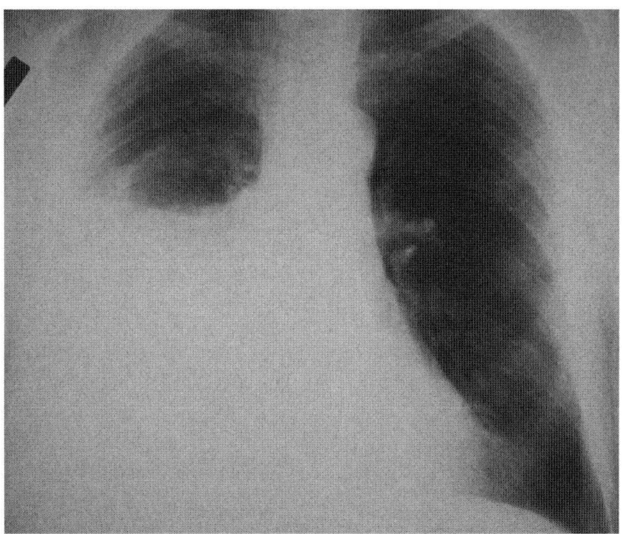

Figure 14.2

X-Ray Report

Compared with a previous film taken 1 year earlier **(left)**, there has been the development of a large right-sided pleural effusion **(above)**. The cardiac silhouette is similar to previous studies. The lung fields demonstrate scarring but no dominant masses.

Differential Diagnosis

The development of new pleural effusion in a person with asbestos exposure is a particularly ominous sign. The differential diagnosis must include mesothelioma, stage IIIB lung cancer (because the risk for development of lung cancer in asbestos-exposed former or present smokers is 40 times higher than in nonsmokers), postpneumonic effusion, pleural metastases from another primary tumor (specifically of gastrointestinal origin), and a traumatic hemithorax. In the absence of a history of injury and other constitutional symptoms, the primary differential must be between lung cancer and mesothelioma.

Discussion

Mesothelioma usually affects older men in their 50s, 60s, and 70s with a 25- to 40-year latency period between occupational asbestos exposure and the development of the tumor. The duration of symptoms will vary from 2 weeks to 2 years, with most series having a median time to diagnosis from symptoms of 2 to 3 months. The right side is affected more than the left side (60% vs 40%) most likely due to its greater volume.

Dyspnea will be present in 50% to 70% of the cases and, indeed, 80% of the patients will present with dyspnea and effusion. In 95% of patients with malignant pleural mesothelioma, a pleural effusion will be documented at some time in the course of the disease.

Nonspecific laboratory findings seen in mesothelioma patients include hypergammaglobulinemia, eosinophilia, and/or anemia of chronic disease. The most striking laboratory abnormality is thrombocytosis (platelet count greater than 400,000), which is seen in 60% to 90% of patients, and approximately 15% of patients will have platelet counts greater than 1,000,000. At present, validated serum markers that are both sensitive and specific for mesothelioma do not exist.

A large, unexplained pleural effusion and minimal or moderate evidence of pleural thickening demands immediate workup, which includes thoracentesis and pleural biopsy or thoracoscopy. Multiple closed pleural biopsies can be performed to avoid sampling error with the Abrams or Cope needle, and this will be able to aid in the diagnosis in 30% to 50% of the cases.

Patients who develop a large effusion and who have negative studies on thoracentesis and pleural biopsy or who recur with effusion after initial thoracentesis should have a video-assisted thoracoscopy. Thoracoscopic examination allows for targeted biopsies, which can then be analyzed with the proper pathologic markers, as well as to determine whether the lung will expand. Thoracoscopy can estimate the amount of disease on the diaphragm, pericardium, chest wall, and nodes. A chest wall mass from seeding of the biopsy site or surgical scar is an uncommon complication (approximately 10%).

Open biopsy (using an incision that can be incorporated into the definitive incision if a major resection is entertained after diagnosis) is required if there is no free pleural space due to previous treatment of pleural effusion and the bulk of the disease in the hemithorax is solid.

Recommendation

Thoracentesis with pleural biopsy and computed tomography (CT) scan.

Case Continued

The thoracentesis revealed 1,000 mL of straw-colored fluid, but only atypical mesothelial cells were seen, and the cytological examination of the cell block using immunohistochemistries was not able to diagnose epithelial malignancy. The pleural biopsy revealed fibrous tissue compatible with a pleural plaque.

Recommendation

Video-assisted thoracoscopy with targeted pleural biopsies.

Endoscopic Images

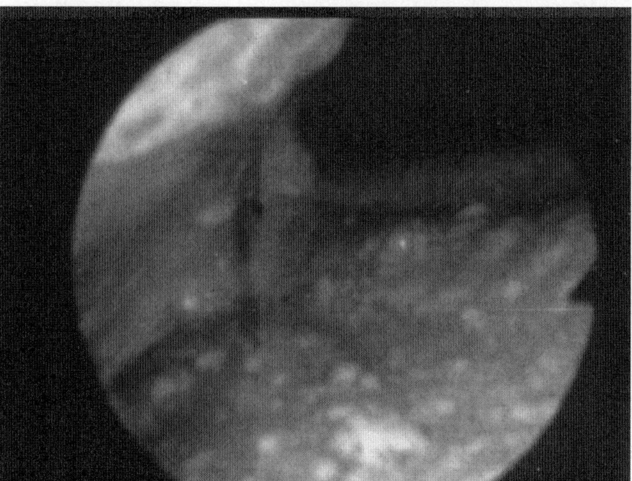

Figure 14.3

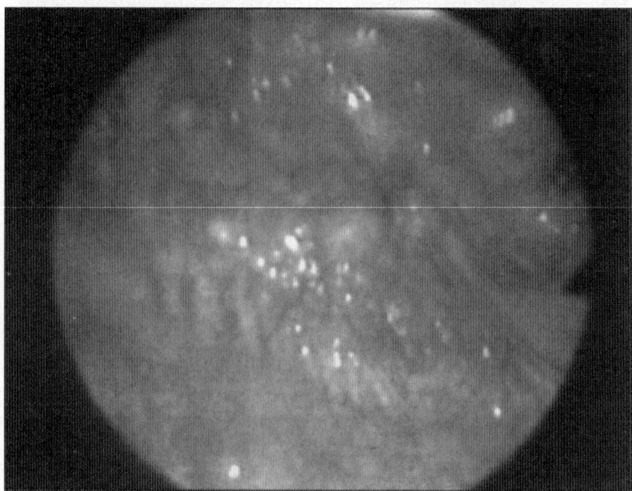

Figure 14.4

Endoscopy Report

Thoracoscopic examination reveals 3 L of straw-colored fluid and multiple nodular densities over the chest wall and diaphragm (**upper image**), as well as the lung and pericardium, along with asbestos plaques. A closer examination of the chest wall and intercostal bundles is provided in the **lower image.** Multiple biopsies were taken of the pleural nodules.

Histopathology Slide

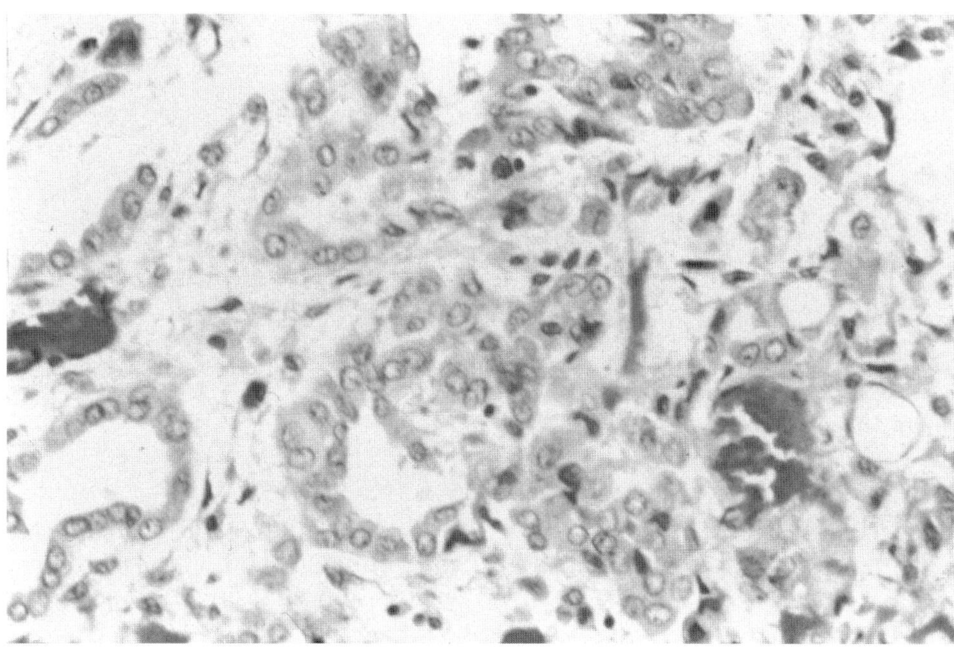

Figure 14.5

Histopathology Report

On immunohistochemical staining, the tumor cells are positive for pankeratin, keratin 5/6, calretinin, and WT-1, and negative for the epithelial markers CEA, LeuM1, B72.3, Ber-EP4, Moc-1, and TTF-1.

Diagnosis

Tubulopapillary neoplasm consistent with epithelial mesothelioma.

Discussion

With the diagnosis of mesothelioma now finalized, it is important to define the extent of disease, the patient's performance status, and his suitability for a multimodality approach using surgery and chemotherapy and/or radiation therapy. Before proceeding with these tests, a discussion with the patient must define his options. The patient is informed that the median survival of patients who select supportive care only for mesothelioma ranges widely from 4 to 13 months. Patients who elect for only chemotherapy will have a median survival of approximately 12 months even with the newest combination of pemetrexed and cisplatin, which has a 41% response rate. Patients who are eligible for multimodality approaches involving a cytoreduction of their disease by pleurectomy decortication or extrapleural pneumonectomy will have median survivals that approach 24 months, depending upon their postoperative pathologic staging status.

Recommendation

Referral to mesothelioma center, chest radiograph, CT scan, pulmonary function tests, quantitative ventilation perfusion scan, and cardiology consultation.

Case Continued

After discharge from the hospital, the patient has a long conversation with his private physician, who had already consulted the Internet regarding referral centers for mesothelioma. The patient elects to have referral to a mesothelioma center that has seen a considerable number of pleural mesotheliomas, after his private physician discusses the case with a mesothelioma expert at the center. The patient brings a new postthoracoscopic chest radiograph, CT scan, pulmonary function test results, quantitative ventilation perfusion scan, and cardiology consultation for his appointment at the mesothelioma center.

▓ Chest X-Rays

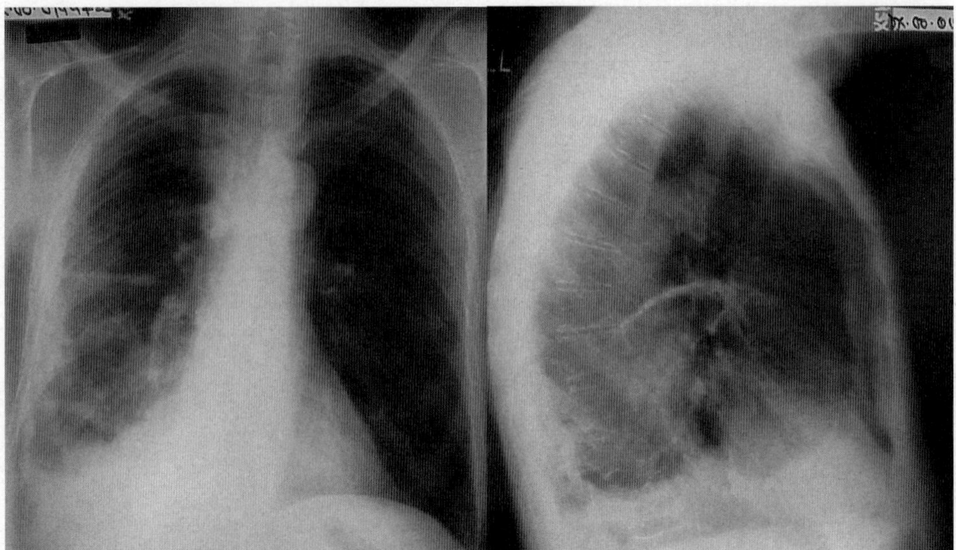

Figure 14.6

Chest X-Ray Report

Fluid/tumor in the fissure, pleural thickening and blunting of the diaphragm, which is new from the previous films.

▓ CT Scans

CT Scan Report

CT scan reveals diffuse thickening of the right pleura with minimal fluid at the posterior diaphragmatic sulcus. Abutment/involvement of the diaphragm, pericardium, and lung is seen. No definitively enlarged lymph nodes in the paratracheal or sub-carinal regions are noted.

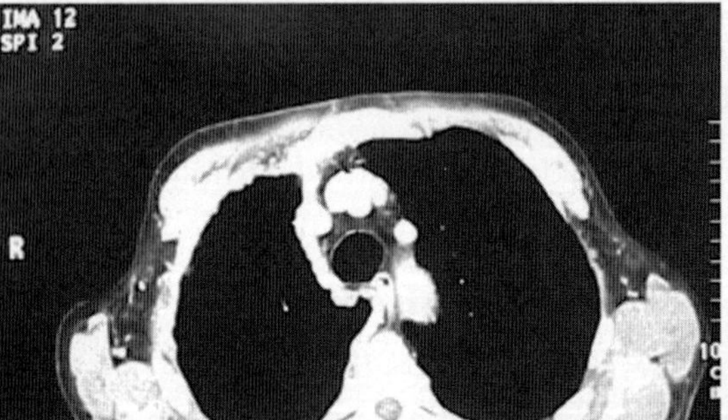
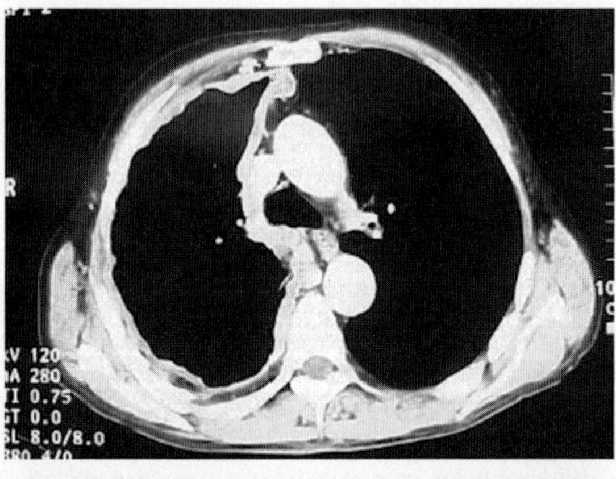
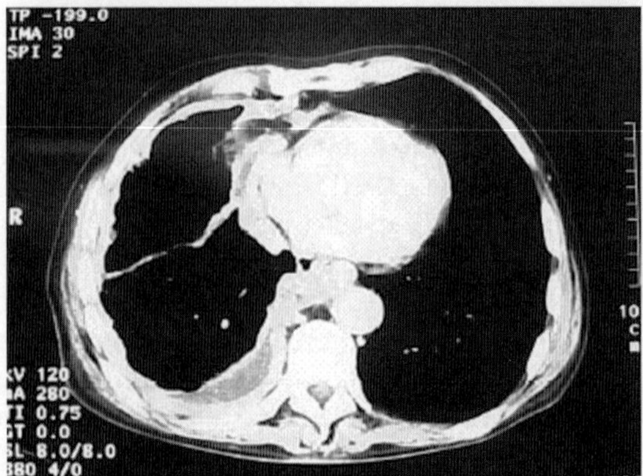
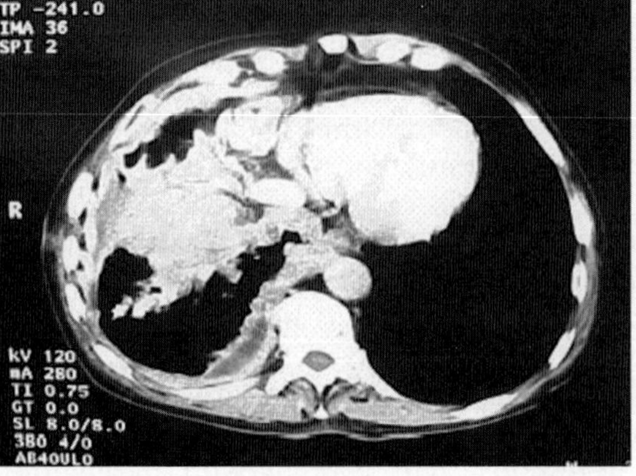

Figure 14.7

Pulmonary Function Test

Table 14-1

	Predicted	Best	% Predicted
FVC (Liters)	4.44	3.14	71
FEV$_1$ (Liters)	3.04	2.70	89
FEV$_1$/FVC (%)	69		86

Pulmonary Function Test Report

Pulmonary function testing revealed mild restriction with otherwise preserved lung function.

Quantitative Perfusion and Ventilation Scans

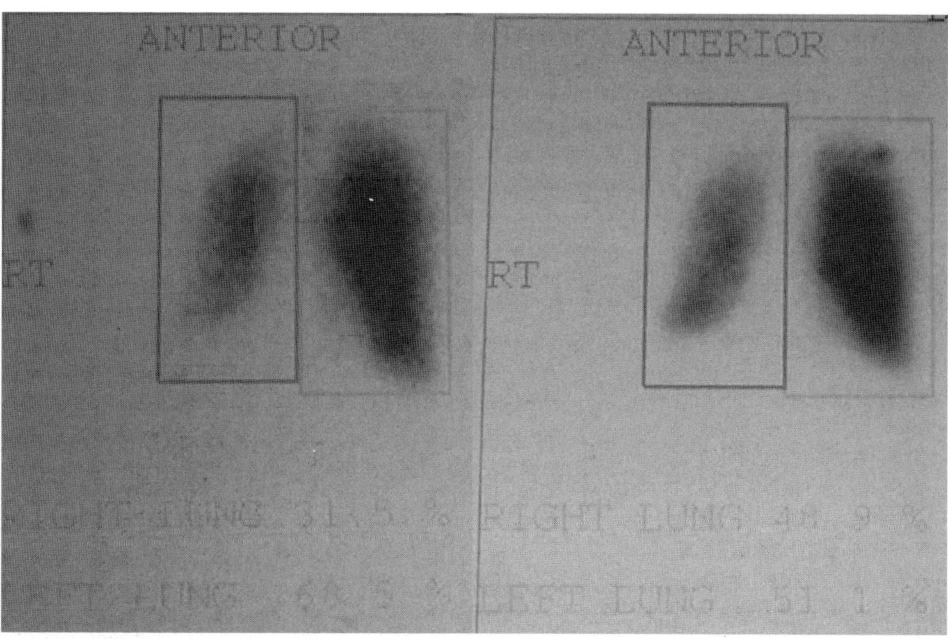

Figure 14.8

Quantitative Perfusion and Ventilation Scan Report

On ventilation-perfusion (V/Q) scan **(left)**, instead of the normal 55% perfusion to the right side, perfusion was reduced to 32%. On Persantine-thallium test **(right)**, there was an ejection fraction of 60%, with no inducible areas of ischemia on nuclear stress testing.

Approach

The patient should also be informed of the ongoing protocols for treatment of mesothelioma, including: (a) induction chemotherapy with pemetrexed and cisplatin followed by extrapleural pneumonetomy and radiation therapy to the hemithorax; (b) extrapleural pneumonectomy followed by chemotherapy and/or radiation therapy; (c) chemotherapy alone; and (d) surgery and novel intraoperative approaches including hyperthermic chemoperfusion, photodynamic therapy, and the use of novel agents postoperatively.

Discussion

Controversy exists regarding the choice of pleurectomy versus extrapleural pneumonectomy (EPP) for this disease. The majority of diffuse malignant mesotheliomas cannot be surgically removed en bloc with truly negative histologic margins because many patients have had a previous biopsy and there is invasion of the endothoracic fascia and intercostal muscles at that site, and/or pleural effusion which, although cytologically negative, may be breached, leading to local permeation of tumor cells either into the residual cavity or into the abdomen. Moreover, involvement of the visceral pleura, and hence the lung, can only be handled with a satisfactory cytoreduction by pneumonectomy. EPP is a more extensive dissection and may serve to remove more bulk disease than a pleurectomy, chiefly in the diaphragmatic and visceral pleural surfaces. Some surgeons, however, will include diaphragmatic resection and pericardial resection *with their pleurectomies* to accomplish removal of all gross disease. For EPP, it is almost a necessity to include pericardiotomy during the resection, for the maneuver aids in the exposure of the vessels and allows intrapericardial control to prevent a surgical catastrophe. The presence of irregular, bulky disease that on the CT scan infiltrates into the fissures probably dictates the necessity for EPP in this particular patient's case, and that was what was recommended as the surgical procedure.

The mortality rate for EPP is approximately 5% to 7%, chiefly from myocardial infarction, adult respiratory distress syndrome (ARDS), and pulmonary emboli. There is a major complication rate of 20% to 40% with EPP, and arrhythmia requiring medical management is the most common complication. The rate for bronchopleural fistula is greater with right-sided EPP, with an overall fistula rate of 3% to 20%; if this occurs, it is handled with open thoracostomy drainage with or without muscle flap interposition. More than 50% of patients undergoing EPP will experience recurrence within 7 to 9 months of the operation either in the chest or at distant sites, and the long-term survival rates depend upon pathologic stage of the disease, with a 30% 5-year survival rate for stage I patients.

▇ Surgical Approach

After comprehensive counseling, the patient elects to have extrapleural pneumonectomy with postoperative chemotherapy to be delivered closer to home by his local oncologist.

A standard posterolateral thoracotomy is made. The dissection is performed in an extrapleural plane with sacrifice of the azygous vein, and is assisted by the intrapericardial dissection of the pulmonary artery and veins. The pulmonary vessels can be transected with a linear stapling device. The bronchial stump is reinforced with a mediastinal fat flap. En bloc resection of the diaphragm and pericardium is performed and reconstructed with Gore-Tex patches, and the pericardial patch is fenestrated to allow drainage. Mediastinal lymph nodes should be resected. A single chest tube is left on closure for 24 hours, and the mediastinum is balanced by establishing negative pressure in the hemithorax upon closure of the chest.

Case Continued

The patient underwent an extrapleural pneumonectomy on the right side where bulky tumor was found completely surrounding the lung and diaphragm, and invading the pericardium. The diaphragm was completely resected, as was the right-sided pericardium, and a complete mediastinal lymph-node dissection was performed. There was minimal endothoracic fascia invasion, mainly at the sites of the previous thoracoscopy.

▇ Intraoperative Images

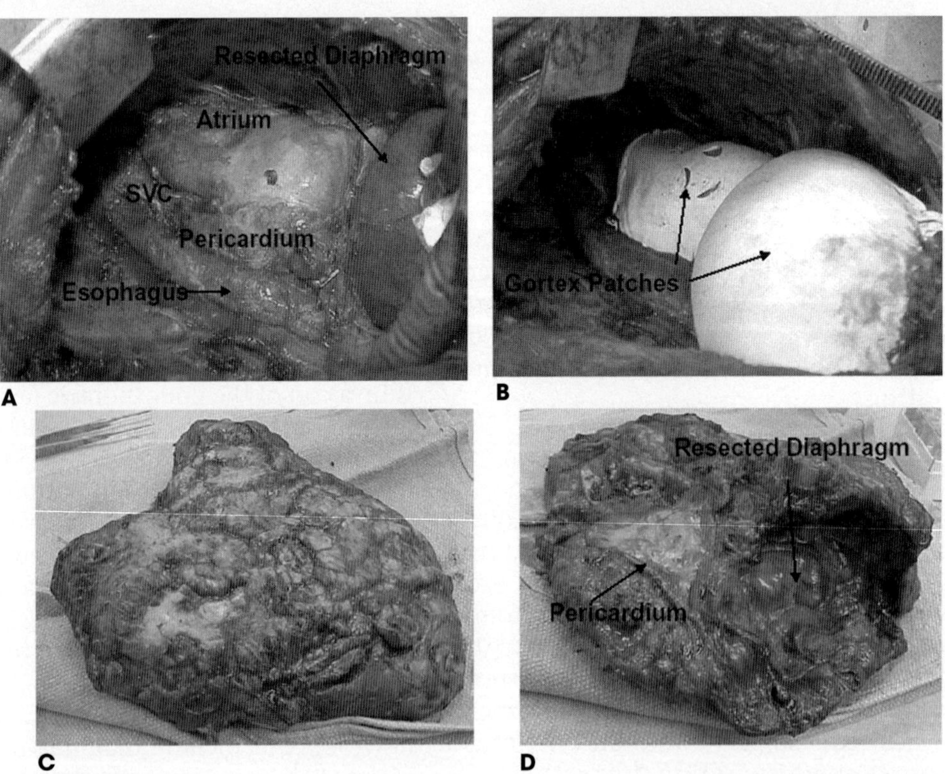

Figure 14.9

Intraoperative Report

Extrapleural pneumonectomy reveals the extent of the tumor (**A**), and Gore-Tex patches are placed (**B**). En bloc removal of the lung, diaphragm, and pericardium is performed (**C, D**).

Case Continued

The pathology report reveals that the patient actually has a biphasic mesothelioma, and all lymph nodes are free of tumor. He is classified as stage II mesothelioma.

The patient is extubated in the recovery room and does well, taking a regular diet on the second postoperative day. His oxygen saturations diminish on the third postoperative day and he has respiratory distress. Sputum culture reveals methicillin-resistant *Staphylococcus aureus* (MRSA). He is intubated, paralyzed with muscle relaxants, given diuresis, and resuscitated with albumin. Antibiotics are added to his postoperative regimen, and his fluid status is monitored with a Swan-Ganz catheter. By the seventh postoperative day his chest radiograph is noted to be improving and his oxygen saturation is remarkably better, allowing extubation. He steadily improves and is discharged on the 15th postoperative day.

Chest X-Rays

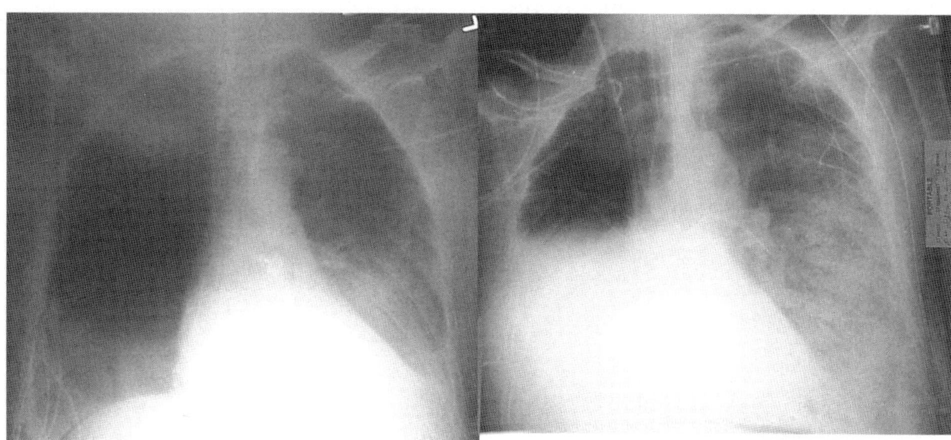

Figure 14.10

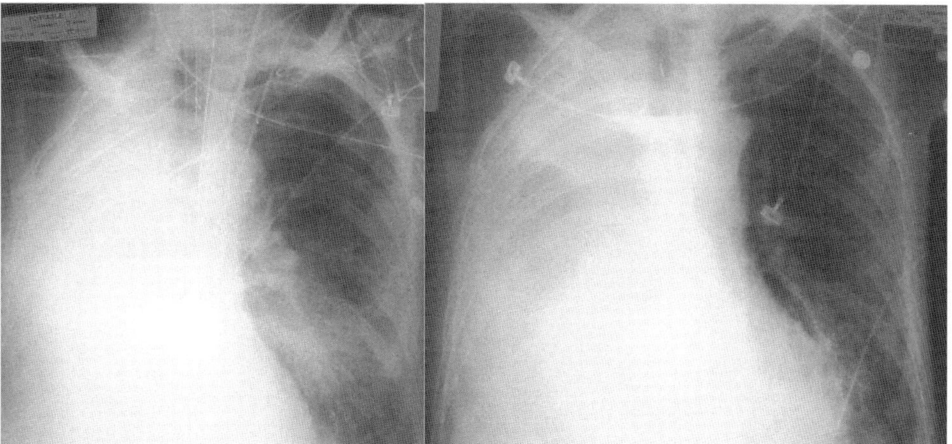

Figure 14.11

Chest X-Ray Report

The immediate postoperative chest radiograph shows no mediastinal shift and clear left lung (**upper left**). Interstitial pneumonitis becomes apparent on the second postoperative day (**upper right**), necessitating critical care measures for his acute respiratory distress syndrome (ARDS) and MRSA. Note the endotracheal tube and Swan-Ganz catheter. With treatment, improvement and clearing of the lung fields is evident (**lower left**). At discharge, his right chest is totally opacified and his left lung is back to baseline (**lower right**).

Case Continued

The patient returned home, where he received four cycles of gemcitabine and cisplatin. His tumor recurred intra-abdominally 20 months after resection, and he died 5 months later.

Suggested Readings

Betta P, Orecchia S, Schillaci F, et al. The present role of immuno-histochemistry in the diagnosis of malignant mesothelioma. *Pathologica* 2003;95:299–300.

Boutin C, Rey F. Thoracoscopy in pleural malignant mesothelioma: a prospective study of 188 consecutive patients. Part 1: diagnosis. *Cancer* 1993;72:389–393.

Boutin C, Rey F, Gouvernet J, Viallat JR, et al. Thoracoscopy in pleural malignant mesothelioma: a prospective study of 188 consecutive patients. Part 2: prognosis and staging. *Cancer* 1993;72:394–404.

Martino D, Pass HI. Integration of multimodality approaches in the management of malignant pleural mesothelioma. *Clin Lung Cancer* 2004;5:290–298.

Maskell NA, Gleeson FV, Davies RJ. Standard pleural biopsy versus CT-guided cutting-needle biopsy for diagnosis of malignant disease in pleural effusions: a randomized controlled trial. *Lancet* 2003;361:1326–1330.

Ordonez NG. Immunohistochemical diagnosis of epithelioid mesotheliomas: a critical review of old markers, new markers. *Hum Pathol* 2002;33:953–967.

Pass HI, Pogrebniak HW. Malignant pleural mesothelioma. *Curr Probl Surg* 1993;30:921–1012.

Pass HI. Malignant pleural mesothelioma: surgical roles and novel therapies. *Clin Lung Cancer* 2001;3:102–117.

Pass HI, Kranda K, Temeck BK, et al. Surgically debulked malignant pleural mesothelioma: results and prognostic factors. *Ann Surg Oncol* 1997;4:215–222.

Pass HI, Vogelzang N, Hahn S, et al. Malignant pleural mesothelioma. *Curr Probl Cancer* 2004;28:93–174.

Rusch VW, Venkatraman ES. Important prognostic factors in patients with malignant pleural mesothelioma, managed surgically. *Ann Thorac Surg* 1999;68:1799–1804.

Sugarbaker DJ, Jaklitsch MT, Buenor, Richards W, et al. Prevention, early detection, and management of complications after 328 consecutive extrapleural pneumonectomies. *J Thorac Cardiovasc Surg* 2004;128:138–146.

Vogelzang NJ, Rusthoven JJ, Symanowski J, Denham C, et al. Phase III study of pemetrexed in combination with cisplatin versus cisplatin alone in patients with malignant pleural mesothelioma. *J Clin Oncol* 2003;21:2636–2644.

Presentation

An 18-year-old man, with no significant past medical history, presented with a 19-months' history of an indolent mass of the anterior right thoracic cage. The mass had slowly increased in size. The neoplasia has a bony consistency, and is fixed to the ribs without signs of cutaneous inflammation.

■ Chest X-Ray

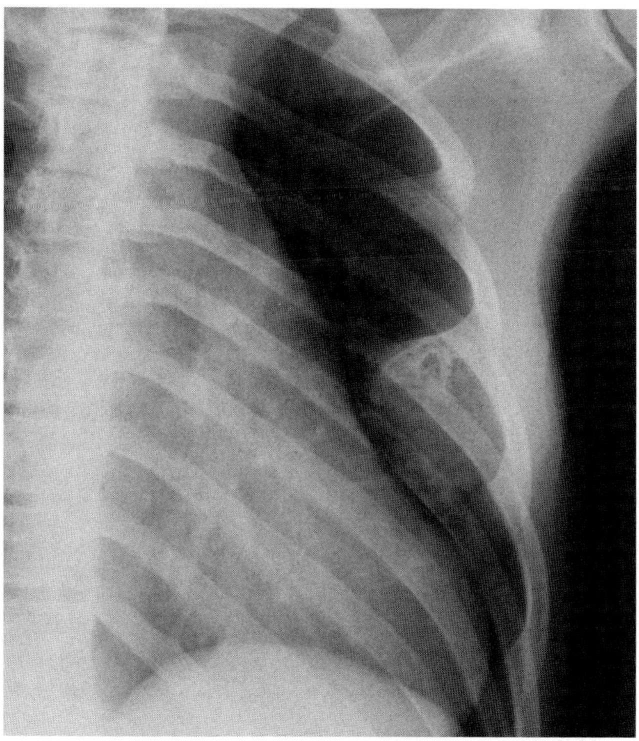

Figure 15.1

Chest X-Ray Report

Opacity of the left anterior thoracic wall with well-defined margins. Osteolysis of the anterior segment of the third left rib.

Differential Diagnosis

The possible diagnoses for this presentation include chondroma, osteochondroma, fibrous dysplasia, desmoid tumor, chondrosarcoma, Ewing's and Askin's sarcomas, osteosarcoma, and solitary myeloma. Each of these pathological entities has unique characteristics and specific radiological features that are of diagnostic value.

Chondroma develops during the pediatric years and becomes clinically evident in the age group of 10 to 50 years. These are usually small and asymptomatic, and are usually localized at the costochondral junction. Radiographically, they appear lobulated and radiodense, without cortical bone invasion or soft-tissue swelling.

Osteochondroma (synonym: solitary exostosis) is rare, appears between 10 and 18 years of age, is usually asymptomatic, and grows slowly during skeletal development. Radiologically, the newly formed bone is represented by cancellous bone, irregularly distributed with "finger-like" evaginations.

Fibrous dysplasia usually arises between the ages of 5 and 20 years as an asymptomatic mass in the posterior part of the thoracic cage. There is usually a history of an antecedent traumatic event. Radiographically, these appear as a central fusiform osteolytic area of the rib, with the cortex eroded from inside. The boundaries are clear or slightly faded, without associated calcification.

Desmoid tumor is observed more frequently in females during the third or fourth decade of life. The clinical presentation is of a slowly growing soft-tissue mass, without any particular radiographic appearance, although magnetic resonance imaging (MRI) may be valuable.

Chondrosarcoma is a tumor of the adult age. It can be associated with mild and intermittent pain and progressive growth with invasion into soft tissues. The radiographic picture represents an osteolytic tumor with interruption of the cortex. Calcifications are evident in the well-differentiated varieties, whereas they are rare or totally absent in the high-degree malignancies (grade 3–4, dedifferentiated). Calcifications are morphologically characterized by irregular granules, nodules, or radiopaque rings. Aggressive varieties are characterized by an interruption of the cortex with invasion of soft tissues by a non-calcified tumor.

Ewing's and Askin's (Primitive Neuroectodermal Tumors) sarcomas are childhood or youth tumors, exceptional before 5 years of age and after 25 years. The first symptom is usually intermittent mild pain that becomes progressively intense, with or without the presence of a mass. Radiologically, these have an onion-peel appearance resulting from periostal bone formation by multiple osteogenetic nuclei infiltrating the medullary spaces and the haversian canals.

Sternal or costal *osteosarcoma* is rare, presenting between the ages of 10 and 30 years. It manifests with intermittent mild pain. Laboratory studies demonstrate an elevated alkaline phosphatase. The radiograph reveals a tumor growing within the cortical and cancellous bones, which are rapidly destroyed. The periosteum is surpassed, and generally there is a neoplastic production of osteoid and bone tissue.

Myeloma (synonym: plasmacytoma) is observed after 40 to 50 years of age. It is localized in ribs, clavicula, and sternum, with diffuse vague symptoms generally associated to asthenia and fever. Laboratory findings show an elevated plasmacellular percentage, immature and atypical elements, a high percentage of globulins with inversion of the albumin/globulin ratio, and Bence-Jones proteinuria. If solitary, the myeloma presents radiologically as multiple large areas of osteolysis, with or without cortical erosion.

Discussion

Primary osseous chest wall tumors are rare (4% to 8 % of all bone sarcomas). The mean age of patients with benign varieties is younger than those with malignant tumors (mean: 26 vs 40). Usually, patients (70% of patients) present with slowly enlarging masses. Pain is more frequent (25% to 50% of patients) in the malignant varieties, but it must be emphasized that one third of patients with benign lesions also complain of pain. At the onset, pain is generalized and nonspecific. The benign tumors demand a diagnostic approach similar to those used for malignant tumors. Radiologic investigations can assist with the diagnosis, but a histologic study is always mandatory.

Recommendation

The diagnosis of thoracic wall tumor requires a careful history and physical examination of the patient, laboratory analysis, a radiologic study of the chest (plain radiography, computed tomography [CT] scan, and MRI), and a total body bone scintigraphy. Tissue diagnosis is established with a biopsy, preferably excisional, when the tumor is small, or incisional, if the tumor is large.

Case Continued

The patient is evaluated with CT scan, MRI, and scintigraphy, followed by an incisional biopsy.

CT Scan

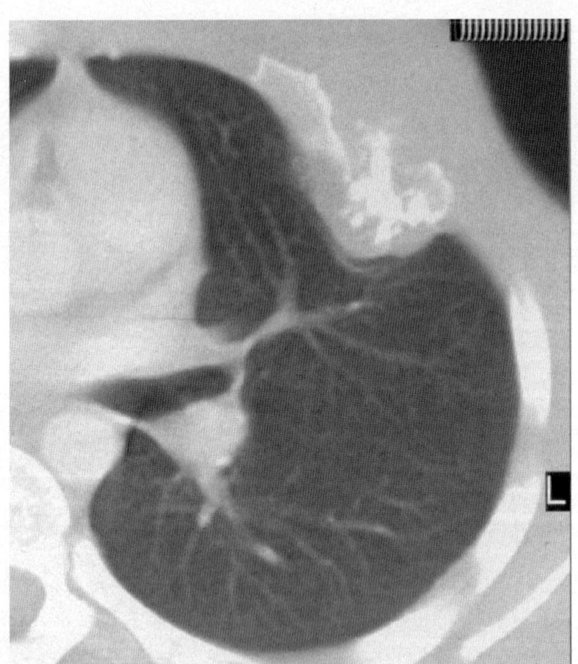

Figure 15.2

CT Scan Report

Mass of the left anterior thoracic wall extending into the thoracic cavity with erosion of the osteocondral portion of the rib associated with diffuse and inhomogeneous calcifications.

■ MRI

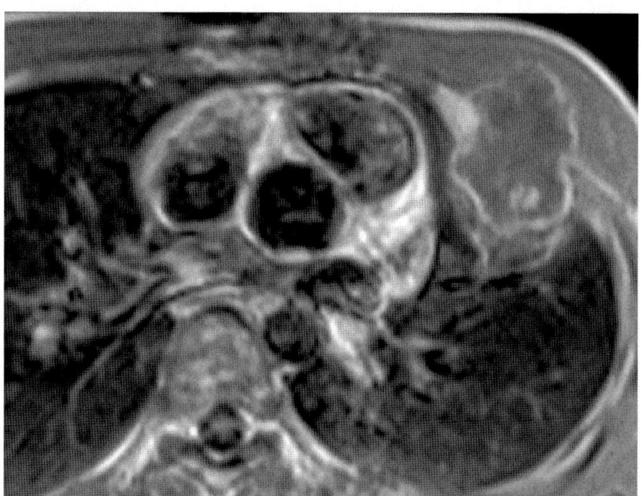

Figure 15.3

MRI Report

Neoplasm penetrating into the thoracic cavity and extending to the skin surface, displacing the pectoralis major muscle without signs of infiltration. There is erosion of the rib osteocondral junction with numerous inhomogeneous calcifications.

Case Continued

Scintigraphy reveals a lesion in proximity to the sternal junction that extends on the third rib with a hyperactive halo. Pathology reveals a central chondrosarcoma (CS). The histopathologic problem is that of distinguishing from a chondroma. The cytologic features of CS include the presence of large, polymorphic double nuclei, and an increase of the cell population.

Diagnosis and Recommendation

The CS is the most frequent malignant tumor of the thoracic wall (50% of malignant tumors and 25% of all primary tumors). The ribs are the predominant site (80%) followed by the sternum (20%). Male: female ratio is 2:1. CS can arise within a preexisting exostosis or, less frequently, it can be secondary to prior radiation therapy. Three grades of malignancy are distinguished: grade I, with rare atypical cells in a context of well-differentiated cartilage; grade II, with greater presence of atypical cells; and grade III, with single isolates of cartilaginous elements within a preponderant background of atypical cells.

CS remains generally asymtomatic for a long time. Radiologically, it appears as an opacity with rib or sternal swelling, together with osteolysis and calcifications, which can be absent in 45% of chest radiographs, but are well defined with CT scan. Cluster calcifications are a pathognomonic diagnostic finding. Bone scintigraphy shows an area of increased activity. CS generally grows slower than osteosarcoma, and can progress to malignancy to behave like osteosarcoma (dedifferentiated CS). In fact, reccurences are frequent (17% to 50%) after marginal or intralesional resections and occur generally within 3 years after resection. Survival after 10 years is 96% after wide local excision, 65% after local excision, and 14% after palliative excision.

■ Approach

The patient must be surgically treated. Radiotherapy and chemotherapy have a therapeutic effect only in the dedifferentiated variety. The surgical treatment is a mandatory wide resection, with 4-cm margins. For a better definition of the superficial and lateral limits of the CS, a preoperative ultrasound examination of the thoracic wall is useful to define the extent of disease, and particularly the presence of micronodules (often seen in recurrent lesions) that would not be clinically evident due to their small size.

■ Surgical Approach

Wide resection of the thoracic wall (16 × 14 × 8 cm) with removal of two rib segments, one of which is deformed by a mass with an irregular-surface, and showed a white, lobular, translucent appearance on transection. The reconstruction of the chest wall is made by fascia lata, anchored to a moldable titanium plate placed on the ribs under and above the resected area.

Discussion

The surgical treatment should follow oncologic principles with particular emphasis on respiratory functions of the thoracic cage. Large chest wall defects require surgical reconstruction to ensure structural stability and to prevent flail chest. The methods of reconstruction are numerous, and they involve the use of biological materials (omentum, fascia lata, latissimus dorsi muscle, pectoralis muscles, serratus anterior muscle, rectus abdominis muscle) or synthetic materials (polypropylene, polytetrafluorethylene, methylmethacrylate). The choice of the material used is often individual and related to personal experience. We prefer a technique of reconstruction using fascia lata, usually from our tissue bank, to diminish the infectious risk, sutured together with one or two moldable titanium plates covered with muscular flap.

Case Continued

At the end of surgery, the patient does not require mechanical ventilation and is transferred to the intensive care unit. A chest x-ray and arterial blood gas sample are obtained.

Postoperative X-Ray

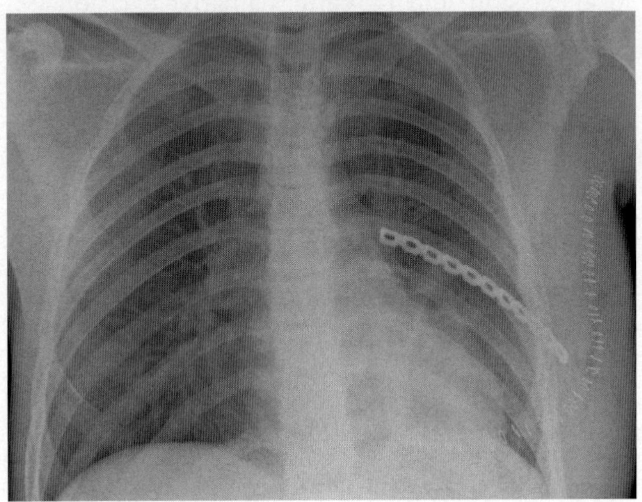

Figure 15.4

Postoperative X-Ray Report

Chest x-ray showing the moldable plate anchored to the anterior segments of the second and fifth ribs.

Case Continued

After discharge, the patient has a follow-up every 3 months for the first 2 years and subsequently every 6 months with ultrasound and CT scan evaluations of the chest. After 4 years, there is absence of local relapse and he has resumed his occupation.

Suggested Readings

Briccoli A, Manfrini M, Rocca M, et al. Sternal reconstruction with synthetic mesh and metallic plates for high grade tumors of the chest wall. *Eur J Surg* 2002;168:494–499.

Campanacci M. *Bone and soft tissue tumors: clinical features, imaging, pathology and treatment.* 2nd ed. Wien, Austria: Springer-Verlag; 1999.

Gordon MS, Hajdu SI, Bains MS, et al. Soft tissue sarcomas of the chest wall. Results of surgical resection. *J Thorac Cardiovasc Surg* 1991;101:843–854.

Graeber GM, Jones DR, Pairolero PC. Primary neoplasms. In: Pearson FG, ed. *Thoracic surgery.* New York: Churchill Livingstone; 1995:1237–1251.

Walsh GL, Davis BM, Swisher SG, et al. A single-institutional, multidisciplinary approach to primary sarcomas involving chest wall requiring full-thickness resections. *J Thorac Cardiovasc Surg* 2001;121:48–60.

Presentation

A 76-year-old man complains of progressive dysphagia for 2 months. He can tolerate only a liquid diet. The hold-up sensation is at the level of the throat; he also frequently regurgitates the fluid that he drinks. He has lost 20 pounds during the same time, and his voice has been hoarse for the past week. He used to be a heavy smoker, but gave up smoking 5 years ago. Physical examination shows a thin man with no cervical lymphadenopathy.

Differential Diagnosis

In an elderly man with symptoms of progressive dysphagia and weight loss, an obstructive malignant growth has to be considered in the upper aerodigestive tract. Cancer of the esophagus is probable; extrinsic compression from cancer of the lung or its associated involved lymph nodes in the mediastinum is also part of the differential diagnosis. Other tumors are less common. A cancer of the larynx with obstruction to the esophagus is a possibility, but hoarseness usually predates the dysphagia. More likely, the hoarseness of voice is related to involvement of the recurrent laryngeal nerve. The level of the complaint of dysphagia does not necessarily equate to the level of the physical obstruction. The hold-up sensation is usually located above, but not below, the actual site of cancer.

Recommendation

A barium contrast swallow and an endoscopy are arranged.

Case Continued

The patient aspirates a small amount of barium with the first swallow, and therefore the procedure is abandoned. On endoscopy, a tumor is found extending from the postcricoid area to the cervical esophagus. It extends to 19 cm when measured from the incisors. The endoscope is advanced through with some negotiation. The rest of the esophagus is normal, and so are the stomach and the second part of the duodenum. Because the patient experiences significant obstruction and has lost a substantial amount of weight, a guide wire is passed and a fine-bore feeding tube is fed down to the stomach for nasogastric tube feeding. At the same setting, a bronchoscopy is also performed to examine the tracheobronchial tree. Right vocal cord paralysis is noted. There is no lesion found inside the airway. Biopsies are taken from the tumor, which proves to be a squamous cell cancer.

Discussion

The diagnosis of cervical esophageal cancer is made. The barium aspiration suggests either high proximal tumor obstruction or that the patient has vocal cord paralysis. The vocal cord palsy is related to either involvement of the right recurrent laryngeal nerve by metastatic lymph node or primary tumor infiltration of the tracheoesophageal groove. It is mandatory to perform a panendoscopy of the upper aerodigestive tract to (a) detect synchronous or metachronous tumors, which can occur in up to 10% of patients due to the phenomenon of field cancerization, and (b) look for tracheal infiltration by the esophageal cancer. Nasogastric tube feeding helps improve the patient's nutritional status since substantial weight loss has occurred, and is preferred over parenteral nutrition. It is customary to consider a weight loss of more than 10% of the usual body weight to be significant, and that may be associated with poor outcome.

Diagnosis and Recommendation

Cervical esophageal squamous cell carcinoma. Further staging and diagnostic workup are needed to establish the extent of the disease, which will determine treatment approach.

▨ PET/CT Scan

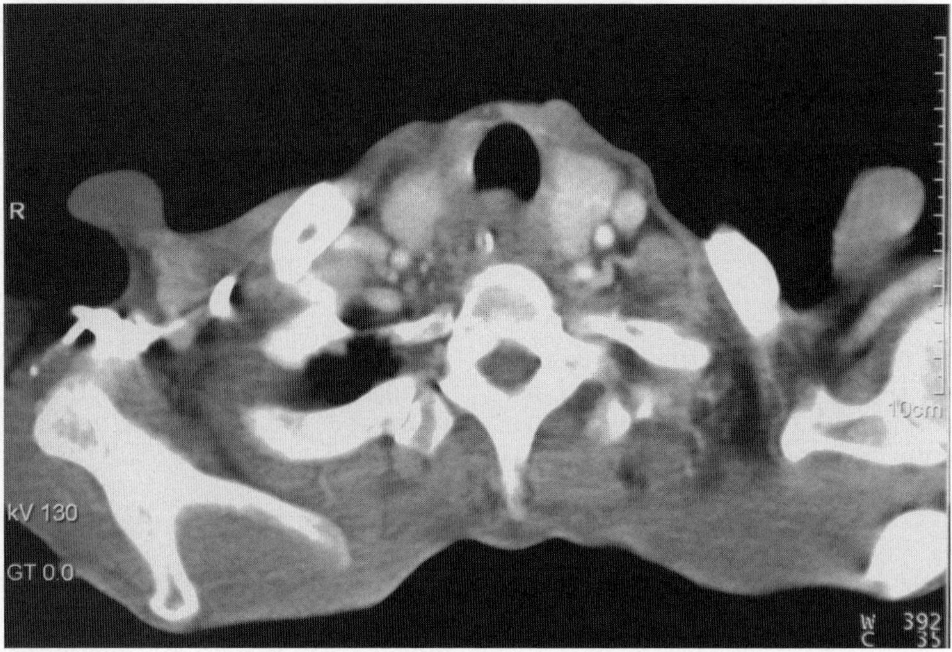

Figure 16.1

PET/CT Scan Report

Mural thickening of the cervical esophagus extends from the cricoid cartilage to just above the sternal notch, measuring 8 cm in length. The plane between the right thyroid lobe and esophagus is unclear, suggestive of infiltration. The standard uptake value (SUV) is 9.8. Some small lymph nodes of less than 5 mm are seen in the paraesophageal region, but all have low SUVs of less than 2.0. No distant metastases are detected. The patient has no contraindication to major surgery.

▨ Approach

A diagnosis of locally advanced cervical esophageal cancer is made. Treatment options include chemoradiation or surgical resection with or without adjuvant therapy. For most patients with significant cervical esophageal involvement, surgical resection involves a pharyngolaryngoesophagectomy. The lack of head-to-head comparisons of the two approaches and evidence-based data should be clearly discussed with the patient in order to formulate a treatment plan.

Discussion

Chemoradiation is increasingly used as primary treatment because the magnitude of surgical resection is substantial and laryngeal preservation is possible. Depending on tumor stage, when chemoradiation is used with a curative intent, good local control has been reported. The main drawbacks of chemoradiation are (a) substantial esophagitis and systemic and local symptoms during treatment; (b) stricture formation; (c) future salvage surgery may be made more difficult due to prior radiation; and (d) laryngeal dysfunction both during and after radiation can lead to aspiration symptoms. Laryngeal preservation surgery is possible in tumors of the distal cervical esophagus where a margin from the cricoid can be obtained, or when downstaging has been obtained with chemoradiation. Preserving the larynx, however, may lead to inadequate oncologic clearance. It also predisposes to aspiration, because of an anastomosis very close to the cricoid, and pharyngolaryngeal dysfunction, especially when the recurrent laryngeal nerves can be injured at surgery. For patients with hypopharyngeal tumors or proximal cervical esophageal tumors, segmental resection with reconstruction by a free jejunal graft can be performed. Alternative voice rehabilitation is required, but aspiration is not problematic because the airway and food passage will be permanently separated.

Case Continued

It is explained to the patient that treatment may be palliative, and the pros and cons of chemoradiation or surgical resection are discussed. The patient opts for primary surgical resection.

Surgical Approach

A pharygolaryngoesophagectomy is performed. The patient is first placed in a left lateral position with one-lung anesthesia. Thoracoscopic esophageal mobilization is performed using a 5-port technique. The patient is next turned to a supine position. A 2-team approach is used, with the abdominal team mobilizing the stomach for a gastric pull-up and the head-and-neck team performing the pharyngo-laryngectomy. A terminal tracheostomy is made. The stomach is then delivered via the posterior medi-astinum to the neck for a pharyngogastric anasto-mosis. Historically, the approach to mobilize the intrathoracic esophagus has been via an open thora-cotomy, or by a transhiatal method. To minimize surgical trauma, minimally invasive techniques, such as thoracoscopy or laparoscopy or their combi-nations, have been explored in dedicated centers.

Case Continued

The tumor at the cervical esophagus is found to be locally advanced with infiltration to the tracheo-esophageal groove on the right side and the right thyroid lobe. The posterior tracheal mucosa is intact, and the tumor, although adherent to the carotid sheath, can be dissected off. No obvious metastatic lymph nodes are seen. Frozen section examinations of all surgical margins are clear. Pharyngogastric anastomosis is performed. At the conclusion of the operation, the patient is extubated and sent to the intensive care unit for monitoring. Initial recovery is uneventful. He is started on oral fluid, but on day 7 after surgery his neck wound becomes erythematous, especially on the left side. A Gastrografin contrast swallow and endoscopy is per-formed.

Gastrografin Study

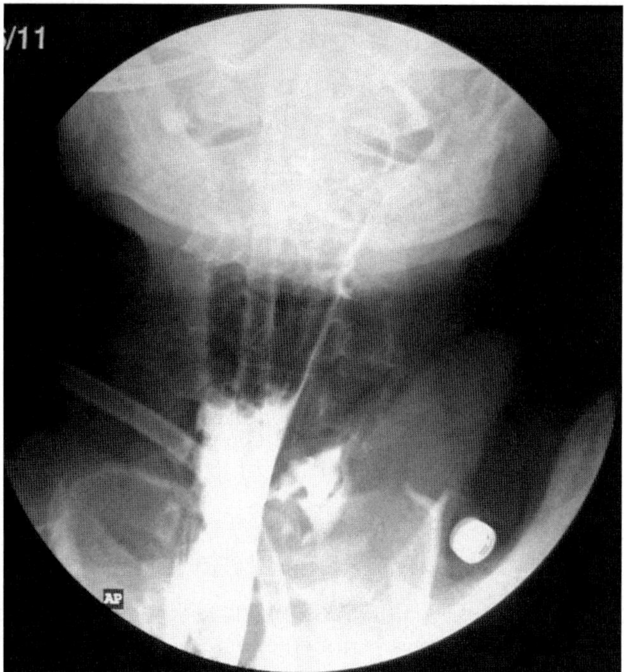

Figure 16.2

Gastrografin Study Report

A loculated pool of contrast is seen at the left-lateral aspect of the stomach in the neck. Anastomotic leak is suspected.

Endoscopic Image

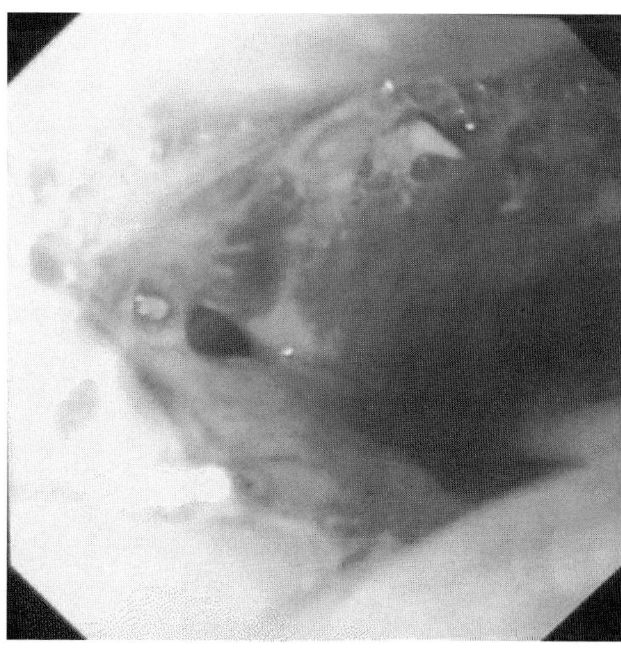

Figure 16.3

Endoscopy Report

A 5-mm defect in the anastomosis facing the left side is noted. The stomach looks healthy otherwise.

Case Continued

Anastomotic leak is diagnosed, which appears small. The left edge of the neck wound is opened for drainage. A suction drain is inserted. After 1 week, however, drainage of saliva shows no sign of reducing, and it becomes apparent that drainage is not effective and the erythema is tracking down to underneath the skin flap above the terminal tracheostomy. A repeat endoscopy shows that the previous leakage site is similar, but another new dehiscence is seen near the mid-anterior portion of the anastomosis.

Diagnosis and Recommendation

It is clear that a major anastomotic leak is encountered and simple drainage is not effective. There is the added danger of saliva tracking down and disrupting the terminal tracheostomy. Exteriorization of the anastomosis is thus recommended, with a view for staged reconstruction when the leak and sepsis are controlled.

◼ Surgical Approach

The neck wound is reopened. The anterior portion of the pharyngogastric anastomosis is taken down, and the separated edges of pharynx and stomach are sutured to the skin edges. A "pharyngogastrostomy" is thus matured like a stoma.

◼ Perioperative Image

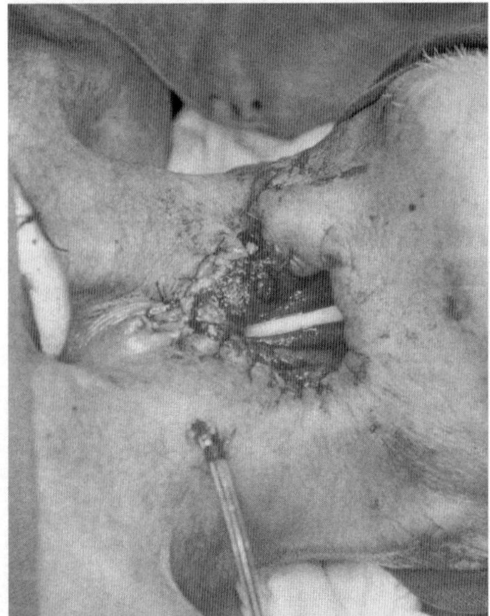

Figure 16.4

Perioperative Report

The anterior wall of the anastomosis is taken down and a stoma is made as described.

Case Continued

The patient's sepsis comes under control, and he is being fed by a nasoenteric tube. After 3 weeks, reconstruction is performed.

◼ Surgical Approach

The patient undergoes left chest wall pectoralis major myocutaneous flap reconstruction of the pharyngogastrostomy.

◼ Perioperative Image

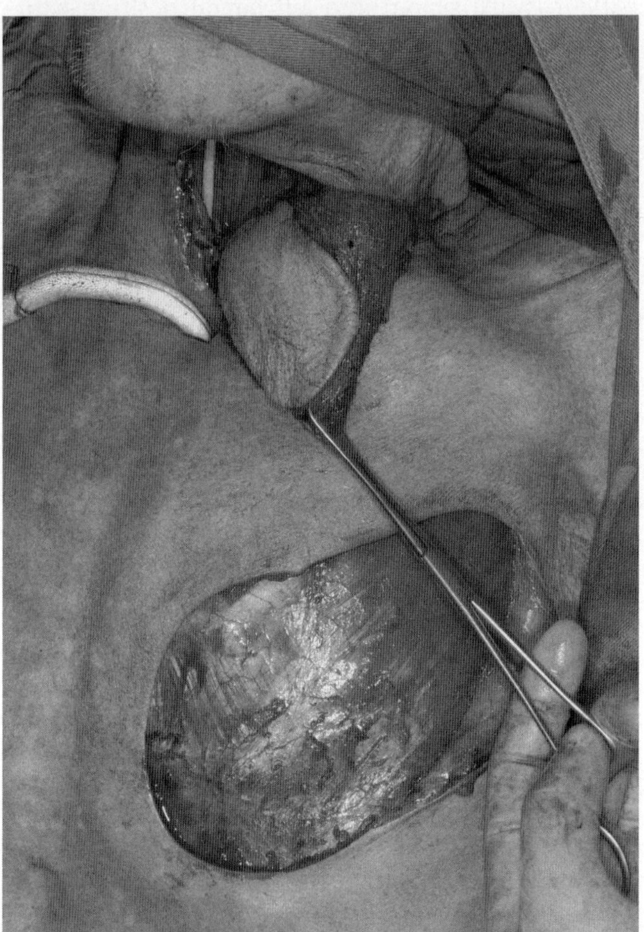

Figure 16.5

Perioperative Report

In order to reconstruct the anterior defect of the stoma, a 6 × 8 cm pectoralis major myocutaneous flap is raised and brought up to the neck through a subcutaneous tunnel.

Surgical Approach

The edge of the stoma is first raised; the skin edge of the pectoralis major flap is sutured to the stomach and pharynx with the skin island facing inward. A split-thickness skin graft is taken from the thigh and used to cover the exterior muscle. The chest wall donor site is closed primarily.

Case Continued

The patient recovers from the operation without complications and is able to resume a full oral diet. The pathology of the surgical specimen from the resection shows a moderately differentiated squamous cell cancer of the cervical esophagus, which has infiltrated to the thyroid (pT4); none of the 55 lymph nodes that are sampled contains metastases (N0). The patient is well, though he suffers occasional regurgitation of acidic stomach contents. He learns to speak with an electrolarynx.

Clinical Photograph

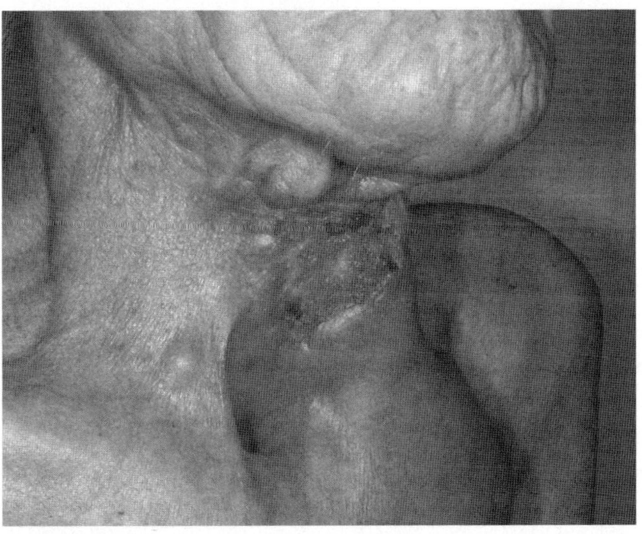

Figure 16.6

Clinical Report

End result with skin graft healed over the muscle. The terminal tracheostomy site can be seen.

Discussion

Given the locally advanced nature of the tumor, although gross tumor clearance with clear resection margins is obtained, it is decided to administer postoperative adjuvant radiotherapy to enhance local disease control. Reconstruction of intestinal continuity with a gastric pull-up has the advantage of relative simplicity. However, most patients will experience some degree of reflux, especially if the cricopharyngeal sphincter has been resected. Some surgeons advocate using a colonic interposition, which has the disadvantage of increasing surgical complexity.

Suggested Readings

Burmeister BH, Dickie G, Smithers BM, et al. Thirty-four patients with carcinoma of the cervical esophagus treated with chemoradiation therapy. *Arch Otolaryngol Head Neck Surg* 2000;126:205–208.

Law SY, Fok M, Wei WI, et al. Thoracoscopic esophageal mobilization for pharyngolaryngoesophagectomy. *Ann Thorac Surg* 2000;70:418–422.

Ong GB, Lee Y. Pharyngogastric anastomosis after esophago-pharyngectomy for carcinoma of the hypopharynx and cervical oesophagus. *Br J Surg* 1960;48:193–200.

Orringer MB. Resection of carcinoma involving the cervicothoracic esophagus: cervical exenteration. In: Pearson FG, Cooper JD, Deslauriers J, et al., eds. *Esophageal surgery*. Philadelphia, PA: Churchill Livingstone; 2002:880–887.

Wei WI, Lam LK, Yuen PW, et al. Current status of pharyngo-laryngo-esophagectomy and pharyngogastric anastomosis. *Head Neck* 1998;20:240–244.

case **17**

Presentation

A 59-year old man with no significant past medical history presents with symptoms of progressive dysphagia lasting 2 months. He can only tolerate a semisolid to liquid diet. The hold-up sensation resides at the thoracic inlet; he also regurgitates sometimes. He used to be a heavy smoker but has given up smoking for about 5 years. He drinks heavily, and has consumed a bottle of whiskey every week for many years. He has lost about 10 pounds in weight. Physical examination is unremarkable.

Differential Diagnosis

In an elderly man with symptoms of progressive dysphagia and weight loss, an obstructive malignant growth has to be considered. In areas where esophageal cancer is common, this should be high on the list of the differential diagnosis. Smoking and alcohol intake are both predisposing factors. Bronchogenic carcinoma with extrinsic compression of the esophagus by the primary tumor or mediastinal metastatic lymph nodes is also possible. The location of the complaint of dysphagia, however, does not necessarily equate to the level of the obstruction. The sensation of hold-up is usually above, but not below, the actual site of cancer.

Recommendation

Barium contrast swallow and endoscopy.

Barium Contrast Study

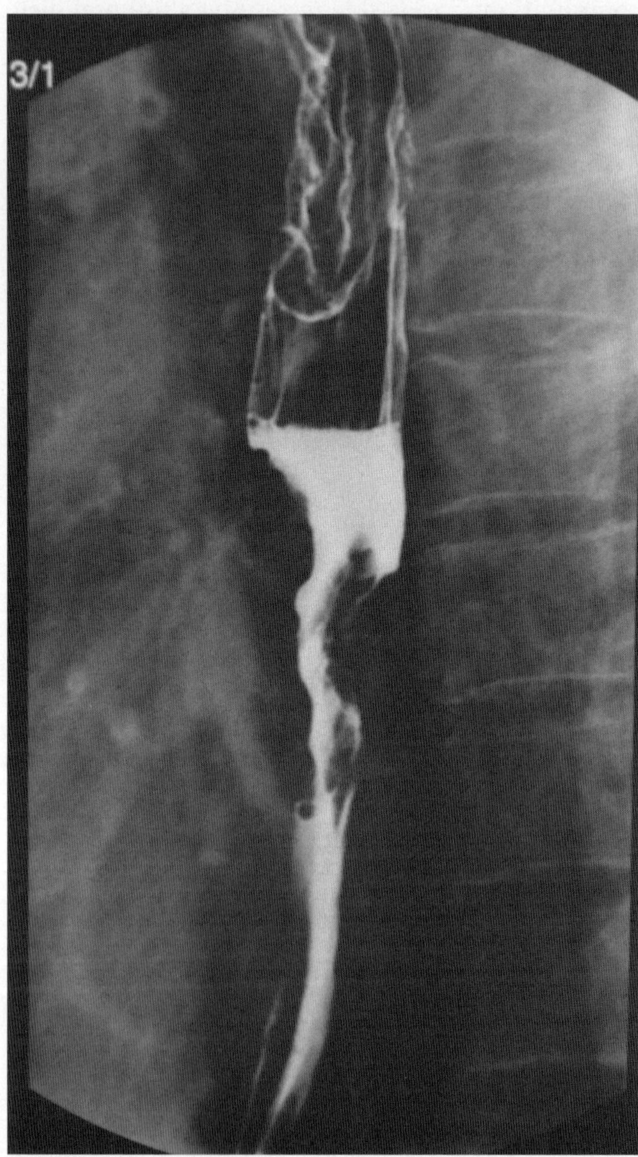

Figure 17.1

Barium Contrast Study Report

Barium contrast study shows mucosal irregularity on the right side of the midesophagus at about the T6-T7 level. Circumferential narrowing is also observed lower down at T9-T10. Proximal hold-up of contrast is demonstrated.

Case Continued

The endoscopy reveals two ulcerative tumors, one measuring 26 to 30 cm from the incisor and the other 31 to –36 cm. The intervening mucosa seems normal. Staining with Lugol's iodine does not reveal other lesions. Biopsies later confirm squamous cell cancers for both tumors. A bronchoscopy is also performed, which shows that both vocal cords are mobile, and there is no mucosal lesion seen in the tracheobronchial tree.

Diagnosis

Squamous cell esophageal cancer.

Discussion

In the West, adenocarcinoma of the lower esophagus and gastric cardia has surpassed squa-mous cell cancer as the predominant cell type, believed to be related to gastroesophageal reflux disease, obesity, and Barrett's esophagus, which are uncommon in Asian populations. When found, squamous cell cancers tend to locate in the midesophagus; they can be multicentric, and have the propensity for submucosal spread. Both are reasons prompting the use of special stains like Lugol's iodine to look for unsuspected lesions in the rest of the esophagus. A panendoscopy is also a necessity to examine the tracheobronchial tree for involvement by the esophageal tumor. This is of particular importance for tumors that are located in the upper or midesophagus because of the close proximity to the airway. Tumor involvement of the tracheobronchial tree contraindicates resection. The rest of the upper aerodigestive tract is also screened for synchronous tumors because of the phenomenon of field cancerization.

Recommendations

Further staging and diagnostic workup are undertaken. Positron emission tomography (PET)/computed tomography (CT) scan and endoscopic ultrasound are carried out.

PET/CT Scan

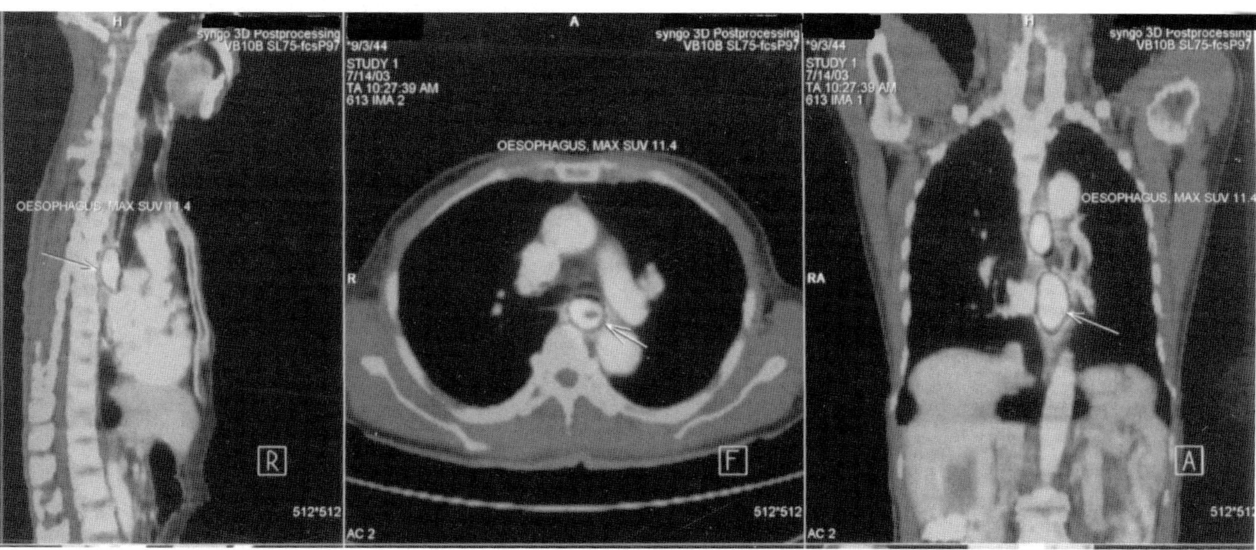

Figure 17.2

PET/CT Scan Report

Two tumor segments corresponding to the barium and endoscopic findings are found. The maximum standard uptake value (SUV) is 11.4. No involved regional lymph nodes or distant metastases are found.

Case Continued

On endoscopic ultrasound (EUS), both tumors are found to involve the full thickness of the esophageal wall. Multiple small lymph nodes, up to 1.5 cm in size, are seen. The celiac lymph node is not enlarged. The staging on EUS is therefore T3 N1. Pulmonary function tests show no contraindication to proceed with major surgery.

Discussion

Accurate staging of esophageal cancer has gained more importance because of stage-directed therapy. The sensitivity and specificity of a conventional CT scan for local tumor infiltration and local-regional lymph node are suboptimal. PET with 18-F-fluoro-deoxy-D-glucose (FDG) is increasingly used, and is of particular use in identifying distant nodal or systemic metastases. Sensitivity, specificity, and accuracy rates for the detection of distant metastases of 88%, 93%, and 91%, respectively, have been reported, but local-regional staging of N1 disease seems much inferior to EUS. On EUS, lymph nodes that are typically identified as harboring metastatic disease usually are larger than 5 mm in size and oval in shape, with an echo-poor pattern and smooth borders. The accuracy of determining T stage ranges between 85% and 90%, while nodal staging accuracy approximates 70% to 90%. When EUS-guided fine-needle aspiration cytology (EUS-FNA) is used, the diagnostic accuracy extends beyond 90%.

Patients with squamous cell cancers often have different operative risks than those with adenocarcinomas. Smoking and alcohol consumption are common, and thus the risks are mostly pulmonary and hepatic. For patients with adenocarcinomas, cardiac risk should be carefully evaluated.

Approach

The patient is suffering from locally advanced stage III esophageal cancer. It is explained to him that although surgical resection is the conventional treatment, the long-term result is suboptimal. If R0 resection can be achieved, a 5-year survival rate of approximately 30% may be expected. The patient opts for neoadjuvant chemoradiation therapy, which consists of cisplatin and 5-fluorouracil for weeks 1 and 4, given concurrently with 40 Gy of external-beam radiotherapy given at 2 Gy/fraction for 4 weeks.

Discussion

Neoadjuvant therapy is increasingly used in an attempt to improve outcome. One large, randomized controlled trial conducted by the Medical Research Council investigating preoperative chemotherapy demonstrated improved survival, but this was contradicted by another equally well-conducted intergroup trial. Preoperative chemoradiation for adenocarcinoma of the esophagus has been shown by one trial to result in better survival in the neoadjuvant group; however, survival in the resection-alone group was unexpectedly poor. Thus, there is as yet no conclusive evidence that these approaches will result in a better outcome than with surgical resection. A pathological complete response to neoadjuvant therapy is likely to lead to longer survival, but the overall effect is neutralized by the nonresponders. A delay in surgical resection could lead to unnecessary side effects and worse prognosis.

Case Continued

The patient tolerates the treatment well, despite some transient neutropenia. His dysphagia improves, and he gains 5 kg in weight. Restaging is performed 3 weeks after completion of chemoradiation.

On endoscopic ultrasound evaluation, good response to chemoradiation is evident. Shallow ulceration at 27 to 29 cm is seen. The lesion involves the full thickness of the esophageal wall, but it is unclear whether this is scarring or tumor. Biopsies later show only necrotic tissue with no evidence of malignancy. Two enlarged lymph nodes of 7 to 8 mm are seen.

PET/CT Scan

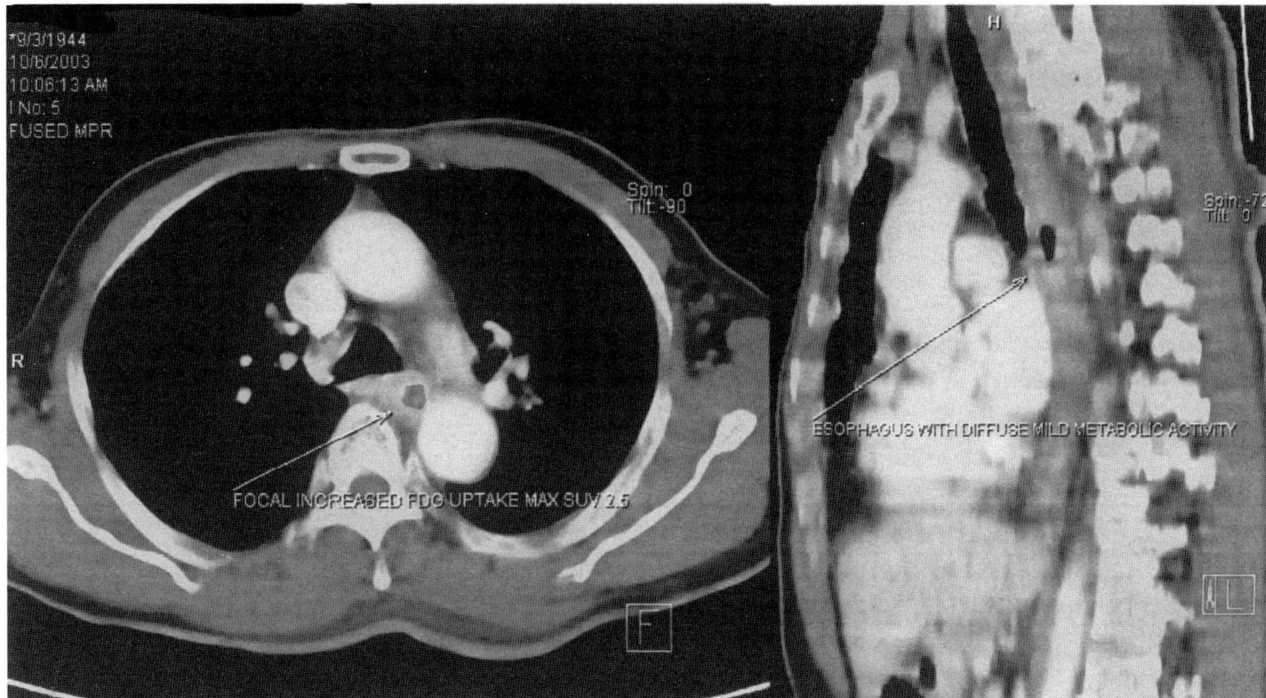

Figure 17.3

PET/CT Scan Report

There is a reduction in size of the original tumors; only a thickening with an SUV of 2.5 (previously 11.4) is seen at the level of the tracheal bifurcation. No regional lymph nodes or distant metastases are evident.

Discussion

Restaging of esophageal cancer after neoadjuvant therapy is difficult. CT scan, endoscopy, and EUS are unreliable in response assessment. PET scan, with its metabolic measurement, has gained some support in recent studies.

Case Continued

Although the investigations cannot demonstrate with certainty the presence of residual tumor, the chemoradiation is given with intent as neoadjuvant therapy. The patient agrees to surgical resection, so a transthoracic Lewis-Tanner esophagectomy is planned.

Intraoperative Image

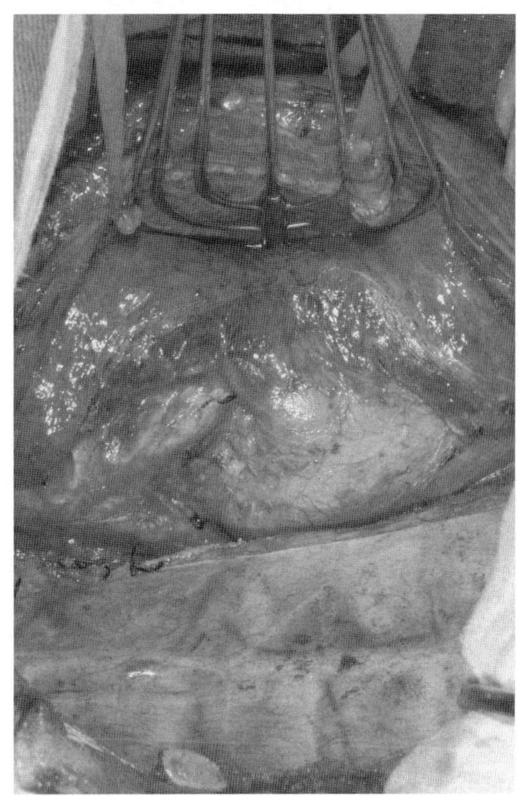

Figure 17.4

Intraoperative Report

The posterior mediastinum after esophageal mobilization. The esophagus is behind the retractor, and the pericardium, tracheal bifurcation, and main bronchi are clearly seen.

■ Surgical Approach

The gastric conduit is first mobilized at laparotomy, its blood supply based on the right gastric and right gastroepiploic vessels. A pyloroplasty is performed. Lymphadenectomy is performed around the celiac trifurcation. The patient is then turned to a left lateral position. Access is gained via a right fifth space posterolateral thoracotomy. The esophagus is removed en bloc with its surrounding connective tissue, with the plane of dissection anteriorly on the pericardium, laterally on the left side pleura, and posteriorly on the thoracic aorta. The periaortic connective tissue, including the thoracic duct, is removed. The thoracic duct is ligated where it emerges from the diaphragmatic hiatus. Bronchial, hilar, and carinal lymph nodes are all resected. Sampling of the superior mediastinal lymph node is performed. The stomach is delivered into the chest, the esophagus is transected near the apex of the thoracic cavity, and an esophagogastrostomy is made. The patient undergoes the operation as planned. Epidural analgesia is employed. Good response is evident in the esophagus, with no extraesophageal infiltration, though significant postirradiation fibrosis is evident. A 2-field lymphadenectomy as described above is performed. The patient is extubated after surgery and is sent to intensive care for monitoring.

Discussion

There are many variables to consider in esophagectomy. The optimal access for esophagectomy and extent of lymphadenectomy are most controversial. Transhiatal esophagectomy without thoracotomy is an alternative, with its theoretical advantages of being less invasive, faster, and resulting in better postoperative recovery. Proponents of the transthoracic approach argue for safer dissection of the tumor under vision and the ability for a more thorough lymphadenectomy leading to better staging and survival. Randomized trials are few, and meta-analyses show that the transthoracic approach probably has a higher perioperative morbidity, but there is a trend for better survival. The issue remains controversial, however. For a locally advanced tumor located in the midesophagus, and the fibrosis associated with preoperative chemoradiation, transhiatal mobilization may be hazardous. Minimal access methods

with combinations of thoracoscopic and/or laparoscopic approaches are practiced in selected centers.

When lymphadenectomy is performed, most surgeons carry out a 2-field lymph-node dissection, with clearance of lymphatic tissue from the tracheal bifurcation down to the celiac axis. Lymph nodes in the superior mediastinum are often sampled only. Some surgeons, notably in Japan, perform 3-field lymphadenectomy, extending the dissection from the superior mediastinum (especially along the recurrent laryngeal nerves) to the bilateral neck. The rationale is a high incidence of lymphatic spread along the recurrent laryngeal nerves up to the cervical lymph nodes. Such surgery, however, is complicated and is associated with higher morbidity rates, especially of recurrent laryngeal nerve palsy, and is practiced only in limited centers outside Japan.

Case Continued

The patient develops sputum retention and pulmonary atelectasis. A tracheostomy is performed on day 3 after surgery to aid sputum suction. Regular bronchoscopic suction is also carried out. He has episodes of atrial fibrillation, which require amiodarone infusion for rate control. A Gastrografin contrast study does not show anastomotic leak. He is advanced on an oral diet and recovers.

Pathology of the surgical specimen shows only fibrosis in the esophageal wall; of 21 lymph nodes sampled, none contains metastases. This is therefore a complete pathological response to neoadjuvant chemoradiation. No further treatment is planned.

Discussion

Cardiopulmonary complications are the most common nonsurgical morbidity after esophagectomy. Postoperative epidural analgesia is an important advance and has been shown to improve outcome. Despite its use, severe pulmonary complications affect up to 20% of patients. Frequent bronchoscopy, early tracheostomy for gaining access for sputum suction, fluid restriction, and active physiotherapy help treat such morbidities. Atrial arrhythmia may not be indicative of cardiac dysfunction, but often signifies underlying pulmonary pathology or sepsis from surgical complications. This should prompt a search for its cause. Surgical complications are operator dependent, and the risk for anastomotic leak is still substantial except in dedicated experienced centers. There is clear evidence that both hospital volume and surgeon volume are related to outcome in complex surgery like esophagectomy.

Cisplatin-based chemoradiation therapy has been shown to result in an average pathological complete response rate of 25%, and these patients usually have good prognoses. The ability to accurately predict response to chemoradiation is useful, because potentially toxic treatments should not be given to nonresponders, with delay to definitive surgery. Unfortunately, this cannot be predicted with reliable accuracy at present, whether by serological or molecular markers. Results of metabolic imaging by PET scan are encouraging, when changes in SUV early in the course of treatment can potentially predict eventual response.

Suggested Readings

Law S, Kwong DL, Kwok KF, et al. Improvement in treatment results and long-term survival of patients with esophageal cancer: impact of chemoradiation and change in treatment strategy. *Ann Surg* 2003;238:339–348.

Law S, Wong J. Esophagogastrectomy for carcinoma of the esophagus and cardia, and the esophageal anastomosis. In: Baker RJ, Fischer JE, eds. *Mastery of surgery*. Philadelphia, PA: Lippincott Williams & Wilkins; 2001:813–827.

Law S, Wong J. Two-field dissection is enough for esophageal cancer. *Dis Esophagus* 2001;14:98–103.

Law SYK, Wong J. Complications: prevention and management. In: Daly JM, Hennessy TPJ, Reynolds JV, eds. *Management of upper gastrointestinal cancer*. London: WB Saunders; 1999:240–262.

Malthaner R, Fenlon D. Preoperative chemotherapy for resectable thoracic esophageal cancer (Cochrane Review). The Cochrane Library. Chichester, UK: John Wiley & Sons; 2004.

Siewert JR, Stein HJ, Feith M, et al. Histologic tumor type is an independent prognostic parameter in esophageal cancer: lessons from more than 1,000 consecutive resections at a single center in the Western world. *Ann Surg* 2001;234:360–367.

Wieder HA, Brucher BL, Zimmermann F, et al. Time course of tumor metabolic activity during chemoradiotherapy of esophageal squamous cell carcinoma and response to treatment. *J Clin Oncol* 2004;22:900–908.

case 18

A 58-year-old, slightly overweight man presents to your office after he is seen by his physician with symptoms of dysphagia. He has a 20-year history of gastroesophageal reflux disease (GERD), which was treated with proton-pump inhibitors. The patient reports that he has problems swallowing meats.

Endoscopic and Endosonographic Images

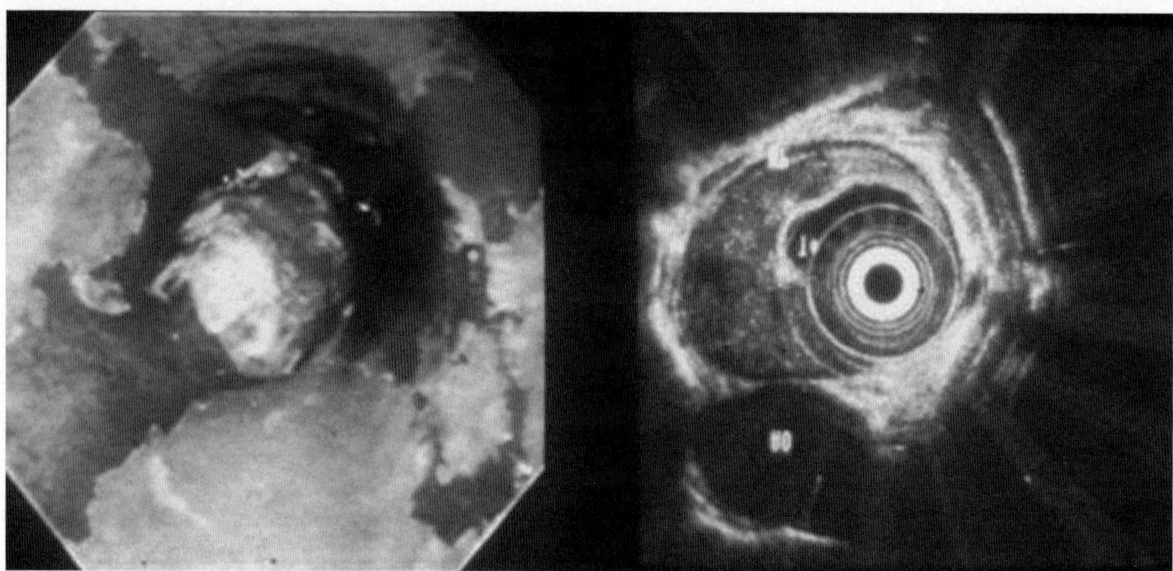

Figure 18.1

Endoscopy and Endosonography Report

Tumor at the distal esophagus, arising within Barrett's mucosa. Endosonography shows that the tumor encompasses the whole wall of the esophagus (T3 category).

Case Continued

The pathology report shows goblet cells as a sign of intestinal metaplasia, that is, Barrett's esophagus, and cells representing intestinal adenocarcinoma. Adenocarcinoma of the distal esophagus based on Barrett's metaplasia is diagnosed.

Differential Diagnosis

The differential diagnosis for dysphagia should first include malignant tumors of the oropharynx or esophagus followed by other causes such as compression by an enlarged goiter, benign esophageal tumors, achalasia of the esophagus, diverticula of the esophagus, and reflux disease complicated by strictures. If a patient presents with dysphagia, upper gastrointestinal (GI) endoscopy is mandatory to exclude malignant disease. With the help of endosonography, early forms of tumor growth (i.e., cT1 categories) can be detected, and these patients can be offered endoscopic treatment or a limited surgical resection (see below).

Discussion

The incidence of adenocarcinoma of the esophagus and gastroesophageal junction rose dramatically in the United States and other Western countries over the last decades of the 20th century. The increase has been particularly impressive in white men, in whom the incidence of adenocarcinoma of the esophagus has risen by more than 350% since the mid-1970s. The causes of this startling increase and its pattern are poorly understood, although intense work on risk factors and etiology has yielded some insights.

The transitional nature of the anatomic gastro-esophageal (GE) junction has added further confusion to the understanding of this disease. Adenocarcinomas of the distal esophagus, GI-junction, and gastric cardia have all increased in incidence, and many studies have grouped tumors at these locations together. A consensus conference of the International Gastric Cancer Association and the International Society of Diseases of the Esophagus in 1998 defined adenocarcinomas of the GE junction as tumors that have their center within 5 cm proximal and distal to the anatomic cardia. Within this area, tumors are differentiated into the following three distinct entities.

Type 1: adenocarcinoma of the distal esophagus usually rising from an area with specialized intestinal metaplasia of the esophagus (Barrett's esophagus); it may infiltrate the esophagogastric junction from above.

Type 2: True carcinoma of the cardia, arising from the cardiac epithelium or short segments of intestinal metaplasia at the GE junction. This entity is often referred to as "junctional carcinoma."

Type 3: Subcardial gastric carcinomas that infiltrate the esophagogastric junction and the distal esophagus from below.

This differentiation is especially of importance for surgeons because these types lead to different resection strategies. Type 2 and type 3 tumors can mostly be operated by a transhiatal approach with total gastrectomy and resection of the distal esophagus. Type 1 tumors have to be operated with a thoracoabdominal approach. In these tumors, subtotal esophagectomy is mandatory.

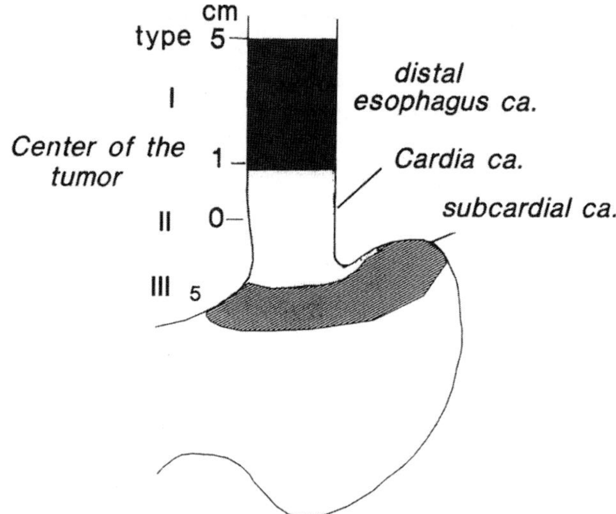

Figure 18.2 Classification of adenocarcinoma of the esophageal gastric junction (AEG) tumors.

CT Scan

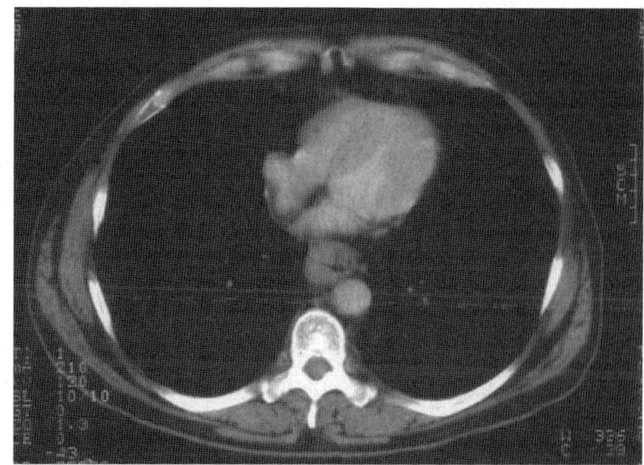

Figure 18.3

CT Scan Report

There is thickening of the distal esophagus, consistent with tumor. There is evidence of enlarged periesophageal lymph nodes.

Diagnosis and Recommendation

After histologic confirmation of adenocarcinoma of the distal esophagus, staging must be performed to exclude distant metastases. Staging consists of computed tomography (CT) scan of the neck, thorax, and abdomen to reveal lymphatic spread and/or metastatic disease. If distant metastases are found (e.g., liver, bone), surgery is not indicated in these patients. The treatment for patients with adenocarcinoma of the GE junction is primarily palliative chemotherapy. In patients with severe dysphagia, insertion of a stent is appropriate.

Approach

As the CT scan of this patient reveals no signs of metastatic disease, surgical resection is considered appropriate.

Discussion

Surgical resection of the adenocarcinoma of the GE junction is a demanding procedure for the patient. Essential in this context is the medical condition of the patient, who should have sufficient cardiopulmonary, hepatic, and renal functional reserves.

The reported surgical approaches to adenocarcinoma of the distal esophagus include abdominothoracic en bloc esophagogastrectomy, subtotal esophagectomy with resection of the proximal stomach, total gastrectomy with transhiatal resection of the distal esophagus, and limited resection of the esophagogastric junction. In our own experience, there is no significant difference in long-term survival between transthoracic and radical transmediastinal esophagectomies, provided the tumor is removed completely.

The experience with systematic lymph-node dissection in patients with adenocarcinoma of the distal esophagus shows that lymph node metastases are virtually never present in patients with tumors limited to the mucosa (pT1a) and are uncommon in patients with tumors limited to the submucosa (pT1b). In patients with more advanced tumors, lymph node metastases occur in decreasing order in the paracardial region, the posterior lower mediastinum, the lesser and greater curvature side of the stomach, along the left gastric artery toward the celiac axis, at the superior border of the pancreas along the splenic artery toward the splenic hilum, and in the area of the left adrenal gland and the left renal vein. Lymph node metastases in the upper mediastinum or cervical region occur only in patients with locally advanced adenocarcinoma who also have numerous positive locoregional nodes.

Mortality rates following esophageal resection range from 2% to 10%. The expectable 30-day mortality rate is approximately 5%. This surgically demanding procedure provides much better results if it is done in high-volume units. Nevertheless, despite these patients being in good medical condition with no underlying medical problems like patients with squamous cell carcinomas of the esophagus (i.e., smoking and drinking), the prognosis even after complete resection continues to be poor. The reported 5-year survival rates range from 10% to 25%.

Surgical Approach

The thoracoabdominal en bloc esophagectomy is performed via a right transthoracic approach. In our opinion, only the right transthoracic approach allows adequate lymphadenectomy in the upper mediastinum. The procedure starts with an inverse abdominal T-shaped incision in the upper epigastrium, mobilization of the stomach, and formation of a gastric tube along the greater curvature. After mobilization of the stomach and tubular transformation, the lymphadenectomy along the celiac axis and parapancreatic region is relatively easy to perform. The gastric tube is placed in the right chest and the abdomen is closed. The patient is then turned to the left for a right-sided posterolateral thoracotomy. An en bloc esophagectomy is performed, including a resection of large portions of both diaphragmatic crura around the esophageal hiatus. The gastric tube can then be easily pulled into the chest. The esophageal transection is always performed clearly above the azygos vein. The reconstruction of the intestinal passage is performed with an esophagogastrostomy (end-to-end) in the tip of the right pleural cavity.

Case Continued

Following esophagectomy, the patient is transferred to the intensive care unit. Early extubation is intended. Oral feeding can be started on the fourth day after surgery. The right chest is drained by chest tubes for at least 6 to 7 days to diagnose anastomotic leakage at an early stage. If an anastomotic leakage is developing, early endoscopy and placement of a stent should be considered.

Discussion

The morbidity associated with extended total gastrectomy and esophagectomy and the compromised quality of life after these procedures have in recent years stimulated efforts to assess more limited forms of resection for adenocarcinoma of the distal esophagus. Based on the virtual absence of lymph node metastases/micrometastases in patients with tumors limited to the mucosa, and the very low prevalence of lymph node metastases found in patients with tumors extending to the submucosa, we have evaluated a limited resection of the distal esophagus, cardia, and proximal esophagus in such patients. To avoid postoperative reflux, reconstruction is performed by interposition of a pedicled jejunal segment. In our experience with tumors staged as cT1 on endoscopic ultrasound, a complete resection (R0) could be achieved in all instances. Quality-of-life assessment showed no evidence of gastroesophageal reflux and good to excellent swallowing function in more than 90% of the patients.

Endoscopic resection techniques have been attempted in patients with early stages of esophageal adenocarcinomas, as they have for patients with high-grade dysplasia. Because a lymphadenectomy is not possible with this technique, endoscopic mucosa resection can only be recommended in patients with pT1a tumors. Indications include small superficial and early tumors in patients at high surgical risk and in those refusing surgery. Tumor destruction can also be accomplished by either Nd:YAG laser or photodynamic therapy. However, due to the frequent multicentric tumor growth, the inaccuracy of current preoperative staging modalities, including high-frequency endoscopic ultrasound, to differentiate mucosal from submucosal tumors, and the persistence of precancerous lesions (Barrett's esophagus), there are currently limits to the broad clinical application of this truly limited procedure. Resection done by endoscopic mucosal resection (EMR) has the advantage of providing tissue for pathologic evaluation.

Prospective studies dealing with preoperative therapy in adenocarcinoma of the esophagus only are rare. The interpretation of these preferentially phase II and few phase III trials is complicated, because most studies include adenocarcinoma of the esophagus (Barrett's carcinoma), adenocarcinoma of the esophagogastric junction (including cardia carcinoma and subcardia carcinoma), and squamous cell carcinoma. Preoperative chemotherapy, generally well tolerated, could not decrease the local failure rate compared with surgery alone, but might delay systemic relapse. Preoperative radiotherapy can enhance local control, but fails to improve overall survival. Neoadjuvant chemoradiation demonstrated a survival benefit only in one randomized trial; however, survival in the surgery-alone group was unusually poor (3-year survival: combined group, 32%; surgery alone, 6%). Generally, survival was better in patients responding to neoadjuvant treatment. In this respect, nonresponding patients have a worse prognosis than responders following resection. However, preoperative chemoradiation was often accompanied by an increase in postoperative morbidity and mortality. In a recently published abstract from a randomized trial of neoadjuvant chemotherapy followed by surgery versus surgery alone (MAGIC trial from Great Britain), there was a higher rate of completely resected patients after preoperative treatment. However, follow-up data are not mature enough and the results of this promising trial will allow conclusions to be drawn regarding the role of neoadjuvant chemotherapy.

Today, there is no proven evidence that neoadjuvant treatment for patients with potentially resectable Barrett's cancer prolongs survival. In patients with locally advanced, presumably not completely resectable, adenocarcinoma of the esophagus, preoperative treatment appears to increase the chance for a curative resection and enhance survival in responding patients. Neoadjuvant treatment of adenocarcinoma of the esophagus, as a consequence, is currently not the standard treatment and has to be performed only within controlled clinical trials.

In contrast to gastric cancer, in which there are numerous phase II and phase III studies performed in recent years, in adenocarcinoma of the distal esophagus there are only two phase II trials investigating the feasibility of adjuvant postoperative treatment after complete resection. In the study from the Royal Marsden Hospital, 29 patients with various adenocarcinomas of the esophageal gastric junction (AEG) and gastric tumors were treated with ECF (epirubicin, cisplatin, 5-FU) after complete resection. Chemotherapy was well tolerated and there were no treatment-related deaths. The encouraging results, especially in stage III patients, support the investigation of this regimen within a prospective, randomized trial. A group from Chicago investigated the feasibility of concurrent chemoradiation in 25 patients (15 patients with adenocarcinoma) after initial esophagectomy. Acute toxicity was common. Control of local disease appeared to be improved, but distant failure was common. From these two pilot studies, no definitive conclusions can be drawn concerning the value of adjuvant treatment in adenocarcinoma of the distal esophagus.

Suggested Readings

Peters JH, Hagen JA, DeMeester SR. Barrett's esophagus. *J Gastrointest Surg* 2004;8:1–17.

Siewert JR, Stein HJ. Barrett's cancer: indications, extent, and results of surgical resection. *Semin Surg Oncol* 1997;13:245–252.

Siewert JR, Stein HJ, Feith M. Surgical approach to invasive adenocarcinoma of the distal esophagus (Barrett's cancer). *World J Surg* 2003;27:1058–1061.

Siewert JR, Stein HJ, Feith M, et al. Histologic tumor type is an independent prognostic parameter in esophageal cancer: lessons from more than 1,000 consecutive resections at a single center in the Western world. *Ann Surg* 2001;234:360–367.

Stein HJ, Brücher BL, Sendler A, et al. Esophageal cancer: patient evaluation and pre-treatment staging. *Surg Oncol* 2001;10:103–111.

Stein HJ, Feith M, Rahden BA, et al. Approach to early Barrett's cancer. *World J Surg* 2003;27:1040–1046.

Zacherl J, Sendler A, Stein HJ et al. Current status of neoadjuvant therapy for adenocarcinoma of the distal esophagus. *World J Surg* 2003;27:1067–1074.

case 19

Presentation

A 60-year-old man presents to his physician with dyspepsia and mild anemia. He is referred to the endoscopic unit. Except for these vague symptoms, the patient is in good condition. The abdominal examination is normal.

Endoscopic and Endosonographic Images

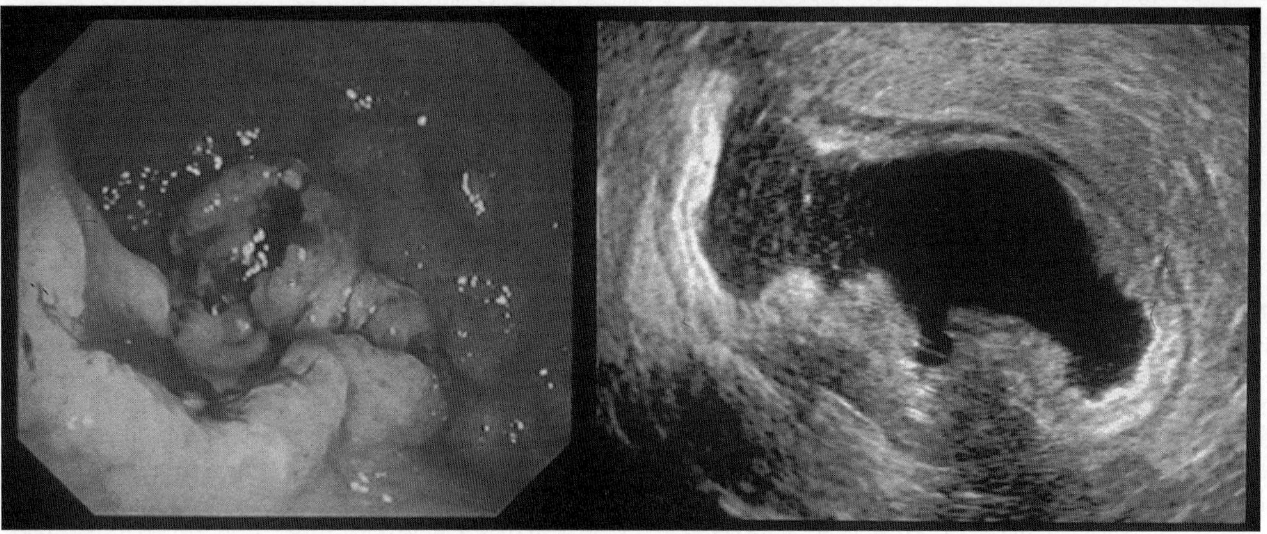

Figure 19.1

Endoscopy and Endosonography Report

The esophagus is normal, but in the body of the stomach (corpus region) there is a tumor with ulceration, with no signs of active bleeding. Endosonography demonstrates that the tumor encompasses the entire gastric wall and is considered as category T3 (Union Internationale Contre le Cancer [UICC]/American Joint Committee on Cancer [AJCC]).

Case Continued

Biopsies are obtained. Histologic study reveals adenocarcinoma of the stomach, intestinal type (Lauren classification).

Differential Diagnosis

Differential diagnosis for a gastric mass includes malignancies such as gastric adenocarcinoma, lymphoma, leiomyomas, leiomyosarcomas, and gastrointestinal (GI) stromal tumors (GISTs). The initial diagnostic modality for gastric cancer is upper GI endoscopy. Following that, endoscopic ultrasound might be used to reveal the depth of tumor infiltration. Endosonography has the advantage of identifying early gastric cancer that can be treated by minimally invasive procedures.

Typically in the development of adenocarcinoma of the stomach, symptoms are minimal until relatively late in the course of the disease. A high index of suspicion must be maintained to avoid delay in diagnosis. Weight loss and abdominal pain are the most frequent initial symptoms. Weight loss often indicates more advanced disease, and patients with weight loss have a shorter survival than those without. Abdominal pain begins as insidious upper abdominal discomfort that ranges in intensity from a vague sense of postprandial fullness to a severe, steady pain. Anorexia and nausea are quite common. Dysphagia may indicate a cancer in the cardia or gastroesophageal junction. Vomiting is more consistent with an antral carcinoma obstructing the pylorus. Patients with scirrhous carcinomas (e.g., linitis plastica) may develop early satiety. Although 20% of patients have melena, massive hemorrhage is more common with leiomyoma or GIST. Physical examination cannot detect an early carcinoma. An epigastric mass, enlarged liver, ascites, jaundice, or palpable supraclavicular lymph nodes indicate extensive and incurable disease.

Identification of asymptomatic patients at high risk for developing gastric cancer is warranted. However, mass screening programs, as in Japan, are not cost-effective in Western countries.

GI lymphomas and especially mucosa-associated lymphatic tissue (MALT) lymphomas have to be ruled out prior to therapy; these patients are treated primarily by chemotherapy. Furthermore, if MALT lymphoma is present, *Helicobacter pylori* status has to be considered.

Discussion

Despite the diminishing prevalence, adenocarcinoma of the stomach still has significant clinical importance. Between 1980 and 2000, the incidence of gastric cancer declined by about 45% and the location of the tumor has changed. The tumors used to be primarily located in the distal part of the stomach, but now they are predominantly present in the subcardial region. Gastric cancer is extremely rare in patients younger than the age of 30; thereafter, it increases rapidly and steadily reaches the highest rates in the oldest age groups, both in males and females (median age: 68 for men and 74 for women).

Case Continued

The patient is admitted to a specialized surgical unit for evaluation. The patient undergoes a staging computed tomography (CT) scan of the abdomen.

■ CT Scan

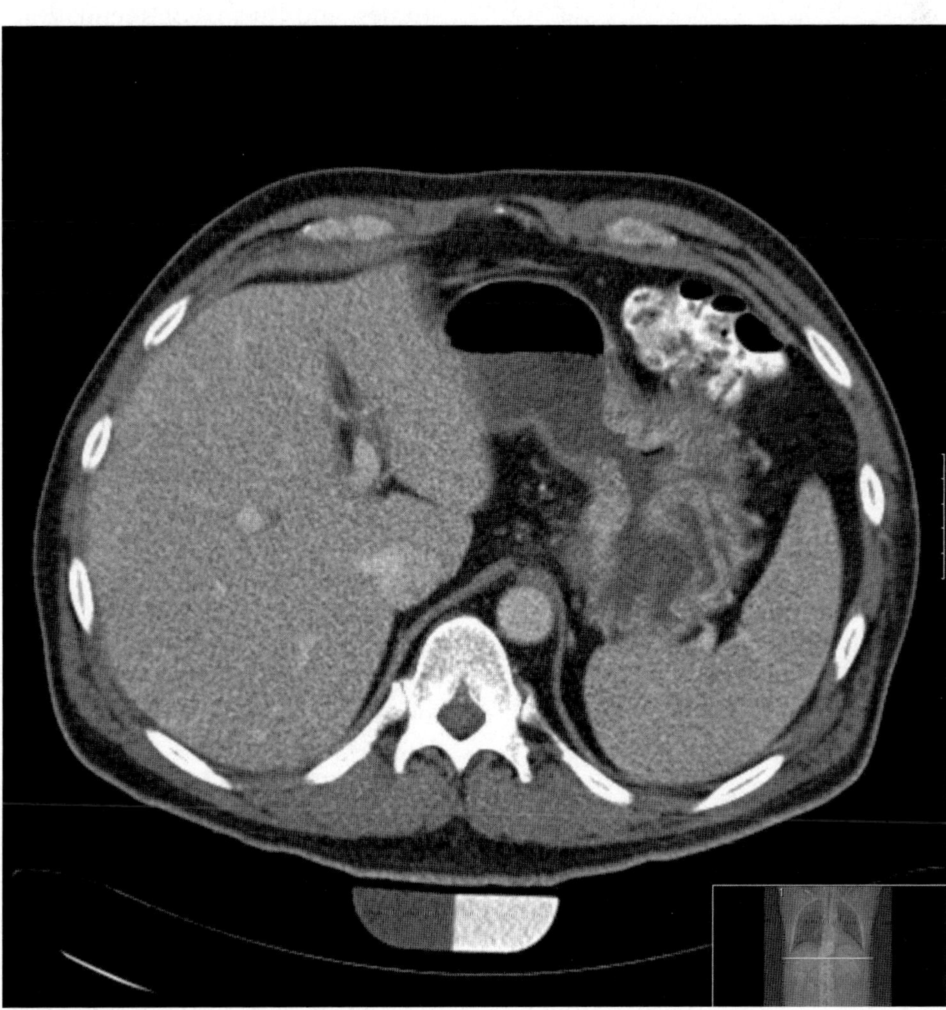

Figure 19.2

CT Scan Report

There is thickening of the gastric wall, with no signs of ascites.

Diagnosis and Recommendation

Using endoscopy and CT scan, locally advanced adenocarcinoma in the body of the stomach is diagnosed. The patient is referred to surgery. Prior to proceeding with surgical exploration, distant metastases have to be excluded. On CT scan, secondary signs of peritoneal carcinomatosis such as ascites may be recognized. If there is any suspicion of peritoneal carcinomatosis, a diagnostic laparoscopy should be performed. If there is evidence of peritoneal spread, prognosis of the patient cannot be altered by surgery. In women, metastases to the ovaries (Krukenberg tumors) must be ruled out by CT scan.

Approach

Surgery is the only curative treatment for gastric cancer. The aim of any surgical approach to gastric carcinoma should be a complete resection with no residual tumor left behind at the end of the operation. This corresponds to the R0 category of the UICC/AJCC, that is, a curative resection. Complete tumor resection in this respect refers to the primary tumor, with no residual tumor at the proximal and distal resection margins and the tumor bed (the so-called third dimension) and the lymphatic drainage (as a minimal requirement, no residual tumor in the peripheral or border lymph nodes).

Discussion

To improve the prognosis of a patient, the tumor must be removed with an adequate safety margin. The extent of this safety margin depends on the growth pattern of the tumor according to the Lauren classification. Gastric carcinoma with a "diffuse-type" growth pattern requires a larger proximal and distal safety margin than tumors with an "intestinal-type" growth pattern. Surgical procedures that do not lead to complete tumor resection will not improve the prognosis of the patient and must be considered "palliative resections."

Three different clinical situations, each with its own therapeutic relevance, must be considered:

(a) Gastric carcinoma stage IA (early gastric cancer, mucosa carcinoma). This subgroup of patients with early gastric carcinoma can be cured by local excision because the probability of lymphatic metastases is well below 5%. Such limited surgery may be best performed with a combined endoscopic or laparoscopic approach (combined endoscopic/laparoscopic wedge resection).

(b) Tumor stages IB (submucosa carcinoma), II, and IIIA. Lymph node metastases can be expected in a high percentage of these patients. Based on presently available published data, these patients receive the most benefit from radical surgery. In this group of patients, it is possible to achieve R0 resection of the primary tumor as well as the lymphatic drainage area when appropriate surgical techniques are used.

(c) Locally advanced gastric tumors that may already have distant metastases (tumor stage IIIB and IV). In this situation, complete tumor removal by surgical resection usually cannot be achieved. Rather, microscopic or macroscopic residual tumor remains in situ after the surgical resection. The procedure is only palliative and cannot improve the prognosis of the patient. Consequently, preoperative therapeutic modalities (neoadjuvant treatment) such as neoadjuvant chemotherapy or chemoradiation are currently being investigated for this group of patients. However, most results are from phase II studies, and thus recommendation for preoperative treatment should still be considered experimental.

In the palliative situation, resection has to be avoided unless there is a complete tumor obstruction or the tumor is bleeding. However, palliative operations bear risk of significant morbidity and mortality.

The selection of the appropriate surgical procedure in patients with resectable gastric carcinoma should be guided primarily by the location of the tumor. Based on the recommendations of the Japanese Research Society for Gastric Cancer, the stomach is divided into thirds. Although the borders between these thirds are not defined exactly, this definition has proven to be useful for determining the extent of resection.

Total Gastrectomy

Standard therapy of gastric cancer in the Western Hemisphere is total gastrectomy. It should be performed along with a systematic lymphadenectomy. Analyses of the quality of life after total gastrectomy support reconstruction using a pouch. Because the advantages observed after pouch reconstruction are only important for long-term outcome, the prognosis of the patient must be taken into account when considering the type of reconstruction. If the prognosis is good, a pouch is recommended. If the prognosis is poor, the easiest reconstruction (Roux-en-Y-esophagojejunostomy) should be performed.

For the construction of a pouch, a side-to-side anastomosis over a distance of 10 to 15 cm between

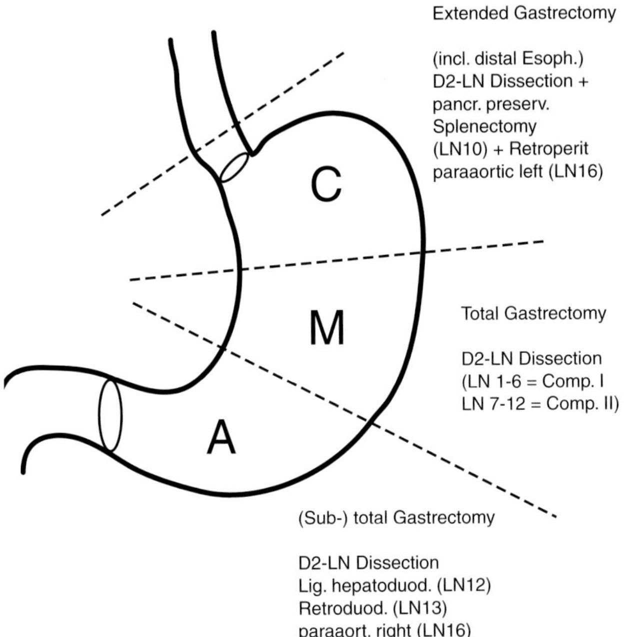

Figure 19.3 Synopsis of resection strategies and lymph node dissection in gastric cancer based on different points of origin.

the ascending and descending portion of the first jejunal loop is usually sufficient (the Hunt-Rodino pouch). A jejunoplication can be added to the pouch. Whether a Roux-en-Y diversion should be added to the pouch to avoid alkaline reflux into the pouch and the distal esophagus is controversial, but is recommended based on our own experience. Furthermore, if the tumor involves the pancreatic tail and the spleen, left-sided extension of the resection that includes distal pancreatectomy and splenectomy may be necessary. Such an extended resection does add additional risks (e.g., pancreatic fistula and abscesses). The insertion of a feeding jejunostomy tube is optional.

Subtotal Gastrectomy

The luminal extent of the subtotal gastrectomy resection specimen comprises about four fifths of the stomach. Along the lesser curvature the resection should reach up to about 2 cm below the anatomic cardia. Along the greater curvature the resection must extend beyond the right and left gastroepiploic veins, extending to the hilus of the spleen. The small remaining fundus is fed through the short gastric vessels from the splenic hilus.

Because subtotal gastrectomy is usually performed for tumors located in the distal third, the resection must be extended as far as possible beyond the pylorus. In any case, the dissection of the duodenum should be extended beyond the gastroduodenal border. Lymphadenectomy must be performed as radically as with a total gastrectomy.

The reconstruction of alimentary tract continuity can be performed with a retrocolic or antecolic jejunal loop, with an isoperistaltic orientation of the gastroenterostomy (oralis partialis). A Roux-en-Y is recommended.

Lymphadenectomy in Gastric Cancer

Both randomized European trials (the Dutch and the British trial) did not demonstrate any advantage for extended lymphadenectomy (D2 lymphadenectomy with dissection of the perigastric nodes, the nodes around the celiac axis, the splenic artery, and the hepatic artery). However, most specialized centers in western Europe and the United States perform extended lymphadenectomies routinely. Both randomized studies, however, bear two inherited problems. There was a very high complication rate after extended lymphadenectomy in both studies. This can be explained by the high number of splenectomies and distal pancreatic resections in the D2 group. Following these, septic complications and pancreatic fistulas were common, leading to unusually high morbidity and mortality in both trials. The training of the operating surgeons in both trials seemed not to be high enough; in the Dutch trial, the aim of the D2 lymphadenectomy was reached only by 49%. In the British trial, 200 extended lymphadenectomies were performed in 31 separate hospitals, that is, six procedures/hospital in 7 years. In nonrandomized trials, there are no demonstrated differences in morbidity and mortality after D2 dissection. However, this demanding procedure has to be done in well-trained, experienced hands in high-volume centers.

Patients in stage II and IIIA show significant survival advantages if the extended lymphadenectomy is performed under specific rules. This means that distal pancreatectomy and splenectomy are avoided, unless the tumor is directly invading these organs (T4).

Surgical Approach

In view of the cancer present in the body of the stomach, a total gastrectomy is performed with a D2 lymphadenectomy. After a midline incision is made, the abdomen is carefully explored to exclude peritoneal and liver metastases. The total gastrectomy begins with first performing an omentobursectomy (removing the lesser sac) and division of the arterial blood supply of the stomach. While mobilizing the entire stomach, the lymph node stations 1 to 6 are resected en bloc. Due to absence of disease extension to the splenic hilum or the pancreas, a pancreas- and spleen-preserving D2 dissection is feasible. The duodenum and next the esophagus are transected, and the surgical specimen is sent to the pathologist for frozen section of the proximal and distal margins. While waiting for these results, a standard D2 lymphadenectomy is performed on the lymph node stations along the celiac axis and its branches. For the construction of a pouch, a side-to-side anastomosis over a distance of 10 to 15 cm between the ascending and descending portions of the first jejunal loop is usually sufficient (the Hunt-Rodino pouch). A Roux-en-Y diversion should be added to the pouch to avoid alkaline reflux into the pouch and the distal esophagus. A feeding jejunostomy is inserted.

Case Continued

The postoperative course of this patient is uneventful, the abdominal drains are taken out after the third day, and the nasogastric tube is removed on the second postoperative day. Enteral feeding was started on the third day after operation. The pathologic examination of the specimen reveals a T3 N1 tumor.

Discussion

Following surgical resection of locally advanced gastric cancer (stage IIIA), the utility of adjuvant therapy has to be discussed. The South West Oncology Group (SWOG) randomized trial, which compared surgery alone with surgery plus adjuvant chemotherapy and chemoradiation therapy, showed a significant survival advantage for the adjuvant group. However, from the surgical point of view, the results of lymphadenectomy in the study population were especially poor, with 54% of patients having only D0 lymphadenectomies. Overall, the indication for adjuvant chemoradiation therapy after gastric resection should be considered if the lymphadenectomy is incomplete. After incomplete resection with microscopic or even macroscopic positive margins, additional treatment does not alter the prognosis.

Suggested Readings

Brennan MF. Lymph-node dissection for gastric cancer [editorial]. *N Engl J Med* 1999;340:956–958.

Hartgrink HH, van de Velde CJ, Putter H, et al. Extended lymph node dissection for gastric cancer: who may benefit? Final results of the randomized Dutch gastric cancer group trial. *J Clin Oncol* 2004;22:2069–2077.

Macdonald JS, Smalley SR, Benedetti J, et al. Chemoradiotherapy after surgery compared with surgery alone for adenocarcinoma of the stomach or gastroesophageal junction. *N Engl J Med* 2001;345:725–730.

Roth AD. Curative treatment of gastric cancer: towards a multidisciplinary approach? *Crit Rev Oncol Hematol* 2003;46:59–100.

Sendler A, Siewert JR. Individualizing therapy in gastric cancer. *Expert Rev Anticancer Ther* 2003;3:457–470.

Siewert JR, Fink U, Sendler A, et al. Gastric cancer. *Curr Probl Surg* 1997;43:837–937.

Presentation

A 42-year-old woman presents to your office with dyspepsia and weight loss. There are no signs of dysphagia, but she reports early satiety. Her vague upper gastrointestinal (GI) complaints have been present for 2 months. She treated the symptoms by herself with proton-pump inhibitors for 2 weeks, which did not resolve the symptoms.

Endoscopic and Endosonographic Images

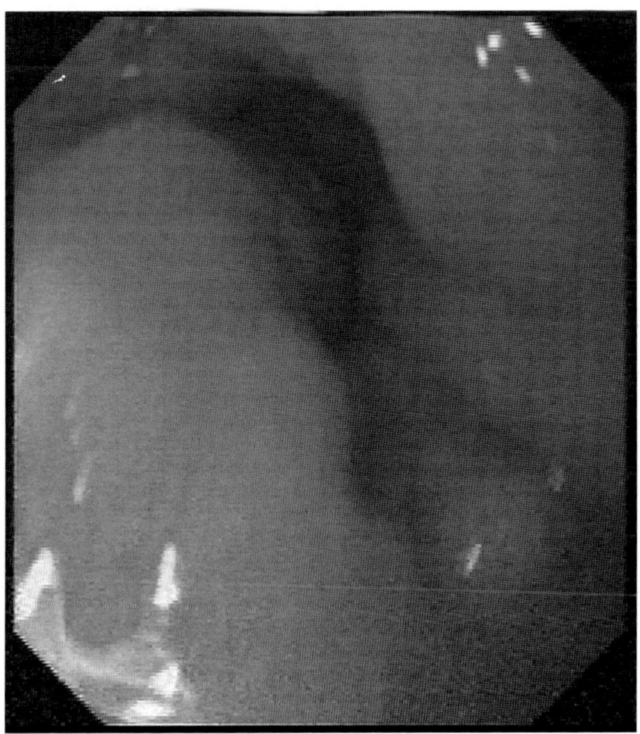

Figure 20.1A

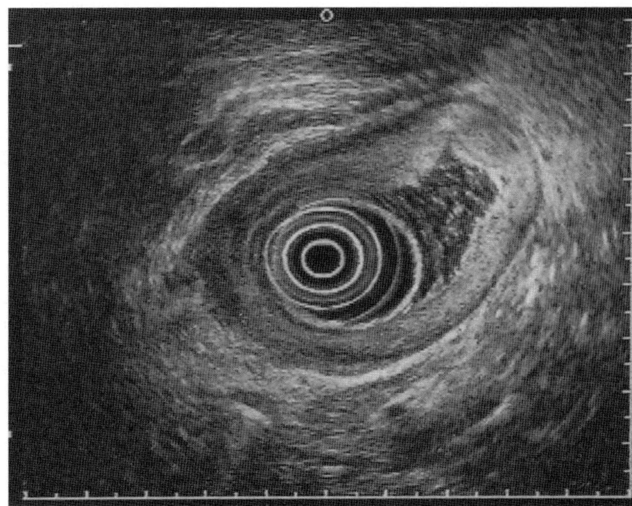

Figure 20.1B

Endoscopy and Endosonography Report

The esophagus is inconspicuous; giant folds in the whole stomach show no signs of tumor growth; and the duodenum is normal. The stomach cannot be unfolded after insufflation during endoscopy. On endosonography, there is thickening of the gastric wall.

Differential Diagnosis

A large variety of problems can lead to upper GI discomfort and/or dyspepsia. These include gastritis with *Helicobacter pylori* infection, peptic ulcers, and gallbladder problems. Not all dyspeptic problems will be completely solved with diagnostic tests. Nevertheless, one has to be very suspicious not to overlook tumors in the upper GI tract, especially in young, apparently healthy individuals. Every upper abdominal discomfort should lead, at least after 2 weeks of unsuccessful medical treatment, to upper GI endoscopy with biopsy. As with other gastric neoplasms, there are no specific signs or symptoms that denote linitis plastica. Initial symptoms are usually nonspecific and well tolerated, and often these patients may develop early satiety.

Diagnosis

Total carcinomatosis of the stomach, suspicious for linitis plastica.

Case Continued

The histology report revealed no signs of adenocarcinoma of the stomach. A second endoscopy with multiple biopsies is ordered. During this endoscopy, 14 deep biopsies are taken. These biopsies reveal adenocarcinoma of the stomach, grading 3, and of the diffuse type according to the Lauren classification.

CT Scan

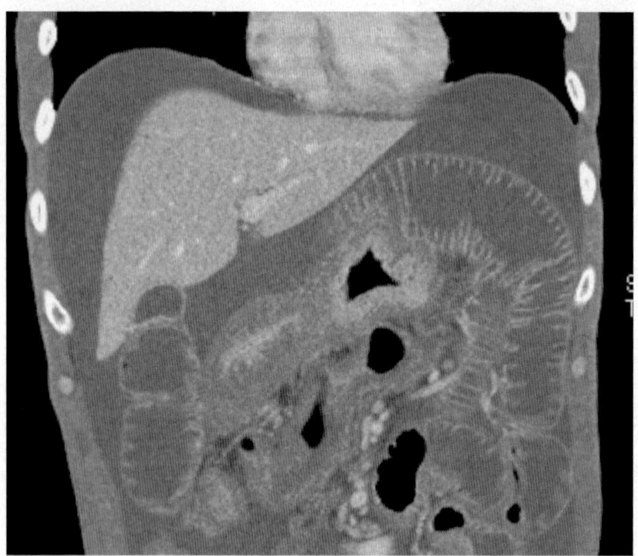

Figure 20.2

CT Scan Report

The gastric wall is very thickened with no obvious distant metastases; notably, the ovaries are not enlarged (Krukenberg tumor). However, there is a large amount of ascites around the liver and spleen, which is suspicious for peritoneal spread.

Recommendation

Diagnostic laparoscopy is essential in these patients, because patients with linitis plastica have peritoneal spread in about 70% to 80% of cases at presentation.

Laparoscopic Image

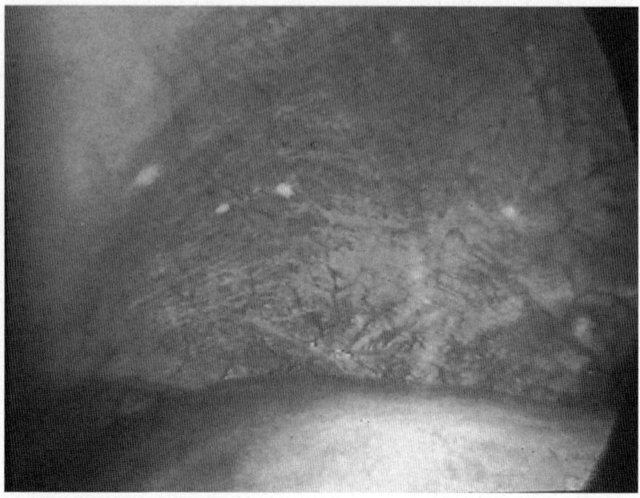

Figure 20.3

Surgical Approach

The patient is placed in the supine position and, after general anesthesia is administered, standard abdominal insufflation is established. A 30 degree camera is inserted through the 10-mm periumbilical port and a careful exploration is performed. Two separate 5-mm ports are placed to perform additional intra-abdominal maneuvering. Any ascitic fluid is aspirated and sent for cytologic examination. Biopsies of peritoneal nodules are sent for frozen section.

Case Continued

The patient has peritoneal seeding at the right abdominal diaphragm (white spots), and the cytologic examination of the ascites is positive for tumor cells. Biopsies of the seeding were taken, and frozen sections show adenocarcinoma.

Discussion

The crucial point in the decision-making process for or against an operation is the exclusion of peritoneal spread and the possibility of infiltration into neighboring organs. Laparoscopy is valuable in these patients. Peritoneal spread of a tumor is easily visualized and confirmed by a biopsy. In addition, laparoscopy also provides the possibility of obtaining abdominal lavage fluid. Using immunocytochemical staining, even small amounts of free tumor cells can be detected.

■ Approach

Linitis plastica of the stomach with peritoneal carcinomatosis is diagnosed. In this case, surgery would be of little value to the patient. Systemic chemotherapy has to start immediately. A resection is only indicated in the case of tumor bleeding (very rare) or in the case of gastric outlet obstruction. In the case of peritoneal spread, reconstruction might be extremely difficult because the mesentery of the jejunum might not be long enough to perform an esophagojejunostomy.

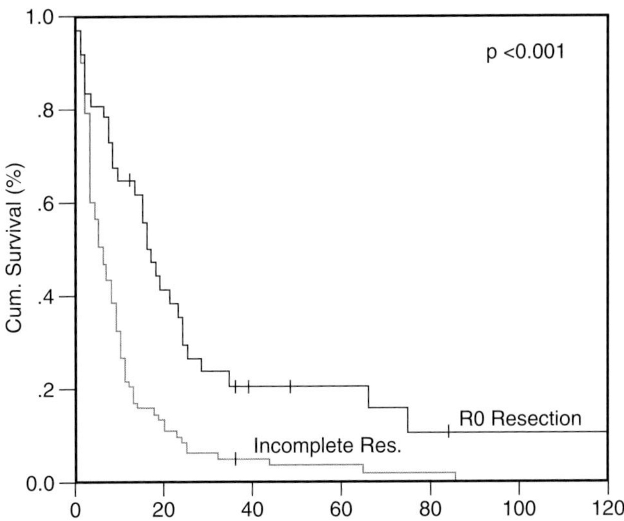

Figure 20.4 Survival after gastrectomy and lymphadenectomy for linitis plastica (n = 120, R0 74 patients).

Discussion

Linitis plastica is a subtype of gastric cancer that is characterized by diffuse infiltrating adenocarcinoma without obvious craters and ulcers. The tumors always belong to the diffuse type according the Lauren classification. Before 1943, it was unclear whether linitis plastica, also called "leather bottle" stomach, was an inflammatory or neoplastic condition. Linitis plastica is thought to originate from the parietal cell portion of gastric mucosa. The tumor cells permeate subsequently into the deeper layer of the stomach wall. This can take place from a very early stage of disease progression.

Because of its diffuse nature, this form of gastric cancer usually involves the whole stomach. Peritoneal seeding and extended lymph node metastasis are relatively common. Furthermore, extension of the tumor into the neighboring organs and serosal implants on the small and large bowel are sometimes observed. All these factors often hinder complete resection. Only about 20% of the patients presenting with linitis plastica are candidates for and benefit from total gastrectomy. Consequently, this type of gastric cancer has a notoriously dismal prognosis. The reasons for such poor results of treatment may be the high scattering activity of the cancer cells, the difficulty of early detection, the high frequency of serosal invasion, and the involvement of distant lymph nodes. These factors result in a high rate of peritoneal and lymph node recurrences even after complete resection.

Treatment decisions for patients with linitis plastica remain difficult. Only meticulous staging can assist with decisions to perform a complete tumor resection, opt for multimodal treatment strategies with secondary surgery, or follow a solely palliative treatment.

If the workup indicates that there is no peritoneal spread and the tumor is still localized in the stomach, a complete resection of the entire stomach and its lymphatic drainage should be performed. In all cases, total gastrectomy, and sometimes transhiatal resection of the distal esophagus, has to be performed. Reconstruction should be a simple esophagojejunostomy with a Roux-en-Y loop.

If the tumor is invading neighboring organs, an extension of the gastrectomy (splenectomy, left-sided pancreatectomy, Whipple procedure, left hemicolectomy) might be performed in patients with good results. These procedures are indicated only if a complete resection can be achieved. The palliative nature of incomplete resections is demonstrated by a median survival time of 7 to 9 months.

If the diagnostic workup indicates that the patient has an advanced tumor and that local tumor eradication cannot be achieved by surgical resection alone, the following options are possible: (a) preoperative chemotherapy in patients with no peritoneal spread, with subsequent surgical resection in those who respond to chemotherapy; and (b) palliative therapy of tumor complications to improve the patient's quality of life only temporarily, such as therapy of gastric outlet obstruction by gastroenterostomy, therapy of dysphagia by tumor stenting, or endoscopic laser therapy of bleeding caused by the tumor.

Based on individual encouraging reports on complete tumor resection or even complete histopathologic response after chemotherapy in patients with locally far advanced gastric cancer, prospective phase II studies have been performed in the past few years to assess the role of chemotherapy and subsequent second attempt at resection in patients with gastric cancer found unresectable at an initial diagnostic laparotomy. The median survival time of these patients ranged between 19 and 24 months, as compared to less than 6 months reported for unresectable gastric cancer in historic series.

If peritoneal dissemination is established by laparoscopy, only palliative chemotherapy might help the patient. There is, so far, no possibility for a curative attempt, even with the use of intraperitoneal chemotherapy. Several randomized prospective trials comparing combination chemotherapy with best supportive care in patients with metastatic gastric cancer have not only shown a significant prolongation of survival but also a marked improvement in quality of life in the chemotherapy group.

Suggested Readings

Barreiro CJ, Lillemoe KD, Koniaris LG, et al. Diagnostic laparoscopy for periampullary and pancreatic cancer: what is the true benefit? *J Gastrointest Surg* 2002;6:75–81.

Feussner H, Omote K, Fink U, et al. Pretherapeutic laparoscopic staging in advanced gastric carcinoma. *Endoscopy* 1999;31: 342–347.

Hamy A, Letessier E, Bizouarn P, et al. Study of survival and prognostic factors in patients undergoing resection for gastric linitis plastica: a review of 86 cases. *Int Surg* 1999;84:337–343.

Roth AD. Curative treatment of gastric cancer: towards a multidisciplinary approach? *Crit Rev Oncol Hematol* 2003;46: 59–100.

Sendler A, Dittler HJ, Feussner H, et al. Preoperative staging of gastric cancer as precondition for multimodal treatment. *World J Surg* 1995;19:501–508.

Siewert JR, Sendler A. The current management of gastric cancer. *Adv Surg* 1999;33:69–93.

Presentation

A 63-year-old man with no significant past medical history is sent from his family physician for evaluation of his epigastric abdominal pain, early satiety, and a 20-pound unintentional weight loss over a 2-month period.

Differential Diagnosis

The differential diagnosis for epigastric pain includes gastritis, gastroparesis, gastroesophageal reflux disease, gastric carcinoma, peptic ulcer disease, Ménétrier's disease, pancreatitis, pancreatic cancer, biliary colic or acute cholecystitis, colon cancer, and inflammatory bowel disease. Given his age, the duration of symptoms, and particularly the history of weight loss, a neoplastic process should be at the top of the differential.

Case Continued

He has no history of ulcer disease and denies tobacco or alcohol use or blood in his stools. His last colonoscopy, performed 18 months ago, was normal. On physical examination, his scleras are anicteric and there is no supraclavicular adenopathy. There is a firm mass occupying the entire left upper quadrant extending across the midline, and the liver is palpable 7 cm below the costal margin. A computed tomography (CT) scan of the abdomen is ordered.

CT Scan

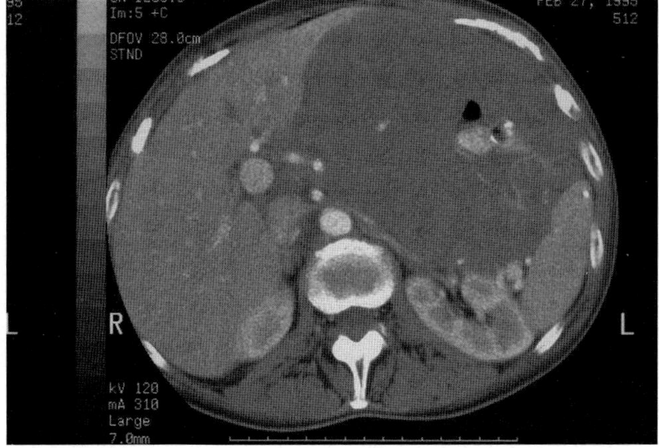

Figure 21.1

CT Scan Report

Extensive thickening and irregularity of the gastric wall with minimal contrast in the lumen and displacement of the left lateral segment of the liver to the right of the midline.

Case Continued

Given the CT scan findings, an endoscopy is performed, which revealed an ulcerated mass. Biopsies from the margins demonstrate sheets of large atypical lymphoid cells infiltrating the lamina propria and submucosa. The cells stain CD20 positive and CD3 negative, and the morphology is consistent with diffuse large B-cell lymphoma.

Diagnosis

Primary intermediate-grade B-cell gastric lymphoma.

Recommendations

Treatment with chemotherapy with or without radiation is recommended, reserving surgery for the complications of the chemotherapy, recurrences, or failure of the primary therapy to achieve a complete response.

Discussion

Historically, any discussion regarding the management of gastric lymphoma has included chemotherapy, radiation, and surgery, either in combination or alone. Recently, however, with improved understanding of the pathophysiology of gastric lymphoma, as well as treatment responses and survival, there has been a shift to treating this disease initially with chemotherapy with or without radiation and reserving surgery for the complications of the chemotherapy, recurrences, or failure of the primary therapy to achieve a complete response. Even in the latter two instances, second-line chemotherapy remains effective and is therefore an option along with surgery.

Clearly advanced disease, defined as penetration through the serosa or spread to adjacent organs (T4 and T5, stage III) or distant metastasis (stage IV), requires chemoimmunotherapy and radiation. On occasion, surgery had been advocated for advanced disease, in the case of bleeding or obstruction, but bleeding can often be treated by endoscopy and only rarely necessitates surgery, while obstruction can be treated with steroids, allowing the commencement of chemotherapy and radiation.

The controversy regarding therapy arises for stages I and II. There have been numerous studies trying to determine the best approach to treating gastric lymphoma, but the protocols have varied widely so the ability to compare effective treatments between studies has been difficult. It is not surprising that there is no consensus, even regarding the most appropriate surgical procedure, particularly, whether a radical lymphadenectomy should be performed. For years, surgery was the treatment of choice because there was a concern for the potential complications associated with chemotherapy (bleeding and perforation), and it was used as a necessary tool for staging. With refinements in chemotherapeutic regimens and with the addition of immune-based therapy for lymphoma, rituximab, a monoclonal antibody against CD20, disease-free survival and overall survival have improved. Additionally, advances in preoperative staging, both with CT scanning and PET imaging, have obviated the need for surgical staging.

Approach

CHOP (cyclophosphamide, doxorubicin, vincristine, and prednisone) with rituximab is given every 3 weeks for six cycles followed by 5 weeks of radiation. Response to therapy is assessed after the second cycle and 1 month after completion of the regimen. Generally, with extensive lymph-node involvement, as in this case, radiation is beneficial. However, if the disease is limited to stage I or if there is a near-complete response after two cycles of chemoimmunotherapy, radiation can be postponed.

Case Continued

Following completion of the chemoimmunotherapy and radiation, a follow-up CT scan is performed, which demonstrates remission of the lymphoma.

CT Scan

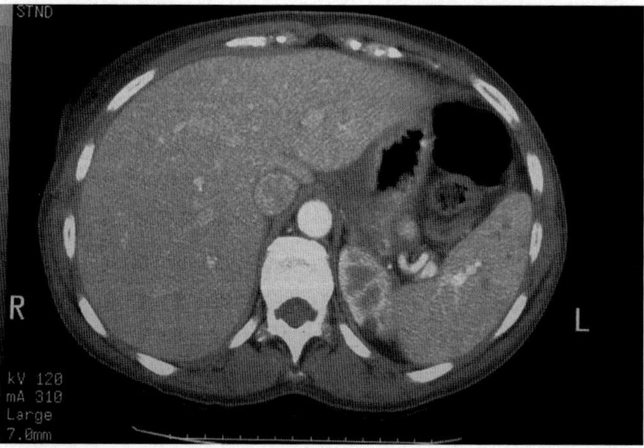

Figure 21.2

CT Scan Report

Remission of disease. Normal-appearing gastric wall.

Case Continued

There are no complications from the chemoimmunotherapy and radiation, and the patient is currently 4 years out from his initial therapy; therefore, operative intervention has not been necessary. If surgery were the primary procedure indicated for complications of therapy, then a total gastrectomy with lymphadenectomy and reconstruction with an esophagojejunostomy would be the operation of choice.

Discussion

Although the incidence of gastric adenocarcinoma has steadily decreased since the 1930s, the incidence of gastric lymphoma has progressively increased. Approximately 22,000 new cases of gastric cancer will be diagnosed this year, and of these, 2% to 7% will be primary gastric lymphomas. Gastric adenocarcinoma and gastric lymphoma share similar symptoms on presentation, as well as CT and endoscopic characteristics, but it is crucial to make the distinction based on pathologic criteria, due to the differences in therapy and prognosis.

An obvious advantage of nonoperative management is retention of the stomach and its function, and maintenance of gastrointestinal continuity. The complications of total gastrectomy, such as dumping, in addition to the morbidity and mortality of a total gastrectomy versus the risk of bleeding and perforation from chemotherapy, have been estimated to be between 2% and 5%, whereas the mortality of the operation is essentially equivalent. Another difference between operative and nonoperative management is the pattern of recurrence. When initial treatment was operative, recurrences have tended to be systemic, whereas in chemotherapy-treated groups, recurrences generally are local. In either case, salvage chemotherapy with or without radiation has proven effective for recurrent disease.

Another variant of gastric lymphoma that warrants discussion is gastric mucosa-associated lymphoid tissue (MALT). Several investigators have established a clear link between *Helicobacter pylori* and MALT lymphoma. It is believed that antigenic stimulation by *H. pylori* promotes proliferation of monoclonal B cells via nonmalignant T cells, and without this stimulation the proliferation ceases. The initial treatment of low-grade MALT lymphoma is to remove the stimulant and therefore eradicate the *H. pylori*. This has been a highly successful approach. However, transformation to high-grade MALT lymphoma can occur and is best treated with systemic chemotherapy.

Suggested Readings

Aviles A, Nambo M, Neri N, et al. The role of surgery in primary gastric lymphoma: results of a controlled clinical trial. *Ann Surg* 2004;240:44–50.

Raderer M, Valencak J, Osterreicher C, et al. Chemotherapy for the treatment of patients with primary high-grade gastric B-cell lymphoma of modified Ann Arbor stages IE and IIE. *Cancer* 2000;88:1979–1985.

Stephen J, Smith J. Treatment of primary gastric lymphoma and gastric mucosal-associated lymphoid tissue lymphoma. *J Am Coll Surg* 1998;187:312–320.

Yoon SS, Coit CG, Portlock CS, et al. The diminishing role of surgery in the treatment of gastric lymphoma. *Ann Surg* 2004;240:28–37.

case 22

Presentation

A 46-year-old woman with no significant medical history visits her primary physician with vague epigastric pain. She is noted to have a large mass in the upper abdomen and is referred to your office. She is a nonsmoker and drinks no alcohol. There is no family history of cancer. On examination, she appears slightly anemic, and a mobile, 1-cm upper abdominal mass is palpable. On rectal examination, the mass is not palpable and there is no clinical evidence of ascites. Upper gastrointestinal imaging (UGI) series and endoscopy are ordered.

Clinical Photograph

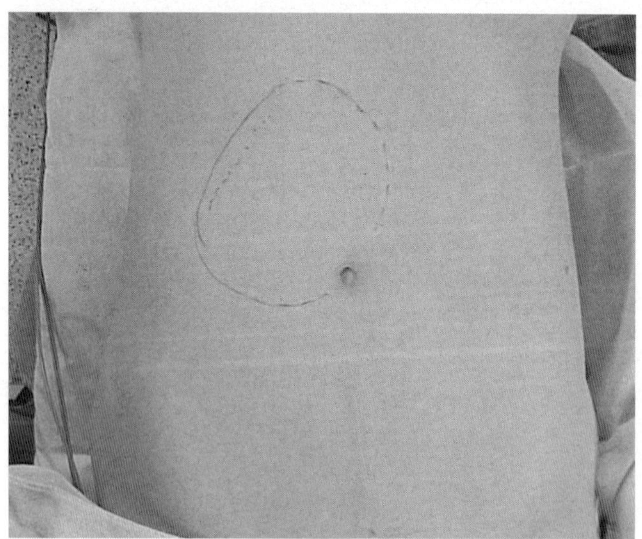

Figure 22.1

Physical Examination Report

A large mass is localized to the upper right abdomen.

UGI Series and Endoscopy

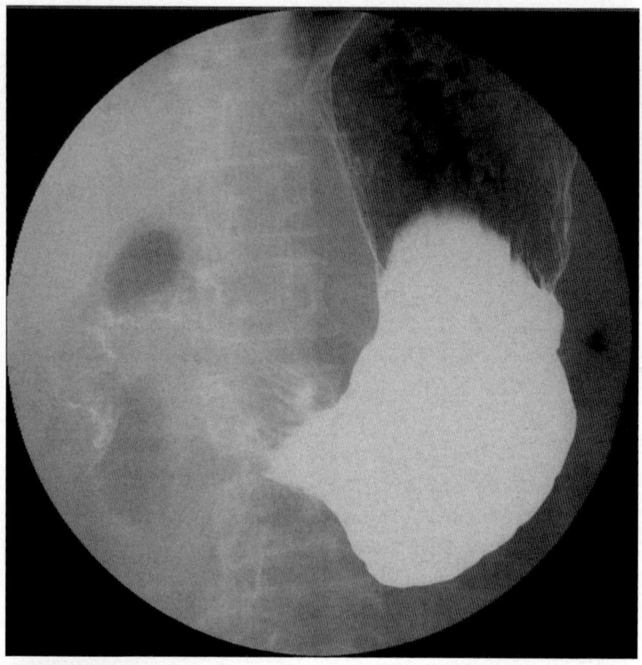

Figure 22.2A

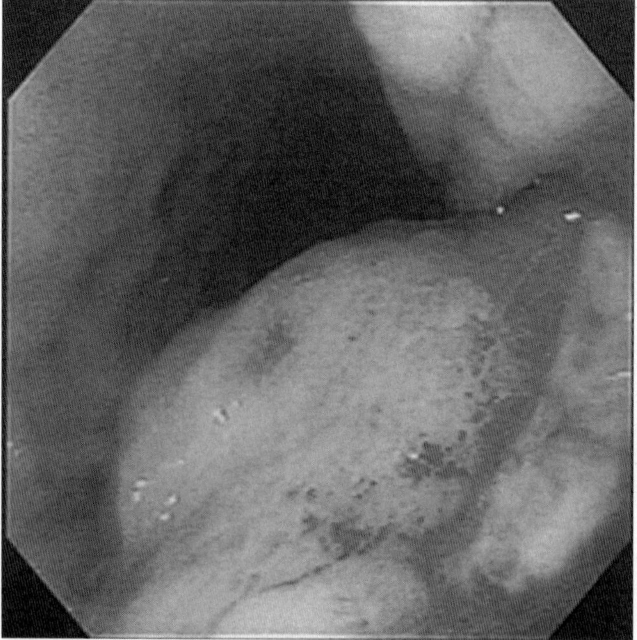

Figure 22.2B

UGI Series and Endoscopy Report

The esophagus is normal. In the stomach, the greater curvature appears to be compressed by a large tumor. There are bridging folds found by the UGI series and no tumor ulcer is found by endoscopic examination. Endoscopic biopsy reveals normal epithelial cells and no malignant cells.

Differential Diagnosis

The differential diagnosis for submucosal tumors (SMTs) in the adult stomach includes (a) mesenchymal tumors; (b) lymphomas (mostly mucosa-associated lymphoid tissue [MALT] lymphomas, such as high-grade MALT and low-grade MALT); (c) epithelial malignancies, such as stomach carcinoma and gastric carcinoid; (d) congenital diseases; (e) inflammation or inflammatory tumors, such as inflammatory fibroid polyp; and (f) extragastric tumors that compress the stomach.

SMTs frequently show bridging folds and a center spot ulcer in the UGI series and endoscopic examinations.

Discussion

Mesenchymal tumors include stromal cell tumors such as gastrointestinal stromal tumors (GISTs), myogenic tumors (leiomyoma or leiomyosarcoma), and neurogenic tumors (mostly schwannomas in the stomach), lipomas, hemangiomas, lymphangiomas, and granular cell tumors. Mesenchymal tumors sometimes form central ulceration, and biopsies of these areas are often nondiagnostic. Lymphomas and carcinomas mimicking SMT-like tumors sometimes demonstrate slight mucosal changes. Most carcinoma-forming SMT-like tumors are poorly differentiated carcinomas. Congenital diseases include aberrant pancreas and gastric duplication, in which ductal components or cystic lesions are sometimes found in the submucosal area. Aberrant pancreas is most frequently found in the lower third, but may also be located in the body, of the stomach. Gastric submucosal tumors are frequently asymptomatic until they become large. When symptomatic, most patients suffer from hematemesis and/or melena, iron-deficiency anemia, a palpable abdominal mass, and dull abdominal pain. Gastric SMTs form three types of growth: intraluminal, extragastric, and combined. Large tumors tend to form extragastric or combined growth.

The most frequent gastric mesenchymal tumors (70% to 80%) forming submucosal tumors are GISTs; the rest are myogenic tumors (leiomyoma or leiomyosarcoma) and schwannomas. GISTs are preferentially located in the upper and middle stomach, myogenic tumors in the upper third of the stomach around the gastroesophageal junction, and neurogenic tumors along the lesser curvature. GISTs demonstrate the most aggressive behavior compared to the other two mesenchymal tumors. These three stromal tumors in the gastrointestinal tract, however, show very similar macroscopic appearances and they cannot be discriminated from each other by conventional radiographic or endoscopic examinations. They can be differentiated primarily by pathologic examination.

Recommendation

A computed tomography (CT) scan of the abdomen and endoscopic ultrasound as well as endoscopic ultrasound-guided aspiration biopsy. Transcutaneous needle biopsy is not recommended because of the risk of peritoneal seeding.

Case Continued

The patient has a CT scan of the abdomen and pelvis. An endoscopic sonography and endoscopic ultrasound-guided aspiration biopsy are performed.

CT Scans

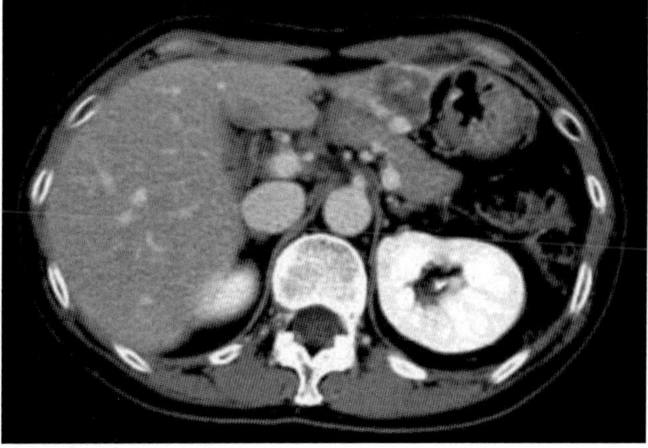

Figure 22.3A

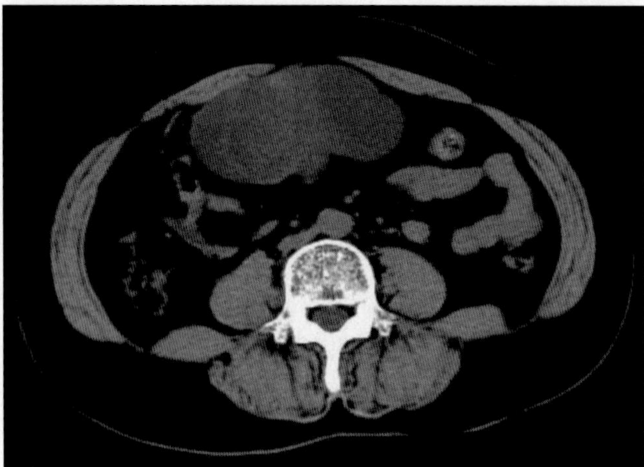

Figure 22.3B

CT Scan Report

A 13-cm inhomogeneously enhancing mass is found in the upper abdomen, which appears to be in continuity with the greater curvature of the stomach and does not involve the other abdominal structures.

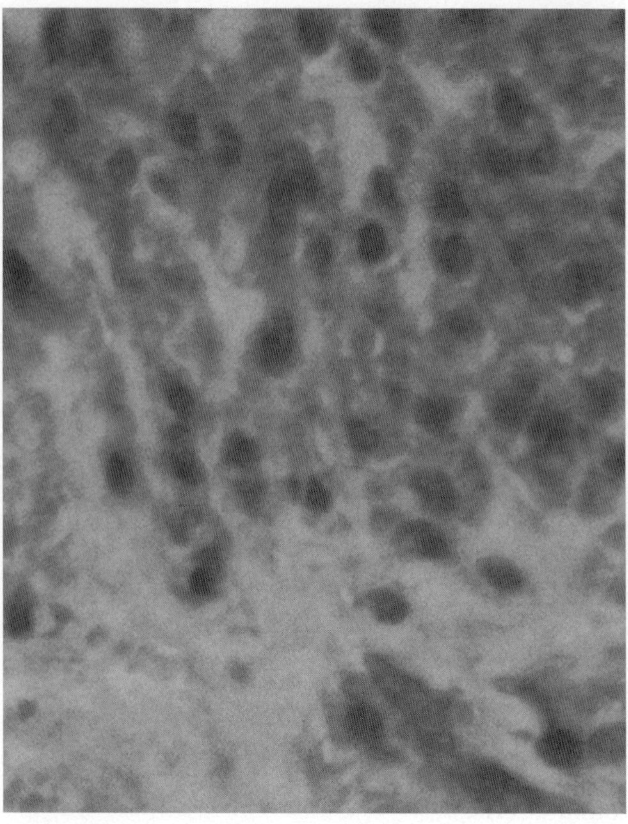

Figure 22.4B

Histopathology Slides

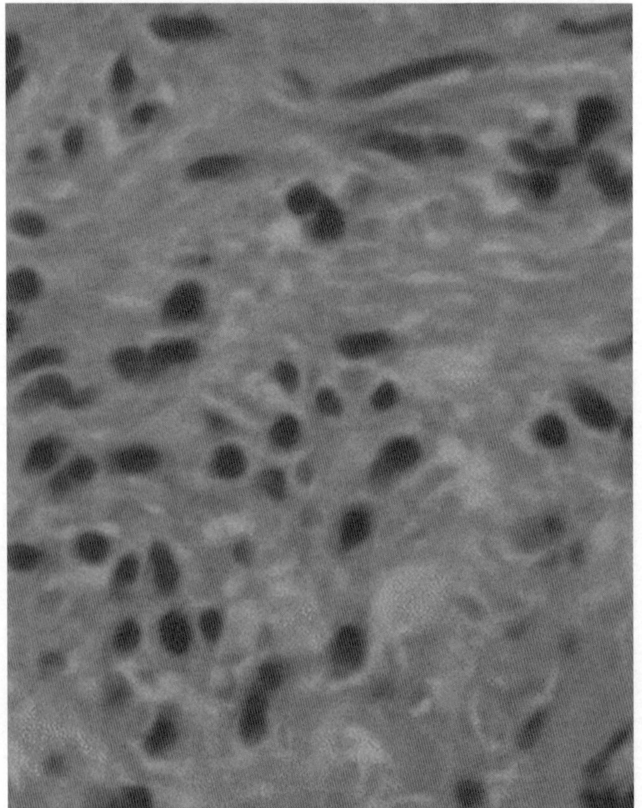

Figure 22.4A

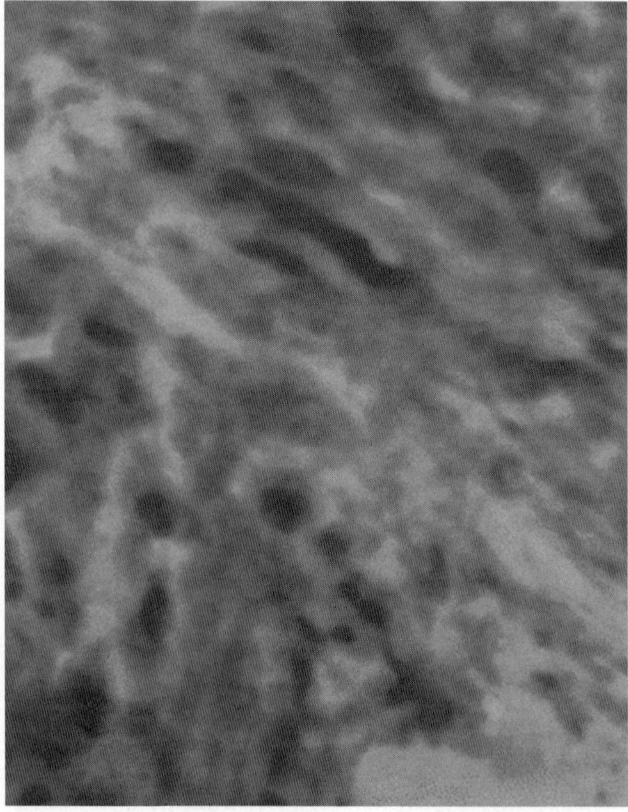

Figure 22.4C

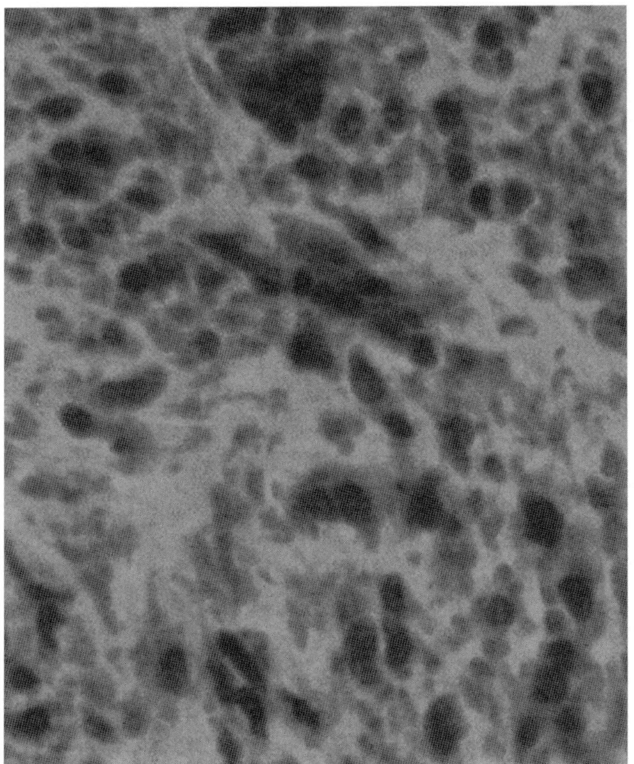

Figure 22.4D

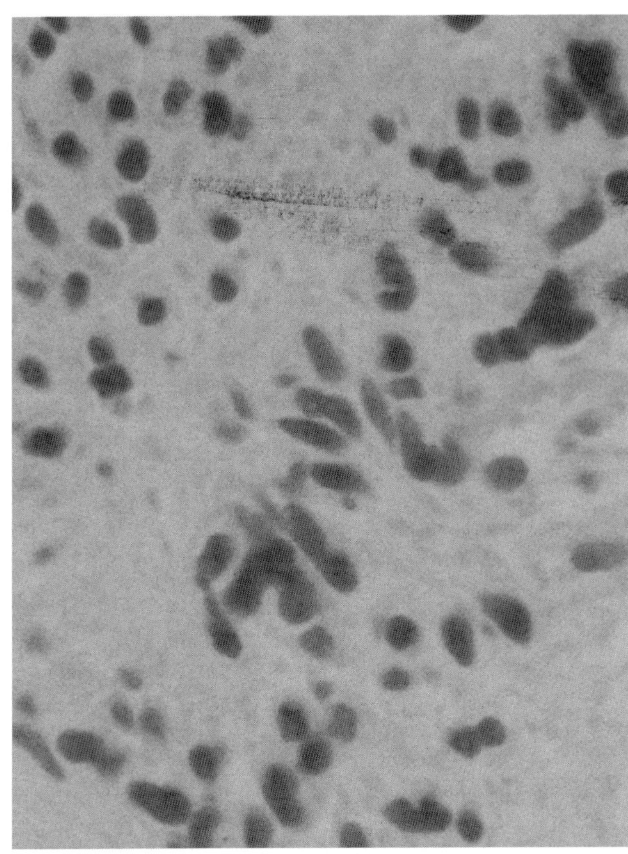

Figure 22.4F

Histopathology Report

Samples obtained by endoscopic ultrasound-guided fine-needle aspiration biopsy show a spindle cell tumor with rare mitotic figures and moderate numbers of cells. Tumor cells are positive for KIT protein **(B)**, CD34 **(C)**, and vimentin **(D)**, and negative for S-100 protein **(E)**, desmin **(F)**, and α-smooth-muscle actin by immunohistochemistry. Cellularity is moderate, and mitotic counts of tumor cells are 8/50 high-power field (HPF). Thus, the tumor would be placed in the high-risk category of the National Institutes of Health (NIH) Risk Classification (Table 22-1).

Table 22-1: Risk classification of GIST

Tumor size		Mitotic count in histologic examination
Very low risk	<2 cm	<5/50 HPF
Low risk	2-5 cm	<5/50 HPF
Intermediate risk	<5 cm	6-10/50 HPF
	5-10 cm	<5/50 HPF
High risk	>5 cm	5-10/50 HPF
	>10 cm	>10/50 HPF

HPF, high-power field.

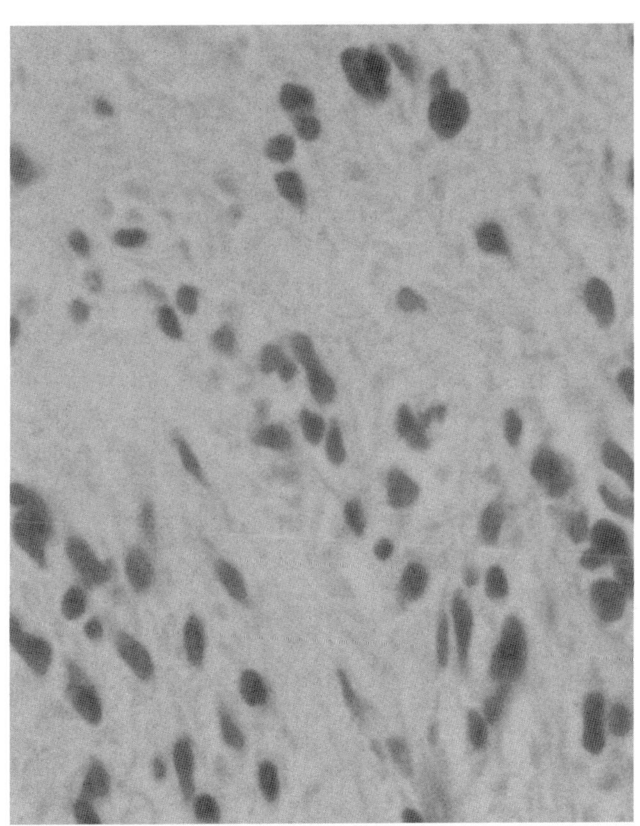

Figure 22.4E

Diagnosis

Histologic diagnosis is GIST.

Approach

This patient is offered open partial resection of the stomach. Surgical removal of the tumor is the most effective treatment modality for GIST. Neither conventional chemotherapy nor radiation is active for GIST. The patient is informed that recurrence or relapse rates of GIST in the 10 years after complete resection are assumed to be 50% to 70% when tumor size is greater than 10 cm. Relapse rates also depend on mitotic rates of tumor cells by postoperative pathologic examinations.

It is critical to perform a complete tumor resection while being particularly careful to avoid tumor rupture. Partial resection of the stomach is a basic principle unless the tumor is huge (requiring distal or total gastrectomy) or involves other structures. Any structures that are involved should be resected. Lymph-node dissection is not required because lymph node metastasis is very rare in stromal tumors of the gastrointestinal tract. Laparoscopic surgery is usually recommended for small size GISTs (<5 cm), especially for GISTs with extragastric growth.

Surgical Approach

An upper midline abdominal incision is performed. There is a 14-cm hypervascular tumor arising from the greater curvature of the stomach without any peritoneal dissemination and liver metastasis. The greater omentum is dissected off, and marginal vasculatures of the stomach are ligated and divided. No macroscopic lymph node metastasis was found. The tumor is removed by partial gastric resection with a 2-cm margin. Postoperative course is uneventful.

Discussion

GIST most frequently occurs in the stomach (60% to 70%), followed by the small intestine (20% to 30%), the colon and rectum (5%), and the esophagus (a few percent). GIST is a potentially malignant tumor, and differentiation of GIST that demonstrates a benign course from one showing malignant behavior is very difficult, even with pathologic examination. NIH consensus recommends certain criteria to allow risk stratification of GIST (see Table 22-1).

Low-risk and very-low-risk GIST relapses are extremely rare after complete resection. Intermediate-risk GIST may recur even after complete resection. High-risk GIST may be associated with more than 50% recurrence rates, thus a careful postoperative surveillance program is required.

GIST is histologically differentiated from other mesenchymal tumors, including leiomyoma, leiomyosarcoma, and schwannoma. Only GIST expresses the KIT protein in the plasma membrane, which is the receptor tyrosine kinase for stem cell factor. Most GISTs (80% to 90%) accompany somatic gain-of-function mutations in the C-KIT gene encoding the KIT protein; 5% of GISTs have gain-of-function mutations in the platelet-derived growth factor receptor alpha gene; and 5% to 10% may have unknown gene mutations. GISTs frequently express other proteins such as CD34 (70%), vimentin (70%), and alpha-smooth muscle actin (30%), but rarely express desmin (a few percent) and S-100 protein (a few percent).

Suggested Readings

Demetri GD, Benjamin R, Blanke CD, et al. Optimal management of patients with gastrointestinal stromal tumors (GIST). Expansion and update of NCCN clinical guidelines. *JNCCN* 2004;2(suppl 1):S1–S26.

Fletcher CD, Berman JJ, Corless C, et al. Diagnosis of gastrointestinal stromal tumors: a consensus approach. *Hum Pathol* 2002;33:459–465.

Greenson JK. Gastrointestinal stromal tumors and other mesenchymal lesions of the gut. *Mod Pathol* 2003;16:366–375.

Joensuu H, Fletcher C, Dimitrijevic S, et al. Management of malignant gastrointestinal stromal tumors. *Lancet Oncology* 2002;3:655–664.

Nishida T, Hirota S. Biological and clinical review of stromal tumors in the gastrointestinal tract. *Histol Histopathol* 2000;15:1293–1301.

Presentation

A 55-year-old male with no significant past medical history is referred with the recent diagnosis of anemia. Physical examination is normal with the exception of stools that are positive for occult hemoglobin. Colonoscopy shows only two benign tubular adenomas. An upper gastrointestinal (GI) endoscopy is performed.

Endoscopic Image

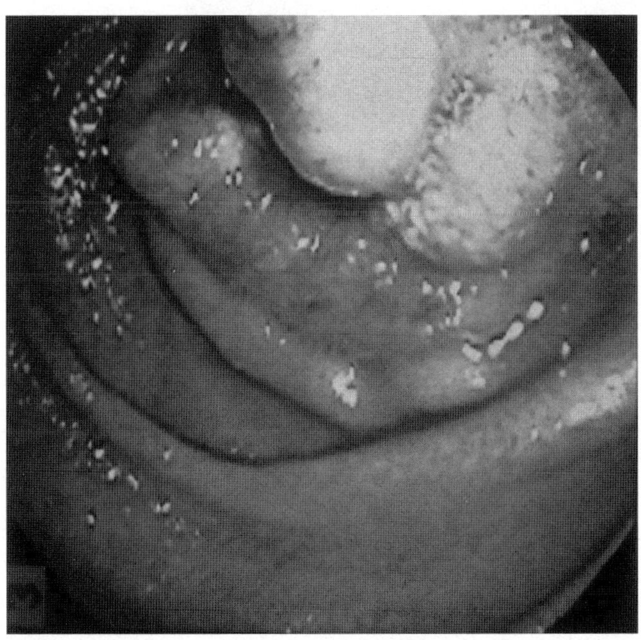

Figure 23.1

Endoscopy Report

Upper GI endoscopy reveals a 3 × 3 cm ulcerated villous tumor in the second portion of the duodenum.

Endoscopic biopsy shows villous adenoma of the duodenum with marked atypia.

Differential Diagnosis

The differential diagnosis for duodenal polypoid lesions includes benign villous adenomas or invasive adenocarcinoma.

Discussion

Villous adenomas, especially those larger than 3 cm, have a malignant potential similar to that of colonic tumors, and total excision is necessary. Up to 50% of such large tumors that are benign on endoscopic biopsy may harbor foci of invasive cancer. Symptoms usually are associated with GI blood loss, although tumors in the periampullary region may obstruct the ampulla of Vater, causing either obstructive jaundice or, rarely, acute pancreatitis. Risk factors for duodenal cancer include familial colonic polyposis syndromes (familial adenomatous polyposis, Gardner's syndrome) and hereditary non-polyposis colon cancer (HNPCC).

Duodenal neoplasms may present with symptoms due to GI blood loss or, if circumferential, duodenal obstruction. Lesions in the periampullary area may present with obstructive jaundice.

Recommendation

Endoscopic ultrasound to determine the presence of invasion.

Endoscopic Ultrasound Image

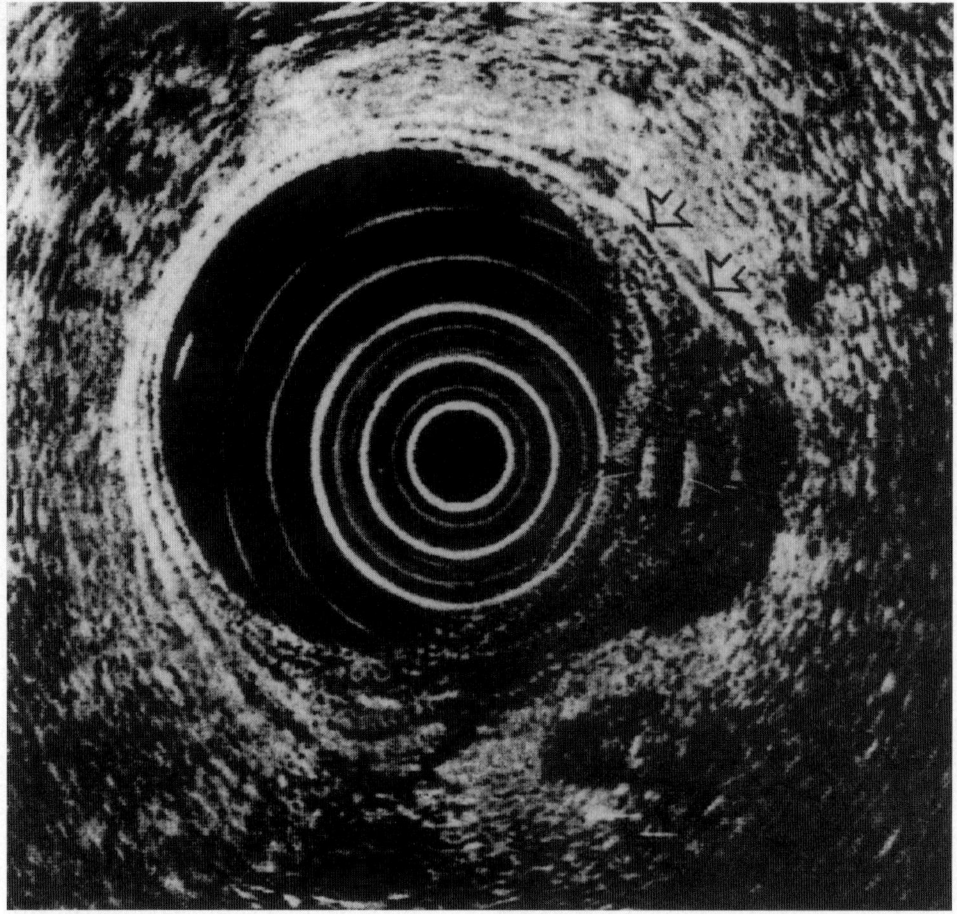

Figure 23.1

Endoscopic Ultrasound Report

Endoscopic ultrasound shows tumor infiltration beyond the muscularis propria of the duodenum with invasion into the pancreas. Repeat biopsies show invasive adenocarcinoma.

Diagnosis and Recommendation

The diagnosis is adenocarcinoma of the duodenum. A computed tomography (CT) scan should be obtained to exclude metastatic disease.

Approach

If staging studies demonstrate that the disease is localized, the patient should be prepared for surgery. The appropriate operative approach is pancreatico-duodenectomy. If endoscopic ultrasound and biopsy suggest benign disease, complete transduodenal resection of smaller (<2 cm) tumors may be possible. If this option is attempted, multiple frozen sec-tions should be obtained to ensure that invasive cancer is not present. If cancer is detected, pancre-aticoduodenectomy should be performed.

Surgical Approach

The surgical approach can include either standard pancreaticoduodenectomy (including antrectomy) or, if an adequate margin can be obtained, the pylorus-preserving modification is appropriate. (See Chapter 49 for details.) There is no role for extended lymph-node dissection. In most cases of duodenal neoplasms, the texture of the pancreas is soft, with a normal, small pancreatic duct. This finding increases the risk of postoperative pancreatic anastomotic leak following pancreaticoduodenectomy.

Discussion

Duodenal carcinoma is the least common of the four periampullary cancers, which also include pan-creatic, distal bile duct, and ampullary carcinomas. Duodenal cancer, however, has the best chance of cure and long-term survival. The 5-year actuarial survival rate reported in most series following pancreaticoduodenectomy for duodenal carcinoma is usually in the range of 50% to 70% versus less than 30% for pancreatic carcinoma. Factors that have been shown to influence survival include tumor size, lymph-node status, resection margin status, tumor differentiation, and depth of invasion.

The role of postoperative adjuvant therapy for resectable duodenal carcinoma is undetermined, with no strong evidence available to address the topic. Options include chemoradiation, which is used frequently for pancreatic cancer, and systemic chemotherapy regimens, used in patients with colon cancer.

Case Continued

The patient is deemed to have a curable duodenal tumor and successfully undergoes standard pancreaticoduodenectomy.

Suggested Readings

Bakaeen FG, Murr MM, Sarr MG, et al. What prognostic factors are important in duodenal adenocarcinoma? *Arch Surg* 2000;135:635–642.

Farnell MB, Sakorafas GH, Sarr MG, et al. Villous tumors of the duodenum: reappraisal of local vs. extended resection. *J Gastrointest Surg* 2000;1:13–21.

Heniford BT, Iannitti DA, Evans P, et al. Primary nonampullary/periampullary adenocarcinoma of the duodenum. *Am Surg* 1998;12:1165–1169.

Kaklamanos IG, Bathe OF, Franceschi D, et al. Extent of resection in the management of duodenal adenocarcinoma. *Am J Surg* 2000;179:37–41.

Ryder NM, Clifford Y, Hines OJ, et al. Primary duodenal adenocarcinoma: a 40-year experience. *Arch Surg* 2000;135:1070–1074.

Sarela AI, Brennan MF, Karpeh MS, et al. Adenocarcinoma of the duodenum: importance of accurate lymph node staging and similarity in outcome to gastric cancer. *Ann Surg Oncol* 2004;4:354–355.

Sohn TA, Lillemoe KD, Cameron JL, et al. Adenocarcinoma of the duodenum: factors influencing long-term survival. *J Gastrointest Surg* 1988;2:79–87.

case 24

A 56-year-old man with no significant past medical history presents to his primary care physician with symptoms of intermittent crampy abdominal pain, nausea, and diarrhea for a few weeks. He denies fever or chills. Physical examination reveals a mildly distended abdomen without any tenderness.

Small Bowel Follow-Through With Barium Contrast

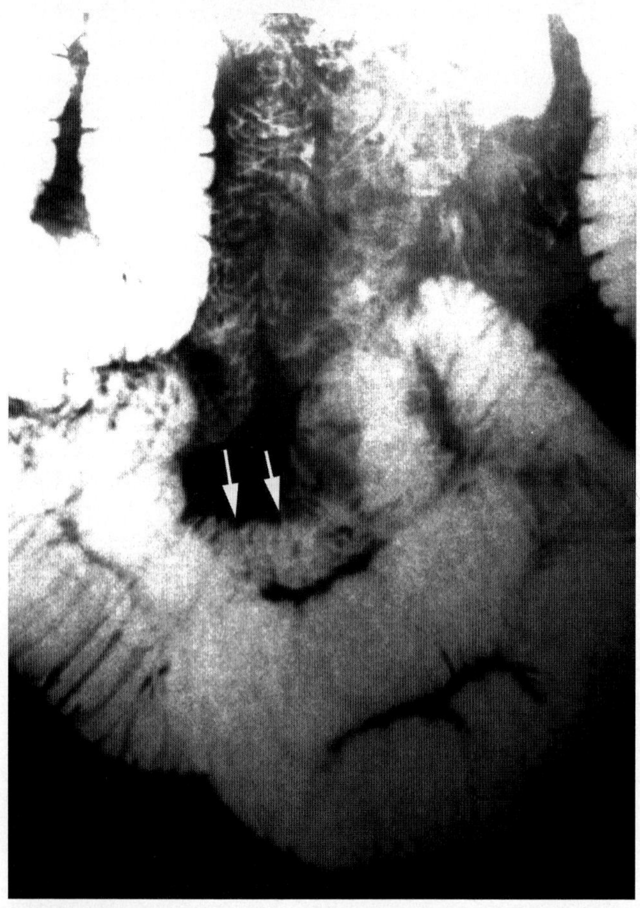

Figure 24.1

No masses or hernias are palpated. His stool is positive for occult blood. His hematocrit is 25%; other laboratory tests are unremarkable. An abdominal series reveals a mildly dilated stomach without evidence of free intraperitoneal air. Workup, including upper gastrointestinal (GI) endoscopy and colonoscopy, is negative. A small bowel follow-through is obtained.

Small Bowel Follow-Through Report

There is a 3-cm apple-core lesion on the proximal jejunum with high-grade obstruction, suggesting malignancy.

Differential Diagnosis

The differential diagnosis for this patient with a jejunal mass includes benign and malignant tumors of the small intestine, in addition to an inflammatory mass secondary to Crohn's disease. The most common benign tumors of the small intestine are leiomyomas, adenomas, and lipomas. Malignant tumors of the small bowel include adenocarcinomas, gastrointestinal stromal tumors (GISTs), lymphomas, and carcinoid tumors. In addition, the small intestine is frequently affected by metastases from cancers originating at other sites. Melanoma, in particular, is associated with a propensity for metastasis to the small intestine. The small bowel follow-through suggests this patient has a malignant lesion, although the diagnosis can be confirmed only by pathology.

Discussion

Primary small bowel malignancies are rare, with an estimated incidence of 5,300 cases per year in the United States. They account for only 1% to 2% of all GI tract malignancies. Most small intestinal neoplasms are asymptomatic until they become large. Partial small-bowel obstruction, with associated symptoms of abdominal pain and distention, nausea, and vomiting, is the most common mode of presentation. Obstruction can be the result of luminal narrowing, the tumor itself, or intussusception, with the tumor serving as the lead point. Bleeding, usually indolent, is the second most common mode of presentation. Physical examination may be unrevealing in the absence of small bowel obstruction. Up to 25% of patients with intestinal cancers are reported to have a palpable abdominal mass. Fecal occult blood tests may be positive. Jaundice secondary to biliary obstruction (in the case of duodenal tumors) or hepatic metastases may be present. Cachexia and ascites may be present with advanced disease.

Because of the nonspecific symptoms associated with most small intestinal neoplasms, these lesions are rarely diagnosed preoperatively. CT scanning has a low sensitivity for detecting mucosal or intramural lesions in the small intestine, but can demonstrate large tumors and is useful in staging malignancies. Upper GI with small bowel follow-through examinations have reported sensitivities ranging from only 30% to 44% for the detection of small intestinal tumors. Enteroclysis is the test of choice for detecting small intestinal neoplasms, particularly those located in the distal small intestine, with a sensitivity of 90%. Angiography or radioisotope-tagged red blood cell (RBC) scans can be used to localize actively bleeding tumors. Tumors located in the duodenum can be biopsied during esophagogastroduodenoscopy (EGD); lesions located in the distal ileum can sometimes be reached during colonoscopy. Intraoperative enteroscopy can be used to localize tumors beyond the reach of standard endoscopic techniques.

Recommendation

Abdominal CT scan for staging.

CT Scan

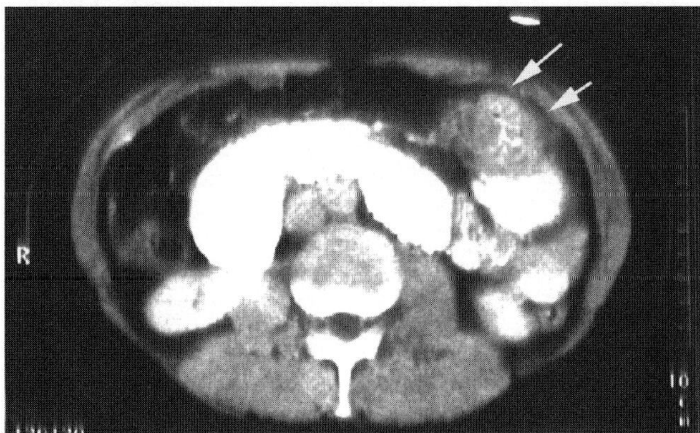

Figure 24.2

CT Scan Report

An obstructing lesion is present in the proximal jejunum resulting in massive gastric and duodenal dilation. Liver, kidney, and pancreas are normal. No ascites is seen.

Approach

Surgical resection is the treatment of choice. This patient is offered exploratory laparotomy with segmental resection of tumor. The risks and benefits were discussed with the patient and his family, and they agree to proceed with surgery.

Surgical Approach

A vertical midline incision is made, and the peritoneal cavity is entered. Careful exploration is performed, evaluating for presence of peritoneal dissemination and liver metastases. A segmental resection of the small intestine harboring the tumor with resection of the associated mesentery should be performed. The amount of small bowel resected should be based on the following goals: (a) to achieve negative microscopic longitudinal resection margins and (b) to allow for adequate lymph node sampling. Overextensive lymph-node dissection may result in devascularization of large lengths of normal small bowel, and should therefore be avoided. Tumors located in the distal ileum are best managed by right hemicolectomy.

Case Continued

At exploration there is no evidence of ascites, peritoneal nodules, or liver metastases. There is a 4- to 5-cm small bowel tumor 15 cm distal to the ligament of Treitz with several hard mesenteric lymph nodes. Radical small bowel resection is performed and intestinal continuity is restored with a side-to-side stapled anastomosis. Postoperatively, the patient is stable. He is discharged on postoperative day 5, tolerating a regular diet without difficulty. One week later, the patient and his family come to the clinic to discuss the pathology findings and expected prognosis.

Pathology Report

Moderately differentiated adenocarcinoma (5.5 cm) of the small intestine, invading through the muscularis propria and extending into perijejunal adipose tissue is diagnosed. The resection margins are free of tumor. Metastatic adenocarcinoma, in 4 of 8 lymph nodes, with extracapsular invasion is found. American Joint Committee on Cancer (AJCC) stage is T3 N1 M0, stage III.

Discussion

The overall prognosis of patients diagnosed with small bowel adenocarcinoma is poor, with reported 5-year survival rates ranging from 5% to 32%. Five-year survival rates according to AJCC stage, as determined on analysis of the National Cancer Database (NCDB), are 65% for stage I, 48% for stage II, 35% for stage III, and 4% for stage IV. Patients with adenocarcinomas of the small intestine are typically diagnosed with advanced disease; as a result, curative resection can be achieved only in 52% to 65% of patients. Reported 5-year survival rates of patients who have undergone curative resection range from 30% to 48%. T and N stage have both been reported to be significant prognostic factors for patients who have undergone curative resection. In the literature, 5-year survival rates of patients with T1/2 cancer and those with T3/4 cancer are 64% to 82% and 32% to 47%, respectively; 5-year survival rates of patients without lymph node metastasis are 48% to 58%, and for those with lymph node metastasis are 25% to 29%. The role of chemotherapy for adenocarcinoma of the small intestine is still undefined. To date, there is no evidence supporting the benefit of adjuvant treatment.

Case Continued

The patient is informed that his tumor has been completely resected. He has stage III disease. The reported 5-year survival rate for patients with stage III disease is 35%. Given that there is no evidence supporting the survival benefit of adjuvant therapies for small bowel adenocarcinoma, no additional therapy is elected.

Suggested Readings

Abrahams NA, Halverson A, Fazio VW, et al. Adenocarcinoma of the small bowel: a study of 37 cases with emphasis on histologic prognostic factors. *Dis Colon Rectum* 2002;45: 1496–1502.

Cunningham JD, Aleali R, Aleali M, et al. Malignant small bowel neoplasms: histopathologic determinants of recurrence and survival. *Ann Surg* 1997;225:300–306.

Howe JR, Karnell LH, Menck HR, et al. The American College of Surgeons Commission on Cancer and the American Cancer Society. Adenocarcinoma of the small bowel: review of the National Cancer Data Base, 1985-1995. *Cancer* 1999;86: 2693–2706.

Ito H, Perez A, Brooks DC, et al. Surgical treatment of small bowel cancer: a 20-year single institution experience. *J Gastrointest Surg* 2003;7:925–930.

Talamonti MS, Goetz LH, Rao S, et al. Primary cancers of the small bowel: analysis of prognostic factors and results of surgical management. *Arch Surg* 2002;137:564–570; discussion 570–571.

Presentation

A 62-year-old man presents to the emergency department with diffuse crampy abdominal pain, bloating, nausea, and vomiting, and obstipation for 2 days. His history is notable for vague abdominal pain for the past 2 years for which he has undergone extensive workup, including esophagogastroduo-denoscopy (EGD), colonoscopy, and abdominal computed tomography (CT) scan, which were all normal. His primary care physician had empirically started him on a proton-pump inhibitor, and he had been scheduled to undergo an outpatient small bowel follow-through the following month. He also has a remote history of an uncomplicated laparo-scopic cholecystectomy.

A plain abdominal radiograph of the kidneys, ureter, and bladder (KUB) reveals moderately dilated loops of small bowel with multiple air fluid levels in the left abdomen, indicating ileal versus small bowel obstruction. Abdominal CT scan shows a 4-cm mass involving the mid-ileum with evidence of proximal small bowel dilatation. Visceral angiography showed mild aortic calcification, but no stenosis of the mesenteric vessels.

Differential Diagnosis

The differential diagnosis for small bowel obstruc-tion related to mural thickening includes mesenteric ischemia, a neoplastic process or, less likely, an infectious process. The patient's lengthy history of vague abdominal pain is characteristic of either of the first two etiologies. Delay in diagnosis of a small bowel tumor is characteristic given the low sensitiv-ities of imaging tests.

Recommendations

Small bowel obstruction from a mechanical cause due to findings on the CT scan of the abdomen is diagnosed. An exploratory laparotomy is necessary after initial resuscitation, placement of nasogastric tube decompression, and Foley catheter for moni-toring of urine output.

Case Continued

At operation, an obstructing distal ileal mass is noted along with several firm masses in the mesen-tery. The small bowel and attached mesentery is resected, and a primary anastomosis is performed. The length of the bowel is inspected, and no further abnormalities are discovered. The liver is likewise palpated with no appreciable masses. The patient tolerates the procedure.

Intraoperative Image

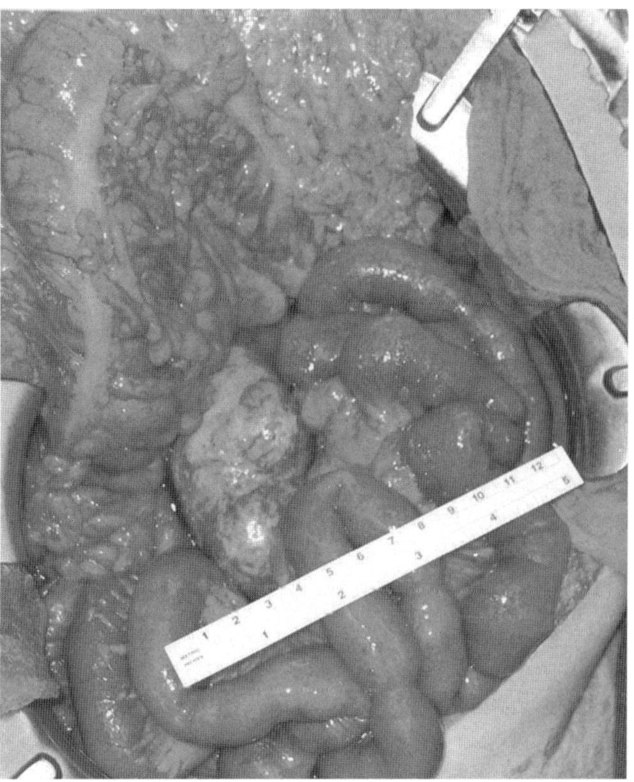

Figure 25.1

Intraoperative Report

Carcinoid tumor in small bowel visible at base of transverse mesocolon. A 25-cm length of small bowel specimen reveals a 4-cm carcinoid tumor invading the muscularis, mesenteric fat, and serosa. Three of 15 lymph nodes reveal carcinoid metastases.

Discussion

Carcinoid tumors are rare neuroendocrine tumors. In 1907, Obendorfer first described these tumors using the term "carcinoid" to denote their slower rate of growth compared to adenocarcinomas. Carcinoid tumors secrete hormones and biogenic amines, the most common of which is serotonin, but also include histamine, kallikrein, and prostaglandins. These substances are responsible for the symptoms of the carcinoid syndrome: episodic flushing, diarrhea, wheezing, and eventual right-sided valvular heart disease. The liver normally metabolizes serotonin, but once metastases occupy the liver, the hormone is released to systemic circulation and the syndrome may occur. Carcinoid syndrome is the initial presentation in 5% to 10% of carcinoids. Small bowel carcinoid tumors occur most commonly in patients in their sixth or seventh decade of life.

The small bowel is the most commonly affected location, containing 25% of all carcinoids. Carcinoid tumors comprise roughly one third of all small bowel malignancies.

Carcinoid tumors may be multicentric. Patients with small bowel carcinoid tumors can present with protean disease manifestations such as abdominal pain, nausea and vomiting, and weight loss. Patients may present with gastrointestinal bleeding, although this is less common given the deep submucosal location of most tumors and their relatively small size. Most tumors are less than 2 cm in diameter, but mass effects are responsible for most symptoms. Acutely they may cause bowel obstruction, as in this case. Additionally, they may be discovered incidentally or may present as a lead point of small bowel intussusception.

Because of their relatively small size and location, many lesions are difficult to identify with conventional imaging. Reported CT scan sensitivities for detecting primary tumors range from rare to 20%. Enteroclysis similarly has a poor rate of detection. Most small bowel carcinoids are located in the distal ileum, beyond the reach of push enteroscopy.

There are little data on the use of magnetic resonance imaging (MRI) for small bowel carcinoids. The sensitivity of capsule endoscopy for detecting these lesions remains to be determined. If the tumors are actively secreting serotonin, an octreotide scan may help to localize them. However, this modality is better suited to identifying hepatic and extra-abdominal metastases. Elevation of urinary levels of 5-hydroxy-indol-acetic-acid (5-HIAA), a serotonin metabolite, may be diagnostic.

Sixty percent of small bowel carcinoids are metastatic at the time of diagnosis. The most common sites of metastasis are lymph nodes, liver, lung, and pancreas.

Primary curative therapy is surgical and consists of resection of the intestinal segment harboring the tumor with its mesentery. Because of the relatively high rate of multicentric and synchronous tumors (as high as 40%), it is important to carefully examine the entire length of the small bowel and mesentery. Primary tumors may appear as little more than a puckering of the serosal surface, but the metastases can typically grow to be much larger and involve the mesentery. Small bowel carcinoids are also associated with noncarcinoid tumors in the gastrointestinal tract in up to 29% of cases, further underlining the need for thorough exploration at the time of surgery.

Diagnosis and Recommendation

Small bowel carcinoid with lymph node metastasis. There were no lesions seen in the liver preoperatively, but the patient should undergo an octreotide scan to look for metastatic disease.

Case Continued

The patient has an uneventful recovery from surgery, and 2 weeks postoperatively undergoes an octreotide scan, which is negative for metastatic disease. He does well until 3 years later, when he begins to develop progressive symptoms of diarrhea and occasional flushing and fevers. Liver function tests are normal. An octreotide scan demonstrates metastatic disease in the liver, which is confirmed by CT scan.

▣ Octreotide Scan

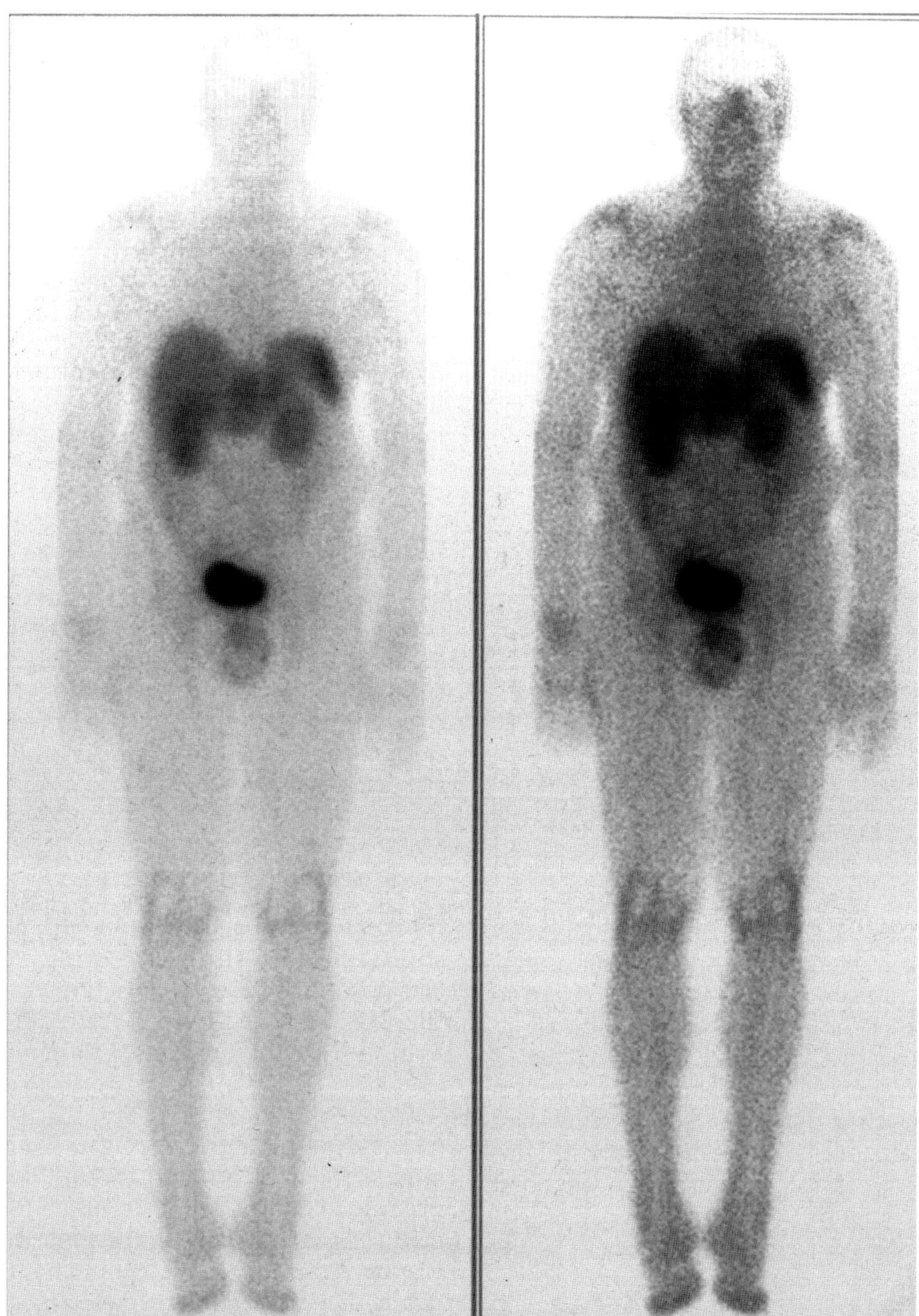

Figure 25.2

Octreotide Scan Report

Abnormal focal uptake of mild intensity in the left hepatic lobe.

Discussion

Patients develop the carcinoid syndrome when tumor metastasizes to the liver and the organ is no longer able to metabolize serotonin. Treatment is directed toward ameliorating the debilitating symptoms of diarrhea, flushing, and abdominal pain. Be cognizant that some symptoms attributed to carcinoid syndrome, such as abdominal cramping or weight loss, may in fact be due to tumor mass effects causing obstruction or ischemia.

The mainstays of medical therapy are the somatostatin analogues, such as octreotide. Although effective for symptom relief, they are not associated with tumor regression or increased survival. The addition of interferon-α may augment the biologic response and has resulted in tumor regression, albeit without a concomitant improvement in survival. Systemic chemotherapy includes streptozotocin with either 5-fluorouracil or cyclophosphamide.

Options for localized therapy for liver metastases associated with carcinoid tumors can include surgical resection, chemoembolization, cryotherapy/radiofrequency ablation, and liver transplantation. No prospective controlled studies comparing these modalities have been performed. However, for good-risk patients with resectable disease, surgical resection is the mainstay of treatment. This may be accomplished by either anatomic or wedge resection. In selected patients, complete tumor resection provides symptom relief and a survival benefit. However, this is most successful in unilobar disease, and most hepatic metastases are bilobar or diffuse. Surgical debulking of liver metastases remains an area of controversy. Although it may improve symptoms, it has an unknown effect on patient survival. Liver transplantation for metastatic carcinoid is of uncertain utility, but may benefit highly selected patients.

For poor-risk patients or those with disease too extensive to allow for complete resection, chemoembolization or ablation is a reasonable palliative option. Multiple or unresectable liver lesions are particularly amenable to hepatic artery occlusion or embolization. Although it has been shown to improve symptoms, the benefit is short-lived, often less than a year. There are no data on the survival benefit of such therapy. Both cryotherapy and radiofrequency ablation have been used with low associated morbidity rates, but their efficacy as compared to surgery remains to be defined.

Approach

The patient has a carcinoid tumor metastatic to the left lobe of the liver. Preoperative octreotide therapy is recommended for symptom relief and potential control of the tumor, followed by resection of the left hepatic lobe.

Discussion

Because of the effects of serotonin on the tricuspid valve, all patients should have a cardiac evaluation, including echocardiography. As many as 45% of these patients may have clinically significant right-sided valvular heart disease requiring perioperative hemodynamic monitoring. Fluid and electrolyte abnormalities related to diarrhea should be corrected. Surgery on patients with known carcinoid disease, whether it is resection of the primary lesion, hepatic metastases, or tumor debulking, should be done with a minimum of tumor manipulation. A carcinoid crisis may be precipitated by the release of bioactive mediators from the tumor. This may result in bronchospasm from histamine or profound hypotension following vasomotor relaxation from bradykinin or kallikrein. Catecholamines may in fact worsen mediator release. Preoperative and intraoperative octreotide treatment is essential. Both surgeon and anesthesiologist should be vigilant for sudden drops in blood pressure.

Case Continued

Given that the patient's metastatic disease is confined to a single lobe of the liver, he is offered hepatic lobar resection. Octreotide is begun, which controlled his symptoms, and this is continued in the operating room. His fluid and electrolyte status is normalized. A cardiac workup reveals no significant valvular disease.

Surgical Approach

A bilateral subcostal incision with a midline extension ("Mercedes incision") or a midline incision can be appropriate for resection of the left lobe of the liver. The abdomen is carefully explored. The liver is carefully palpated bimanually and then evaluated with intraoperative ultrasound. For a lesion in the left lateral lobe, the liver is mobilized by dividing the falciform ligament and the left triangular ligament, being careful not to injure the phrenic vessels. A vessel loop is placed around the porta hepatic for the Pringle maneuver. The Glisson's capsule, just 1 cm medial to the falciform ligament, is scored with electrocautery and the parenchyma is divided to expose vascular pedicles to segment II and III, which can be transected with a linear stapling device. Any major veins are also ligated, and the resection surface is inspected for hemostasis.

Case Continued

At operation, tumor is present in the left lateral lobe, and thus a left lateral segmentectomy (segment II and III) is performed. The patient remains hemody-

namically stable throughout the operative procedure. The abdomen is explored for further evidence
of metastatic disease with particular attention to the
small bowel and mesentery. No additional lesions are
discovered. The patient tolerates the procedure well.

Discussion

The clinical course of patients with metastatic
carcinoid tumors is highly variable. Patients may
develop bowel obstruction or impingement of the
mesenteric vessels related to the extensive desmo-
plastic tumor response. Although metastatic disease
is incurable, debulking of tumor may provide
symptom relief and some survival benefit in certain
patients. Recent studies indicate 5-year survival rates
between 40% and 69% when patients' metastatic
disease is treated. The protracted course of the

disease warrants an aggressive surgical approach,
which may confer survival benefit.

Suggested Readings

De Vries H, Verschueren RC, Willemse PH, et al. Diagnostic, surgical and medical aspects of the midgut carcinoids. *Cancer
Treat Rev* 2002;28:11–12.
Goede AC, Winslet MC. Surgery for carcinoid tumors of the lower
gastrointestinal tract. *Colorectal Dis* 2003;5:123–128.
Gourtsoyiannis N, Grammatikakis J, Prassopoulos P. Role of conventional radiology in the diagnosis and staging of gastrointestinal tract neoplasms. *Semin Surg Oncol* 2001;20:91–108.
Kulke M. Medical progress: carcinoid tumors. *N Eng J Med*
1999;340:858–868.
Modlin IM, Lye KD, Kidd M. A 5-decade analysis of 13,715 carci-
noid tumors. *Cancer* 2003;97:934–959.
Ohrvall U, Erikson B, Juhlin C, et al. Method for dissection of
mesenteric metastases in mid-gut carcinoid tumors. *World J
Surg* 2000;24:1402–1408.

case 26

Presentation

A 45-year-old white man presents with a 9-month history of central abdominal pain and an abdominal mass that has increased in size gradually over the past month. He denies changes in bowel habits or constitutional symptoms (i.e., weight loss, fatigue, fever, night sweats). On examination, there is an abdominal mass that is somewhat mobile. No generalized lymphadenopathy or testicular mass is felt.

Clinical Photograph

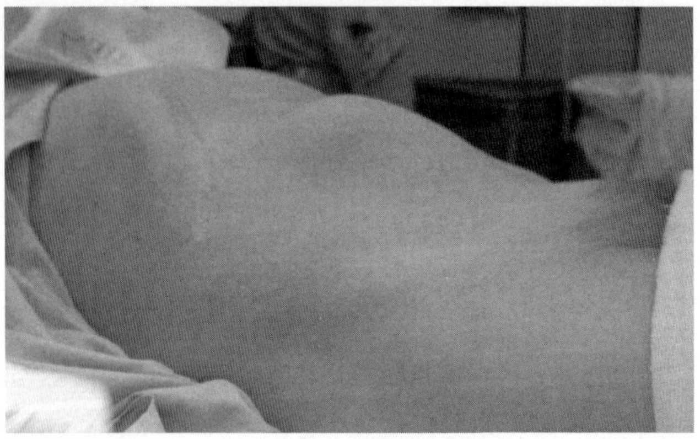

Figure 26.1

Physical Examination Report

A visible abdominal mass is present.

CT Scans

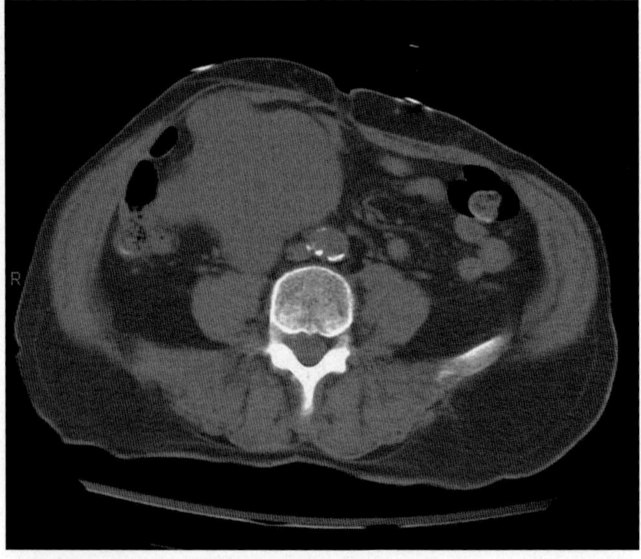

Figure 26.2A

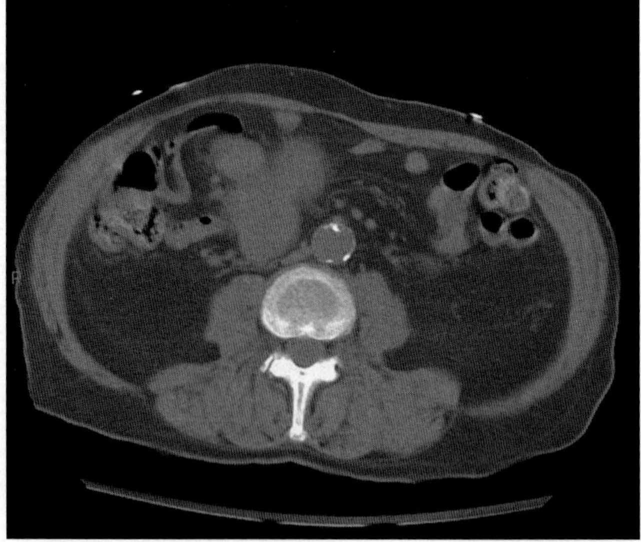

Figure 26.2B

CT Scan Report

A large, solid, well-circumscribed, multilobulated mass in the midabdomen in proximity to loops of small bowel with clear delineation from the retroperitoneal and psoas muscle. The distal ileum is in proximity to the lobulated mass.

Differential Diagnosis

Based on the clinical findings of a mobile abdominal mass, and with the computed tomography (CT) scan demonstrating a lobulated mass in proximity to the small bowel, this most likely represents a small bowel neoplasm. The abdominal mass is clearly delineated from the retroperitoneal structures; therefore, it is unlikely to be a retroperitoneal sarcoma. Though a large mesenteric cyst may present as a palpable abdominal mass, the solid nature on the CT scan would argue against this diagnosis. Given the clinical presentation and the accompanying imaging findings, a mesenchymal tumor of the small intestine is very likely.

Discussion

Leiomyomas, leiomyosarcomas, and gastrointestinal stromal tumors (GISTs) of the small intestine often enlarge with extraluminal orientation and thus may reach considerable, even palpable, size before causing symptoms. The mean duration of symptoms before diagnosis can be as long as 1 year. Unlike adenocarcinomas, these neoplasms tend to grow extrinsically and obstruct the small intestine late in their course. Obstruction occurs from external compression, and less commonly from circumferential growth, and very rarely from intussusception. A palpable abdominal mass may be evident in up to half of patients. Many of these tumors eventually outgrow their highly vascular blood supply, leading to central necrosis and occasional calcification that would be evident on a CT scan (although this was not present in the patient in this case). Due to their highly vascular nature and large size, ischemia within the tumor and areas of tumor necrosis are common, leading to hemorrhage in two thirds of patients, and intestinal perforation resulting in an acute abdomen in 10% of patients. The hemorrhage can be intra-abdominal, gastrointestinal, or within the tumor, leading to rapid enlargement in size.

Adenocarcinomas (accounting for 30% to 50% of all small bowel cancers) occur more frequently in the duodenum and the proximal jejunum. Adenocarcinomas almost always present with a slowly progressive intestinal obstruction; in contrast to leiomyosarcomas, a palpable mass or perforation is unusual. Primary carcinoid tumors (accounting for approximately 30% of small bowel tumors) are often 1 to 2 cm in size; however, when locally invasive, primary carcinoid tumors metastasize via regional lymph nodes and are often associated with fibrotic reaction that foreshortens the adjacent small bowel mesentery. This may cause kinking of the bowel and obstruction, or intestinal ischemia as a result of encasement of mesentery blood vessels.

Diagnosis and Recommendation

When the clinical features and imaging studies are suggestive of a small bowel GIST, an exploratory laparotomy is required for both diagnosis and treatment. In addition to the CT scan of the abdomen and pelvis, a radiograph or CT scan of the chest is obtained to exclude metastatic disease. Preoperative biopsy is unnecessary because it carries the theoretical risk of peritoneal seeding or tumor rupture; biopsy is indicated only for clearly unresectable disease, or when treatment would be altered (e.g., if the mass proved to be lymphoma or germ cell tumor).

Approach

Surgery is the mainstay of the therapeutic approach to patients with nonmetastatic GISTs. These tumors are resectable in two thirds of cases, on average, but present a high recurrence rate (40% to 90%), an overall survival rate ranging from 28% to 43%, and a median survival time of 50 months. At present, adjuvant radiation therapy has no role, because it does not have any impact on the natural history of these tumors; furthermore, any benefit is outweighed by the toxicity to the intra-abdominal structures. Radiation should be reserved for palliation of pain and bleeding.

Case Continued

The patient undergoes an exploratory laparotomy where a multilobulated mass is seen arising from the small bowel, with no invasion of adjacent organs. There is no palpable small bowel lymphadenopathy or liver metastasis. A complete en bloc resection of the tumor with a segmental small bowel resection with primary anastomosis is performed.

Intraoperative Images

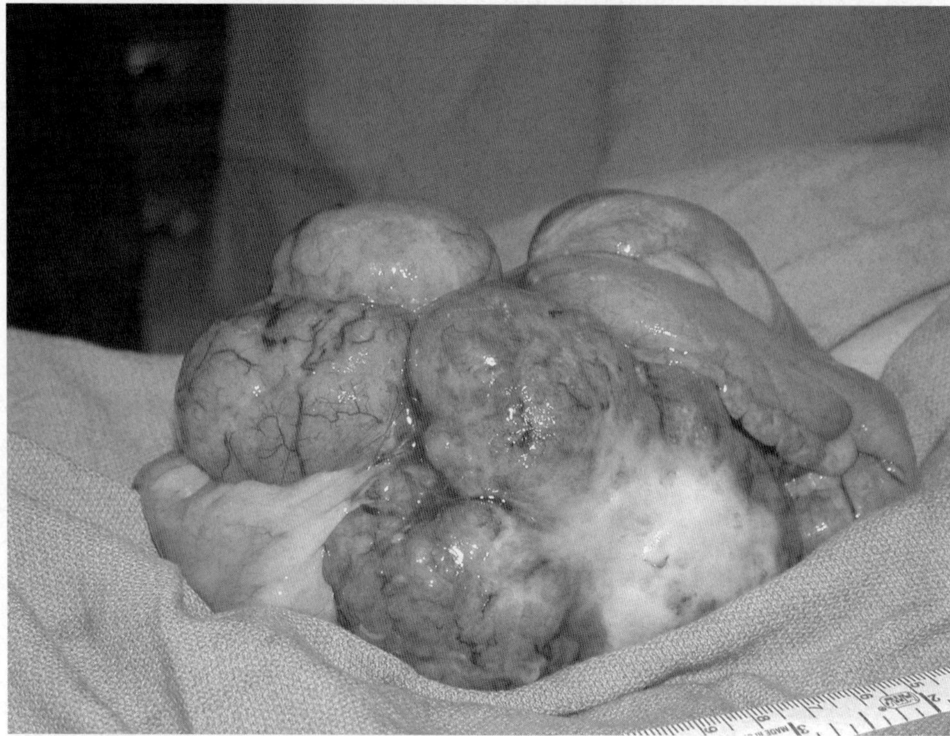

Figure 26.3A

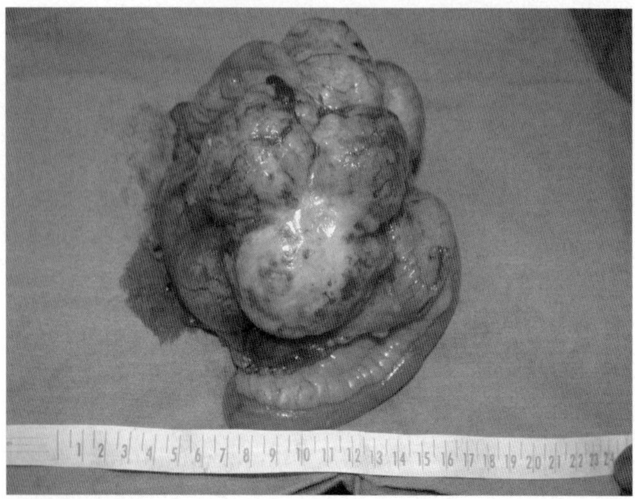

Figure 26.3B

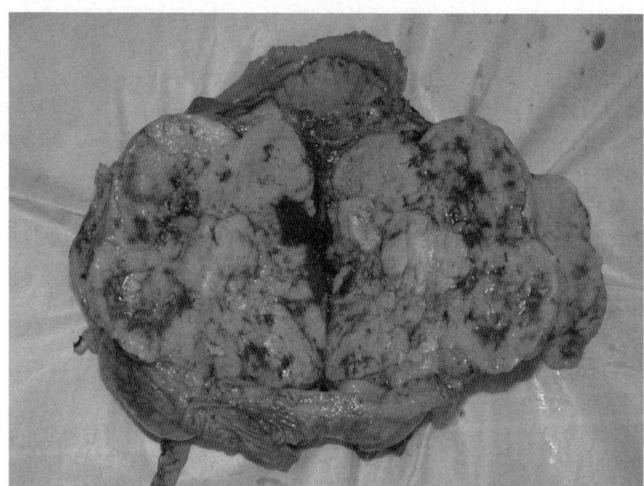

Figure 26.3C

Surgical Approach

Celiotomy is performed through a standard midline incision, which allows careful exploration and assessment of the extent of the disease. Meticulous handling of the tumor is imperative to avoid intraoperative tumor rupture, which has been demonstrated to be an independent adverse prognostic factor. Presence of liver metastasis should be evident from the preoperative CT scan of the abdomen; however, a careful bimanual palpation and biopsy of any suspicious lesion should be performed. Once distant metastases have been excluded, attention is directed toward performing a complete en bloc resection of the tumor with a margin of normal tissue. Most often, a wedge or a segmental resection of the adjacent organ is adequate, because GISTs tend to protrude from the tissue of origin and displace surrounding structures, unlike carcinomas, which are often locally infiltrative. An extensive mesenteric lymphadenectomy is not required in patients with GISTs because lymph node metastases are rare. The extent of surgery to produce complete resection does not appear to influence survival; however, the optimum width of the tumor-free margin remains to be defined.

Case Continued

Gross pathologic examination reveals a multilobulated 13-cm fleshy tumor with considerable surface vascularity. Histologic examination establishes a diagnosis of a small bowel GIST, with 5 to 10 mitoses per high-power field and negative surgical margins. The tumor stains strongly for the CD117 antigen. The tumor is also positive for CD34 and smooth muscle actin, but is negative for S-100.

Discussion

Despite adequate local surgery, more than two thirds of patients later present with recurrent intra-abdominal disease in the liver (50%), local disease (33%), or combined local and liver (19%) disease.

The lung is an uncommon site of metastasis. Less than one third of all recurrent cases are amenable to gross resection; median survival is approximately 15 months. Conventional chemotherapeutic agents have minimal activity in patients with metastatic GISTs, and radiation only serves to palliate symptoms. Knowledge that over 90% of GISTs expresses the C-KIT receptor has allowed investigators to target this tyrosine kinase with a specific inhibitor, imatinib mesylate (Gleevec). Imatinib is a powerful, yet relatively selective and competitive, inhibitor of tyrosine kinase by a mechanism that involves binding to the ATP site of the tyrosine kinase, thus preventing transfer of phosphate from the ATP to the tyrosine residues of the substrates. This inhibits downstream signaling from the tyrosine kinase, which thereby switches the balance toward reduced proliferation and increased apoptosis. In a U.S./Finnish study group, a partial response rate of 59% was noted, with stable disease experienced in 26%. Because complete responses have not been observed with imatinib therapy, patients with stable disease or partial responses should be considered for surgical resection or in situ reduction.

GISTs constitute less than 1% of gastrointestinal malignancies, with an annual incidence of 2,000 to 5,000 cases per year in the United States. The anatomic distribution of the tumors is as follows: stomach (60% to 70%), small bowel (20% to 30%), colon/rectum (10%), and esophagus (<5%). More than 95% of patients present with a solitary primary tumor, and two thirds of those in the stomach, small bowel, and colorectum are considered malignant. In 10% to 40% of cases, these tumors directly invade the surrounding organs.

It is important to differentiate between GISTs, which constitute about 80% of gastrointestinal mesancomal tumors, and the less common gastrointestinal nonepithelial neoplasms, such as leiomyomas, leiomyosarcomas (10% to 15% of mesenchymal tumors), and schwannomas (5%). Characteristically, GISTs stain strongly for the CD117 antigen, an epitope of the C-KIT receptor tyrosine kinase. Conversely, smooth leiomyomas, leiomyosarcomas, schwannomas, and desmoid tumors typically do not show this part of expression of CD117. Thus, CD117 immunostaining is an important method for diagnostic distinction. CD117 antigen is an epitope of the KIT-receptor tyrosine kinase.

KIT is a transmembrane tyrosine kinase, and binding of its natural ligand, stem cell factor, to the extracellular domain causes dimerization, and autophosphorylation of intracellular tyrosine residues, which creates docking sites for signal transduction molecules. The result is activation of a cascade of intracellular proteins that promote cell survival and proliferation. Mutation leads to ligand-independent dimerization, activation, and thus, uncontrolled cell proliferation. Activating mutations of KIT seem to have a central role in GIST pathogenesis.

Generally, almost all incidental GISTs are small (<1 cm) and are clinically benign, whereas tumors larger than about 5 cm in diameter are generally malignant. Apart from tumor size, the other morphologic feature that has emerged as a fairly reliable predictor of outcome is the mitotic rate. Based on these two predictive factors, the National Institutes of Health (NIH) consensus provided an approach for assigning risk for aggressive behavior in GISTs.

Table 26-1: Prognostic Criteria for GIST

Histopathology	Size	Mitosis
Benign	<5 cm	<1/10 HPF
Borderline	>5 cm	<1/10 HPF
Malignant	Any size	>1/10 HPF

HPF, high-power field.

Case Continued

The patient is carefully followed, and 1 year later, a CT scan is obtained for surveillance.

■ CT Scans and Histopathology Slide

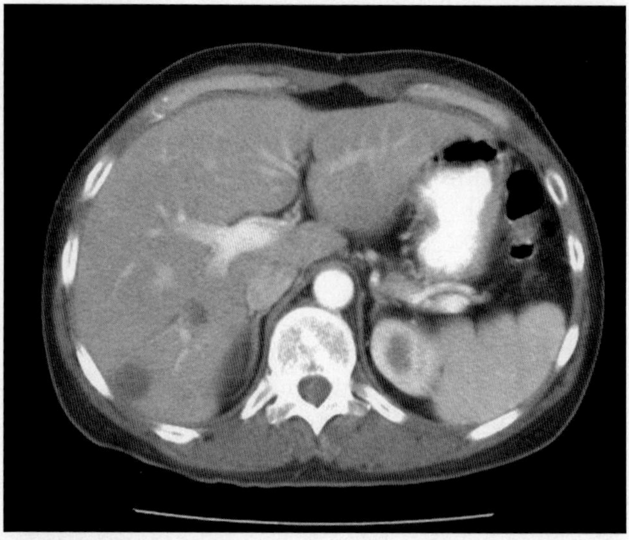

Figure 26.4C

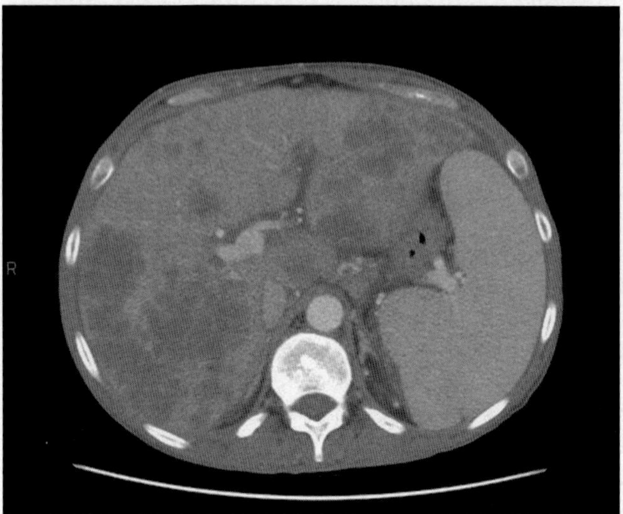

Figure 26.4A

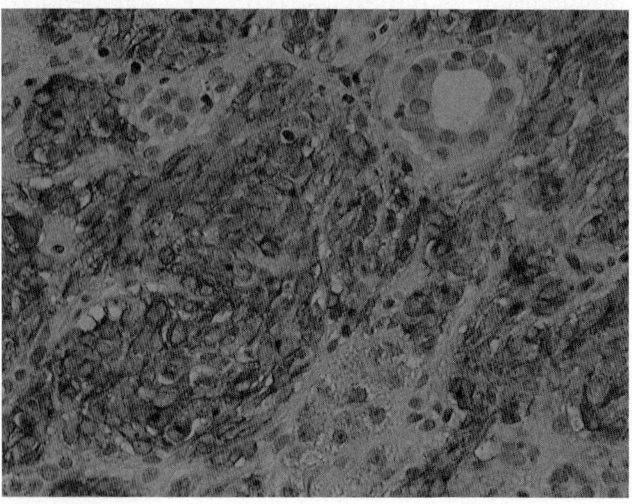

Figure 26.4B

CT Scan and Pathology Report

Multiple liver metastases are noted in both lobes. CT-guided biopsy shows metastatic GIST, which stained positive for CD117. Therefore, the patient was placed on imatinib mesylate at a daily dose of 400 mg, which resulted in a considerable reduction in the size and number of liver metastases. The patient is currently alive with the disease.

Suggested Readings

Clary BM, DeMatteo RP, Lewis JJ, et al. Gastrointestinal stromal tumors and leiomyosarcoma of the abdomen and retroperitoneum: a clinical comparison. *Ann Surg Oncol* 2001;8:290–299.

DeMatteo RP, Lewis JJ, Leung D, et al. Two hundred gastrointestinal stromal tumors: recurrence patterns and prognostic factors for survival. *Ann Surg* 2000;231:51–58.

Eisenberg BL. Imatinib mesylate: a molecularly targeted therapy for gastrointestinal stromal tumors. *Oncology (Huntingt)* 2003;17:1615–1620; discussion 1620, 1623, 1626 passim.

Fletcher CD, Berman JJ, Corless C, et al. Diagnosis of gastrointestinal stromal tumors: a consensus approach. *Hum Pathol* 2002;33:459–465.

Franquemont DW. Differentiation and risk assessment of gastrointestinal stromal tumors. *Am J Clin Pathol* 1995;103:41–47.

Pidhorecky I, Cheney RT, Kraybill WG, et al. Gastrointestinal stromal tumors: current diagnosis, biologic behavior, and management. *Ann Surg Oncol* 2000;7:705–712.

Presentation

An 11-year-old girl presents with acute appendicitis. An emergency appendectomy is performed, and an acutely inflamed, thickened, and perforated appendix is found. Macroscopic examination of the inflamed appendix reveals a solid tumor obstructing the proximal lumen with a maximum diameter of 14 mm.

Differential Diagnosis

The incidental finding of a tumor in an acutely inflamed appendix at histologic examination is a well-recognized presentation of an appendiceal carcinoid tumor. Carcinoid is regarded as the most common tumor of the appendix, though highly unusual in this age group. Postmortem studies have demonstrated a high incidence of appendiceal carcinoid (up to 1%) tumors that are not clinically apparent.

The pathologist should differentiate between benign and malignant carcinoid tumors. Benign carcinoids are no longer included in cancer registries. When considering primary malignancies of the appendix in all age groups (excluding benign carcinoids), mucinous adenocarcinomas are the most common (37%), followed by colonic-type adenocarcinomas (25%), malignant carcinoid tumors (20%), goblet cell carcinoids (adenocarcinoids; 14%), and rarely signet ring cell carcinomas (4%) (Surveillance, Epidemiology, and End-Results [SEER] Program data, 1973–1998).

Malignant carcinoids occur at a mean age of 38 years, and goblet cell carcinoids at 52 years, whereas adenocarcinomas occur at 60 years of age or later. Histologic examination of the removed appendix is performed.

Histopathology Slides

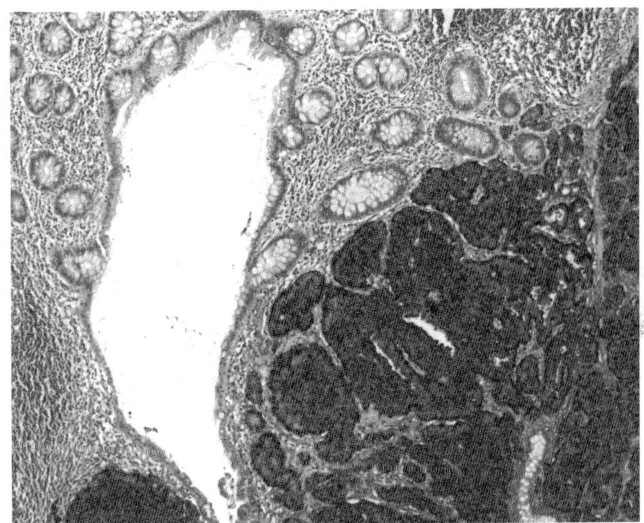

Figure 27.1

Histopathology Report

The morphological appearances on histology are those of a malignant carcinoid tumor. Immunohistochemistry confirms the diagnosis, with strong staining with chromogranin A (Fig. 27.1), synaptophysin, and serotonin. The tumor extends through the muscularis and serosa out to the surrounding fat and is present on the serosal surface. A distinct mesoappendix could not be identified, and it is not clear if the fatty infiltration constitutes mesoappendiceal involvement. The proximal resection margin is clear. No vascular invasion is identified.

Very few mitoses are seen, and the cycling rate using Ki67/MIB-1 is less than 3%. Ki67 staining demonstrates the low cycling index of the tumor cells and the higher proliferation index of the normal mucosal cells.

Diagnosis

A 14-mm appendiceal neuroendocrine tumor with carcinoid features.

Discussion

Carcinoid tumors are neuroendocrine tumors originating from endodermal neuroendocrine cells. These cells originate from the same progeny cells as other gastrointestinal cells and are endogenous to the gut, producing important gut hormones such as serotonin and gastrin.

Appendiceal carcinoid tumors used to be regarded as the most common appendiceal tumor, with a prevalence of up to 0.9% in patients undergoing appendectomy. However, because a large proportion of these lesions do not demonstrate any malignant features, reporting tendencies and inclusion in cancer registry databases have changed. Recent data show that appendiceal carcinoids represented only 2.43% of the 4,989 carcinoid tumors diagnosed between 1992 and 1999, compared to 44% of the 1,867 carcinoid tumors registered between 1950 and 1969. True malignant carcinoid tumors of the appendix, therefore, have become an extreme rarity. It remains important, however, to deal appropriately with a pathology report of an incidental carcinoid tumor in an appendix specimen, because these are still common.

Malignant carcinoids present most commonly at a mean age of 38 years, although earlier diagnoses of smaller "benign" lesions occur commonly in teenagers and those in their early twenties.

A female predominance is still evident, although not as pronounced as originally thought. Asymptomatic carcinoids may be found coincidentally at laparoscopy for pelvic disease in women; however, even when this is taken into account, a true higher incidence is still evident in females.

Carcinoid tumors of the appendix present as an asymptomatic incidental finding in up to 60% of cases, and very rarely present with metastases. Luminal obstruction may result in acute appendicitis, although this is not common because two thirds are located at the tip of the organ.

Goblet cell carcinoids, or adenocarcinoids, are a distinctly different and rare variant of carcinoid tumors. They originate from pluripotent cells that differentiate into both mucinous and neuroendocrine cells, and behave very differently from typical carcinoids.

Recommendation

Further investigations to determine the extent of disease should be performed because presence of systemic disease may alter the preoperative and surgical approaches.

Case Continued

A computed tomography (CT) scan of the abdomen is normal and demonstrates no evidence of intraabdominal, mesenteric lymph node, or liver metastases. Serum chromogranin A levels are within normal limits, and 24-hour urinary 5-hydroxyindoleacetic acid (5-HIAA) secretion is not increased. At this stage of investigation, with no evidence of systemic metastases and given the patient's young age, an octreotide scan is not performed.

Approach

Due to the proximal location on the appendix, the intermediate size, and the infiltration into adjacent fat, a right hemicolectomy is advised.

Discussion

The surgical management of appendiceal carcinoid tumors is based primarily on tumor size, histologic subtype, and mesoappendiceal involvement.

Tumors less than 1 cm in diameter require no further treatment after complete resection with an appendectomy.

Lesions between 1 and 2 cm in the distal appendix, with typical carcinoid histology, no angiolymphatic or mesoappendiceal invasion, and a low proliferative index will generally not require further surgery because the metastatic risk is low.

Other factors that may influence decision making when the lesion is between 1 and 2 cm include positive resection margins and location at the base of the appendix. Tumor features that should also be taken into account are raised mitotic or Ki67 indices (indicative of high-grade malignant carcinoids), mucin production, angioinvasion, and goblet cell carcinoids. Patient factors may also influence management, because the risk of metastatic disease overall is regarded as low. In younger patients, one may prefer surgery, whereas in patients with associated comorbid conditions, the risks of a right hemicolectomy may be regarded as unacceptable.

Lesions larger than 2 cm have a significant risk for metastasis, and warrant a right hemicolectomy. Because appendiceal carcinoids usually spread primarily by the lymphatic route, an oncological resection is indicated.

Surgical Approach

A right hemicolectomy is performed through a midline incision. After mobilization of the cecum, ascending colon, and hepatic flexure, the vascular pedicles (ileocolic branch of the superior mesenteric and right colic vessels) are transected and ligated. Attention is paid to identifying the right ureter and the second part of the duodenum. An ileocolic hand-sewn or side-to-side stapled anastomosis is performed. Hemostasis is achieved and the abdomen is closed.

Case Continued

Histologic examination of the right hemicolectomy specimen demonstrates no residual carcinoid tumor in the appendicular stump or cecum. There is no evidence of lymph node metastases.

The patient recovers well with no postoperative complications. Follow-up serum chromogranin A and 24-hour urinary 5-HIAA screen are all negative. CT scan of her liver at 1-year follow-up demonstrates no evidence of metastases.

Discussion

Recurrence in this case in highly unlikely, and this may well be said for the vast majority of appendiceal carcinoid tumors smaller than 2 cm in diameter. Carcinoid tumors may be indolent and slow growing; however, those that do metastasize are often more aggressive and often behave like true carcinomas.

In all reported series of appendiceal carcinoid tumors, the significance of associated malignancies is noticeable. It is estimated that up to 18% of patients with appendiceal malignant carcinoids may develop or have coexisting neoplasms, the most common site being colorectal. The exact nature of this risk is unknown, but a high index of suspicion should prevail.

Treatment of advanced disease is generally considered to be as for other midgut carcinoid tumors, although limited evidence for tumors originating in the appendix is available.

Suggested Readings

Goede AC, Caplin ME, Winslet MC. Carcinoid tumor of the appendix. *Br J Surg* 2003;90:1317–1322.

McCusker ME, Cote TR, Clegg LX, et al. Primary malignant neoplasms of the appendix: a population-based study from the surveillance, epidemiology, and end-results program, 1973–1998. *Cancer* 2002;94:3307–3312.

Moertel CG, Weiland LH, Nagorney DM, et al. Carcinoid tumor of the appendix: treatment and prognosis. *N Engl J Med* 1987;317:1126–1701.

Sandor A, Modlin IM. A retrospective analysis of 1570 appendiceal carcinoids. *Am J Gastroenterol* 1998;93:422–428

Syracuse DC, Perzin KH, Price JB, et al. Carcinoid tumors of the appendix. Mesoappendiceal extension and nodal metastases. *Ann Surg* 1979;190:58–63.

case 28

Presentation

A 48-year-old man with no significant past medical history presents with a new-onset right inguinal hernia. Increasing abdominal distention was noted over approximately 1 year. He is taken to the operating room for a hernia repair under local anesthesia. As the hernia sac is opened, a large volume of mucoid fluid is released into the operative field.

Differential Diagnosis

The presence of profuse mucoid drainage from the abdominal cavity is highly suggestive of pseudomyxoma peritonei syndrome arising from an appendiceal epithelial tumor. This clinical entity has a perforated appendiceal adenoma or villous adenoma as its primary site. Hyperplastic polyps, adenomatous polyps, and villous polyps within the appendix that have resulted in an appendiceal perforation will also cause the pseudomyxoma peritonei syndrome. The mucus accumulations that are distributed in a characteristic fashion around the peritoneal cavity are referred to as adenomucinosis. Histologically, epithelial cells in single layers are surrounded by lakes of mucin. These epithelial cells show little atypia and absent mitosis, and result in mucinous tumor accumulations that follow the flow of peritoneal fluid within the abdomen and pelvis.

A second morphologic type of appendiceal epithelial cancer that may cause mucus ascites is the mucinous adenocarcinoma. This more invasive tumor type tends to involve the appendix diffusely. Also, Ronnett et al. in their histologic description of mucinous appendiceal tumors found a proportion of patients with pseudomyxoma peritonei syndrome with small foci of mucinous adenocarcinoma within the large volume of adenomucinosis. These tumors presented with the typical pseudomyxoma peritonei syndrome, but had a reduced prognosis similar to that of patients with mucinous carcinomatosis. Tumors with a predominant histology of adenomucinosis but foci (<5% of fields) of muci-nous adenocarcinoma are referred to as hybrid or intermediate histologic type.

Discussion

The most common symptom in both men and women with pseudomyxoma peritonei syndrome is a gradually increasing abdominal girth. In women, the second most common symptom is an ovarian mass, usually on the right side and frequently diagnosed during a routine gynecologic examination. In men, the second most common symptom is a new-onset hernia. The hernia sac is found to be filled by mucinous tumor. In both men and women, the third most common presenting feature is appendicitis. This is the clinical manifestation of rupture of an appendiceal mucocele that contains intestinal bacteria.

The most common varieties of epithelial malignancy within the appendix are mucinous adenomas or mucinous adenocarcinomas. Mucinous tumors from the appendix are many times more common than the intestinal type of adenocarcinoma. In contrast, only approximately 15% of colonic adenocarcinomas are of the mucinous variety. The preponderance of mucinous tumors is probably related to the high proportion of goblet cells within the appendiceal epithelium.

At the time of exploratory laparotomy or laparoscopy, it may be difficult or impossible to distinguish a mucinous tumor of the appendix from a benign mucocele. Both benign and malignant tumors of the appendix are likely to cause symptoms, and there may be mucin collections within the right lower quadrant or throughout the abdominopelvic space. Two features should be sought that will histopathologically separate tumors that are inconsequential with complete removal from those capable of causing death from progressive pseudomyxoma peritonei syndrome. The first is invasion through the appendiceal wall by neoplastic glands. The second is atypical epithelial cells found within the extra-appendiceal mucin collection. If these clinical features occur, the diagnosis of pseudomyxoma peritonei syndrome is made and aggressive treatments are required.

Diagnosis and Recommendation

Pseudomyxoma peritonei syndrome. Intraoperatively, the fluid in the sac of a new-onset hernia and the hernia sac should be sent for frozen section examination to determine if this represents a malignant process.

Case Continued

The hernia sac is sent for histopathologic examination and shows a low-malignant-potential mucinous tumor thought to be of gastrointestinal origin. The hernia sac is closed, results of paraffin-section permanent section are awaited, and postoperative computed tomography (CT) scans of the chest, abdomen, and pelvis are obtained.

CT Scans

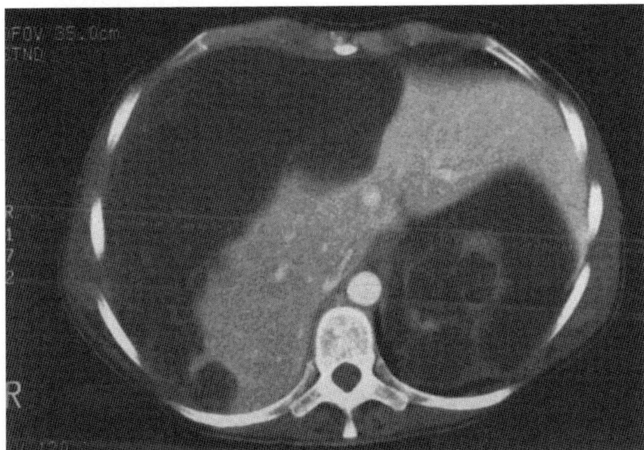

Figure 28.1A

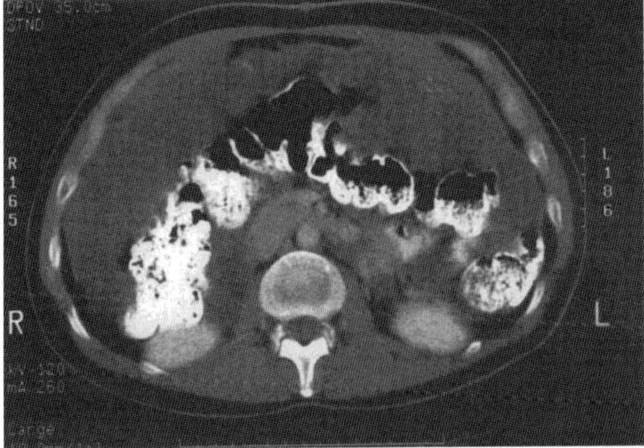

Figure 28.1B

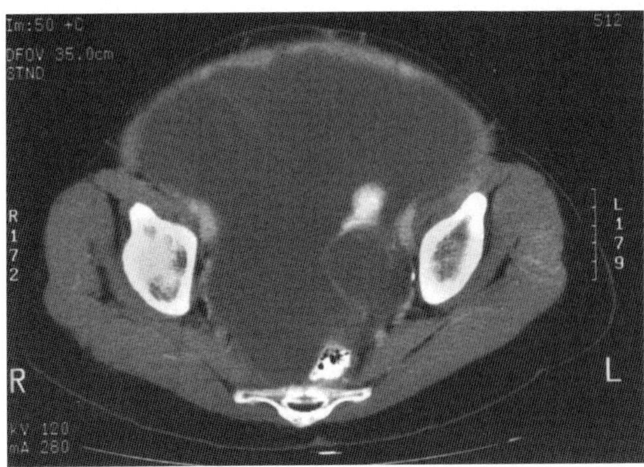

Figure 28.1C

CT Scan Report

The chest CT scan was normal. The abdominal CT scan showed mucoid tumor accumulation beneath the right and left hemidiaphragm. The mid-abdomen showed copious mucinous ascites, and the omentum was replaced by mucoid tumor (omental cake). The small bowel was displaced posteriorly and appeared to have normal function. The pelvic CT scan revealed that the pelvic structures were obscured by a large mass of mucinous tumor.

Approach

Due to the pattern of spread of pseudomyxoma peritonei, removal of the involved parietal and visceral peritoneal surfaces by visceral resections and peritonectomy procedures combined with intraperitoneal chemotherapy would be an appropriate option to provide this patient long-term, disease-free survival.

Discussion

In the pseudomyxoma peritonei syndrome, the peritoneal cavity becomes filled in a characteristic pattern with mucinous tumor and mucinous ascites. The greater omentum is greatly thickened (omental cake) and extensively infiltrated by tumor. The dependent parts of the abdomen that tend to accumulate malignant cells are also filled by tumor. Also, the undersurface of the right and left hemidiaphragms trap tumor cells moved along by the flow of intraperitoneal fluid. An important clinical feature of pseudomyxoma peritonei is the relative sparing of the small bowel by this process.

A caveat should be mentioned regarding the "benign mucocele" of the appendix. If a mucocele of the appendix is found during a planned laparoscopic appendectomy, then the laparoscopic procedure should be aborted and an open appendectomy should be performed. Laparoscopic resection of a mucocele is likely to cause rupture of that structure, and pseudomyxoma peritonei syndrome will then result within months or years.

A second caveat regarding the use of laparoscopy in patients with ascites must be noted. When a patient presents with increasing abdominal girth as a result of presumed malignant ascites, a paracentesis or laparoscopy with biopsy is usually performed to establish a diagnosis. In many female patients, an ovarian neoplasm will be found. In both women and men, a perforated adenocarcinoma from the colon, stomach, gallbladder, or appendix will be found. The remainder of these patients will have a peritoneal surface tumor such as peritoneal mesothelioma, papillary serous tumor, or mucinous peritoneal adenocarcinoma of unknown site. In all instances, paracentesis or laparoscopy with biopsy should be performed directly within the midline and through the linea alba. These sites can be excised as part of a midline abdominal incision. No lateral puncture sites or port sites should be used, because these will seed the abdominal wall with tumor and greatly interfere with disease eradication. Cytoreductive surgery and intraperitoneal chemotherapy are not effective for tumors within the abdominal wall.

Surgical Approach

The cytoreductive procedure begins by performing an exploration through a wide midline incision. A greater omentectomy and splenectomy followed by peritonectomy to strip tumor from the abdominal gutters, pelvis, right subhepatic space, and right and left subphrenic spaces are carefully undertaken. Any involved viscera are also resected. After the resection is completed, the peritoneal space are extensively irrigated and followed by heated mitomycin C intraperitoneal chemotherapy. A Tenchkoff catheter is placed for perioperative intraperitoneal 5-fluorouracil (5-FU) chemotherapy. The abdomen is closed, and the patient is monitored carefully for fluid management.

Intraoperative Images

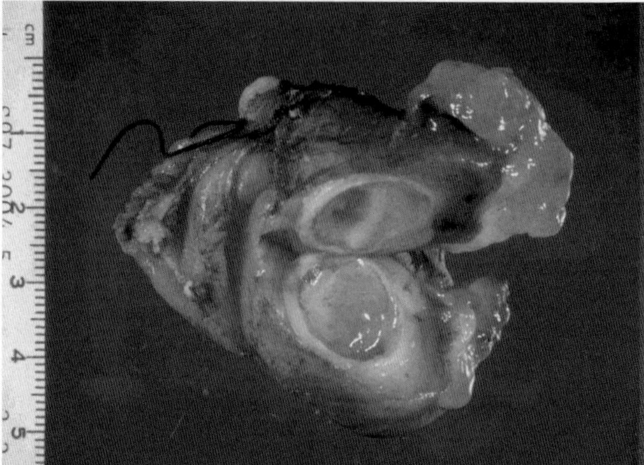

Figure 28.2A

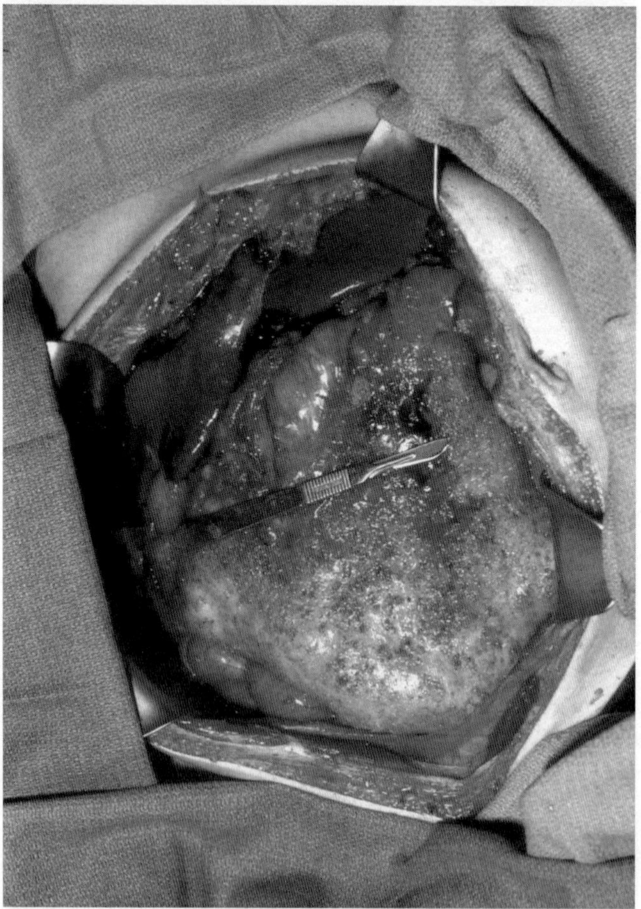

Figure 28.2B

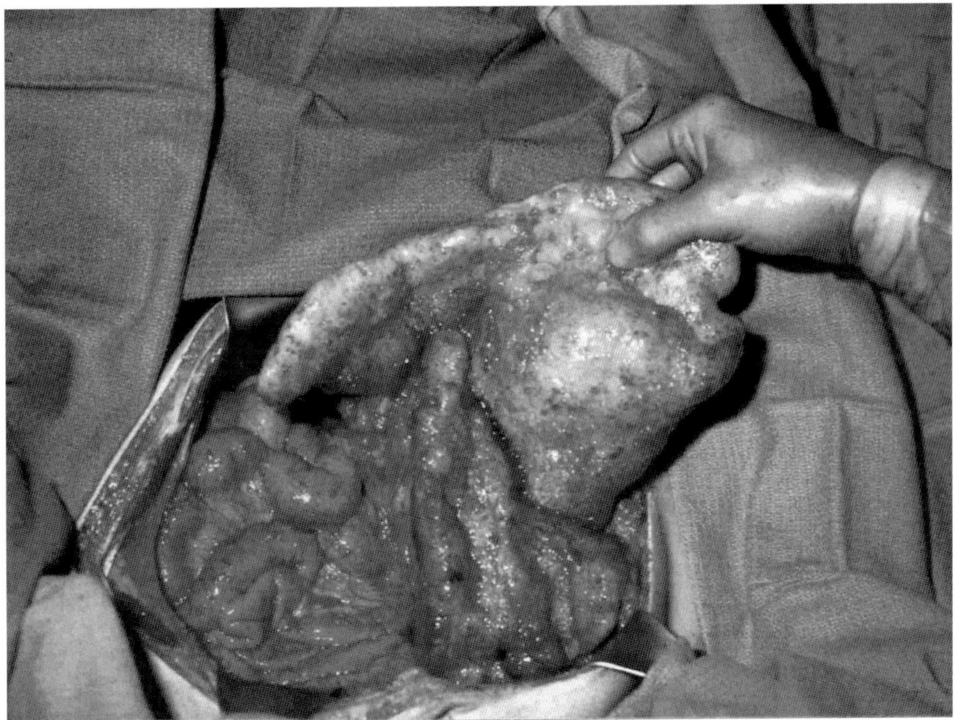

Figure 28.2C

Case Continued

During the cytoreductive surgery, as expected, omental caking was present and there was small bowel sparing. Peritonectomy was performed along with intraoperative warm mitomycin C intraperitoneal chemotherapy using the Coliseum technique, in which the skin edges are suspended on a self-retaining retractor and warm (41°C to 42°C) chemotherapy solution is perfused while being manually distributed throughout the abdomen and pelvis. Postoperatively, the patient is treated with perioperative 5-FU chemotherapy and recovers well without complications.

Discussion

A window of time exists in which all intraperitoneal surfaces are available for intraperitoneal chemotherapy utilizing 5-FU in the early postoperative period. Uniformity of treatment with intraperitoneal chemotherapy to all peritoneal surfaces, including those surfaces dissected by the surgeon, can be achieved if the intraperitoneal chemotherapy is used during the first postoperative week. As the chemotherapy is dwelling, distribution is facilitated by the patient turning alternately onto their right and left side as well as into the prone position.

This perioperative intraperitoneal chemotherapy (combination of heated intraoperative mitomycin C and early postoperative 5-FU) has been utilized in more than 750 patients, and has not been associated with an increased incidence of anastomotic disruptions. In patients who have had extensive prior surgical procedures, who require many hours of lysis of adhesions, there is an increased incidence of postoperative small bowel perforation. This is presumably a result of the combined effects of damage to small bowel from electrosurgical dissection of adhesions (seromuscular damage), and systemic effects of intraperitoneal chemotherapy on the intestine (mucosa and submucosal damage).

It is important that definitive treatment of peritoneal carcinomatosis or pseudomyxoma peritonei be instituted in a timely fashion. Each nondefinitive (debulking) surgical procedure makes potentially curative cytoreductive surgery more difficult. The relative sparing of the small bowel is only seen early in the natural history of peritoneal carcinomatosis and pseudomyxoma peritonei. After several surgical procedures have been performed, the fibrous adhesions that inevitably result become infiltrated by tumor. This leads to extensive involvement of the small bowel by the malignant process. Eventually it becomes impossible to cytoreduce the tumor safely, and the effects of the intraperitoneal chemotherapy by itself are not adequate to keep the patient disease free.

Suggested Readings

Esquivel J, Sugarbaker PH. Clinical presentation of the pseudomyxoma peritonei syndrome. *Br J Surg* 2000;87:1414–1418.

Jacquet P, Averbach AM, Stephens AD, et al. Cancer recurrence following laparoscopic colectomy: report of two patients treated with heated intraoperative chemotherapy. *Dis Colon Rectum* 1995;38:1110–1114.

Ronnett BM, Shmookler BM, Sugarbaker PH, et al. Pseudomyxoma peritonei: new concepts in diagnosis, origin, nomenclature, and relationship to mucinous borderline (low malignant potential) tumors of the ovary. In: *Anatomic Pathology*. Chicago: ASCP Press; 1997:197–226.

Stephens AD, Alderman R, Chang D, et al. Morbidity and mortality of 200 treatments with cytoreductive surgery and hyperthermic intraoperative intraperitoneal chemotherapy using the Coliseum technique. *Ann Surg Oncol* 1999;6:790–796.

Sugarbaker PH. *Intraperitoneal Chemotherapy and Cytoreductive Surgery: A Manual for Physicians and Nurses.* 3rd ed. Grand Rapids, MI: The Ludann Company; 1999.

Sugarbaker PH. Observations concerning cancer spread within the peritoneal cavity and concepts supporting an ordered pathophysiology. In: Sugarbaker PH, ed. *Peritoneal Carcinomatosis: Principles of Management.* Boston: Kluwer; 1996:79–100.

Sugarbaker PH. Peritonectomy procedures. *Ann Surg* 1995;221: 29–42.

Sugarbaker PH. Results of treatment of 385 patients with peritoneal surface spread of appendiceal malignancy. *Ann Surg Oncol* 1999;6:727–731.

Presentation

An 80-year-old woman presents to your office with a 4-month history of change in bowel habit: dark red blood per rectum following defecation. On several occasions, the patient noticed that the blood was mixed with the stool and was associated with mucus discharge. She has no tenesmus, fecal urgency, or weight loss, and no family history of colon cancer. She suffers from hypertension and is taking an oral anticoagulant for atrial fibrillation. On examination the abdomen is soft with no palpable masses. Rectal examination is unremarkable, rigid sigmoidoscopy shows normal rectal mucosa, and anoscopy reveals small first-degree hemorrhoids.

Differential Diagnosis

The differential diagnosis for bleeding per rectum in an adult includes hemorrhoidal disease, fissure-in-ano, inflammatory bowel disease, rectal or colonic polyp, large bowel malignancy, diverticular disease, and colonic angiodysplasia. In this patient, with symptoms of mixed altered blood and mucus per rectum, one must exclude colorectal malignancy and benign polyps.

Case Continued

Following full bowel preparation and cessation of the oral anticoagulant 3 days prior to the procedure, an outpatient colonoscopy is performed. Good views are obtained to the cecum, which was identified by the presence of the ileocecal valve.

▧ Colonoscopic Image

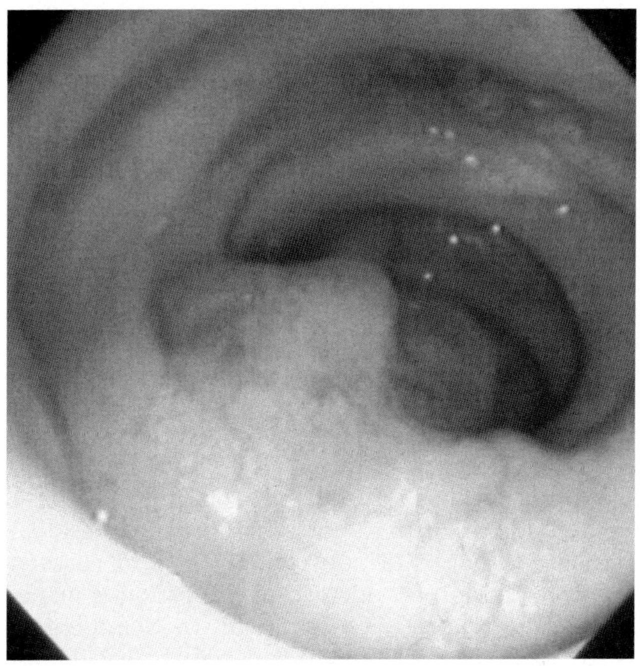

Figure 29.1

Colonoscopy Results

Three polyps are present. The most proximal polyp is 25 cm from the anal verge and is broad based, appearing to occupy up to one third of the circumference of the bowel and measuring 30 mm in size.

Case Continued

Using submucosal infiltration with India ink, the polyp base is elevated off the muscularis propria and snared in three pieces. The two additional polyps, measuring 4 mm each, in the proximal sigmoid colon are snared and retrieved.

Histologic examination of the two smaller polyps reveals moderately dysplastic tubular adenomas. The larger lesion is a tubulovillous adenoma with a focus of moderately differentiated adenocarcinoma infiltrating into the submucosa, reaching within 1 mm of the deep resection margin. There is no evidence of lymphovascular or perineural invasion.

Recommendation

To determine disease stage, obtain a chest x-ray and computed tomography (CT) scans of the abdomen and pelvis. If the chest x-ray shows any abnormality, then further evaluation can be performed with CT scan of the chest.

Case Continued

In this patient, CT scans of the chest, abdomen, and pelvis are obtained to exclude evidence of metastatic disease. There was a small area of scarring in the left lung, the liver was normal, and there was no evidence of abdominal or pelvic lymphadenopathy.

Approach

The risk of death, based on the patient's comorbidity, for oncologic bowel resection is estimated to be on the order of 5%. The risk of lymph node metastases is calculated to be 7.2% based on the St. Mark's Lymph Node Positivity model. The risk of residual tumor is thought to outweigh the risk of surgery, and the decision for open radical resection is made. Radiation therapy has no place in the treatment of early malignant colonic polyps, and the role of chemotherapy as an adjuvant treatment for endoscopically resected colonic polyps is doubtful. In patients with carcinoma near the margins, follow-up endoscopic examination every 6 months is necessary for at least 5 years.

Surgical Approach

It is critical that the tumor is completely removed together with the regional lymph nodes up to the root of the inferior mesenteric artery. Under a general anesthetic, the patient is placed in the Lloyd Davies position to allow the distal rectum to be washed out prior to the anastomosis. The abdomen is entered through a lower midline incision and a complete exploration is performed to exclude liver metastases and locally advanced disease. The sigmoid, descending colon, and splenic flexure are mobilized along the "white line" of Toldt, in the plane anterior to the gonadal vessels and left ureter, which are identified and preserved. A sigmoid colectomy is performed by dividing the colon at the rectosigmoid junction and proximally at the level of the descending colon. A stapled end-to-end colorectal anastomosis is performed and tested under water by air insufflation through the rectum.

Case Continued

The patient has an uneventful recovery and is discharged home on the seventh postoperative day.

Histopathology Slide

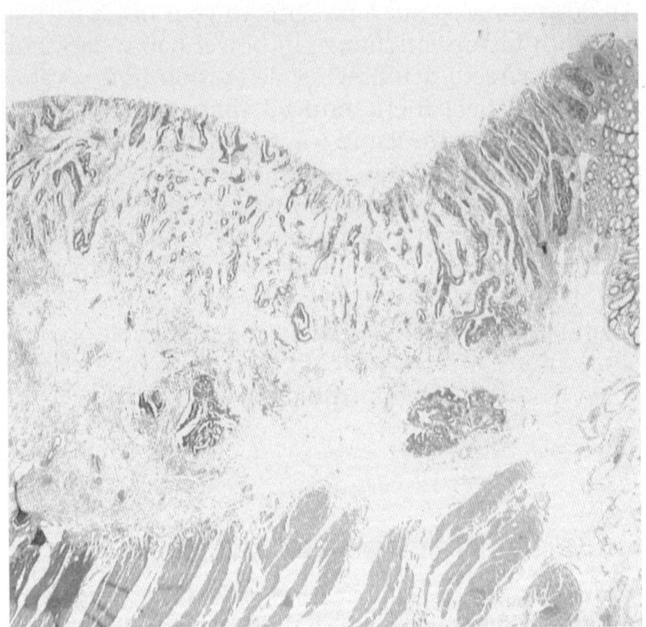

Figure 29.2

Histopathology Report

Histologic examination of the resected specimen reveals a focal area of residual moderately differentiated adenocarcinoma, which extends to the middle third of the submucosa (Haggitt level 4, Sm2). There is no evidence of vascular or perineural invasion, and none of the 13 lymph nodes examined contained tumor.

Discussion

The incidence of malignancy in colorectal adenomas increases with the diameter of the polyp: 2% for adenomas 0.6 to 1.5 cm, 19% for adenomas 1.6 to 2.5 cm, 43% for adenomas 2.6 to 3.5 cm, and 76% for adenomas larger than 3.5 cm. Malignant polyps of the colon and rectum can be broadly classified as pedunculated or sessile.

The risk for lymph node metastases is dependent on the depth of submucosal invasion, for sessile lesions, and on the morphological classification proposed by Haggitt et al. in 1985, for pedunculated polyps. The risk for lymph node metastases for Haggitt level 1, 2, or 3 is less than 1%, and for level 4 pedunculated lesions it is similar to that of the sessile lesions. Haggitt level 4, in which the invasion is into the base of the pedunculated polyp, has a risk for lymph node metastasis on the order of 12% to 25%. Kikuchi et al. reported no lymph node metastases among patients with Sm1 cancers, 5% for Sm2 lesions, and 25% for Sm3 lesions. Information on the adverse factors for lymph node metastases vary among authors because most studies have small numbers of patients, and many only use univariate analyses. In general, involvement of the muscularis propria (T_2), inadequate excision (within 1 mm of the resection margin), the presence of lymphovascular invasion, poor differentiation, and lesions sited in the lower third of the rectum have been reported as risk factors for lymph node metastases.

In our experience, the likelihood of lymph node metastases, based on histopathologic data collected from 303 early malignant lesions of the rectum (T_1 and T_2), is similar for all Sm levels (12.1% to 14.3%) of submucosal invasion and higher for T_2 lesions (19.9%). Poorly differentiated lesions are associated with a higher risk of lymph node metastases in comparison with well-differentiated lesions (45.0% vs. 8.3%). Similar rates were recorded for lesions with extramural (62.5%) or intramural (22.5%) vascular invasion compared with no vascular invasion (15.5%, $p = 0.002$). Cooper et al. also observed that, among 140 polyps examined, the high risk in poorly differentiated lesions coexisted with other unfavorable features, such as tumor at or near the resection margins and/or lymphatic and/or venous invasion. Patients with unfavorable histologic features had a higher rate of local recurrence or lymph node metastases, in comparison with patients with no risk factors (19.7% versus 0%). In contrast to these findings, Nascimbeni et al., in a cohort of 353 patients with sessile T_1 colorectal lesions, found that the degree of tumor differentiation was associated with lymph node metastases only on univariate analysis but not on multivariate analysis. Independent predictors of lymph node involvement were Sm3 lesions ($p = 0.001$), lymphovascular invasion ($p = 0.005$), and the location of the tumor in the lower third of the rectum ($p = 0.007$). The latter is in agreement with recent authors reporting high recurrence rates (5% to 28%) after transanal full-thickness resection of malignant polyps despite favorable parameters. Other risk

Table 29.1: Classification systems for the depth of invasion of pedunculated and sessile polyps in the colon and rectum.

Haggitt Classification (Pedunculated Polyps)

Level 0	Carcinoma in situ or intramucosal carcinoma, not invasive
Level 1	Carcinoma invading through the muscularis mucosa into the submucosa but limited to the head of the polyp
Level 2	Carcinoma invading the level of the neck of the adenoma
Level 3	Carcinoma invading any part of the stalk
Level 4	Carcinoma invading into the submucosa of the bowel wall below the stalk of the polyp but above the muscularis propria

St Mark's Classification (Sessile Polyps)

Sm1	Invasion into the upper third of the submucosa (200–300 μm)
Sm2	Invasion into the middle third of the submucosa
Sm3	Invasion into the lower third of the submucosa near the inner surface of the muscularis propria

Data from Haggitt RC, Glotzbach RE, Soffer EE, et al. Prognostic factors in colorectal carcinomas arising in adenomas: implications for lesions removed by endoscopic polypectomy. *Gastroenterology* 1985;89:328–336, and St Mark's Lymph Node Positivity Model. Available at: www.riskprediction.org.uk/index-lnp.php. Accessed July 20, 2004.

factors such as age, size of tumor, extent of residual adenoma, and histologic type (mucinous vs. nonmucinous lesions) did not seem to have any adverse prognostic significance.

In view of the low risk for lymph node metastases, pedunculated lesions of Haggitt levels 1, 2, and 3 may be safely removed by complete endoscopic polypectomy provided there are no adverse prognostic factors. Level 4 pedunculated lesions should be treated as sessile lesions, and their risk for lymph node metastasis is dependent on the polyp size, depth of invasion, tumor grade, and the presence of lymphovascular and perineural invasion. Sessile Sm1 or Sm2 lesions of less than 2 cm in diameter, which are well differentiated with no evidence of vascular or perineural invasion, may be adequately snared endoscopically. Sessile or pedunculated lesions with adverse prognostic factors (i.e., Sm3 level of submucosal invasion, poor differentiation, larger than 2 cm diameter, vascular or perineural invasion, or uncertain margin involvement) should be considered for radical bowel resection. In borderline cases, such as Sm2 lesions with moderate differentiation, the risk for lymph node metastasis should be balanced against the risk for postoperative mortality following radical bowel resection. The patient should be given the risks and benefits of each alternative treatment in order to make an informed choice of the type of treatment received.

Suggested Readings

Bowley DM, Tekkis PP, Sadat, et al. Depth of tumor invasion and lymph node positivity: implications for local excision of rectal cancer. *Colorectal Dis* 2004;6(suppl 1):2.

Cooper HS, Deppisch LM, Gourley WK, et al. Endoscopically removed malignant colorectal polyps: clinicopathologic correlations. *Gastroenterology* 1995;108:1657–1665.

Haggitt RC, Glotzbach RE, Soffer EE, et al. Prognostic factors in colorectal carcinomas arising in adenomas: implications for lesions removed by endoscopic polypectomy. *Gastroenterology* 1985;89:328–336.

Kikuchi R, Takano M, Takagi K, et al. Management of early invasive colorectal cancer. Risk of recurrence and clinical guidelines. *Dis Colon Rectum* 1995;38:1286–1295.

Nascimbeni R, Burgart LJ, Nivatvongs S, et al. Risk of lymph node metastasis in T1 carcinoma of the colon and rectum. *Dis Colon Rectum* 2002;45:200–206.

Nivatvongs S. Surgical management of malignant colorectal polyps. *Surg Clin North Am* 2002;82:959–966.

Nusco G, Mansmann WO, Artzsch W, et al. Invasive carcinoma in colorectal adenomas: multivariate analysis of patients and adenoma characteristics. *Endoscopy* 1997;29:626–631.

St Mark's Lymph Node Positivity Model. Available at: www.riskprediction.org.uk/index-lnp.php. Accessed July 20, 2004.

Tekkis PP, Thompson MR, Poloniecki JD, et al. Risk-adjusted postoperative mortality in colorectal cancer. *BMJ* 2003;327:1196–1201.

Presentation

A 62-year-old man presents with a recent episode of bright red blood per rectum. He denies any weight loss, anemia, obstructive symptoms, or change in bowel habits. There is no family history of colon carcinoma. The abdomen is soft with no apparent masses. Digital rectal examination reveals no palpable lesion. The patient undergoes a colonoscopy.

Colonoscopic Images

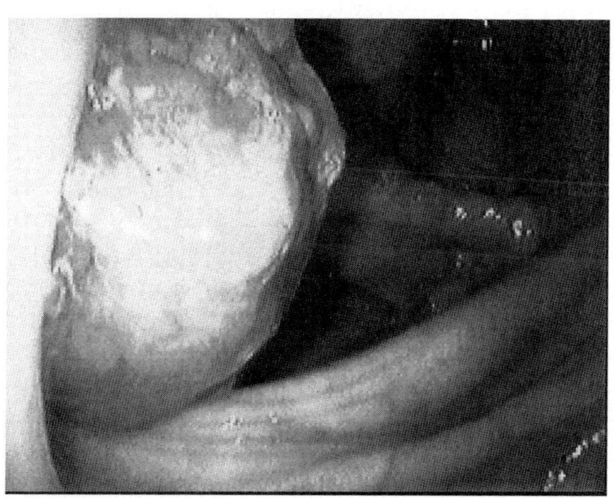

Figure 30.1

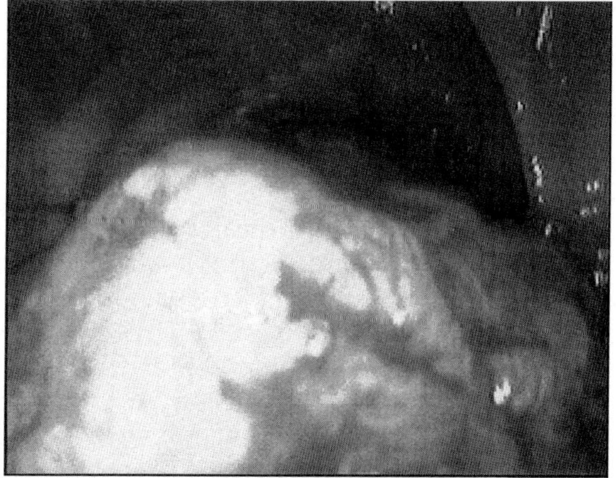

Figure 30.2

Colonoscopy Report

A sessile multilobulated 4-cm polyp is found in the ascending colon. The polyp is not amenable to complete polypectomy; therefore, piecemeal polypectomy is attempted. The site of the polyp is marked with 1 mL of India ink; no other polypoid lesions are identified.

Pathology Report

Tubulovillous adenoma with foci of moderately differentiated adenocarcinoma.

Differential Diagnosis

The differential diagnosis for early colon carcinoma is adenomatous polyps of the colon. The risk of adenocarcinoma arising in these polyps is relative to the size of the polyp. A sessile lesion has a greater risk of malignancy than a pedunculated polyp. In this patient, with a large sessile polyp, adenocarcinoma in an adenomatous polyp is highly probable.

Discussion

Colonoscopy is regarded as the most effective screening modality for the detection of early colon carcinoma. It enables a visualized surveillance of the entire colon as well as biopsy or removal of grossly abnormal lesions. Synchronous or metachronous carcinoma can also be excluded during this procedure.

It is generally accepted that the majority of colorectal cancer tracks an adenoma-carcinoma sequence. An adenoma smaller than 1 cm has an approximately 1% risk of malignancy. Conversely, polyps larger than 2 cm have a 35% to 50% incidence of associated carcinoma. The histologic presentation of adenomatous polyps consists of tubular, tubulovillous, and villous. The malignant potential augments with increased villous glandular formation. The malignant potential also correlates with histologic degree of dysplasia. Polyps with severe dysplasia have about a 50% incidence of malignancy. Other adverse risk factors of malignant polyps are lymphovascular invasion, poorly differentiated or mucinous adenocarcinoma, tumor budding, a flat or depressed lesion, and depth of tumor invasion into the lower third of the submucosal level, although these characteristics may be difficult to determine.

Sessile polyps have a reportedly higher incidence of lymph node metastasis than pedunculated polyps, ranging from 12% to 25%. Therefore, sessile polyps often require more aggressive surgical treatment for curability than pedunculated polyps.

Diagnosis and Recommendation

Adenocarcinoma within a tubulovillous adenoma. Computed tomography (CT) scan is recommended to assess the presence of clinically undetectable distant metastases as well as for staging of the primary lesion. Carcinoembryonic antigen (CEA) level may be useful in assessment of prognosis, early recurrence, and depth of invasion, although it has limited value in screening for colon cancer.

Case Continued

The patient has a serum CEA level of 1.49 ng/mL (normal level: 0 to 3.4) and CT scan with the following results. The liver, spleen, and kidney appear unremarkable. There is no retroperitoneal lymphadenopathy and no evidence of bowel obstruction.

Approach

The patient has an endoscopically irretrievable tubulovillous polyp with adenocarcinoma. There is no evidence of distant liver metastasis or regional lymphadenopathy. This patient is offered a laparoscopic colonic resection. The risks, benefits, and alternative procedures, including an open colectomy, are discussed prior to the surgery.

Surgical Approach

A 30-degree laparoscope is introduced using the Hasson technique with two to three subsequent ports inserted for instrumentation. The entire abdominal cavity must be inspected to determine curability and resectability. It is crucial to intraoperatively localize the tumor site. Preoperative tattoo marking is advisable because it allows extraluminal recognition of the anatomic location of the lesion. It is essential to perform sufficient mobilization of the right colon to extracorporealize the diseased segment with adequate resection margins. The speci-

men is exteriorized through a small midline incision with an extracorporeal anastomosis. Care must be taken to avoid potential tumor implantation throughout the surgery. A laparoscopic-assisted right hemicolectomy is performed without any complications. If at any time during the procedure difficulty is encountered, particularly in identifying important structures, or there are concerns regarding intra-abdominal injury, the procedure should be converted to an open one.

Discussion

Although laparoscopic colectomy has not been acknowledged as the standard management of colorectal cancer, it appears to be oncologically reasonable to perform laparoscopic resection from a technical standpoint. In the short term, it may provide advantages over conventional laparotomy, including less pain, lower incidence of postoperative ileus, shorter hospital stay, faster perioperative recovery, and superior cosmesis. Port site metastasis has been an issue in laparoscopic colon cancer surgery because small series of studies have reported incidences as high as 21%. However, recent prospective trials have revealed a less than 1% incidence of wound recurrence. This suggests that port site metastasis is associated with technical advances and surgeon experience and is associated with a learning curve. Recent clinical trials have reported similar or more favorable results regarding tumor recurrence and long-term survival with laparoscopic colectomy compared with conventional open colectomy, suggesting that the laparoscopic approach for colon cancer can be an alternative to open surgery from an oncologic perspective.

Case Continued

The patient tolerates the procedure well and the postoperative course is uneventful. His wound is clear and dry and the abdomen is not distended throughout the hospital stay. The patient is discharged on postoperative day 5.

The pathology report indicates invasive moderately differentiated adenocarcinoma arising in association with tubulovillous adenoma. The greatest dimension of the polyp is 3.5 cm. The tumor invasion is confined to the submucosa and is negative for vascular and lymphatic invasion. All pericolonic lymph nodes are negative for malignancy. Proximal and distal resectional margins are negative for metastasis.

Diagnosis

This patient is finally diagnosed with T1 N0, stage I colon carcinoma

Recommendation

The patient undergoes a curative resection. The local recurrence and survival rates following laparoscopic resection for stage I colon cancer have not been well estimated, while in several reported series, the recurrence rate is approximately 7% and the 3-year survival rate is 93%. At present, postoperative surveillance should include the following: a history and physical examination, CEA level measurement, colonoscopy, and chest x-ray. If there is suggestion of recurrence, diagnostic imaging, including CT or magnetic resonance imaging (MRI) scan, should be obtained. Positron emission tomography (PET) is the most current imaging modality that may be helpful in detecting recurrence for patients in whom other methods remain indeterminate.

Case Continued

A history and physical examination will be performed every 3 to 6 months for the first 3 years, and annually thereafter. This patient is scheduled for follow-up colonoscopy at 1 year, and then every 3 to 5 years thereafter.

Suggested Readings

Chorost MI, Datta R, Santiago RC, et al. Colon cancer screening: where have we come from and where do we go? *J Surg Oncol* 2004;85:7–13.

Clinical Outcomes of Surgical Therapy Study Group. A comparison of laparoscopically assisted and open colectomy for colon cancer. *N Engl J Med* 2004;350:2050–2059.

Longo WE, Johnson FE. The preoperative assessment and postoperative surveillance of patients with colon and rectal cancer. *Surg Clin North Am* 2002;82:1091–1108.

Nivatvongs S. Surgical management of malignant colorectal polyps. *Surg Clin North Am* 2002;82:959–966.

Paraskeva PA, Purkayastha S, Darzi A. Laparoscopy for malignancy: current status. *Semin Laparosc Surg* 2004;11:27–36.

Williams CB, Saunders BP, Talbot IC. Endoscopic management of polypoid early colon cancer. *World J Surg* 2000;24:1047–1051.

A 65-year-old woman with no significant past medical history presents to the emergency department with a several-week history of increasing abdominal pain, vomiting, distension, bloating, and worsening constipation. She admits to a 20-lb weight loss over the past 2 months.

Clinical Photograph

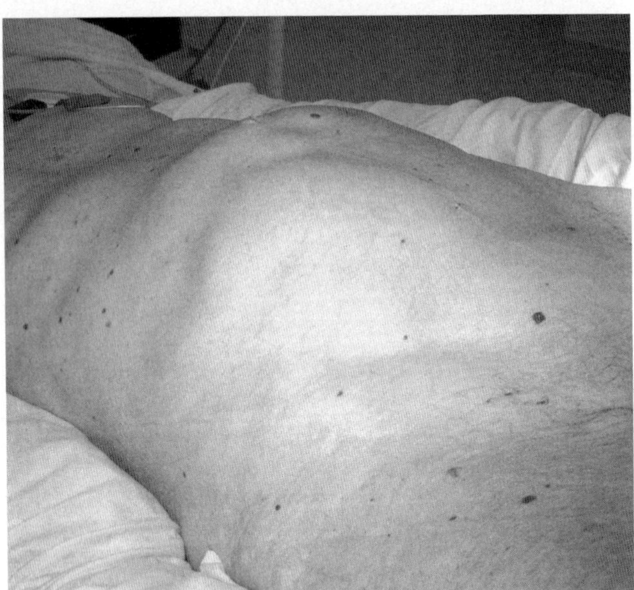

Figure 31.1

Abdominal X-Rays

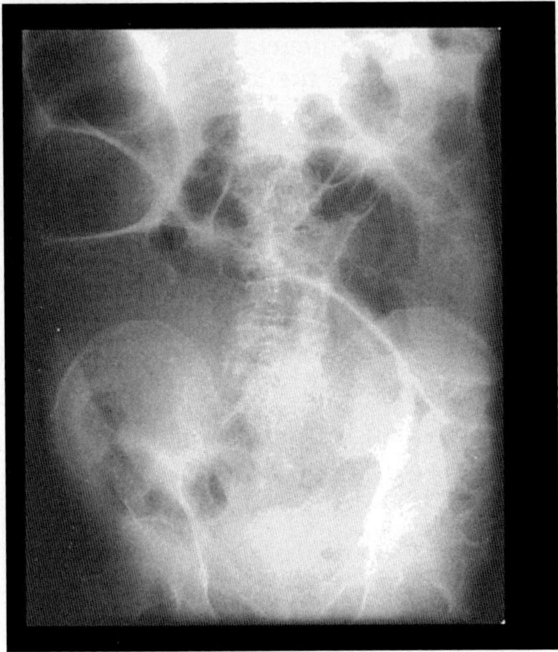

Figure 31.2A

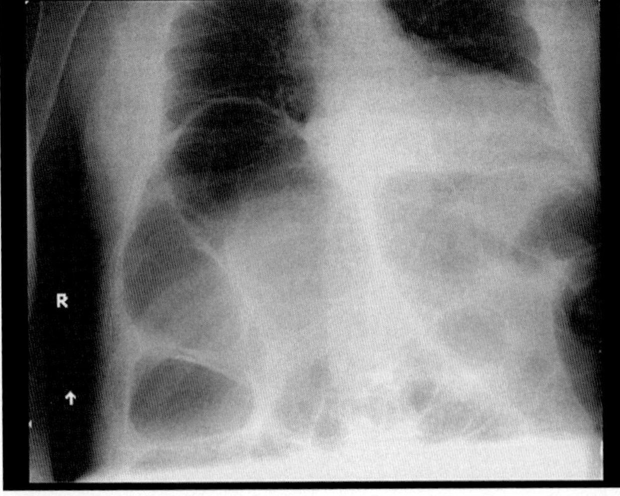

Figure 31.2B

Physical Examination Report

On physical examination, she has no tenderness but her abdomen is markedly distended. Her vital signs are normal and she is afebrile. She denies a family history of colon carcinoma or polyps and has never undergone a colonoscopy.

Abdominal X-Ray Report

Markedly dilated cecum and transverse colon.

Differential Diagnosis

The differential diagnosis of left-sided colonic obstruction includes carcinoma, incarcerated hernia, inflammatory bowel disease, extrinsic compression from noncolonic pathology (i.e., ovarian cancer), volvulus, fecal impaction, anastomotic stricture, colonic pseudo-obstruction, constipation with megacolon, intussusception, and stricture from diverticulitis or ischemic colitis. In this case, the insidious onset of symptoms over several weeks indicates a chronic process involving neoplasia, stricture, or megacolon. The most common cause (78%) of large bowel obstruction in adults is adenocarcinoma of the colon or rectum.

Discussion

Patients with chronic large bowel obstruction complain of pain, distension, and constipation over several weeks. The distension is progressive dilation of the proximal large bowel by the closed-loop obstruction formed by a competent ileocecal valve. Because of the chronicity of this process, ischemia and gangrene of the cecum in association with tenderness and leukocytosis are usually absent. Vomiting is a late manifestation accompanying complete obstruction or involvement of the small bowel. Peritonitis may result from perforation at the site of the obstruction or of the cecum.

An abdominal radiograph is a simple and effective method of diagnosing large bowel obstruction. The proximal colon is often distended with air and a cutoff is seen at the level of the obstruction. The next step is to determine the degree, partial versus complete, and location of the obstruction using a water-contrast enema (with Hypaque or Gastrografin). Partial obstructions are amenable to endoscopic dilation (for strictures), endoscopic stenting (for strictures or carcinoma), and preoperative bowel preparations. Complete obstructions require early surgical intervention for proximal decompression. Location with respect to right colon, left colon, or rectum is important in planning any therapeutic intervention. In addition, length of the obstruction and presence of mucosal irregularities give clues to the etiology and candidacy for stenting.

Following the water-soluble enema, a computed tomography (CT) scan is performed, which provides extraluminal information about the cause and nature of the obstruction and associated pathology, such as extrinsic compression, tumor size, presence of metastases, perforation, or signs of diverticulitis. However, if the patient requires an exploratory laparotomy, then a CT scan of the abdomen and pelvis is unnecessary because the time can be spent resuscitating. Any pathology present can be evaluated intraoperatively, and appropriate decisions can be made at that time.

Recommendation

Gastrografin enema; CT scan of the abdomen and pelvis.

Gastrografin Enema

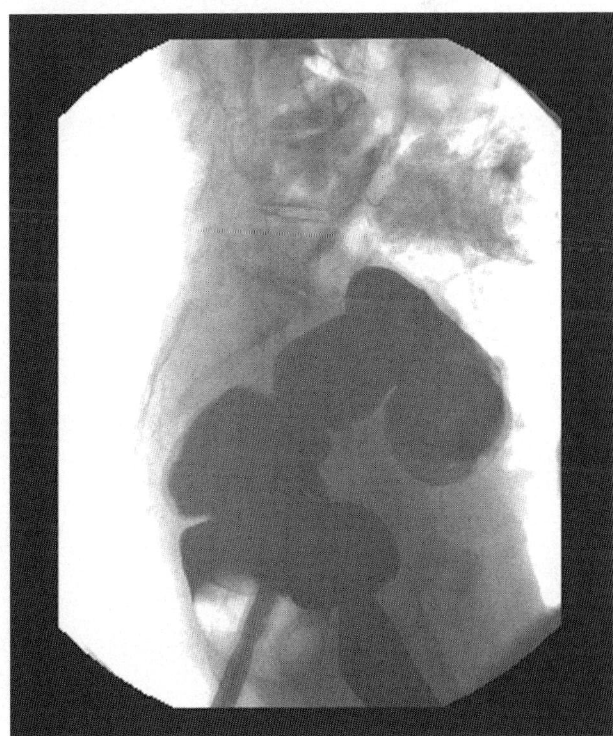

Figure 31.3

Gastrografin Enema Report

Complete obstruction of the sigmoid colon.

▌ CT Scan

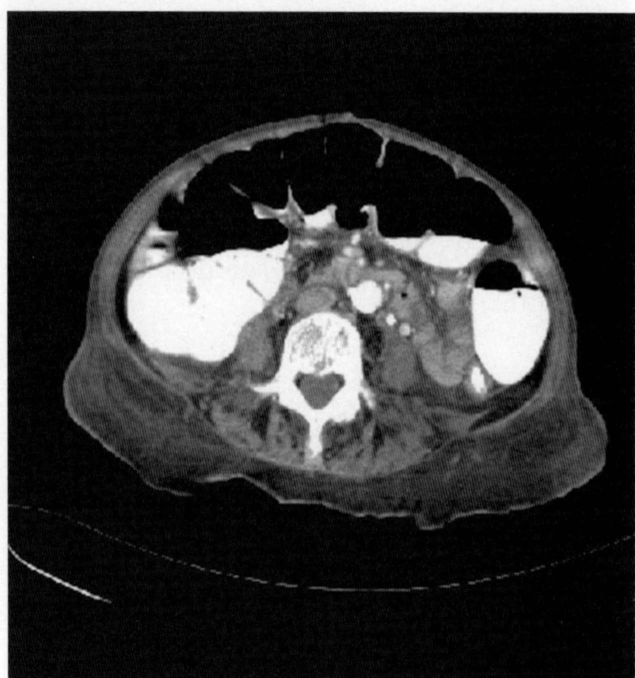

Figure 31.4A

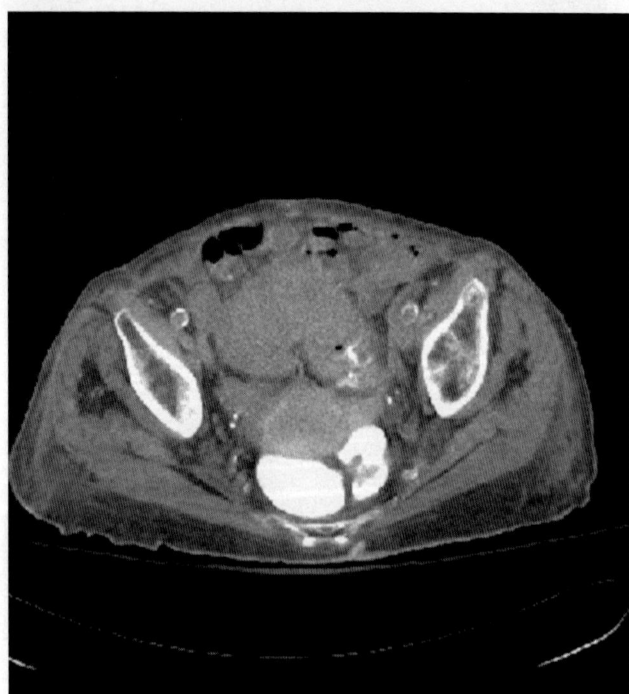

Figure 31.4B

CT Scan Report

The right and transverse colon are distended (see Fig. 31.4A). A 7-cm mass is identified in the sigmoid colon. The distal colon and rectum are decompressed. Thickening in the wall of an adjacent loop of small bowel is present anterior to the tumor. No identifiable plane can be discerned between the tumor and the adjacent lateral pelvic wall. The liver is normal.

Diagnosis and Recommendation

The patient has a completely obstructing colon carcinoma of the sigmoid colon with possible invasion into the small bowel and adjacent abdominal wall. Colonoscopy is unnecessary because the diagnosis is apparent on CT, and decompression with a colonic stent is only an option for partial high-grade colonic obstructions. Optimal treatment involves curative en bloc resection of the tumor with the secondarily involved structures, though the feasibility of a curative resection will be made at the time of surgery. At minimum, the obstruction requires proximal decompression, which can be accomplished with tube cecostomy or diverting ileostomy in patients with prohibitively high operative risk for more extensive procedures or who are found to have carcinomatosis.

▌ Surgical Approach

Surgical options include segmental resection with primary anastomosis, subtotal colectomy with primary anastomosis, segmental resection with colostomy, or segmental resection with primary anastomosis and proximal fecal diversion (loop colostomy or ileostomy). Because of the obstruction, this patient cannot undergo preoperative bowel preparation or colonoscopic evaluation of the proximal colon. Although on-table lavage is an option when segmental resection and anastomosis are considered, significant dilation of the proximal bowel and poor nutritional status associated with the recent weight loss in this patient preclude safe restoration of bowel continuity, with or without on-table lavage. Subtotal colectomy with ileosigmoid anastomosis would address the dilated proximal colon and any unidentified proximal lesions, but requires a more extensive procedure with associated risk of chronic diarrhea. In this patient, en bloc resection of the tumor with colostomy is planned. A preoperative carcinoembryonic antigen (CEA) level is obtained. An enterostomal therapist is consulted for preoperative counseling and stoma marking of both lower quadrants in preparation for a colostomy or diverting ileostomy. When an emergency surgery needs to be performed, an enterostomal therapist may not be available and the surgeon will need to assess the optimal site for possible stoma placement.

Case Continued

At exploration, no evidence of carcinomatosis or liver metastasis is identified. The tumor in the descending colon invades the small bowel and has perforated into the pelvic lateral sidewall. An abscess cavity is identified and evacuated. The tumor is mobilized en bloc by resecting a short portion of small intestine and a portion of the pelvic sidewall. A 1-cm margin of normal tissue is ensured circumferentially. The tumor does not grossly invade the kidney or ureter, and the integrity of the ureter is confirmed by lack of extravasation of indigo carmine after intravenous injection. A primary anastomosis of the small bowel is performed. Because of massive distension of the proximal large bowel, mobilization of the left colon and splenic flexure can be performed only after decompression of the transverse colon using a purse-string suture and soft rubber catheter. Once the bowel is mobilized, the descending colon containing the tumor is resected.

Operative Images

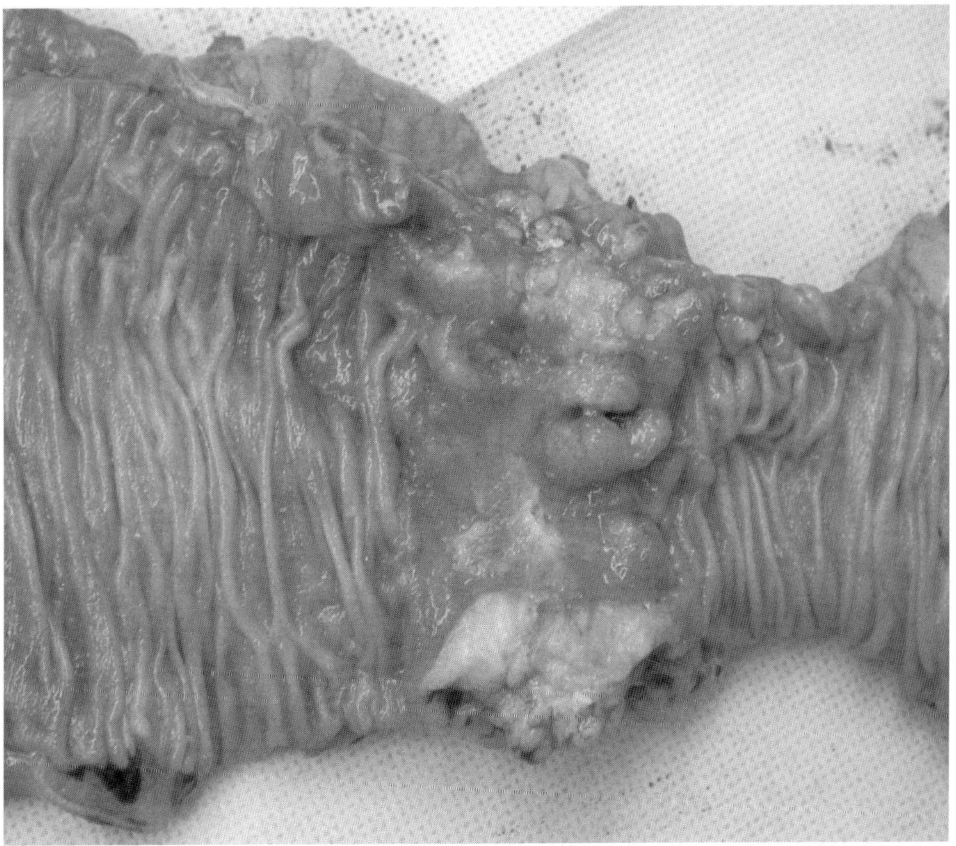

Figure 31.5A

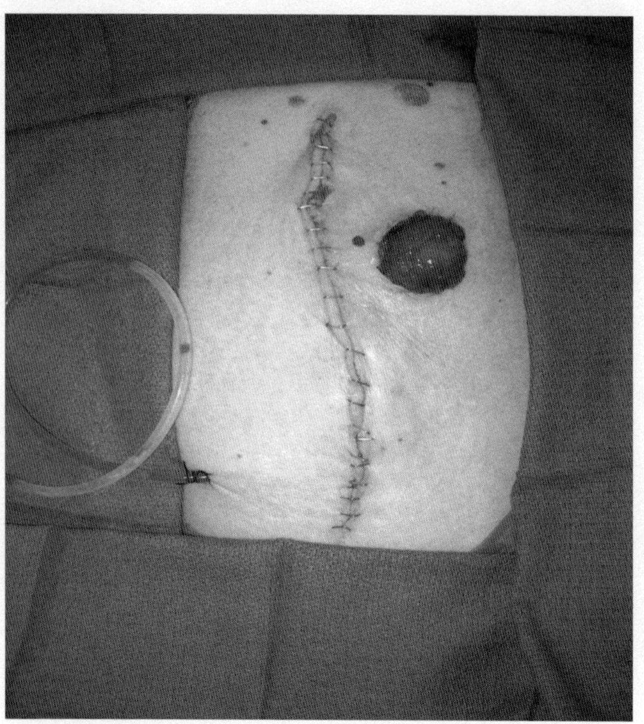

Figure 31.5B

Operative Report

Clips are used to outline the involved area of abdominal wall and retroperitoneum, should the margins be microscopically positive and radiation needed. A colostomy is created, and the distal stump is sutured to the abdominal wall adjacent to the colostomy to facilitate future colostomy reversal.

Pathology Report

A moderately well-differentiated adenocarcinoma with invasion of the adjacent abdominal muscles. The margin of resection is free of tumor. There was no involvement of the small bowel. Pathology examination showed that 4 of 12 nodes were positive for metastatic disease.

◼ Approach

Staging, prognosis, and adjuvant treatment are based on the tumor-node-metastasis (TNM) classification system. In this patient, the pathology report indicates involvement of four associated lymph nodes, classifying this as a T4 N2 M0 or stage III lesion. The margins of the tumor are negative and thus radiation to the pelvic sidewall or retroperitoneum is not needed. Because of the invasion into surrounding structures and positive lymph nodes, the patient is a candidate for adjuvant chemotherapy, which currently would consist of 5-fluorouracil (5-FU), leucovorin, and oxaliplatin. Toward the end of the convalescence period and prior to induction of the chemotherapy, the patient will be advised to undergo colonoscopy to evaluate the proximal colon.

Case Continued

Six weeks after the surgery, the patient undergoes colonoscopy through the colostomy and via rectum. No other polyps or tumors are found. The patient successfully completes adjuvant 5-FU, leucovorin, and oxaliplatin. Repeat CT scan, chest x-ray, CEA level, and liver function tests (LFTs) are normal. The patient undergoes successful colostomy reversal.

Suggested Readings

Buechter KJ, Boustany C, Caillouette R, et al. Surgical management of the acutely obstructed colon. A review of 127 cases. *Am J Surg* 1988;156:163–168.

Deans GT, Krukowski ZH, Irwin ST. Malignant obstruction of the left colon. *Br J Surg* 1994;81:1270–1276.

Scotia Study Group. Single-stage treatment for malignant left-sided colonic obstruction: a prospective randomized clinical trial comparing subtotal colectomy with segmental resection following intraoperative irrigation. *Br J Surg* 1995;82:1622–1627.

Wong SK, Eu KW, Lim SL, et al. Total colectomy removes undetected proximal synchronous lesions in acute left-sided colonic obstructions. *Tech Coloproctol* 1996;4:87–88.

Presentation

You are called to the emergency department to evaluate a 44-year-old white man who presents with a 2-month history of intermittent lower abdominal pain, which became acutely worse over the last 24 hours with associated abdominal distention. He also had nausea and vomiting with absence of bowel movements for at least 1 week. He is passing flatus, but much less than normal. He describes a change in bowel habit as constipation intermixed with diarrhea for the last 2 months, and he had an episode with hematochezia. He describes a 10-lb weight loss with a fair appetite. Upon examination, the patient appears pale and in some discomfort, but there is no evidence of jaundice. His abdomen is distended with tenderness in the right lower quadrant, but no guarding or rigidity. Bowel sounds are high pitched and hyperactive. Rectal examination reveals no masses.

Differential Diagnosis

The clinical presentation is suggestive of acute on chronic large bowel obstruction. When faced with suspected bowel obstruction, the surgeon needs to address three specific issues:

Is this obstruction simple or strangulated? Physical examination in conjunction with basic laboratory tests is indispensable in determining whether there is any evidence of jeopardy to the blood supply to the involved bowel. The presence of localized guarding, rigidity, and absent bowel sounds associated with elevated white blood cell (WBC) count and elevated amylase and lactate acid levels is indicative of compromised bowel. In this case, the tenderness in the right lower quadrant is concerning, and it may be due to a grossly distended or compromised cecal wall resulting perhaps from a distal large bowel obstruction.

What is the level of obstruction? The level of obstruction can often be ascertained from plain radiographs of the abdomen taken in the supine and erect positions. A Gastrografin enema or, even better, a computed tomography (CT) scan of the abdomen and pelvis in a stable patient can provide valuable information regarding the cause of intestinal obstruction.

What is the cause for the obstruction? In an adult, the etiology of obstruction is usually obvious from the clinical history and physical examination. Important causes include external hernia, adhesions from previous abdominal surgery, carcinoma of the colon, diverticular stricture, and volvulus. Given the history of change of bowel habit with hematochezia and weight loss, the diagnosis of left-sided colon carcinoma should be strongly considered.

Recommendation

Obtain complete blood cell count (CBC), Chem 7 (tests for glucose, blood urea nitrogen, creatinine, potassium, sodium, chloride, and carbon dioxide), amylase level, lactic acid level, and radiograph of the abdomen in supine and erect positions. Initiate fluid resuscitation and decompression of the bowel with nasogastric tube.

Case Continued

Intravenous fluid consisting of lactated Ringer's solution is commenced, and nasogastric tubing and Foley catheter are placed. His laboratory tests reveal the following: WBC count 14,000, hemoglobin 10, hematocrit 33, and serum amylase and lactic acid levels are normal. After physical examination, 4 mg of morphine is administered intravenously for pain control.

Abdominal X-Ray

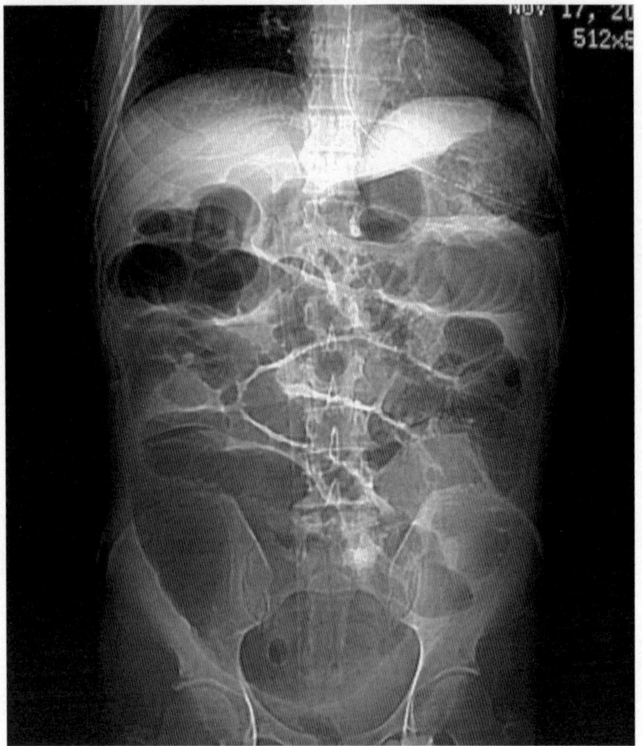

Figure 32.1

Abdominal X-Ray Report

There are dilated loops of small bowel as well as a grossly distended large bowel, which appears to abruptly end near the descending colon. There is no air in the rectum. The cecum is dilated and measures 7 cm at its widest dimension.

Recommendation

The clinical presentation and plain radiographs are highly suggestive of an obstruction in the left colon. Because there is no clinical evidence of acutely compromised bowel and no peritonitis, a CT scan of the abdomen and pelvis may be valuable.

CT Scan

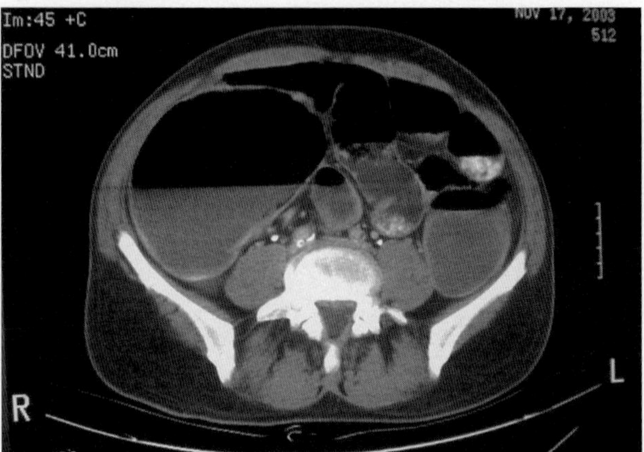

Figure 32.2A

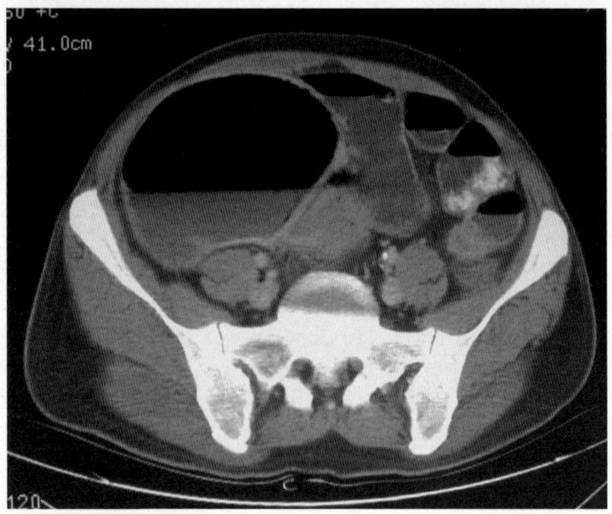

Figure 32.2B

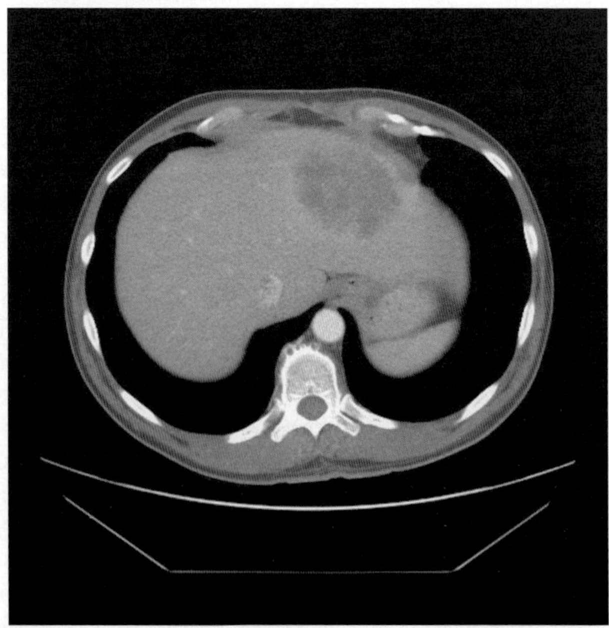

Figure 32.2C

CT Scan Report

An 8-cm complex liver lesion is seen in the left lateral lobe, which is highly suggestive of a metastatic lesion. The dilated small and large bowels are seen, with a 3-cm area of thickening and associated narrowing in the sigmoid colon. There is no evidence of suspicious periaortic lymphadenopathy.

Approach

The clinical presentation and the findings on imaging studies strongly suggest the presence of a colon carcinoma presenting as acute large bowel obstruction with a synchronous liver metastasis. A serum sample should be sent to establish a preoperative carcinoembryonic antigen (CEA) level, which, if elevated, would be useful for comparison during postoperative follow-up.

Obstructing or near-obstructing colon carcinomas present a special treatment challenge. Although right or transverse colon-obstructing malignant lesions are amenable to resection with primary ileocolonic anastomosis, the management of an obstructing left-sided lesion is more controversial. The options available to the surgeon include the following:

1. A three-staged approach involving an initial diversion, a subsequent resection, and ultimately an anastomosis is the most conservative option. This approach is not used very frequently except for patients with significant comorbid conditions that would prohibit a major operative intervention.

2. The safest and most common approach is to perform a resection of the tumor with an end-descending colostomy with either a distal mucus fistula or Hartmann pouch. A second-stage procedure is subsequently required for reversal of the colostomy.

3. A subtotal colectomy can be performed followed by an ileorectal anastomosis, particularly if the proximal colon is massively distended and there is evidence of impending cecal perforation. This approach is also necessary if the patient has a synchronous colon carcinoma in another segment.

4. Following resection of the colon carcinoma, the proximal bowel can be cleaned with intraoperative colonic lavage, followed by creation of a primary anastomosis. If necessary, this anastomosis can be protected with a diverting loop ileostomy.

5. In the absence of signs suggestive of compromised bowel, the obstructing carcinoma can be recanalized either with laser electrocoagulation or by placement of an internal stent, which can sufficiently relieve bowel obstruction to facilitate a bowel preparation and thus allow a single-stage procedure.

6. If at exploration the tumor is unresectable, the patient can be given a diverting colostomy for palliation.

The approach to synchronous liver metastasis is also somewhat controversial. The safest approach would be to perform a liver biopsy to establish a tissue diagnosis of liver metastasis and to perform colectomy only. The presence of synchronous liver metastasis represents a poor prognostic factor, and to determine the natural history of the metastatic process, the alternative "biologic" approach would be to treat the patient initially with systemic chemotherapy. If the patient demonstrates progressive disease during chemotherapy, an unnecessary hepatic resection would be avoided. For patients presenting with synchronous metastatic disease, the literature is somewhat mixed regarding the increased morbidity and mortality associated with performing both colectomy and hepatic resection at the initial operation; concerns about the increased operative risk may be particularly valid in patients who present emergently with either malignant bowel obstruction or perforation.

Case Continued

At exploration, the carcinoma is bulky but shows no evidence of perforation. The proximal bowel is viable and a hard 8-cm liver metastasis is felt. Following sigmoid colectomy, the proximal bowel is noted to be loaded with solid stool; therefore, an end colostomy with a Hartmann pouch is performed. A liver biopsy is performed and sent for frozen section, which is reported as metastatic adenocarcinoma of colonic origin.

Pathology Report

A moderately differentiated adenocarcinoma with near complete luminal obstruction with complete invasion through the muscularis propria with infiltration of the subserosal tissue. Metastatic adenocarcinoma was found in one of nine regional lymph nodes. Therefore, the patient has stage IV disease (T3 N1 M1).

Case Continued

The patient undergoes complete restaging with CT scan of the chest, abdomen, and pelvis prior to commencing chemotherapy. Apart from the large single lesion seen in the left lobe of the liver, no additional metastatic disease is present. The patient receives two cycles of FolFox-4 (5-fluorouracil [5-FU], leucovorin, and oxaliplatin). A repeat CT scan of the liver demonstrates stable disease. He continues to complete a total of nine cycles of FolFox-4. Cycle 10 is delayed because of myelosuppression (moderate thrombocytopenia). Oxaliplatin-associated neuropathy has not significantly affected his quality of life.

Discussion

Recent years have seen a surge in agents active against colorectal cancer. The combination of 5-FU/ leucovorin is the most widely used chemotherapeutic treatment of colorectal cancer both in the adjuvant and in the metastatic setting. As a first-line treatment for metastatic colon carcinoma, the objective response rate for 5-FU/leucovorin is in the range of 15% to 20%, leaving substantial room for improvement. The response rate has been enhanced with continuous 5-FU infusion (22% vs. 14%), but without a significant improvement in time to progression or survival. Irinotecan was introduced in the second-line setting, and demonstrated improved quality of life compared with best supportive care or infusional 5-FU and leucovorin, which led to testing of its efficacy in the first-line setting in combination with 5-FU/leucovorin. A phase III trial comparing standard 5-FU/leucovorin with 5-FU/leucovorin/irinotecan demonstrated that the latter regimen was associated with a significantly longer median progression-free survival and median survival, and a significantly higher objective response rate. These results were mirrored by a similar European study by Douillard. This led to the adoption of 5-FU/leucovorin/irinotecan as the standard treatment for first-line metastatic disease. Oxaliplatin is a third-generation platinum agent, which, in combination with 5-FU/leucovorin, has been shown to be superior in terms of response rate, time to progression, and survival time to both 5-FU/leucovorin and 5-FU/leucovorin/irinotecan. Two studies have demonstrated the success of oxaliplatin-based combination chemotherapy in patients with initially unresectable metastatic disease. Following administration of a neoadjuvant chemotherapeutic regimen, more than 50% of patients were able to undergo hepatectomies with a resulting 5-year survival rate of 40% to 50%. Other agents that have enhanced response rates in combination with cytotoxic chemotherapy are cetuximab (Erbitux) and bevacizumab (Avastin).

Case Continued

With the systemic therapy, CEA level normalizes, and the patient's disease is restaged with a CT scan of the chest, abdomen, and pelvis as well as positron emission tomography (PET) imaging.

CT Scan

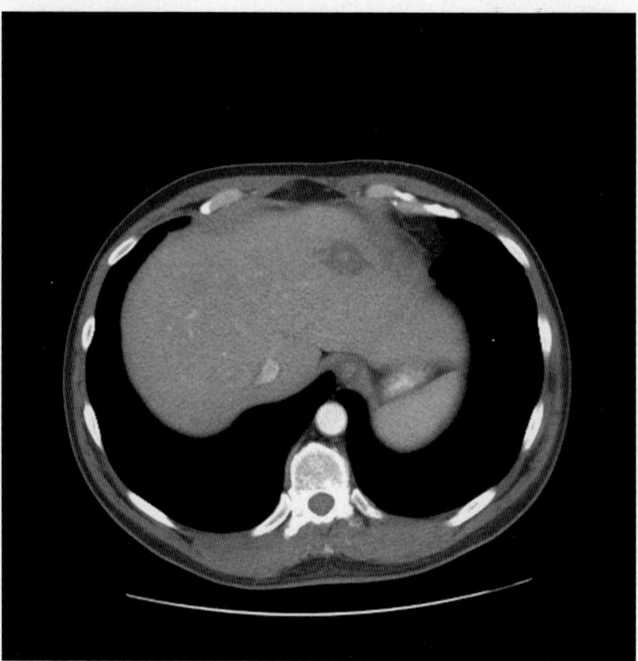

Figure 32.3

CT Scan Report

There is no evidence of pulmonary metastasis. There is a decrease in the hypodense left lateral lobe metastasis, which now measures 4 × 2.5 cm.

Recommendation

Because the patient has shown a response in the liver with no evidence of extrahepatic metastases, hepatic resection should be offered.

Surgical Approach

The patient is counseled regarding the risks, benefits, and complications of hepatic resection, and informed consent is obtained. Any anemia or coagulopathy present is corrected, and a medical evaluation is sought if there is a history of comorbid conditions. Because this patient has had a prior laparotomy, a preoperative bowel preparation would be valuable in case dense adhesions are encountered.

Central venous, Foley, and epidural catheters are placed. Perioperative antibiotics are administered. An anesthetic technique that provides a low central venous pressure (<5 mm Hg) with judicious use of intravenous fluids, intravenous nitroglycerin, and epidural infusion of narcotics and anesthetic agents is preferred. The abdomen is opened through a subcostal incision with midline extension. Any adhesions to the liver are initially divided to avoid avulsion of the capsule and subsequent bleeding. The falciform ligament is divided proceeding to the suprahepatic vena cava. The lesser omentum is incised and a vessel loop is placed around the porta hepatis. A careful evaluation of the abdomen is performed to exclude extrahepatic disease, including biopsy of any suspicious porta hepatis lymph nodes. The liver is bimanually palpated. The liver is further investigated with intraoperative ultrasound scan. A self-retaining retractor that allows elevation of the costal margin is crucial. In preparation for the left lateral hepatic lobectomy, the left triangular ligament is divided, keeping in mind the left phrenic vein and its branches. This dissection is carried to the level of the left hepatic vein. The liver is elevated to reveal the undersurface where, if present, the bridge of tissue between segment IV and the left lateral lobe should be divided with electrocautery. Dissection is carried out within the umbilical fissure to the left of the ascending portion of the left portal vein. The pedicles to segments II and III can usually be found within a depth of 5 to 10 mm; the pedicles are dissected and then transected with an endovascular stapler. The liver capsule is scored approximately 5 mm to the left of the falciform ligament. Parenchymal transection ensues, and any one of many techniques can be used to facilitate this (Kelly clamp, Cavitron ultrasonic aspirator [CUSA], tissue link). During the trisection phase, the porta hepatis can be clamped (Pringle maneuver) intermittently. The surgeon needs to be cognizant of avoiding injury to the ascending portion of the left portal pedicle and to the branches of segment IVA and B. The left hepatic vein or one of its branches is then identified and transected with an endovascular stapler. Hemostasis is achieved along the surface of the transected liver. Leaking biliary radicals are controlled with figure-of-eight sutures using polypropylene.

Case Continued

At exploration, in the absence of extrahepatic disease, the patient successfully undergoes lateral hepatic lobectomy. Intraoperative ultrasound scan reveals no additional metastatic lesions. Gross examination by pathologists reveals a 2.5-cm metastatic lesion close to the surface of the liver. Microscopic examination demonstrates metastatic adenocarcinoma of colonic origin 2.7 cm from the surgical margin, which is negative. The patient recovers well from the hepatic resection and is placed on surveillance.

Suggested Readings

Chua HK, Sondenaa K, Tsiotos GG, et al. Concurrent vs staged colectomy and hepatectomy for primary colorectal cancer with synchronous hepatic metastases. *Dis Colon Rectum* 2004;47:1310–1316.

Fujita S, Akasu T, Moriya Y. Resection of synchronous liver metastases from colorectal cancer. *Jpn J Clin Oncol* 2000;30:7–11.

Lambert LA, Colacchio TA, Barth RJ Jr. Interval hepatic resection of colorectal metastases improves patient selection. *Arch Surg* 2000;135:473–479.

Lyass S, Zamir G, Matot I, et al. Combined colon and hepatic resection for synchronous colorectal liver metastases. *J Surg Oncol* 2001;78:17–21.

Tygidakis NJ, Singh G, Bardaxoglou E, et al. Two-stage liver surgery for advanced liver metastasis synchronous with colorectal tumor. *Hepatogastroenterology* 2004;51:413–418.

Martin R, Paty P, Fong Y, et al. Simultaneous liver and colorectal resections are safe for synchronous colorectal liver metastasis. *J Am Coll Surg* 2003;197:233–241; discussion 241–242.

Tanaka K, Shimada H, Matsuo K, et al. Outcome after simultaneous colorectal and hepatic resection for colorectal cancer with synchronous metastases. *Surgery* 2004;136:650–659.

Weber JC, Bachellier P, Oussoultzoglou E, et al. Simultaneous resection of colorectal primary tumour and synchronous liver metastases. *Br J Surg* 2003;90:956–962.

case 33

Presentation

A 52-year-old healthy man complains of recurrent colicky abdominal pain following an infectious gastroenteritis 6 months ago, and reports hematochezia, mucinous diarrhea, and changes in stool habit for several weeks. His medical history includes a transurethral resection of a urinary bladder tumor 7 years ago. Current nicotine abuse has been present for many years. Family history is devoid of colorectal cancer (CRC). Abdominal and rectal examinations are unremarkable.

Differential Diagnosis

A history of changes in bowel habit associated with hematochezia in a 52-year-old patient is highly suspicious for CRC. However, hematochezia may be the dominant symptom in several other diseases, such as inflammatory bowel disease, infectious colitis, telangiectasias, diverticular disease, and hemorrhoids, which must also be considered. Changes in stool habit, especially the presence of pencil-shaped stool, may indicate advanced colonic obstruction and may be accompanied by colicky pain.

Recommendation

Colonoscopy, including biopsies.

Case Continued

Colonoscopy reveals a circular stenosis caused by a rectal mass 15 cm from the anal verge. The tumor shows firm central parts with bleeding ulcerations and peripheral areas with softer adenoma-like growth patterns. The stenosis cannot be overcome and colonoscopy is incomplete. The exact distance from the lower border of the tumor to the anal verge is determined by rigid proctoscopy and is found to be 14 cm. Histologic examination of the biopsies reveals a moderately differentiated colorectal adenocarcinoma.

Discussion

The risk for developing CRC rises exponentially with increasing age, starting at about age 45 and ending with an incidence of 400 to 500 in 100,000 at the age of 80. The average incidence in Western countries of CRC is about 50 in 100,000. More than 90% of CRC cases are thought to be sporadic CRC, and less than 10% are found in the context of hereditary syndromes such as hereditary nonpolyposis colorectal cancer (HNPCC) syndrome, familial adenomatous polyposis (FAP) syndrome, Gardner syndrome, Turcot syndrome, Peutz-Jeghers syndrome, juvenile polyposis, and inflammatory bowel disease (ulcerous colitis and Crohn disease).

Rectal cancer is the most common abdominal malignancy and accounts for 35% to 40% of all large bowel cancers. Rectal bleeding and anemia are the most common symptoms associated with rectal cancer (60%). Changes in bowel habit and stool shape are frequently reported, too, and may be present in up to 40% of patients. Patients may experience constipation in obstructive disease as well as mucous diarrhea from villous components of the tumor. Digital rectal examination is of limited value in proximal rectal cancer, as the investigator cannot reach the tumor. However, digital rectal examination allows exclusion of a tumor within the distal third of the rectum, estimation of the prostate's size in men (important for rectal cancer surgery), and clinical examination of anal resting and squeeze pressures with regard to postoperative functional results. Exact measurement of the distance from the tumor to the anal verge is mandatory and is best done by rigid proctosigmoidoscopy. Rectal cancer is defined as a carcinoma within 15 cm from the anal verge, even if only the lower border of the tumor is still within this margin. Therapeutic strategies strongly depend on this definition.

Complete colonoscopy is indicated to exclude synchronous colon cancer (3% to 5%) and to search for underlying large bowel diseases. If the endoscope cannot be passed through the stenosis, as in this case, preoperative double-contrast enema can be performed to exclude additional colonic polyps. However, the stenosis usually prevents a proper large bowel preparation, limiting the diagnostic value of the contrast enema.

Abdominal/pelvic multislice triple-contrast-enhanced computed tomography (CT) or magnetic resonance imaging (MRI) is performed to investigate locoregional tumor spread (i.e., depth of invasion of the primary tumor and presence or absence of enlarged or inhomogeneous lymph nodes) and to scan for liver metastasis as well as signs of peritoneal carcinomatosis (difficult to visualize with CT scan). Additional ultrasonography of the liver may clarify doubtful liver lesions detected on the CT scan. Workup for distant metastasis also includes chest x-ray or chest CT scan. Positron emission tomography (PET) is generally not used in a standard workup, but may be helpful before treatment of distant metastasis. The tumor markers carcinoembryonic antigen (CEA) and cancer antigen (CA) 19-9 should not be used as screening tools, but have proved valuable in monitoring for tumor recurrence during routine follow-up if the markers were elevated preoperatively.

Diagnosis and Recommendation

A proximal rectal moderately differentiated adenocarcinoma. Perform multislice triple-contrast-enhanced CT scans of the pelvis, abdomen, and chest. Determine preoperative CEA level for comparison in follow-up examinations. Perform colonoscopy of remaining colon 3 months postoperatively.

Case Continued

The patient had an abdominal/pelvic and chest CT scan. His CEA value was 2.0 µg/L (normal <4.6 µg/L) and his CA 19-9 value was 7.6k U/L (normal <20 kU/L).

CT Scans

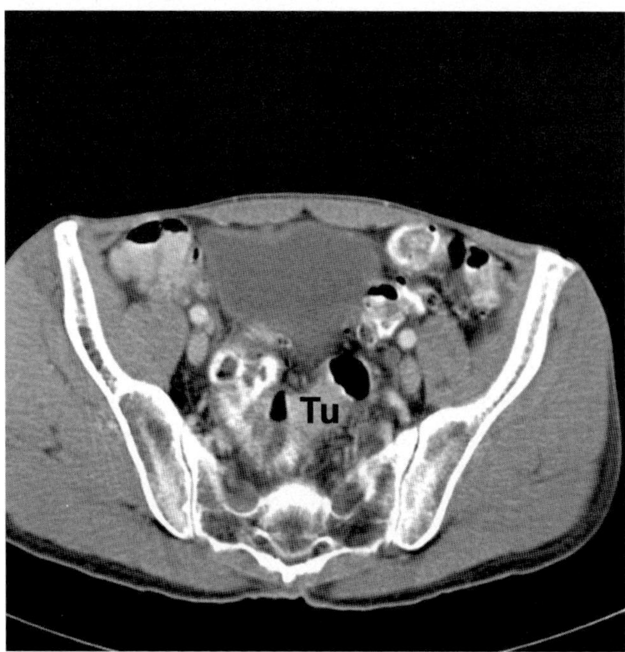

Figure 33.1A

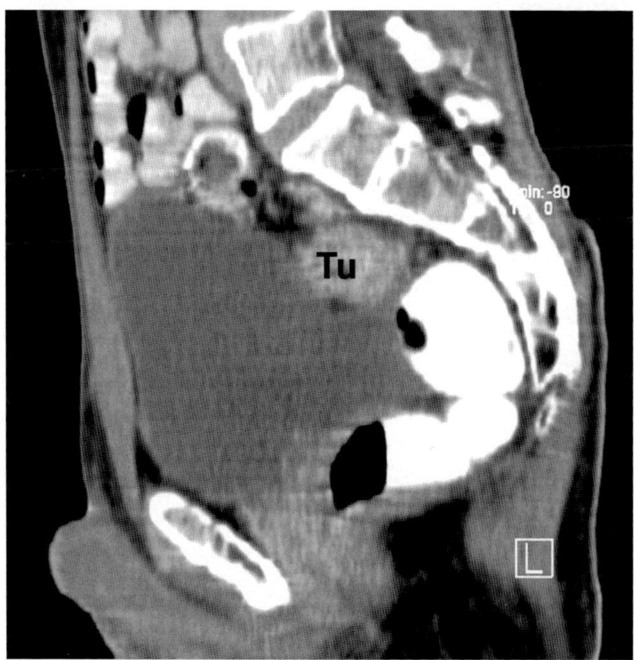

Figure 33.1B

CT Scan Report

Multislice triple-contrast-enhanced CT scan of the chest, abdomen, and pelvis show an obstructive intraluminal mass *(Tu)* with a diameter of 5.5 cm at the rectosigmoidal transition. Prestenotic fecal impaction is seen, without obvious large bowel dilatation. There is suggestion of local tumor infiltration into the mesocolon/mesorectum, but not into neighboring organs, and multiple enlarged lymph nodes within the mesorectum/mesocolon. Minor diverticulosis of the sigmoid colon is seen, but there is no evidence of diverticular inflammation. Multiple liver cysts are seen, but no evidence of liver or peritoneal metastasis. Lung fields appear without suspicion of metastasis.

Approach

After completion of the staging, the patient is found to have proximal rectal carcinoma with perirectal tumor infiltration and local lymph node metastases with incomplete large bowel obstruction, but without evidence of distant metastasis, according to the Union Internationale Contre le Cancer (UICC) staging system: cT3 cN1-2 cM0 G2, UICC stage III.

The patient should be offered a radical anterior resection of the rectum, including the left hemicolon and the locoregional lymphatic drainage area.

Discussion

The Dukes staging system and its modifications should no longer be used because the UICC staging system is uniform and is now accepted worldwide. In the United States, the American Joint Commission on Cancer (AJCC) staging system is commonly used.

If the surgeon performing the operation is experienced and familiar with CRC treatment, no preoperative radiotherapy or chemotherapy is recommended because no infiltration of neighboring organs is shown and the tumor is localized within the upper third of the rectum. In such a case, the surgeon with special interest in colorectal surgery is able to perform a sharp mesorectal excision to remove any potential locoregional lymph node metastasis and direct tumor spread.

Surgical Approach

With the patient in a supine position, the abdomen is explored by a median laparotomy after a standard combination of an antibiotic single shot has been given. Inspection and bimanual palpation are not suspicious for metastasis. The primary tumor is mobile, and at the peritoneal reflection, a careful palpation of the colon reveals no synchronous second colon neoplasm and no evidence of peritoneal carcinomatosis. No lymph node involvement is grossly suspected, especially not at the root of the inferior mesenteric artery or along the aorta. According to the no-touch isolation technique, the inferior mesenteric vein is dissected at the lower border of the pancreas, and the sigmoid lumen is closed by a tie. The left hemicolon including the left colonic flexure is completely mobilized, detaching the omentum from the transverse colon, and dissected at the left colonic flexure. The corresponding left mesocolon including the inferior mesenteric artery is dissected about 1.5 cm distant from its origin at the aorta, after identification of the left ureter. Further sharp dissection of the rectosigmoid follows the mesorectal fascia exactly. The autonomous superior hypogastric plexus and the hypogastric nerves on both sides are carefully preserved. The mesorectum is dissected transversely at least 5 cm below the rectal tumor without conning the mesorectum. The rectum is closed distal to the tumor with a right-angle clamp, and then rinsed with a cytotoxic solution (e.g., 10% povidone-iodine solution). The rectum is then transacted with a TA-stapling device. Using the double-stapling technique, a transverse-rectal end-to-end anastomosis about 8 cm from the anal verge is performed. The omentum is placed into the presacral cavity (pelvic omentoplasty). Drains are placed in the pelvic cavity, and the abdomen is closed. A transanal tube is inserted for 5 days.

Discussion

No preoperative mechanical bowel preparation (orthograde lavage or enema) is performed because the present incomplete obstruction increases the risk of completing the obstruction and inducing abdominal pain. Furthermore, recent data from the literature question the value of a preoperative bowel preparation.

For carcinomas of the upper third of the rectum, a partial mesorectal excision (5 cm of mesorectum below the primary) is adequate from the oncological point of view, because distal lymphatic spread occurs rarely and never beyond 4 cm distally to the primary.

Cytotoxic washout of the rectal stump cleans the remaining rectum of tumor cells and tumor pieces mobilized during the surgical manipulation, and thus may prevent anastomotic recurrence. Because the anastomosis has good blood supply with no tension or air leakage and is located at about 8 cm from the anal verge, no protective ileostomy is created. The pelvic omentoplasty may reduce the occurrence of clinically evident anastomotic leaks, and hence, the necessary re-exploration. The same is true for transanal tube drainage.

Finally, it is important to preserve the autonomic hypogastric nerves and the superior hypogastric plexus, especially in this young patient, because damage may result in retrograde ejaculation.

Surgical Specimen

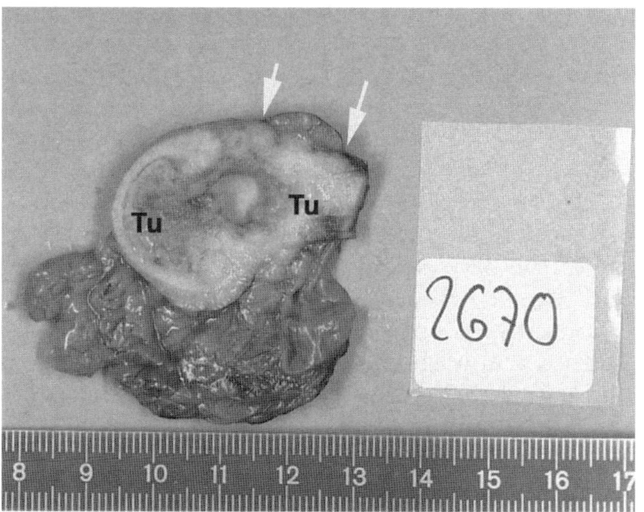

Figure 33.2

Pathology Report

Poorly differentiated adenocarcinoma of the rectum with central ulceration; circular growth pattern, diameter 4.4 cm. Tumor *(Tu)* has infiltrated through all layers of the colonic wall and into the perirectal fat tissue. Tumor invasion has also occurred in small veins and arteries. Resection margins are free of tumor. The distal safety margin at the large bowel wall is 4.4 cm, in an unstretched and formalin-fixed specimen, corresponding with about 7 cm in the native stretched state of the same specimen. Lymph node metastases are seen in 1 of 36 lymph nodes. Left hemicolon with multiple small tubulovillous adenomas (low grade) and minor diverticular disease are noted.

Case Continued

The postoperative recovery is uneventful. He suffers from slight diarrhea, which is treated by dietary meas-

ures. Final histologic analysis reveals adenocarcinoma pT3, pN1 (1/36), cM0, (AJCC stage III). In the United States, the standard management involves adjuvant 5-fluorouracil-based chemoradiation. A standard follow-up is recommended as suggested by various national guidelines (e.g. NCCN, National Cancer Care Network).

Discussion

Definitive histologic analysis confirmed that any local excision of the rectal cancer would have been insufficient, and that with regard to the encountered stage III disease, adjuvant chemoradiation is indicated. In addition to the lymph node involvement, the poor differentiation of the tumor and the microscopic invasion of veins are risk factors for tumor recurrence. In Europe, adjuvant radiotherapy may not be offered if a total mesorectal excision and an R0-resection have been achieved in rectal cancer of the upper third of the rectum. Complete colonoscopy should be done 3 months after the initial surgery to exclude further neoplastic lesions.

Suggested Readings

Leung KL, Kwok SP, Lam SC, et al. Laparoscopic resection of rectosigmoid carcinoma: prospective randomised trial. *Lancet* 2004;363:1187–1192.

Maurer CA, Renzulli P, Meyer JD, et al. Rectal carcinoma. Optimizing therapy by partial or total mesorectum removal [in German] [review]. *Zentralbl Chir* 1999;124:428–435.

Maurer CA, Z'Graggen K, Renzulli P, et al. Total mesorectal excision preserves male genital function compared with conventional rectal cancer surgery. *Br J Surg* 2001;88:1501–1505.

Nelson H, Petrelli N, Carlin A, et al, for the National Cancer Institute Expert Panel. Guidelines 2000 for colon and rectal cancer surgery. *J Natl Cancer Inst* 2001;93:583–596.

Sobin LH, Wittekind C, eds. *TNM Classification of Malignant Tumors, UICC International Union Against Cancer.* 6th ed. New York: Wiley-Liss; 2002.

Wiggers T, Jeekel J, Arends JW, et al. No-touch isolation technique in colon cancer: a controlled prospective trial. *Br J Surg* 1988; 75:409–415.

Presentation

A 38-year-old otherwise healthy white man who has suffered from constipation, painful defecation, and anal/rectal bleeding for several months is referred to your clinic. At admission he complains about weight loss and fatigue for over a month. There is no family history of colorectal cancer (CRC).

Digital rectal examination is painful, and allows detection of a solid and fixed rectal mass 4 cm above the anal verge (i.e., at the upper border of the anal canal). Anal sphincter pressures at rest and under squeezing are clinically within the normal range. A slight anemia is present.

Differential Diagnosis

Constipation is a common complaint, but when associated with symptoms such as painful defecation, anorectal tenesmus, anal bleeding, or sudden change in bowel habits, it should promptly lead to a diagnostic workup. In many patients, hemorrhoidal disease may be found to be the source of bleeding, with constipation having developed secondary to painful defecation. CRC does usually present with occult blood loss rather than hematochezia, but rectal carcinoma or advanced primaries of the colon can also lead to lower intestinal bleeding. In young patients without a family history of CRC or other risk factors, symptomatic therapy may be considered; however, in patients over the age of 45 years, especially with a change in bowel habits, colorectal cancer must be excluded.

Discussion

Because sporadic CRC rarely occurs before the age of 45 (see also Case 33), hereditary CRC should be considered in the present case. Therefore, family history must be carefully assessed. The Amsterdam criteria may help to identify families with hereditary non-polyposis colorectal cancer (HNPCC). These criteria are fulfilled if three first-degree relatives experienced CRC, if at least two generations are involved, and if one of these three patients is younger than 50 years

old. Any suspicion should be verified by genetic testing of the patient and, if genetic testing results are positive, all first-degree relatives. The consequence of a positive genetic test in relatives is colonoscopy starting at the age of 25 and repeated within short intervals (1 to 2 years). If HNPCC or multiple polyps are present, subtotal or total colectomy should be recommended. In our case, the family history and the Amsterdam criteria are negative.

In distal rectal carcinoma, changes in stool form, anorectal tenesmus, or painful defecation are typical. Other symptoms such as pelvic or back pain, malaise, or total mechanical obstruction are less frequent and often indicate advanced disease.

Digital rectal examination is the initial diagnostic tool and is crucial to estimate tumor size, location, and relation to the surrounding structures such as the sphincter muscle. Rigid or flexible proctosigmoidoscopy is used to visualize the tumor, to take biopsies for histologic confirmation of the suspected diagnosis, and to give an accurate measurement of the distance of the tumor from the anal verge.

To determine local tumor margins and the depth of infiltration as well as to evaluate mesorectal lymph node metastases, patients should undergo endorectal ultrasound examination (EUS) or magnetic resonance imaging (MRI), including endorectal MRI. Computed tomography (CT) is less accurate than EUS and MRI for assessing locoregional tumor spread, especially when the primary is located in the distal part of the rectum. However, CT scan is the best means of evaluating distant metastasis, with special attention to the liver, the lungs, the locoregional lymph nodes, and the peritoneal cavity. Liver ultrasound is a reliable alternative to detect liver metastasis, particularly if any question remains after reviewing the CT scan. However, the liver can also be evaluated effectively with intraoperative ultrasound. In distal (and mid-) rectal cancer, pulmonary metastasis may be present as the sole distant metastasis because venous drainage does not entirely follow the splanchnic pathway but may bypass the portal vein through the hemorrhoidal venous plexus and the iliac veins. The tumor markers carcinoembryonic antigen (CEA) and cancer antigen 19-9 should not be used as screening tools, but have proved valuable in monitoring for tumor recurrence during routine follow-up if the markers were elevated preoperatively.

Recommendation

Biopsies of the primary tumor should be sent for histologic analysis. Complete flexible colonoscopy should be performed to exclude a synchronous secondary colon cancer.

Case Continued

Histology of the biopsies of the rectal primary reveals moderately differentiated carcinoma of the rectum. Colonoscopy reveals a polypoid, partially ulcerated tumor that involves one third of the rectal circumference and is located on the left side. Apart from the known rectal carcinoma, the remaining colonic mucosa is normal.

Diagnosis and Recommendation

Distal rectal adenocarcinoma. Perform endorectal ultrasound, and CT scans of the chest, abdomen, and pelvis for local staging and to exclude distant metastases. Determine preoperative CEA level for comparison in follow-up examinations.

Endorectal Ultrasonographic Image

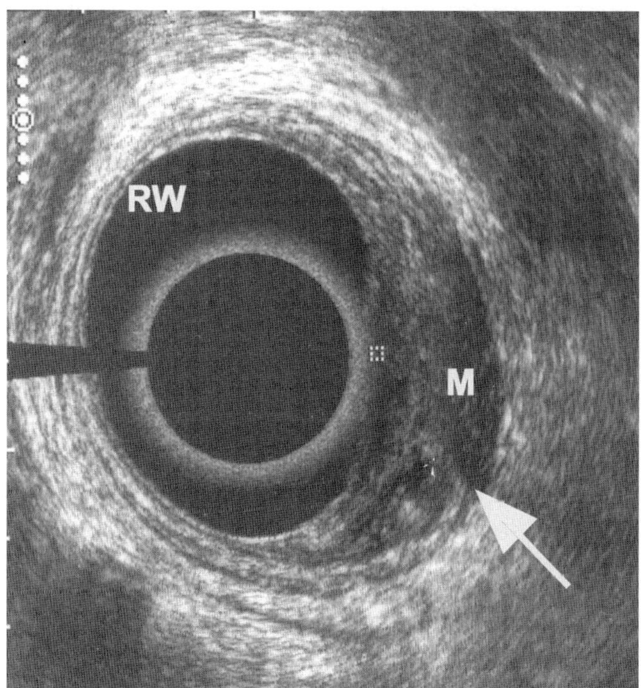

Figure 34.1A

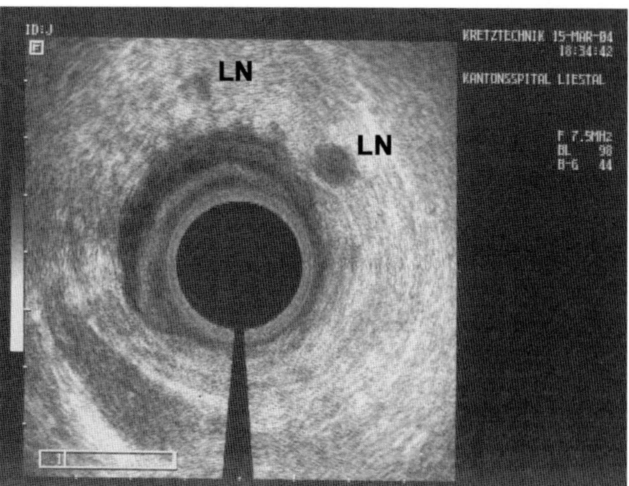

Figure 34.1B

Endorectal Ultrasonography Report

Hypodense 4-cm large rectal tumoral mass *(M)* penetrating all layers of the rectal wall *(RW)* and infiltrating the mesorectum *(arrow)*. No evidence of tumor spread into the prostate, vesicles, pelvic floor, or anal sphincter. Several enlarged mesorectal lymph nodes *(LN)* up to larger than 10 mm, suspicious for lymph node metastasis.

CT Scans

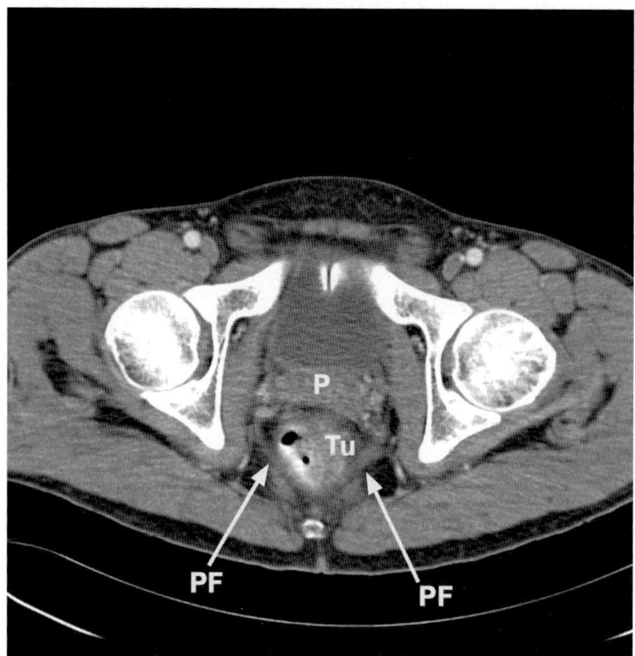

Figure 34.2A

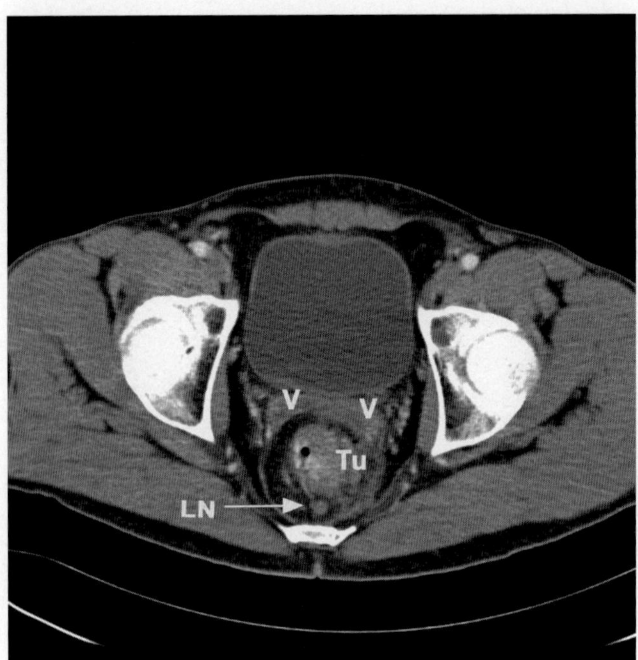

Figure 34.2B

CT Scan Report

Multislice triple-contrast-enhanced CT scan section through the pelvis reveals left-sided tumor *(Tu)* of the distal part of the rectum, immediately above the anal sphincter without evidence of infiltration of the prostate *(P)* or the pelvic floor *(PF)*. At the level of the vesicles *(V)*, distal rectal tumor *(Tu)* with tumor infiltration into the mesorectum, on the left-hand side close to the mesorectal fascia (visceral fascia of the pelvis). There is clear separation from the vesicles. Several enlarged lymph nodes *(LN)* within the mesorectum and at the right and left internal iliac arteries; no ascites, no suspicion of peritoneal carcinomatosis; two small liver cysts, no evidence of liver or pulmonary metastases.

Tumor Marker

CEA level is within normal range.

Approach

After complete evaluation, the patient is found to have a distal rectal adenocarcinoma 4 cm from the anal verge (cT3 cN2 cM0 G2) without infiltration of the anal sphincter or neighboring organs. Because the tumor is close to the dentate line, an adequate distal margin cannot be achieved and abdominoperineal resection would be necessary. To offer a sphincter-sparing approach to the rectal cancer, the patient is presented with the option of neoadjuvant chemoradiation therapy over 6 weeks (50.4 Gy combined with a continuous systemic infusion of 5-fluorouracil [5-FU]), followed by rectal resection 6 to 8 weeks later.

Discussion

There is increasing acceptance that patients with stage III (and stage II) rectal cancer should be irradiated preoperatively rather than postoperatively because functional results and long-term oncologic results are better. The recently published randomized German rectal cancer trial comparing the standard U.S. preoperative versus postoperative 5-FU-based chemoradiation demonstrated a significantly lower local recurrence rate, and lower immediate and late complication rates for the preoperative arm. There was no difference in the overall survival. Although the hypofractionated 1-week schedule of irradiation (5 × 5 Gy over 1 week) with immediate surgery is the favorite preoperative treatment in Europe, in this case we decided to choose a conventional long irradiation protocol (50.4 Gy over 6 weeks, combined with continuous chemotherapy), because the aim was not only tumor sterilization, but also downsizing/downstaging of the tumor, facilitating a complete excision of the mesorectum and increasing the chance of anal sphincter preservation.

Surgical Approach

Following a mechanical bowel preparation the day before surgery, the abdomen is explored by a median laparotomy with the patient in a supine position with straddled legs. Perioperative antibiotics are administered. Inspection and bimanual palpation of the liver is not suspicious for metastasis. As expected, the primary tumor is below the peritoneal reflection and therefore not detectable yet. A careful palpation of the colon reveals no synchronous second colon neoplasia and there is no peritoneal carcinomatosis. Lymph node involvement is grossly suspected along the inferior mesenteric artery, but not along the aorta. The left hemicolon, including the left colonic flexure, is completely mobilized, detaching the omentum from the transverse colon, and dissected at the left colonic flexure. The corresponding left mesocolon, including the inferior mesenteric artery, is dissected about 1.5 cm distant from its origin at the aorta, after identification of the left ureter. Further sharp dissection of the rectosigmoid follows the mesorectal fascia (visceral pelvic fascia) exactly down to the pelvic floor and the anorectal junction. The autonomous superior hypogastric nerve plexus, the hypogastric nerves, and the inferior hypogastric nerve plexus on both sides are visualized and carefully preserved. The puborectal muscle sling is not infiltrated by the tumor. To increase the distal safety margin on the bowel wall, we have to enter the intersphincteric space, dissecting the anococcygeal ligament. Then, the rectum is closed distally to the tumor by means of a rectangular clamp, the anal canal is rinsed with a cytotoxic transanal solution (e.g., 10% povidone-iodine solution), and the specimen is removed by transecting, distally to the rectangular clamp, at the dentate line. Grossly, the tumor is less than 1 cm away from the distal resection margin. However, a frozen section from the distal resection margin is free of tumor. A transverse coloplasty is constructed at the proximal colonic stump by an 8-cm-long antimesenteric colostomy and transverse closure by a two-layer running suture.

Intraoperative Images

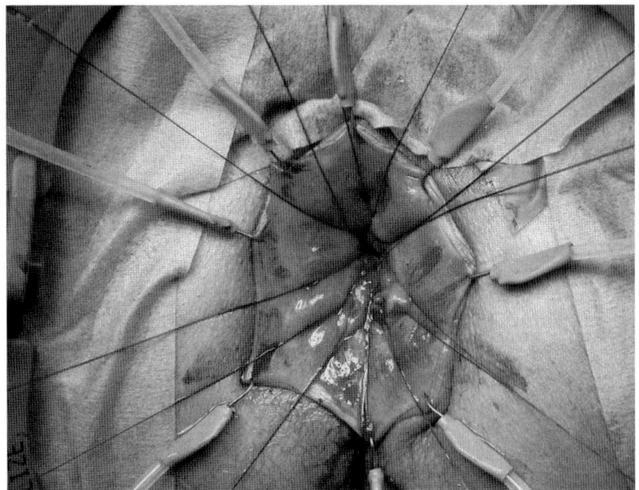

Figure 34.3B

Surgical Approach

The anocutaneous border is everted using a special elastic cord retractor. The cutting level at the dentate line becomes visible (*arrow*). For the transanal anastomosis, 12 sutures are put as preparation for the coloanal hand-sewn suture, grasping the inner sphincter muscle and the anoderm. A transanal tube is inserted and left for 5 days. The omentum is placed into the presacral cavity (pelvic omentoplasty). Drains are put in the pelvic cavity, a protective Brook ileostomy is created, and the abdomen is closed.

Specimen Photographs

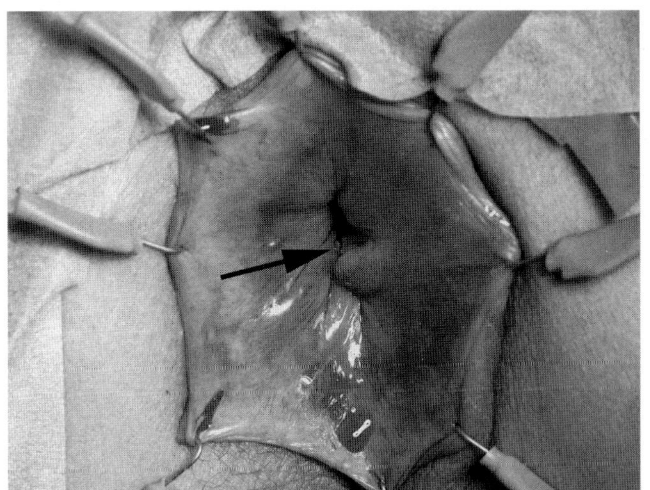

Figure 34.3A

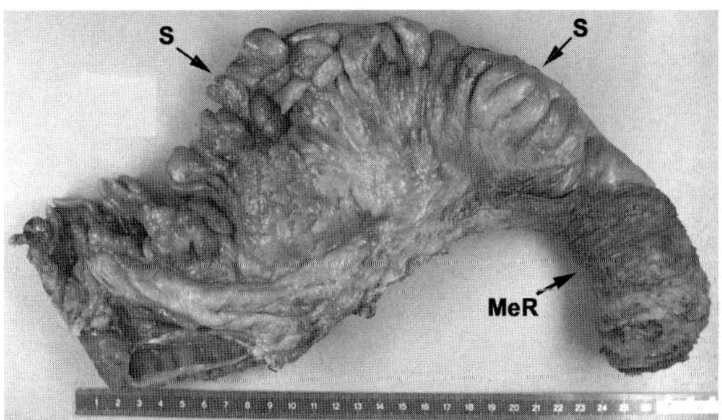

Figure 34.4A

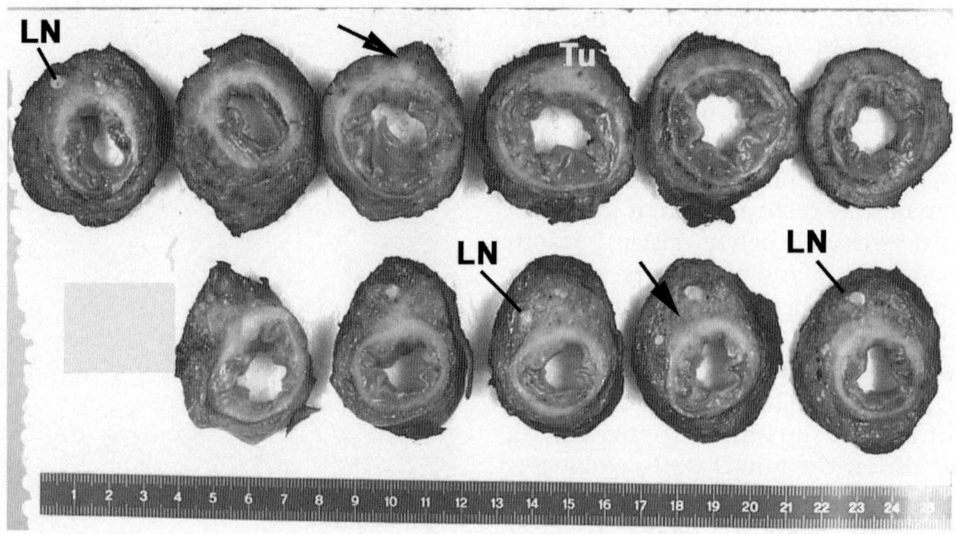

Figure 34.4B

Pathology Report

Note that the mesorectum shrank substantially due to preoperative combined radiochemotherapy. The specimen, consisting of the sigmoid *(S)* and the rectum surrounded with mesorectum *(MeR)*, is not opened and is sent to pathology for ink marking of resection margins. Following formalin fixation, the specimen is cut into slices about 1 cm thick. Photographs are taken as quality control for the surgeon regarding completeness of mesorectal excision. Minimal distances from the tumor to the circumferential resection margin and the distal resection margin are assessed histologically. Transverse slices of the specimen show a thickened rectal wall with primary tumor *(Tu)* and infiltration of the primary into the mesorectum *(arrows)*, but without penetration of the ink-marked resection margin; multiple enlarged lymph nodes *(LN)* in the mesorectum are highly suspicious for lymph node metastasis.

Discussion

Some of the details of the surgical technique are discussed in the chapter on proximal rectal cancer (Case 33). Rectal tumors of the distal third of the rectum are dissected radically with a minimal bowel resection margin, as long as a total mesorectal excision has been performed and the frozen section of the distal margin is negative for tumor spread. Following preoperative chemoradiation therapy a 1 cm distal margin should be adequate as long as frozen section is negative for tumor. Hence, abdominoperineal resection (amputation of the anus) is of no additional benefit with regard to oncologic radicality. The rationales for this circumstance are the following: lymphatic tumor spread almost exclusively occurs in a cranial direction within the mesorectum (and the mesorectum always must be removed completely in rectal cancers of the distal and middle third); distal intramural tumor spread is rare, and if present usually occurs over a distance of only a few millimeters. Mesorectal excision does not include excision of the lateral lymph nodes (i.e., the lymph nodes along the internal iliac arteries). However, the value of routine lateral lymph node dissection is questioned because prognosis seems not to be influenced by this measure.

The rectum never should be transected distally without first closing the bowel lumen because of the risk of tumor cell spillage into the pelvic wound. In our case, a double-stapling technique was not feasible without almost complete resection of the inner sphincter muscle. Therefore, we used a rectangular clamp distal to the tumor to close the lumen, and hence, had no additional loss of inner sphincter muscle by the stapling donut that the double-stapling technique would have brought along.

The formation of a neorectal reservoir, such as our proposed transverse coloplasty, helps to improve postoperative bowel habits when compared with a straight coloanal anastomosis.

Stool frequency, urgency, incontinence, the time to defer defecation, and quality of life are significantly better with a coloplasty. The other commonly used neorectal reservoir, the colonic J-Pouch, gives similar functional results, but is sometimes not feasible, especially in a narrow pelvis of obese male patients or following intersphincteric resection. In such cases, the transverse coloplasty fits better in the pelvis and in the muscular anal funnel.

Protective stoma formation is recommended because even experienced surgeons with a special interest in colorectal surgery encounter leak rates of 15% to 20% at the coloanal anastomosis. The stoma does not help to reduce the leak rates, but reduces the clinical consequences of the leaks and the rate of reintervention.

Case Continued

The patient recovers well from his major surgery. The daily output of his protective ileostomy is closely monitored to prevent dehydration and disturbance of electrolyte concentrations in case of a high output.

Histologic classification of the tumor is pT3 pN2 (16/40) cM0 G2 L1 V1 R0 according to the Union Internationale Contre le Cancer (UICC) classification system. Adjuvant systemic chemotherapy is given for 6 months (oxaliplatin, 5-FU, and leucovorin) due to the encountered UICC stage III and the additional risk factors for recurrence, such as L1 (carcinomatous lymphangiosis) and V1 (microscopic tumor infiltration of veins). Three months after rectal resection, the ileostomy is taken down, following verification of healing of the coloanal reconstruction by contrast enema. The patient is fully continent even for flatus and liquid stools. Six months after stoma closure, the patient has two to three bowel movements per day, no significant urgency, and no evacuation problem.

Suggested Readings

Eriksen MT, Wibe A, Syse A, et al, The Norwegian Rectal Cancer Group and the Norwegian Gastrointestinal Cancer Group. Inadvertent perforation during rectal cancer resection in Norway. *Br J Surg* 2004;91:210–216.

Kapiteijn E, Marijnen CA, Nagtegaal ID, et al, The Dutch Colorectal Cancer Group. Preoperative radiotherapy combined with total mesorectal excision for resectable rectal cancer. *N Engl J Med* 2001;345:638–646. Summary for patients in *Can J Surg* 2003;46:54–56 and *Med J Aust* 2002;177:563–564.

Kapiteijn E, van de Velde CJ. The role of total mesorectal excision in the management of rectal cancer [review]. *Surg Clin North Am* 2002;82:995–1007.

Maurer CA, Z'graggen K, Zimmermann W, et al. Experimental study of neorectal physiology after formation of a transverse coloplasty pouch. *Br J Surg* 1999;86:1451–1458.

Moslein G. Clinical implications of molecular diagnosis in hereditary nonpolyposis colorectal cancer [Review]. *Recent Results Cancer Res* 2003;162:73–78.

Nagtegaal ID, van de Velde CJ, van der Worp E, et al, The Cooperative Clinical Investigators of the Dutch Colorectal Cancer Group. Macroscopic evaluation of rectal cancer resection specimen: clinical significance of the pathologist in quality control. *J Clin Oncol* 2002;20:1729–1734.

Shirouzu K, Isomoto H, Kakegawa T. Distal spread of rectal cancer and optimal distal margin of resection for sphincter-preserving surgery. *Cancer* 1995;76:388–392.

Presentation

A 55-year-old man presents with a 3-year history of intermittent bleeding per rectum. He denies weight loss, nausea, or vomiting. Recently he had noted decreased caliber of stool, increasing episodes of liquid stool, and diminished force of the urinary stream. He had never undergone screening colonoscopy.

The patient's past medical and surgical history is negative. Family history is positive for breast cancer in the patient's mother. The patient worked as a jeweler and had a 17-pack-year history of cigarette smoking.

Auscultation of the lungs reveals scattered wheezing. The abdomen is soft without intra-abdominal masses or hepatosplenomegaly. Colonoscopy performed by the referring physician had revealed a narrowed rectosigmoid colon with a malignant-appearing polyp at 15 to 22 cm. Biopsies showed adenoma with high-grade dysplasia but no evidence of carcinoma. Rigid proctoscopy showed an apparent tumor at 10 cm above the dentate line, which extended for a minimum length of 5 cm. There was no evidence of hemorrhoids, anal fissure, or other anorectal pathology. Laboratory examination is remarkable for a carcinoembryonic antigen (CEA) level of 24.3 ng/mL (normal: <5 ng/mL).

Differential Diagnosis

The patient's history of rectal bleeding, coupled with a recent change in stool caliber and consistency, is strongly suggestive of rectal cancer. The elevated CEA level corroborates this. In addition, the history of recent voiding difficulties suggests the possibility of a locally advanced pelvic tumor. The differential diagnosis also includes colitis of diverse etiologies, arteriovenous malformation, hemorrhoids, and anal fissure. However, no anorectal pathology was identified at proctoscopy. Therefore, the first step after physical examination should be to repeat the colonoscopy and biopsies.

Colonoscopic Image

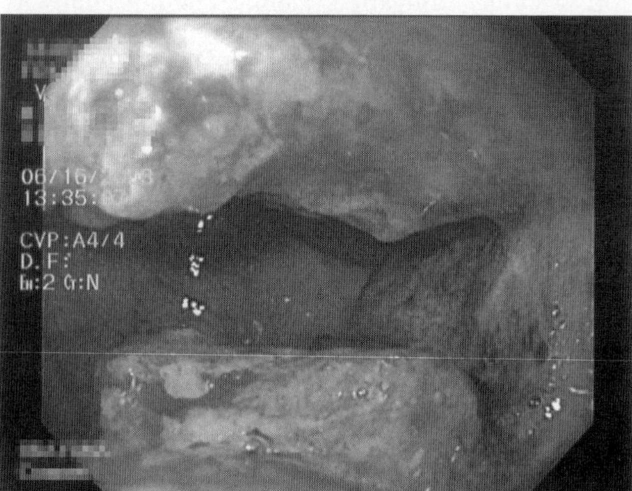

Figure 35.1

Colonoscopy Report

Repeat colonoscopy confirmed a malignant-appearing mass, 11 cm above the dentate line.

Pathology Report

Pathologic examination revealed a villoglandular polyp with moderate to severe dysplasia. No definitive evidence of malignancy was seen.

CT Scan

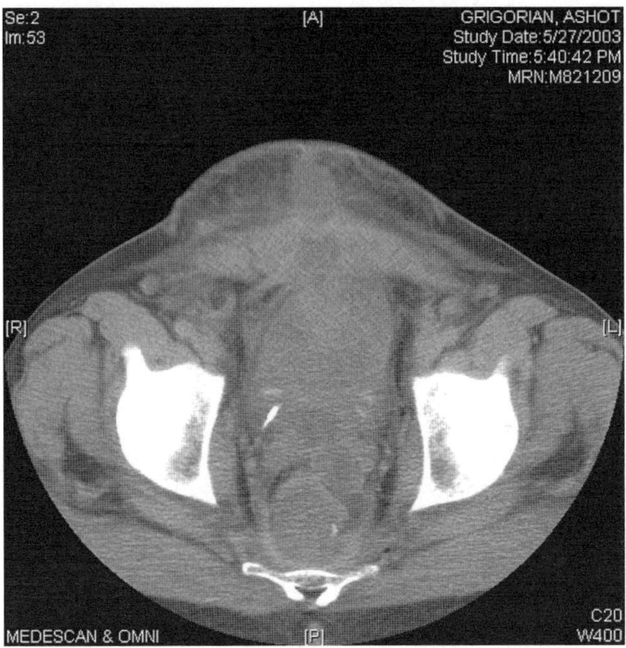

Figure 35.2

CT Scan Report

Computed tomography (CT) scan of the abdomen and pelvis with intravenous and oral contrast agents reveals a 7-cm, heterogenous, irregular mass arising from the rectosigmoid junction, adjacent to the prostate. No clear plane is apparent between the tumor and the prostate/base of bladder. No suspicious adenopathy or ascites is seen. A 2.5-cm hypodense mass with peripheral enhancement, consistent with hemangioma, is seen in the dome of the liver. CT scan of the chest shows no evidence of pulmonary metastasis.

Diagnosis

This patient presents with presumed locally advanced rectal cancer, albeit without tissue diagnosis of malignancy.

Recommendation

The goal of surgical management is complete resection of all gross disease. Adhesions to adjacent organs are malignant in up to 80% of cases and should not be divided; instead, en bloc resection with a rim of normal tissue of the involved organ(s) is required. Neoadjuvant chemoradiation followed by surgical resection is the optimal treatment for this patient presenting with locally advanced rectal cancer. In addition, the use of neoadjuvant chemoradiation increases the likelihood of performing a successful sphincter-sparing procedure for primary resection (rather than abdominoperineal resection). The addition of intraoperative radiotherapy (IORT) to chemotherapy and external beam radiation therapy (EBRT) may significantly improve local control and provide further survival advantage over neoadjuvant chemoradiation followed by surgical resection; however, IORT is available only at select centers.

Discussion

Multiple studies have shown that the use of neoadjuvant chemoradiation increases the resectability rate, and in a defined percentage of patients may induce a complete response. Patients for whom R0 resection (no gross or microscopic residual disease) can be achieved clearly have a better prognosis than those for whom it cannot. Recent studies report decreased local recurrence rates and improved survival with the use of preoperative radiation in patients undergoing total mesorectal excision of rectal cancer. Following total pelvic exenteration for patients with locally advanced rectal cancer, the reported 5-year survival rate is in the range of 30% to 64%.

The use of transrectal ultrasound (TRUS) in the staging of rectal cancer has become standard; accuracy for tumor stage (T) is excellent, though accuracy is somewhat less optimal for assessment of possible nodal involvement (N). The routine use of TRUS in rectal cancer staging allows appropriate use of neoadjuvant chemoradiation in patients with advanced disease. For patients whose tumor is proximal or not well imaged by TRUS for other reasons (e.g., obstructing lesion), magnetic resonance imaging (MRI) is probably the best imaging technique.

Case Continued

Unfortunately, the patient refuses to undergo neoadjuvant chemoradiation. He is taken directly to surgery to attempt primary resection. In the operating room, cystoscopy with bilateral ureteral stenting is performed. At laparotomy, a near-obstructing mass is found 6 cm above the levator ani muscles, occupying the pelvic outlet and appearing to invade the bladder. Although the tumor is extensive, it remains mobile; there is a free plane between the tumor and the prostate. There is palpable lymphadenopathy associated with the rectosigmoid colon. Because of the extent of the tumor, it cannot be safely removed, and a diverting colostomy is performed.

An MRI scan performed to further evaluate the lesion in the liver confirmed multiple benign hemangiomata. Continuous 5-fluorouracil (5-FU) with concomitant EBRT is initiated. The patient develops a severe, confluent rash that resolved after cessation of the 5-FU. EBRT is completed (4,500 cGy in 25 fractions, with a 540-cGy lateral boost).

Approach

Six weeks following completion of chemoradiation, the patient should undergo exploratory laparotomy and proctectomy. Preoperatively, a detailed discussion should be undertaken with the patient regarding the possible need for a pelvic exenteration. Urologic consultation should be obtained for the possibility of needing an ileal conduit, and a convenient site for the stoma should be marked.

Surgical Approach

Initially a cystoscopy should be performed and bilateral ureteral stents placed to allow intraoperative identification of the ureters. Next a rectal washout is performed, followed by a careful examination of the tumor to assess fixation and presence of adenopathy. After opening the abdomen, a careful exploration is performed to exclude evidence of peritoneal and hepatic metastases. In the absence of distant metastases, attention should be directed at evaluating the resectability of the rectal cancer. If there is no plane between the tumor and the bladder, either a partial or a complete cystectomy may need to be performed depending on whether the trigone is involved. After opening the pelvic peritoneum laterally, involvement of the pelvic sidewall is assessed. The goal of the surgical approach should be to achieve complete resection with negative margins. The mesorectum is resected while sparing the pelvic nerve. If a low primary anastomosis is performed, strong consideration should be given to creating a diverting loop ileostomy, particularly as the patient had undergone chemoradiation. If abdominoperineal resection is necessary to achieve negative margins, it should be performed. At completion, a closed suction drain is placed in the pelvis.

Case Continued

At laparotomy, there is no evidence of hepatic metastases. Upon dissection of the tumor, a tight plane was encountered laterally. Anteriorly, the tumor appears to abut or invade into the posterior wall of the prostate. The mesorectum is abnormally thickened down to the levator ani muscles. Because of the extent of tumor and the difficult lateral dissection, no attempt at anastomosis is made; instead, a Hartmann pouch is created and the previous colostomy is left in situ.

Pathology Report

Pathologic examination revealed a 4.8-cm, ulceroinfiltrative, mucinous adenocarcinoma extending through the muscularis propria into the perirectal soft tissue. Surgical margins were negative. There is no evidence of lymphovascular or perineural invasion. Seven of 23 lymph nodes were positive for adenocarcinoma (pathologic T3 N2 M0, stage IIIC).

Recommendation

Based on the type of tumor (mucinous adenocarcinoma, associated with poor prognosis), advanced stage, and presence of residual disease in the resected specimen, the patient should receive adjuvant chemotherapy.

Case Continued

Unfortunately, the patient's postoperative course is complicated by a pelvic abscess that failed an initial attempt at percutaneous drainage. Two months after proctectomy, the patient undergoes operative drainage via transabdominal and transanal approaches. Again, 1 month later, the patient requires operative drainage. One week afterward, he develops a small bowel obstruction and undergoes exploratory laparotomy with lysis of adhesions, terminal-ileum-to-ascending-colon bypass, and peristomal hernia repair. Ten weeks later, the patient presents with recurrent pelvic abscess and is taken to the operating room for drainage. At this time, biopsy-proven adenocarcinoma involving the lower pole of the abdominal incision is identified and excised. Two weeks later, the patient begins chemotherapy with the FolFox regimen (5-FU,/leucovorin, and oxaliplatin).

◼ CT Scan

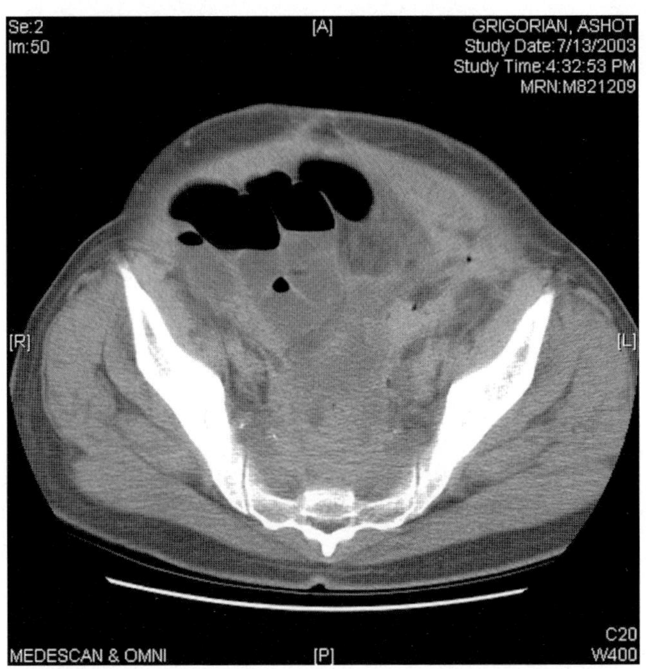

Figure 35.3

CT Scan Report

After four cycles of chemotherapy, a CT image of the abdomen with oral and intravenous contrast shows progression of disease, revealing a massive tumor arising from the pelvis and extending up to the abdominal wall inferior to the umbilicus.

Case Continued

In addition, the patient's CEA level has risen from 43.5 ng/mL to 64.0 ng/mL. His chemotherapy regimen is changed to irinotecan/capecitabine salvage, but the patient continues to experience disease progression.

Acknowledgment

The authors acknowledge Jorge Lagares-Garcia, MD, FACS, FASCRS, Rhode Island Colorectal Clinic, LLC, Providence, RI, for his contributions to content and revision of this manuscript.

Suggested Readings

Crane CH, Skibber J. Preoperative chemoradiation for locally advanced rectal cancer: rationale, technique, and results of treatment. *Semin Surg Oncol* 2003;21:265–270.

Crane CH, Skibber JM, Feig BW, et al. Response to preoperative chemoradiation increases the use of sphincter-preserving surgery in patients with locally advanced low rectal carcinoma. *Cancer* 2003;97:517–524.

Gunderson LL, Nelson H, Martenson JA, et al. Locally advanced primary colorectal cancer: intraoperative electron and external beam irradiation +/− 5-FU. *Int J Radiat Oncol Biol Phys* 1997;37:601–614.

Janjan NA, Crane C, Feig BW, et al. Improved overall survival among responders to preoperative chemoradiation for locally advanced rectal cancer. *Am J Clin Oncol* 2001;24:107–112.

Law WL, Chu KW, Choi HK. Total pelvic exenteration for locally advanced rectal cancer. *J Am Coll Surg* 2000;190:78–83.

Luna-Perez P, Rodriguez-Ramirez S, Hernandez-Pacheco F, et al. Anal sphincter preservation in locally advanced low rectal adenocarcinoma after preoperative chemoradiation therapy and coloanal anastomosis. *J Surg Oncol* 2003;82:3–9.

case 36

The patient is a 38-year-old man who initially presented 8 years previously with rectal bleeding. He had a strong family history of colon cancer: both his paternal aunt and his paternal uncle had died of colon cancer, and his father had known colonic polyps. Physical examination was unremarkable. Colonoscopic evaluation revealed a sessile polyp at 15 cm; biopsies confirmed moderately to poorly differentiated adenocarcinoma. The patient underwent low anterior resection followed by adjuvant chemoradiation. Pathologic examination revealed one of six pericolonic nodes positive for adenocarcinoma (pathologic stage III; T3, N1, M0).

The patient did well for 7 years postoperatively, and then returned to his oncologist with a 6-month history of chronic sacral discomfort and sciatica-like pain in the left lower extremity. He denies any history of trauma to the back or lower extremities.

Differential Diagnosis

The differential diagnosis for sciatica includes spinal stenosis, herniated disc, cauda equina syndrome, and traumatic injury to the spine. Given the patient's history of rectal cancer, recurrent rectal cancer (specifically, tumor involving the sacrum) must be foremost on the list of differential diagnoses. This suspicion is corroborated by the newly elevated carcinoembryonic antigen (CEA) level.

Case Continued

Physical examination reveals a robust young man. Abdominal examination is unremarkable except for a well-healed midline incision, and examination of the back and lower extremities is normal. The CEA level is 10.2 ng/mL (normal: <2.5 ng/mL). After treatment of his rectal cancer 7 years previously, the patient's CEA level had been 1.3 ng/mL. Magnetic resonance imaging (MRI) of the lumbar spine and left hip are normal. Bone scan further confirms abnormal uptake in the area overlying the sacrum. Colonoscopy confirms an anastomotic recurrence at 15 cm; pathologic examination reveals moderately to poorly differentiated adenocarcinoma. In the interim, the patient's CEA level has risen to 12.0 ng/mL.

Computed tomography (CT) scan of the abdomen and pelvis reveals a slight increase in soft tissue density in the retrorectal area, with loss of the normal fat plane between the rectum and the sacrum. There is no evidence of hepatic metastases or retroperitoneal/mesenteric adenopathy. On positron emission tomography (PET), there is a large area of intense, irregular ^{18}F-labeled fluorodeoxyglucose uptake in the presacral area, correlating with the abnormal area on CT.

MRI

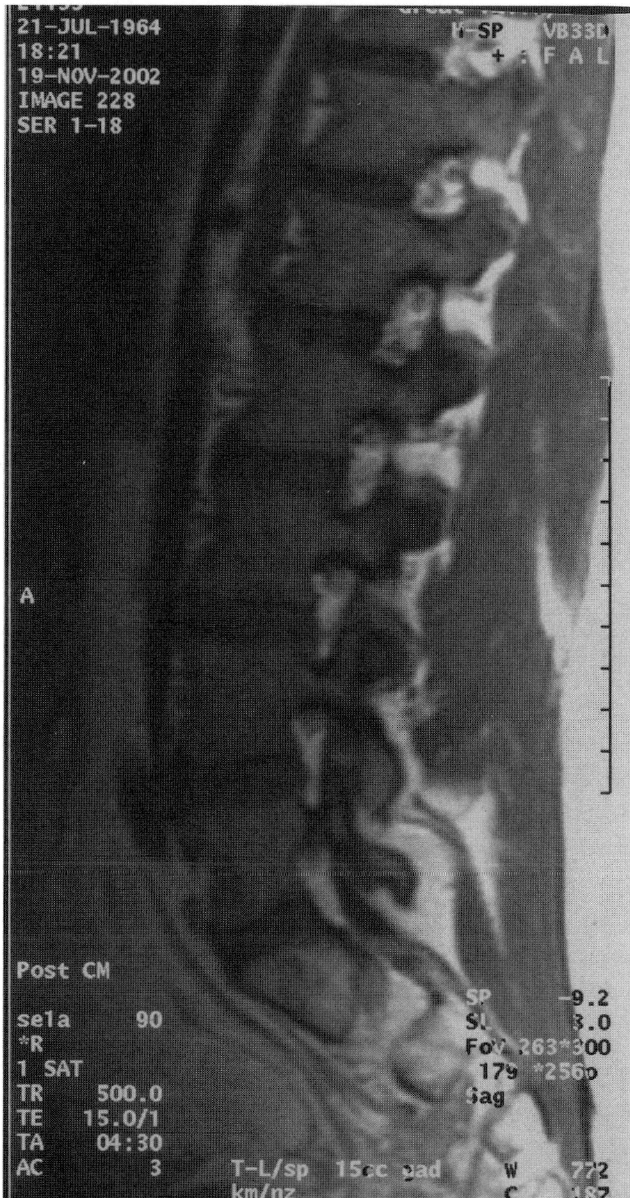

Figure 36.1

MRI Report

Sagittal cuts confirm abnormal signal in the presacral soft tissue with loss of the normal fat plane and probable involvement of the sacral bone at multiple sacral foramina.

Diagnosis and Recommendation

A young, healthy man with locally advanced, recurrent rectal cancer. The patient's performance status and general medical condition are excellent. There is no evidence of systemic metastatic disease.

Optimal treatment of locally recurrent rectal cancer is surgical resection. Imaging studies to fully assess the extent of local disease and to rule out metastatic disease should be performed prior to surgical intervention.

Approach

Complete surgical resection, if possible, offers the best chance of long-term cure of recurrent rectal cancer. Resection will involve total pelvic exenteration with en bloc resection of the tumor and involved sacrum (abdominosacral resection, or ASR).

Case Continued

The patient is treated with a neoadjuvant chemotherapy regimen (5-fluorouracil, leucovorin, and irinotecan) to induce potential tumor shrinkage. He had received the maximum tolerable dose of external beam radiation therapy (EBRT) after his original low anterior resection; thus, further EBRT at this point is not a viable alternative.

Surgical Approach

Preoperative workup including evaluation of cardiac, pulmonary, and renal functions is performed. The patient undergoes mechanical and antibiotic bowel preparation and then is taken to the operating room for exploratory laparotomy. The presence of extrapelvic disease, including hepatic metastases, serosal deposits, or para-aortic lymphadenopathy, should be ruled out. Pelvic node dissection including the obturator nodes is performed and frozen sections are obtained to exclude malignancy. Involvement of the bladder necessitates cystectomy. After en bloc resection of the bladder, rectum, and the associated tumor, an ileal conduit with bilateral ureteral anastomoses and an end colostomy are formed. The patient is then placed in the prone position. Through a presacral incision, the perineal dissection is completed, with mobilization of the sacrum from the gluteus muscles, sacral laminectomy with preservation of the nerve roots, and osteotomy of the sacrum. En bloc resection of the tumor with contiguous abdominal viscera and involved sacrum is then completed. Initial sacral margin tissue was positive for malignancy; this was re-excised to a clear margin 48 hours later, at which time the posterior wound was closed with gluteus myocutaneous flaps.

Intraoperative Image

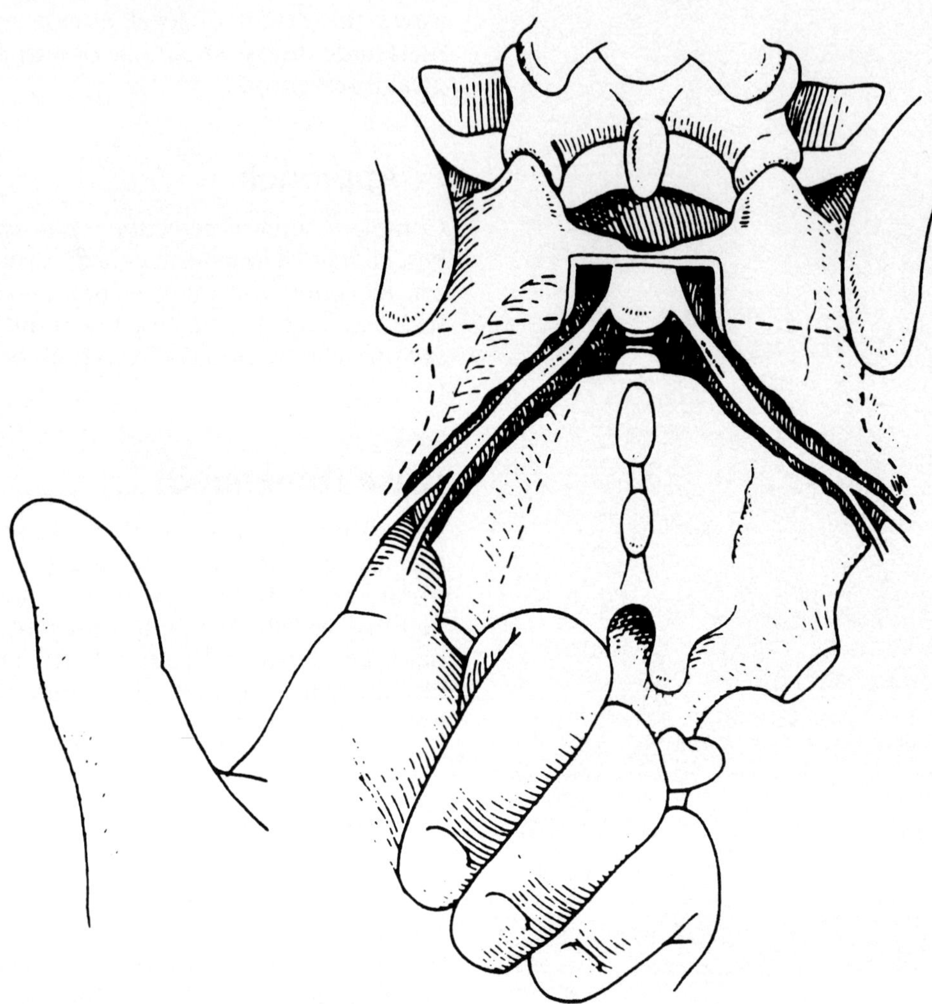

Figure 36.2 (From Wanebo HJ, Turk PS: Abdominal sacral resection for recurrent cancer of the rectum. In: Bauer JJ, ed. *Colorectal Surgery Illustrated*. St. Louis: Mosby; 1993:241. Used with permission from Elsevier.)

Surgical Approach

The patient undergoes a two-stage en bloc resection of the tumor with contiguous abdominal viscera and involved sacrum. Division of the sacrum is achieved with an oscillating saw. Note that the surgeon's finger is positioned anteriorly, protecting the underlying intra-abdominal contents. Initial sacral margin tissue was positive for malignancy; this was re-excised to a clear margin 48 hours later, at which time the posterior wound was closed with gluteus myocutaneous flaps.

Case Continued

Because of the initial positive sacral margin and the patient's previous exposure to the maximal dose of EBRT, he is treated with brachytherapy to 30 Gy. He also receives adjuvant chemotherapy consisting of two cycles of 5-fluorouracil and irinotecan, which due to toxicities is changed to 5-fluorouracil and oxaliplatin for four more cycles.

The patient initially did well, with a decrease in his CEA level to 0.7 ng/mL 5 months after the ASR.

His functional status is excellent, and he returns to work without difficulty. Unfortunately, the patient again begins experiencing sciatica-like pain radiating down his left leg. Eleven months after the ASR, his CEA level rises to 4.2 ng/mL.

MRI

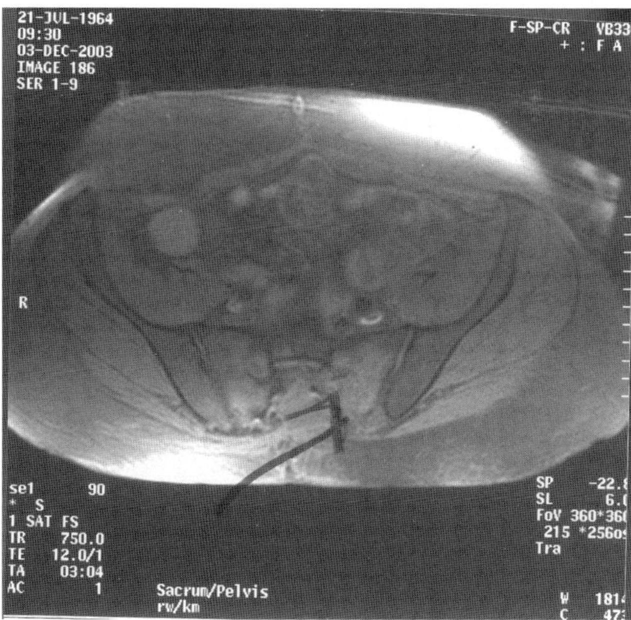

Figure 36.3

MRI Report

Contrast-enhanced MRI shows an intense hypermetabolic focus in the left sacral ala. Percutaneous CT-guided biopsy of the left sacral ala confirms recurrent metastatic adenocarcinoma.

Diagnosis and Recommendation

The patient has developed a second local recurrence of rectal cancer involving the sacral bone. Treatment options at this point are limited. Radiation therapy has been used in such instances for palliation; however, the maximum tolerable dose of EBRT, as well as brachytherapy, has been given. The patient has received multiple courses of chemotherapy using the best available agents for recurrent or metastatic rectal cancer.

Our group and others have shown excellent palliation of pain and occasional significant regression of disease, allowing resection. Using transfemoral access and intraoperative fluoroscopy, balloon occlusion catheters and infusion catheters are inserted into the inferior vena cava and the aorta. Bilateral thigh tourniquets are inflated, thereby isolating the pelvic circulation, and chemotherapeutic agents are infused in a serial fashion using the extracorporeal circuit. We have tested a variety of protocols prior to identification of the current regimen of 5-fluorouracil, eloxatin, mitomycin C, and paclitaxel.

Clinical Photograph

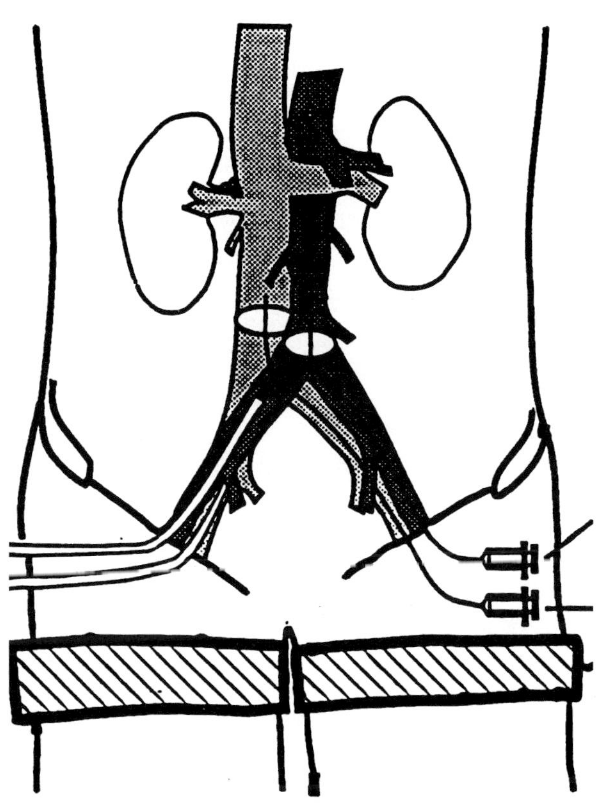

Figure 36.4 (From Turk PS, Belliveau JF, Darnowski JW, et al. Isolated pelvic perfusion for unresectable cancer using a balloon occlusion technique. *Arch Surg* 1993;128: 533–539. Used with permission.)

Approach

The patient undergoes two isolated pelvic perfusion treatments, approximately 1 month apart, using transfemoral access and vascular isolation, with the extracorporeal circuit and standard hemodialysis technology. Based on the response, he may be a candidate for future radiofrequency ablation of remaining disease at the sacral ala, or even possibly resection.

Discussion

Despite improvements in adjuvant therapy regimens and the virtually universal adoption of total mesorectal excision (TME) for middle and lower third rectal cancers, recurrent rectal cancer remains a significant clinical problem. Nonsurgical management options may provide transient palliation, but offer no hope of long-term survival. Surgical resection of pelvic recurrence can provide 5-year survival rates of up to 30%, similar to those seen after resection of solitary metastases to the lung, liver, or brain, and is justified in highly selected patients.

Treatment options are limited for the patient who experiences locoregional recurrence after the above therapeutic maneuvers have been exhausted. We have found isolated pelvic perfusion to be useful in such cases, offering excellent palliation of pelvic pain and occasionally serving as a bridge to surgical resection.

Suggested Readings

Beart RW Jr. New success with management of recurrent rectal cancer: a reason to follow patients. *Ann Surg Oncol* 1999;6:131–132.

Turk PS, Belliveau JF, Darnowski JW, et al. Isolated pelvic perfusion for unresectable cancer using a balloon occlusion technique. *Arch Surg* 1993;128:533–539.

Wanebo HJ, Koness RJ, Vezeridis MP, et al. Pelvic resection of recurrent rectal cancer. *Ann Surg* 1994;220:586–597.

Wanebo HJ. Commentary on: Zacherl J et al. Abdominosacral resection of recurrent rectal cancer in the sacrum. *Dis Colon Rectum* 1999;42:1039–1040.

Wong CS, Cummings BJ, Brierley JD, et al. Treatment of locally recurrent rectal carcinoma—results and prognostic factors. *Int J Radiat Oncol Biol Phys* 1998;40:427–435.

Presentation

A 47-year-old white woman presents with a recent onset of anorectal discomfort and bright red blood per rectum. Digital rectal examination reveals a 1- to 1.5-cm lesion in the rectum, on the anterior aspect just proximal to the anal sphincter.

Differential Diagnosis

The differential diagnosis of a 1.5-cm rectal lesion in this age group commonly includes an adenomatous polyp. The most common malignant cause is a rectal adenocarcinoma (possibly within a tubulovillous adenoma). More rare causes include benign lymphoma, lipoma, leiomyoma, fibroma or hemangioma, and malignancies such as carcinoid, malignant lymphoma, and leiomyosarcoma.

Recommendation

Fresh blood per rectum always requires a full history and thorough clinical examination, including a digital rectal examination, proctoscopy, and flexible sigmoidoscopy in the first instance. The initial management of a rectal polyp is primarily aimed at complete removal of the lesion, obtaining tissue for a histologic diagnosis, and exclusion of other colonic polyps.

Case Continued

The lesion is biopsied for histologic examination, and further investigations are arranged, including colonoscopy and subsequent transanal resection of the lesion. Colonoscopy demonstrates a normal colon beyond this lesion.

Histopathology Slides

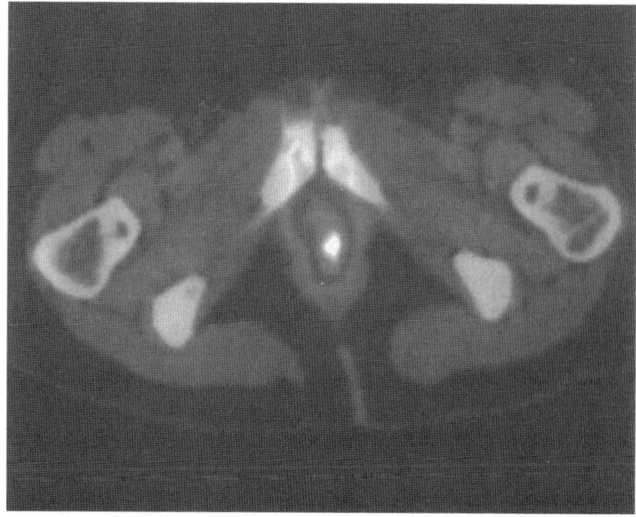

Figure 37.1A

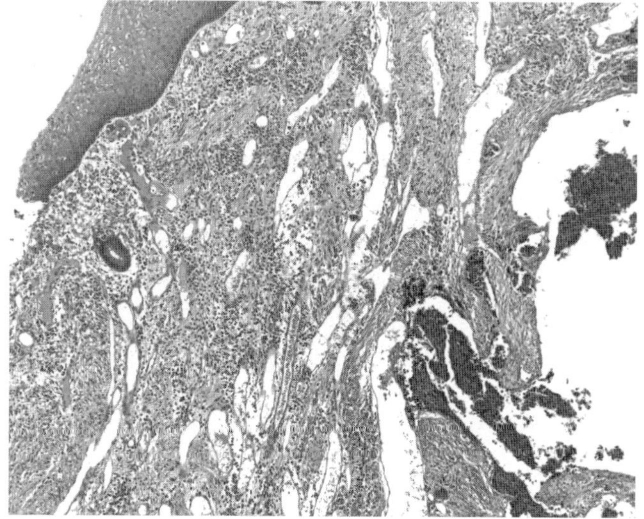

Figure 37.1B

Histopathology Report

Histology of the removed lesion reveals a deeply invasive (beyond muscularis propria) neuroendocrine tumor or carcinoid, 1.8 cm in diameter, with positive stains for chromogranin A and synaptophysin, moderate atypia, angioinvasion, 1 mitosis in 10 high-power fields (HPF) and a tumor proliferative index (TPI) up to 30%, as assessed by Ki67 immunostaining (World Health Organization [WHO] well-differentiated endocrine carcinoma, or malignant carcinoid). Squamous epithelium at the anorectal margin can be visualized in relation to the distal edge of the resected tumor.

▌ PET Scans

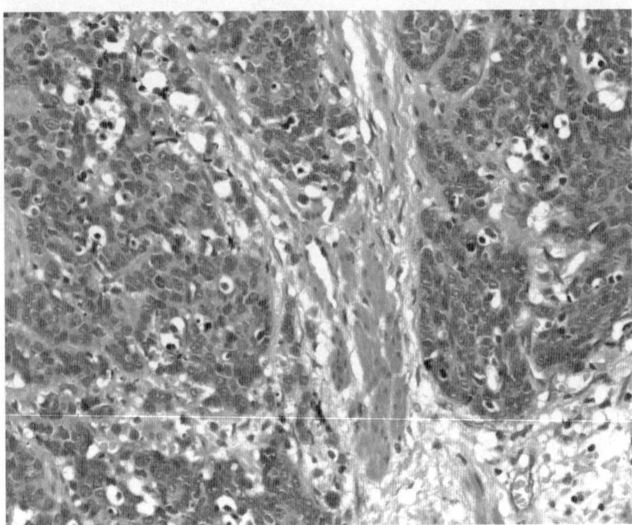

Figure 37.2A

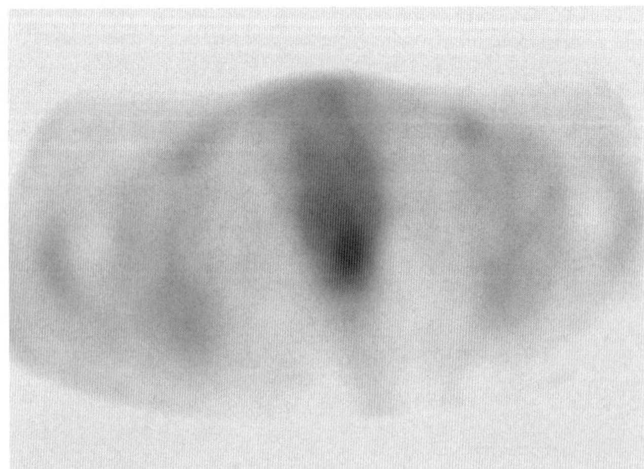

Figure 37.2B

PET Scan Report

Neuroendocrine tumor is seen extending beyond the muscularis propria. The lesion is located very close to the anorectal junction. The deep resection margin is positive, indicating incomplete removal.

Discussion

The endoscopic features of rectal neuroendocrine tumors are well described, and these findings should be detailed and carefully reported. Central mucosal depression or ulceration suggests high metastatic potential.

Rectal carcinoid tumors are of neuroendocrine origin and, unless particularly poorly differentiated, they contain the typical dense-core secretory granules in the cytoplasm, and small clear vesicles. Synaptophysin is associated with the small vesicles, a sensitive marker for neuroendocrine tumors. Chromogranin A is localized to the secretory granules and is regarded as a powerful universal marker for neuroendocrine tumors.

New classification systems and nomenclature now refer to neuroendocrine tumors (NETs) rather than carcinoids, although this term is still commonly used both in histology reports and the literature. Gastrointestinal NETs may be classified by the site of origin (i.e., foregut, midgut, or hindgut embryologically). The majority of hindgut NETs are found in the rectum.

Three types of neuroendocrine tumors have been identified in the hindgut, L cell tumors, EC cell tumors, and small cell tumors. Rectal tumors are usually L cell tumors, producing glicentin-related products and PP-PYY peptides. The tumors may contain subsets of other neuroendocrine cells among the L cells. Argentaffin EC tumors with typical serotonin production are extremely rare in the rectum.

Clinicopathological staging and classification are as follows: (a) *benign nonfunctioning tumor* of small size (<2 cm), within the mucosa or submucosa, without angioinvasion; (b) *uncertain behavior nonfunctioning, greater than 2 cm diameter, within the mucosa or submucosa,* or angioinvasive tumors; (c) *low-grade malignant tumor,* well-differentiated endocrine carcinoma; deeply invasive tumors extending beyond the submucosa, usually functioning; and (d) *high-grade malignant* poorly differentiated neuroendocrine carcinoma (i.e., small cell carcinoma).

The incidence of carcinoid tumors of the rectum is on the increase in clinical practice. Rectal carcinoids are diagnosed in relatively young patients, at an average age of 56 years, and have a three fold higher incidence in the black population than in the white population in the United States.

The majority (75% to 85%) of rectal carcinoids are localized at diagnosis. Around 1.7% of the 925 carcinoids in the latest subset of the Surveillance, Epidemiology, and End Results (SEER) program had distant metastases and 2.2% had regional metastases (lymph node involvement), but 14.4% were classified as unstaged. The shift toward unstaged and purely localized tumors may reflect the common use of endoscopic resection for diagnosis and treatment of early disease.

Patients with rectal carcinoids have an overall 5-year survival rate of 75% to 88%. If localized at diagnosis, the 5-year survival rate is 84% to 91%. This decreases to 36% to 49% with regional disease and to 21% to 32% in the presence of distant metastatic disease. The vast majority therefore has a survival expectancy in excess of 80% at 5 years, comparing favorably with the overall survival for all gastrointestinal carcinoids of 67%.

Diagnosis

This patient has a 1.8-cm deeply invasive neuroendocrine tumor of the lower rectum, with positive resection margins.

Recommendation

Complete resection of the rectal lesion is necessary. Preoperative imaging and biochemical tests are obtained preoperatively for staging purposes.

Approach

Imaging investigations that are important for determining the local extent of the disease and excluding the presence of distant metastases include the following. *Endorectal ultrasound (EUS)* is valuable in assessing depth of invasion and the presence or absence of pararectal lymph node metastases. In conjunction with other investigative techniques and endoscopy, EUS provides important information with respect to choice of therapy. *Computed tomography (CT) scans of the abdomen and pelvis* are used to assess local extent and involvement of other pelvic structures and to exclude hepatic metastases.

Perform *111-Indium octreotide scanning.* Hindgut lesions may be negative for 111-indium uptake, and other modalities such as positron emission tomography (PET) or PET-CT and meta-iodobenzyl guanidine I 123 (MIBG) scanning have to be used if there is suspicion of distant metastases.

Biochemical tests that should be obtained include the following.

Serum chromogranin A is a neuroendocrine marker that is present in the majority of carcinoid tumors irrespective of origin. Serum chromogranin A is the most sensitive screening marker for carcinoid tumors, and serum levels correspond to tumor load and prognosis.

Because rectal tumors may produce peptides other than serotonin, a *fasting serum gut hormone profile* might be helpful, particularly when metastatic disease is expected [pancreatic polypeptide (PP) and glucagon particularly].

Obtain levels of *24-hour urinary 5-hydroxyindoleacetic acid (5-HIAA),* even though the sensitivity is low due to the rarity of serotonin production in rectal carcinoids.

Serum acid phosphatase levels may be raised in prostatic-specific acid phosphatase-positive tumors.

Obtain levels of *human chorionic gonadotropin (β-HCG)*. β-HCG levels may be increased and may correlate with malignant potential.

Case Continued

EUS identifies presence of residual tumor in proximity to the anal sphincter. Magnetic resonance imaging (MRI) of the abdomen/pelvis shows some scarring but no evidence of any residual tumor or metastases. Octreotide scanning is negative. MIBG scanning is negative. All biochemical investigations are normal.

The patient refuses to undergo an abdominoperineal resection (APR), and therefore a transanal excision of the tumor bed is performed. The re-excision reveals residual tumor present in the base, but also multiple foci of tumor up to and including the new resection margins.

Recommendation

In view of the potentially local aggressive behavior, lack of evidence of systemic disease, and positive margins abutting the anal sphincter in a young healthy patient, laparoscopic APR is recommended.

Discussion

Lesions smaller than 1 cm have a low risk of metastatic disease (<3%) and should be completely resected endoscopically or by a transanal technique. Transanal resection using a variety of techniques and equipment offers the ability to resect higher lesions and a full-thickness resection. Aggressive surgery such as anterior resection carries a higher risk than the metastatic potential of the lesion, whereas adequate local resections carry a comparatively low risk. Exceptions do apply, because some small lesions may demonstrate features suggesting high metastatic potential.

A lesion between 1 and 2 cm is a controversial area. The metastatic risk is considered to be between 10% and 15%. Some studies demonstrated no benefit with aggressive management. Other authors have reported successful treatment with local or radical surgery, with disease-free survival in several, but not all, cases. Assessment of tumors endoscopically and by endoanal ultrasound should also guide treatment in this group of patients.

Lesions larger than 2 cm have a significantly higher metastatic risk (60% to 80%), and invasion of the muscularis propria, which is common in this group, indicates a high metastatic potential.

Surgical Approach

Laparoscopic APR is performed, and is begun by initially inspecting the entire abdominal cavity, the peritoneum, and the liver. A complete total mesorectal excision is performed with ligation of the inferior mesenteric vessels. The dissection is continued anteriorly in the rectovaginal plane. An elliptical perineal incision is made, and great care is taken to ensure that clear macroscopic margins are achieved in the region of the tumor. The whole specimen is delivered through the perineum. The colostomy is created in the standard fashion.

Case Continued

The patient recovers well postoperatively. Histologic examination reveals tumor in the area of the resected tumor and two lymph node deposits in the mesorectum. The main tumor mass shows up to 10 mitoses in 10 high-power fields (HPF), while one of the lymph nodal tumor deposits demonstrates a very high mitotic index (up to 50 mitoses in 10 HPF). Circumferential resection margins are clear.

Recommendation

Given the radioinsensitivity of carcinoids, and the resection of the mesorectum, radiotherapy is not offered. Carcinoid tumors are generally not very chemosensitive, and this option, usually streptozocin-based regimes, should be reserved for advanced cases. High mitotic index tumors and poorly differentiated tumors may respond to cisplatin-based chemotherapy. Although its role is controversial, interferon treatment is another therapeutic option. Close follow-up is advisable, with repeat PET-CT or MRI for local disease, and liver ultrasound scan for metastatic disease. Biochemical markers such as chromogranin A should be performed at regular intervals.

Suggested Readings

Koura AN, Giacco GG, Curley SA, et al. Carcinoid tumors of the rectum: effect of size, histopathology, and surgical treatment on metastasis free survival. *Cancer* 1997;79:1294–1298.

Matsushita M, Takakuwa H, Nishio A. Management of rectal carcinoid tumors. *Gastrointest Endosc* 2003;58:641–642.

Modlin IM, Lye KD, Kidd M. A 5-decade analysis of 13715 carcinoid tumors. *Cancer* 2003;97:934–959.

Rindi G, Bordi C. Highlights of the biology of endocrine tumors of the gut and pancreas. *Endocr Relat Cancer* 2003; 10:427–436.

Sauven P, Ridge JA, Quan SH, et al. Anorectal carcinoid tumors. Is aggressive surgery warranted? *Ann Surg* 1990;211:67–71.

Schindl M, Niederle B, Hafner M, et al. Stage-dependent therapy of rectal carcinoid tumors. *World J Surg* 1998;22:628–633.

Solcia E, Kloppel G, Sobin LH. Histological typing of endocrine tumors. *WHO International Histological Classification of Tumors.* 3rd ed. Berlin: Springer Verlag; 1999.

Presentation

A 57-year-old man who has a past medical history of hypertension and hyperlipidemia presents to your office after he was seen by his primary medical doctor for symptoms of occasional anal bleeding and changes in defecation. He is a nonsmoker and has no constipation. On physical examination, there is neither ascites nor a palpable abdominal tumor. On digital rectal examination, a 5-cm firm tumor is palpable on the left side of the rectal wall and 3 cm from the anal verge. The tumor is not movable and appears to be covered by the intact mucosa. No apparent bleeding is noted.

▊ Barium Enema and Colonoscopy

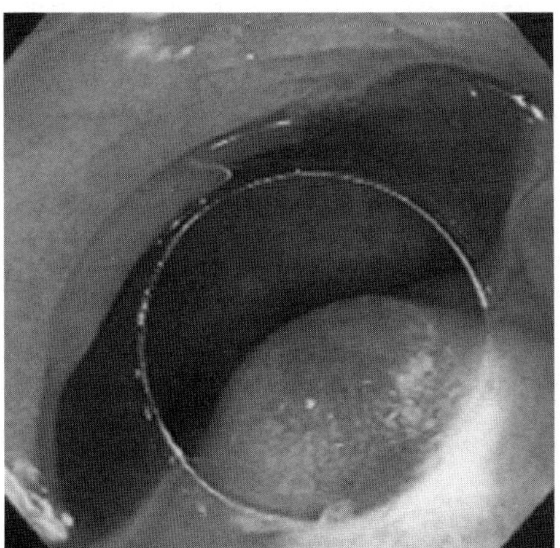

Figure 38.1A

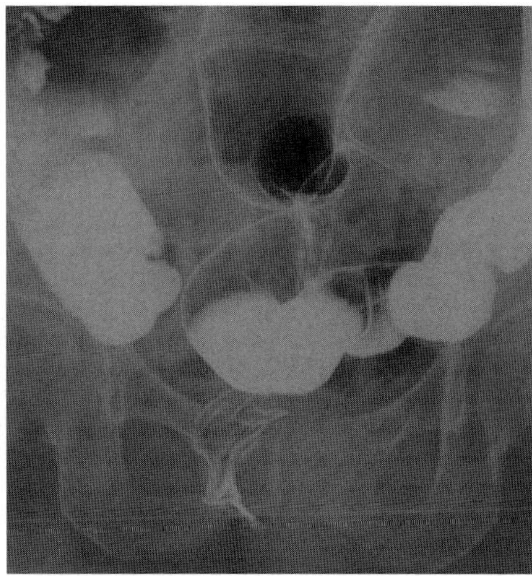

Figure 38.1B

Barium Enema and Colonoscopy Report

The rectum is compressed from the left side by a round tumor. On endoscopy, there is a submucosal tumor on the left sidewall of the rectum with an intact mucosa. The tumor appears to be 5 cm in diameter.

Differential Diagnosis

The differential diagnosis for rectal submucosal masses in the adult include: mesenchymal tumors, lymphomas, submucosal extension of rectal and/or anal carcinomas, melanomas, and genitourological tumors. Mesenchymal cell tumors are mainly composed of gastrointestinal stromal tumor (GISTs), leiomyomas, and leiomyosarcomas. Submucosal extension of rectal or anal carcinoma is relatively frequent in the poorly differentiated type of rectal adenocarcinoma or anal squamous cell carcinoma, respectively, and sometimes accompanies an increase in tumor markers, including carcinoembryonic antigen (CEA), cancer antigen (CA) 19-9, and squamous cell cancer (SCC). In this patient, CEA, CA 19-9, and SCC levels are within the normal range. Based on the location of the tumor, and with no increase in CEA and SCC, one must consider stromal tumor in the rectum to be the primary diagnosis. In radiographic evaluation of a pelvic mass, magnetic resonance imaging (MRI) is superior to computed tomography (CT) scan in discrimination of each structure. The biopsy of the rectal tumor is usually not difficult. Histologic examination is the most reliable test for submucosal tumors.

Recommendation

CT scan of the pelvic region as well as a fine-needle biopsy.

CT Scan

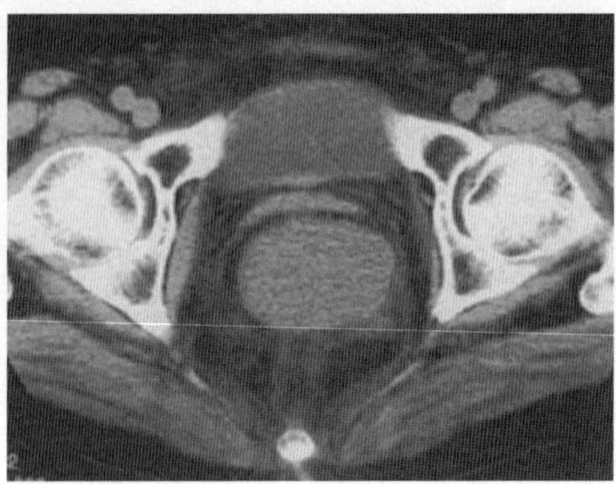

Figure 38.2A

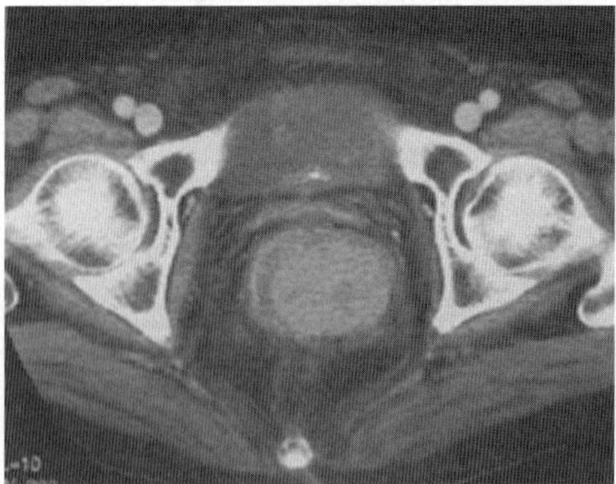

Figure 38.2B

CT Scan

A 5-cm, round, homogenously slightly enhancing mass with clear margin located on the left wall of the rectum. The tumor does not involve the bladder or prostatic gland.

Histopathology Report

Biopsy specimen reveals an epithelioid and spindle cell-type tumor with a few mitoses.

Approach

Stromal tumors of the rectum are usually either GIST or leiomyosarcoma. The patient is offered an abdominoperineal resection (APR) of the rectum. In some cases, local excision or sphincter-sparing operations, including lower anterior resection (LAR), may be recommended if the tumor has adequate distance from the anal sphincter muscles. In this case, the lower border of the tumor is located just above the sphincter muscles. Complete resection by APR is expected in more than 90% of cases; after complete resection, there is an estimated 30% to 40% incidence of local recurrence or hepatic metastasis. The possibility of bladder and sexual dysfunction after APR is relatively less frequent than when performed for rectal or anal carcinoma because no lymph node dissection is required for a stromal tumor and the pelvic nerve plexus innervating to the bladder and penis can be preserved.

Surgical Approach

It is critical to perform a complete tumor resection with a 1- to 2-cm margin. A lower abdominal incision is performed for mobilization of the rectum and preparation of the sigmoid colon for colostomy. Laparoscopic-assisted abdominal procedures may also substitute for an open laparotomy. A synchronous perineal incision and dissection is performed for en bloc resection of the anorectum. A single closed drain is placed in the pelvic cavity at the end of the operation; the drain is usually removed on the second or third postoperative day.

Case Continued

The patient undergoes bowel preparation and receives psychological care for permanent colostomy. A lower median incision is performed and the rectum is mobilized, then, the tumor is found to be in the left lower rectal wall just above the sphincter muscles. No apparent invasions into surrounding tissues are found and the patient undergoes APR. Postoperative course of the patient is uneventful, and he is discharged from the hospital on the sixth postoperative day.

Surgical Specimen and Histopathology Slides

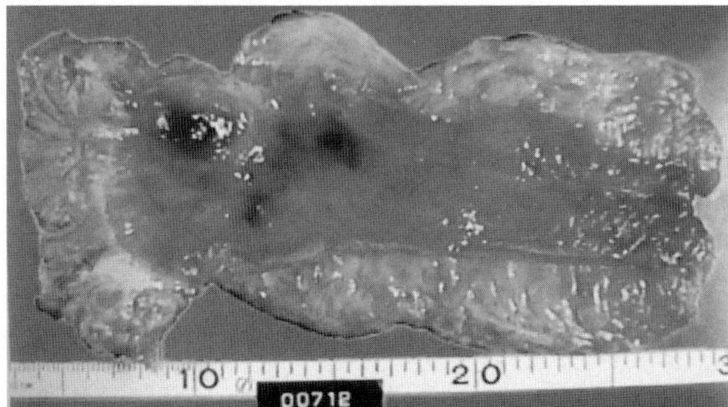

Figure 38.3A

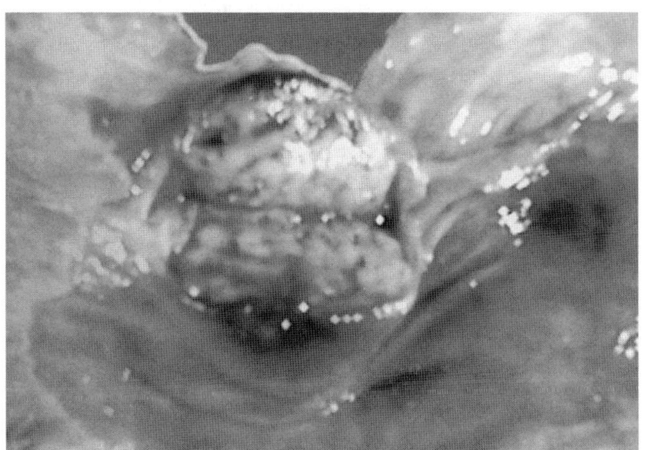

Figure 38.3B

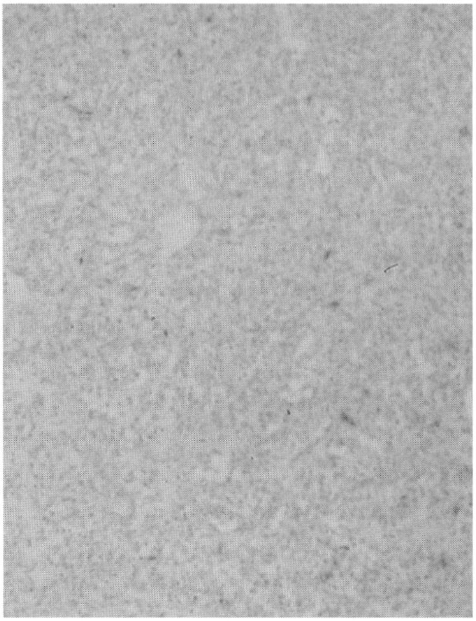

Figure 38.4B

Figure 38.4A

Figure 38.4C

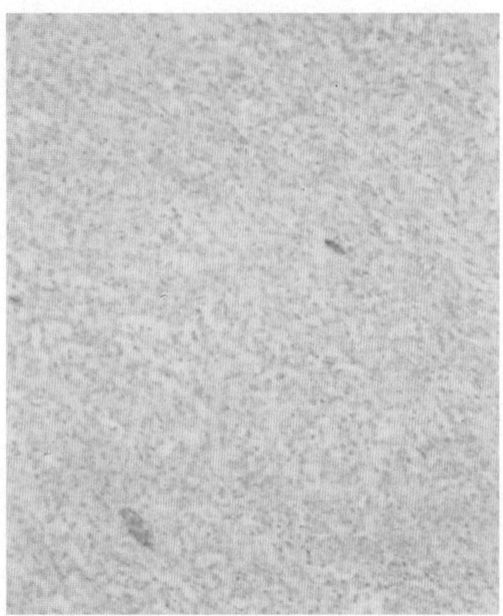

Figure 38.4D

Pathology Report and Genetic Analysis

The pathology report describes a 5-cm tumor located on the lower rectum without invasion into the sphincter and surrounding structures; the tumor is a high-grade GIST with epithelioid-spindle cell type. The report further describes 6 to 7 mitoses per 50 high-power fields (HPF), with immunostaining strongly positive for KIT and partly positive for alpha-smooth muscle actin, but principally negative for CD34 and S-100 proteins, and desmin. Genetic analysis of the tumor reveals inframe deletion mutation in exon 11 of the C-KIT gene.

Discussion

Stromal tumors of the colon and rectum are mainly composed of myogenic tumors (leiomyoma or leiomyosarcoma) and GISTs. Most of the myogenic tumors that originate from muscularis mucosae appear as polypoid lesions and are benign. They can be resected by endoscopic polypectomy. The lesions are typically small and located predominantly in the rectum and sigmoid. All colonic and rectal myogenic tumors are composed of well-differentiated, eosinophilic smooth muscle tumor cells that are seen immediately beneath the mucosa obliterating the muscularis mucosae layer. Only a small portion of myogenic tumors shows malignant features. In contrast to myogenic tumors, GISTs occur predominantly in older adults (median age, 60) and are histologically and clinically malignant. The colonic GISTs are typically transmural tumors with frequent intraluminal and/or outward bulging components. Histologically, most of them are spindle cell tumors

(90%), whereas 10% are epithelioid. Most colorectal GISTs are positive for CD117 (KIT) and less frequently positive for CD34 protein. Some colorectal GISTs coexpress alpha-smooth muscle actin, but none show desmin or S-100 protein.

GISTs are considered to be caused by gain-of-function mutations in the C-KIT (80% to 90%) or platelet-derived growth factor receptor alpha (PDGFR-α) gene (about 5%). Most mutations are found in exon 11 of the C-KIT gene, followed by exon 9 mutations. In 5% to 10% of GISTs, there is no mutation in either gene.

Case Continued

After the operation, the patient has visited your office every 6 months. One year following the APR, he presents with a 2-week history of progressively worsening anal pain. On physical examination, a 5-cm firm fixed subcutaneous mass is palpable on his left hip.

Recommendation

The mass in the patient's left hip is suspicious for recurrent GIST. Thus, CT or MRI is strongly recommended to evaluate disease distribution and progression. A chest x-ray should be obtained to exclude pulmonary metastases.

CT Scan

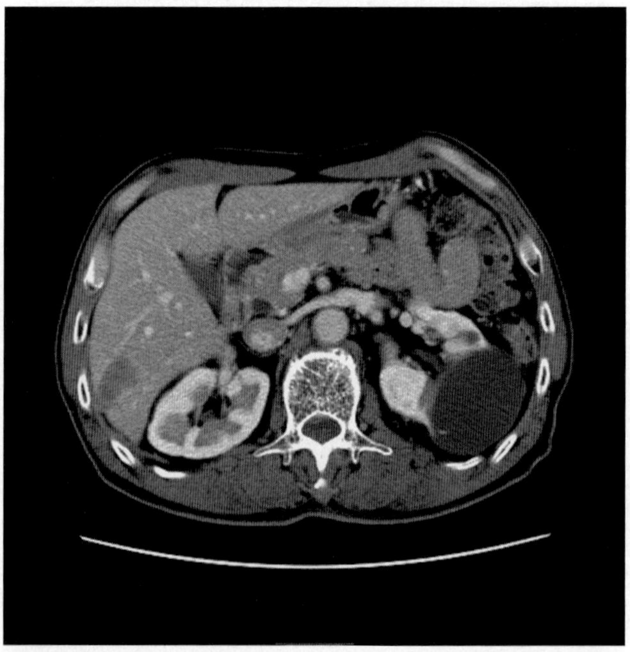

Figure 38.5A

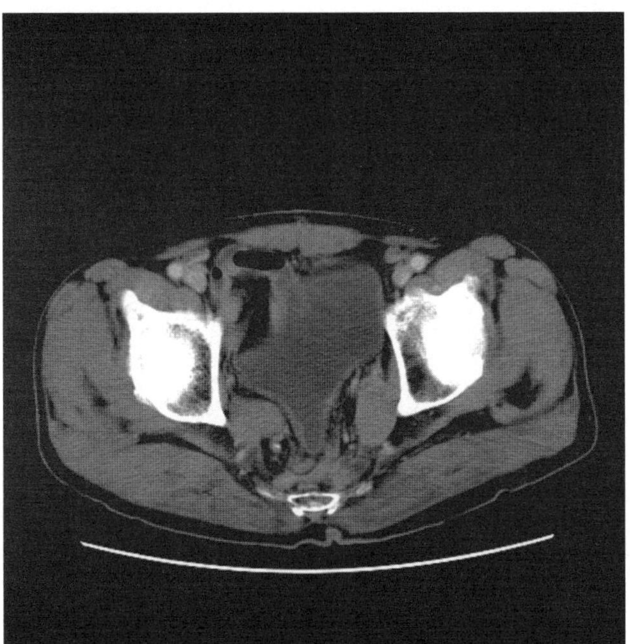

Figure 38.5B

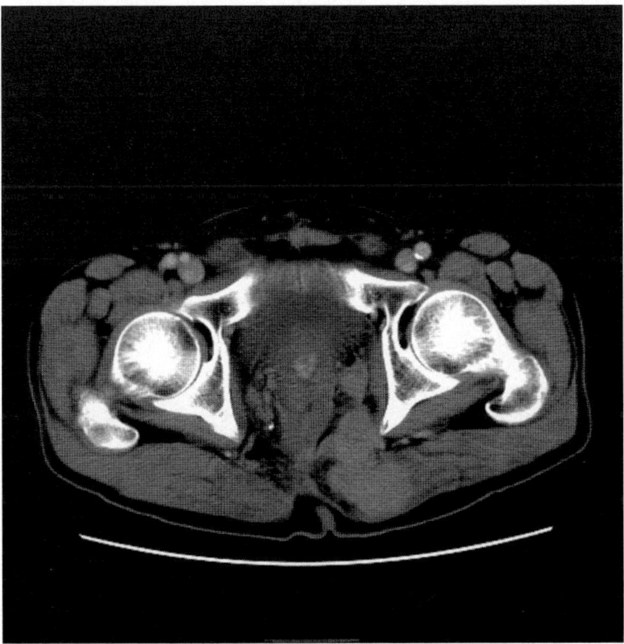

Figure 38.5C

CT Scan Report

The CT scan demonstrates a low-density tumor in segment VI of the liver, which is slightly enhanced with contrast medium, and tumors in the pelvic cavity invading into hip muscles and with suspected invasion to pelvic nerves. No peritoneal dissemination is noted. Chest x-ray shows no pulmonary metastatic lesion.

Case Continued

The patient is offered the option of surgical resection of the solitary liver metastasis and the pelvic tumors. Another strategy for metastatic GIST is imatinib mesylate. The patient decides on the option of imatinib.

Discussion

In GIST, the most important and reliable therapeutic strategy is surgical removal of the tumor if it is resectable. When it is not resectable, treatment with imatinib is recommended. Imatinib has excellent activity in advanced and metastatic GISTs with good tolerability. Drug-related adverse events are very frequent but are manageable, and serious adverse effects are, fortunately, infrequent (each less than 10%). Disease control (stable disease with partial response) is expected in about 80% to 90% of patients with advanced GISTs and is confirmed by CT or MRI evaluation. By 18-month follow-up, two thirds of patients with advanced GISTs treated with imatinib remained free of tumor progression, and 1- and 2-year survival was improved by imatinib compared with conventional chemoradiotherapy. Imatinib is most active against GISTs with mutations in exon 11 and exon 13 of the C-KIT gene and exon 12 of the PDGFR-α gene, followed by GISTs with mutations in exon 9 of the C-KIT gene. GISTs without any mutations in the C-KIT and PDGFR-α genes and those with kinase domain mutations (exon 17 in the C-KIT gene and exon 18 in the PDGFR-α gene) are frequently resistant to imanitib. The GIST of this patient has an inframe-deletion mutation in exon 11 of the C-KIT gene, so the disease control rate of the drug is expected to be more than 90%.

Case Continued

The patient starts 400 mg/day of imatinib. The CT scan and fluorodeoxyglucose-positron emission tomography (FDG-PET) scan are used to evaluate response to the drug. Within a few days, anal pain has rapidly disappeared after initiation of the drug. At 1-month follow-up, the CT scan reveals that hepatic metastasis has become low density compared with baseline, and the pelvic tumor is shrinking and also has become low density. Effects of imatinib are more obviously demonstrated by the FDG-PET scan, in which incorporation of FDG is completely inhibited by the drug.

Discussion

With imatinib, complete response is rare, and most responses are partial responses or long stable disease, suggesting that resistance to the drug will appear in the future. In fact, after 2 years, more than half the patients receiving imatinib suffer from disease progression. Local resistance may be managed by surgery, radiofrequency ablation, or arterial chemoembolization; controlling systemic resistance may be attempted by increasing the dosage of imatinib, or by trials of new drugs.

Suggested Readings

Dematteo RP, Heinrich MC, El-Rifai WM, et al. Clinical management of gastrointestinal stromal tumors: before and after STI-571. *Hum Pathol* 2002;33:466–477.

Demetri GD, Benjamin R, Blanke CD, et al. Optimal management of patients with gastrointestinal stromal tumors (GIST). Expansion and update of NCCN clinical guidelines. *JNCCN* 2004;2(suppl 1):S1–S26.

Heinrich MC, Corless CL. Targeting mutant kinases in gastrointestinal stromal tumors: a paradigm for molecular therapy of other sarcomas. *Cancer Treat Res* 2004;120:129–150.

Kitamura Y, Hirota S, Nishida T. Gastrointestinal stromal tumor (GIST): a model for molecule-based diagnosis and treatment of solid tumors. *Cancer Science* 2003;94:315–320.

Miettinen M, Majidi M, Lasota J. Pathology and diagnostic criteria of gastrointestinal stromal tumors (GISTs): a review. *Eur J Cancer* 2002;38(suppl 5):S39–S51.

Presentation

A 59-year-old man presents with a 4-month history of intermittent bright red bleeding per rectum treated as hemorrhoidal disease. For the last 2 months, he complained of pain with defecation, incontinence, and weight loss.

He was diagnosed 10 years ago with human immunodeficiency virus (HIV) and hepatitis C and had hemorrhoid banding 5 years ago. He has no allergies. Current medications include stavudine (Zerit), lamivudine (Epivir), nelfinavir (Viracept), and an antidepressant. He is homeless and is enrolled in a detox program for alcohol, cocaine, and tobacco (40-pack-year) addiction. There is no known family history of cancer.

He is alert with normal vital signs, is thin but not cachetic, and sits with some discomfort. He has moist mucous membranes with no icterus, pallor, or generalized lymphadenopathy. He has a palpable liver 3 cm below the costal margin.

Clinical Photograph

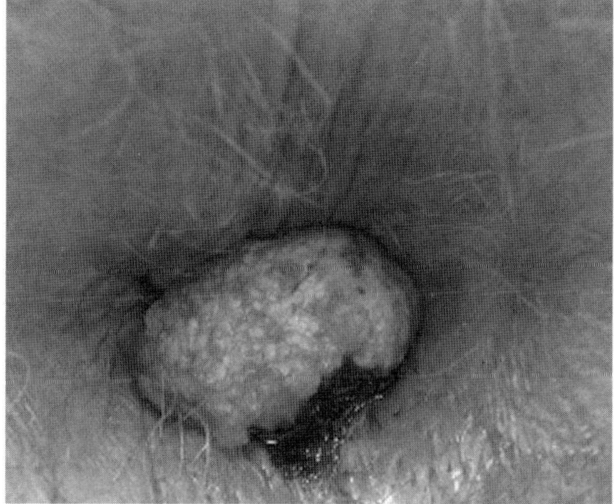

Figure 39.1

Physical Examination Report

Rectal examination shows a 2-cm exophytic mass at the right lateral anal margin with a 5 × 3-cm firm, tender, lobulated, and fixed intra-anal mass. The surrounding skin is erythematous due to pruritus. No enlarged inguinal lymph nodes are palpated.

Differential Diagnosis

Given the appearance and intra-anal component, a neoplastic growth would be on top of the list, most commonly epidermoid carcinoma, anal adenocarcinoma, or amelanotic melanoma. The external component could be mistaken for thrombosed fibrotic hemorrhoids, or hypertrophied and prolapsing anal papilla.

Discussion

The anal canal is defined as extending from the anorectal ring to the intersphincteric groove corresponding to the length of the internal sphincter. The anal verge is the junction of the keratinized hair-bearing squamous epithelium and the anoderm. The mucosa of the anal canal varies from rectal columnar to the anal transitional zone (extending variably above the dentate line, usually 5 to 10 mm) to squamous nonkeratinized anoderm without hair or other skin appendages. The anal transitional zone has the most varied epithelium including basal, columnar, cuboidal, and squamous cells in four to nine layers. In addition, this zone may have endocrine cells and melanocytes. It is this layer that is most susceptible to human papilloma virus (HPV) infection and is where most anal canal cancers arise.

Anal canal squamous cell carcinoma is defined as a tumor between the intersphincteric groove and the anorectal ring. It accounts for about 1.5% of all gastrointestinal tract tumors; however, it has been rising in incidence over the past 25 years, especially in HIV-positive male homosexuals.

Current major known etiological factors are HPV infection and smoking. Smoking increases the risk (relative risk 7 to 9) of anal cancer, and patients with anal cancer have a higher risk of cervical, vulvar, and other smoking-related cancers (i.e., oral cavity, larynx, lung, bladder, and breast cancers). HPV is important in the etiology of anal cancer. There is a strong association among genital warts known to be caused by HPV, low-grade and high-grade squamous intraepithelial lesions and anal cancer, and sexual promiscuity and anal-receptive intercourse. Patients with HIV disease, especially those with CD4 counts less than 200/mm^3, have a higher incidence of HPV infection that is more likely to be persistent compared with patients who do not have HIV disease. HIV infection may also predispose to a greater progression of low-grade to high-grade dysplasia. The incidence of anal cancer has increased in both men and women, but especially in HIV-positive male homosexuals. The relative risk in patients with acquired immunodeficiency syndrome (AIDS) may be as high as 84 for homosexual patients compared with 37 for non-homosexual patients. Transplant patients have been shown to have a tenfold to 100-fold increased risk of HPV infection, anal intraepithelial neoplasia (AIN 1-3), and anogenital cancer. Benign anal disease (e.g., fistulas) is more often a complication of the neoplasm rather than the cause, though very rarely a long-standing fistula in ano can develop adenocarcinoma.

Recommendation

Perform examination under anesthesia, and obtain biopsy to establish tissue diagnosis.

Case Continued

Routine laboratory results show a hemoglobin level of 11.7 g/dL, down from 15 g/dL 6 months ago. Serum chemistry, liver function tests, and chest roentgenogram are normal. His CD4 count is 764 and HIV viral load is less than 50 copies/mL.

The patient undergoes examination under anesthesia, proctoscopy, transrectal ultrasound, and biopsy of the mass.

Histopathology Slide

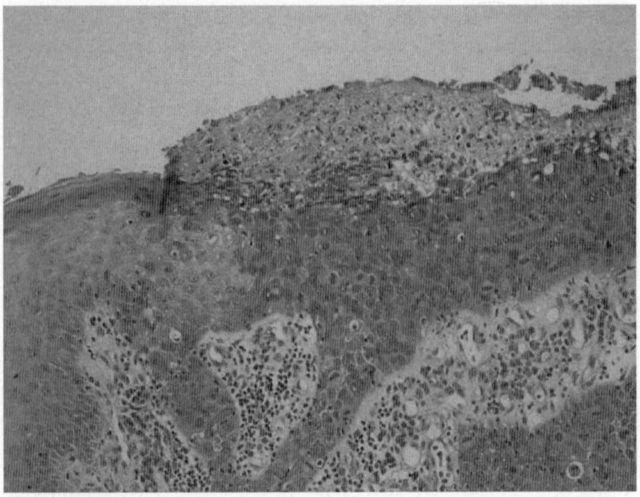

Figure 39.2

Histopathology Report

Photomicrograph showing junction of normal skin and invasive squamous cell carcinoma. The pathologic diagnosis is moderately differentiated squamous cell carcinoma, clinical stage T2 N0 M0. Higher power reveals HPV cytopathologic changes with crumpled crenated nuclei and perinuclear clearing.

Diagnosis and Recommendation

Squamous cell cancer of the anal canal. Computed tomography (CT) scans of the abdomen and pelvis are obtained to exclude abdominal lymph node and liver metastasis. Local tumor staging is best performed with an examination under anesthesia and with endoanal ultrasound. This approach is especially useful because anal canal cancers are often too painful to allow a satisfactory examination in the clinic. Suspicious groin lymph nodes should be evaluated with fine-needle aspiration cytology at the same time.

Discussion

Size, location of the anal cancer, depth of penetration, and lymph node involvement are important prognostic factors. In a study comparing endoanal ultrasound (EAUS) with clinical staging in 50 patients, two thirds of patients with clinical stage 1 and 2 had evidence of muscle penetration ultrasound T staging (UT) 3-4. Overall, there was good correlation among tumor size, depth of penetration, and tumor volume. Depth of penetration has not been incorporated in the recent tumor, node, metastasis (TNM) staging system. In a multicenter study, EAUS staging of anal cancer was more accurate in predicting tumor recurrence and survival after treatment than traditional clinical staging using tumor height. The ultrasonic T stage was the only significant factor in survival using multivariate analysis. In the presence of nodal metastasis, invasion and grade do not influence survival. Staging the tumor has no therapeutic value because most patients are treated with chemoradiation irrespective of stage. Chemoradiation successfully treats 90% of groin disease; therefore, inguinal node staging is more useful for prognosis rather than for change in therapy.

The roles of sentinel node biopsy, positron emission tomography (PET) scan, and magnetic resonance imaging (MRI) scan are unclear. The advantage of accurately staging lymph node disease is to allow selective groin radiation. PET scan is useful in helping differentiate postradiation fibrosis from recurrent tumor in the pelvis. MRI with phased array coil is more useful than endorectal coil due to difficulty in placement of the endorectal coil and similar accuracy. Ultrasound is useful in follow-up of patients after chemoradiation, to assess the response to therapy as well as to help direct postchemoradiation biopsies. The ultrasound in this case showed invasion of the sphincter muscles.

Case Continued

The patient undergoes staging endorectal ultrasound and a CT scan of the abdomen and pelvis.

Endorectal Ultrasonogram

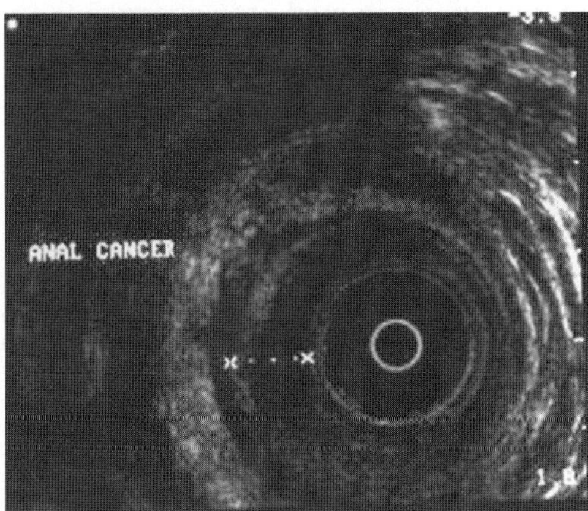

Figure 39.3

Endorectal Ultrasound Report

Endorectal ultrasound reveals invasion of sphincter muscles.

Case Continued

CT scans of the abdomen and pelvis reveal a 4.9 × 5.7-cm mass in the right lateral wall of the rectum. There are no enlarged perirectal, retroperitoneal, or inguinal nodes. There is nonspecific stranding of perirectal fat without definitive invasion.

Approach

The current standard of care for the anal canal margin is to treat definitively with chemoradiation therapy based on the Nigro regimen. The role of post-therapy biopsy in the management of patients with no clinical disease after treatment is controversial. Close clinical follow-up to detect clinical recurrence may be a reasonable approach. The alternate approach to excise residual scar is not beneficial in most patients, and there is a risk of delayed healing in a radiated field. EAUS may help by directing the area of the scar to sample. In patients with large tumors that respond well to therapy but do not completely regress, it may be reasonable to allow 10 to 12 weeks before a decision of salvage therapy is made.

Discussion

The treatment of anal cancer was revolutionized by Norman Nigro of Wayne State University in 1974. The Nigro protocol consisted of 30 Gy of radiation from a cobalt-60 source with continuous infusion of 5-fluorouracil (5-FU) at 1,000 mg/m^2 on days 1 to 4 and 29 to 32 and mitomycin C at 15 mg/m^2 in an intravenous bolus on day 1. The primary lesion disappeared in 40 patients, and only five patients had abdominoperineal resection (APR), four for persistent and one for recurrent disease. It was suggested that bulky tumors larger than 5 cm should have additional chemoradiation or routine APR. Treatments were well tolerated, despite frequent thrombocytopenia, neutropenia, and proctitis, with no treatment interruption from hematologic toxicity. The treatment of anal cancer was dramatically altered. Today the 5-year survival rate has increased from approximately 55% after primary APR to 82% with chemoradiotherapy, with preservation of anal function in the majority of patients in the latter group.

The three trials listed in Table 39.1 have confirmed that the current standard of care for invasive anal cancer is a combined modality approach consisting of radiotherapy, 5-FU, and mitomycin C chemotherapy.

Table 39-1: Clinical Trials Evaluating Chemoradiation Therapy for Anal Canal Squamous Cell Carcinoma

Study	Study Arms	Number of Patients	Complete Tumor Regression (%)	Local Failure (%)	Colostomy-Free Survival (%)	Overall Survival (%)
(UKCCCR)	RT (45 Gy + 15–25 Gy boost)	279	30	59		58
	RT + 5-FU + MitC	283	39	36		65 (NS)
(EORTC)	RT (45 Gy + 15–20 Gy boost)	52	54	69	22	56
	RT + 5-FU + MitC	51	80	42	41 ($p = 0.002$)	56 (NS)
(ECOG/RTOG)	RT + 5-FU	145	86	36	59	67
	RT + 5-FU + MitC	146	92	18	71 ($p = 0.0019$)	76 (NS)

ECOG/RTOG, Eastern Cooperative Oncology Group/Radiation Therapy Oncology Group; EORTC, European Organization for Research and Treatment of Cancer; 5-FU, 5-fluorouracil; MitC, mitomycin C; RT, radiation therapy; UKCCCR, United Kingdom Coordinating Committee on Cancer Research.

The original Nigro protocol was limited to 30 Gy of radiation. Subsequently, higher doses of radiation have been advocated to improve response rates. Although cure rates are more frequent with more than 54 Gy of radiation, complications such as anal ulcers, stenosis, bleeding, necrosis, bowel obstruction, and incontinence lead to colostomy rates of 6% to 12% despite good tumor control. The optimum dose is probably somewhere between 30 and 60 Gy.

Cisplatin has been substituted for mitomycin C due to good efficacy and a better safety profile, with reports of a colostomy-free survival rate of 86% and local control rates of 89% to 94%. A phase III randomized intergroup trial (RTOG-98-11) in which the current standard of care (5-FU, mitomycin C, and radiotherapy) will be compared with induction and concurrent 5-FU and cisplatin with radiotherapy will help define the role of cisplatin.

Case Continued

The patient is treated with combined modality therapy consisting of 5-FU at 1,000 mg/m^2 by continuous infusion on days 1 to 4 and 29 to 32 with mitomycin C at 10 mg/m^2 on day 1. The concomitant radiation therapy regimen consists of 5,040 cGy over 55 days in 180-cGy fractions (3,060 cGy is delivered to the whole pelvis and inguinal lymph nodes at 180 cGy/day utilizing 18-MV photons in three fields with custom blocking, 1,440 cGy to the true pelvis and inguinal lymphatics, and 540 cGy boost to the primary lesion).

Surgical Approach

Eight weeks later, the patient is symptom free and is taken to the operating room. The patient is placed in the lithotomy position. A very careful examination of the anal canal is performed and the groin is palpated for any enlarged lymph nodes, which, if present, should undergo fine-needle aspiration. Anal canal evaluation can be further enhanced with endorectal ultrasound. The tumor has completely regressed except for a 1-cm left lateral anal canal nodule. The nodule is then excised and the margins are carefully approximated with absorbable sutures.

Histopathology Slide

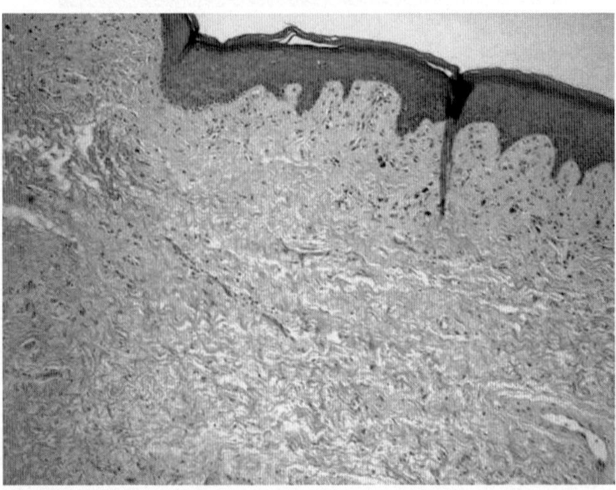

Figure 39.4

Histopathology Report

Postchemoradiation anal canal biopsy shows atrophy and fibrosis only, without carcinoma.

Discussion

It is now believed that cloacogenic, transitional, basaloid, epidermoid, and squamous cell cancers are variants of squamous cell carcinoma with similar prognosis. Tumors of the anal margin (below the anal verge and involving the perianal hair-bearing skin) are classified with skin tumors.

Despite being readily accessible to physical examination, the diagnosis is often delayed by patients as well as physicians because the symptoms mimic common benign anorectal disease. Bleeding is the most common presentation, often associated with pruritus, anal pain, and discharge.

Involvement of adjacent organs such as the prostate and bladder is rare, though vaginal septal invasion has been reported in 12% of cases. Hematogenous metastasis to liver (5% to 8%), lung (2% to 4%), or bone (2%) is more common from tumors above the dentate line. The incidences of synchronous and metachronous inguinal node metastases are 15% and 25%, respectively.

The treatment of anal cancer in HIV-positive patients is limited to small retrospective studies using different treatments. If successfully completed, combined modality treatment is equally effective as in non-HIV–positive patients. HIV-positive patients with CD4 counts less than $200/mm^3$ have been shown to have poor tolerance to combined modality therapy and worse outcome with a higher incidence of grade 3 or 4 acute toxicity, such as diarrhea, moist desquamation, mucositis, and neutropenia. These complications lead to treatment breaks, reduction in doses, or discontinuation of treatment, adversely affecting disease control.

Reducing the radiation dose and using shrinking fields has been reported to be better tolerated with good response. Induction chemotherapy is used prior to radiation in patients who present with abscess or fistula. Cisplatin may be substituted for mitomycin C to reduce hematologic toxicity. Meticulous skin care, monitoring of blood counts, and narcotic pain medications are essential. Preliminary colostomy may be essential in patients with severe pain, sepsis, and incontinence. APR is advocated for patients who are unfit for combined modality therapy, or those who have recurrent disease. Primary radiation alone is also an option. The addition of highly active antiretroviral therapy (HAART) may improve the tolerance to chemoradiation with fewer treatment breaks, although this is controversial.

Case Continued

The patient's follow-up consists of digital rectal examination and anoscopy every 3 months for 1 year, then every 6 months for 2 years, and then annually. He also receives EAUS and CT scan of the abdomen every 6 months for 2 years, and then annually for 2 years. He has remained tumor free as of the last follow-up.

Suggested Readings

Bartelink H, Roelofsen F, Esohwege F, et al. Concomitant radiotherapy and chemotherapy is superior to radiotherapy alone in the treatment of locally advanced anal cancer: results of a phase III randomized trial of the European Organization for Research and Treatment of Cancer Radiotherapy and Gastrointestinal Cooperative Groups [see comment]. *J Clin Oncol* 1997;15:2040–2049.

Bendell JC, Ryan DP. Current perspectives on anal cancer. *Oncology (Huntingt)* 2003;17:492–497, 502-503; discussion 503, 507–509.

Berry JM, Palefsky JM, Welton ML. Anal cancer and its precursors in HIV-positive patients: perspectives and management. *Surg Oncol Clin N Am* 2004;13:355–373.

Chawla AK, Willett CG. Squamous cell carcinoma of the anal canal and anal margin. *Hematol Oncol Clin North Am* 2001; 15:321–344, vi.

Eng C, Abbruzzese J, Minsky BD. Chemotherapy and radiation of anal canal cancer: the first approach. *Surg Oncol Clin N Am* 2004;13:309–320, viii.

Epidermoid anal cancer: results from the UKCCCR randomized trial of radiotherapy alone versus radiotherapy, 5-fluorouracil, and mitomycin. UKCCCR Anal Cancer Trial Working Party. UK Coordinating Committee on Cancer Research. *Lancet* 1996; 348:1049–1054.

Klencke BJ, Palefsky JM. Anal cancer: an HIV-associated cancer. *Hematol Oncol Clin North Am* 2003;17:859–872.

case 40

Presentation

A 52-year-old man presents with perirectal pain, firm area, and bleeding that has worsened over the last 6 months. He was treated for a "boil" on the right anterior cheek 1 year ago. He had a hemorrhoidectomy 5 years ago. He has a 30-pack-year smoking history, and uses alcohol socially.

Clinical Photograph

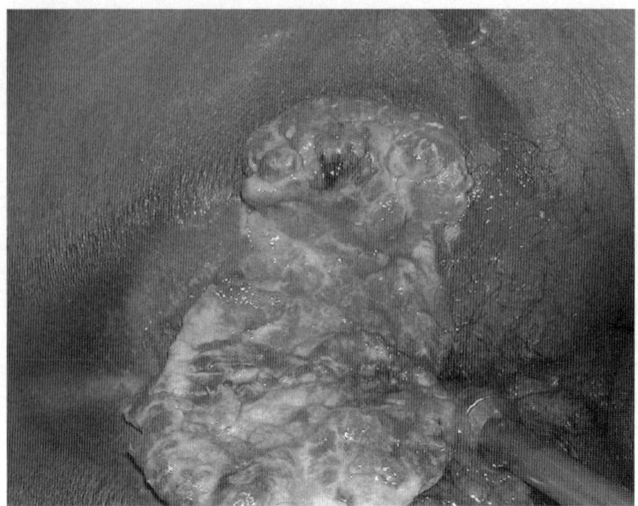

Figure 40.1

Physical Examination Report

An extensive 10 × 15-cm destructive lesion posterior to the anal verge is visible, and there is no suspicious inguinal lymphadenopathy.

Differential Diagnosis

At the time of initial presentation with suppuration, a chance to make an early diagnosis with a biopsy was probably missed. Given the appearance, a neoplastic process is most likely a squamous or basal cell carcinoma. Extensive hidradenitis or Crohn disease are less likely.

Discussion

Anal margin cancers arise from skin lateral to the intersphincteric groove and are usually well-differentiated, keratinized variants of squamous cell carcinoma, which rarely metastasize, compared to anal canal cancers. Other lesions in this area are Bowen disease, basal cell carcinoma, melanoma, verrucous carcinoma, and Paget disease. Bowen disease and Paget disease can present as a persistent pruritic rash. Basal cell carcinoma has raised edges with central ulceration and is often mistaken for a fissure or chancre. Verrucous carcinoma may present as a slowly growing invasive cancer in long-standing large condyloma acuminata. Melanomas in the perianal area are frequently amelanotic and carry a very poor prognosis, with most patients succumbing to distant disease. The differential diagnosis includes numerous benign diseases and dermatoses like fungal infection and psoriasis. The importance of a high index of suspicion is critical to prevent the frequent delay in diagnosis. A biopsy is diagnostic.

Recommendation

Perform examination under anesthesia to evaluate the extent of disease and obtain biopsy for tissue diagnosis. Obtain computed tomography (CT) scans of abdomen and pelvis for staging purposes.

Case Continued

The patient is taken to the operating room for examination under anesthesia because pain and tenderness preclude satisfactory examination in the clinic. CT scans of the abdomen and pelvis with intravenous (IV) and rectal contrast did not show any liver lesions or pelvic or groin lymphadenopathy.

Surgical Approach

Under spinal anesthesia, the patient is placed in the prone jackknife position. Digital examination of the anus and rectum is performed followed by proctoscopy. A transanal ultrasound is performed for local staging. Multiple biopsies are obtained.

Case Continued

Anal mucosa is intact, and proctoscopy to 25 cm reveals no abnormality. Pathologic examination reveals moderately differentiated squamous cell carcinoma, clinical stage T3 N0 M0.

◼ Endorectal Ultrasonogram

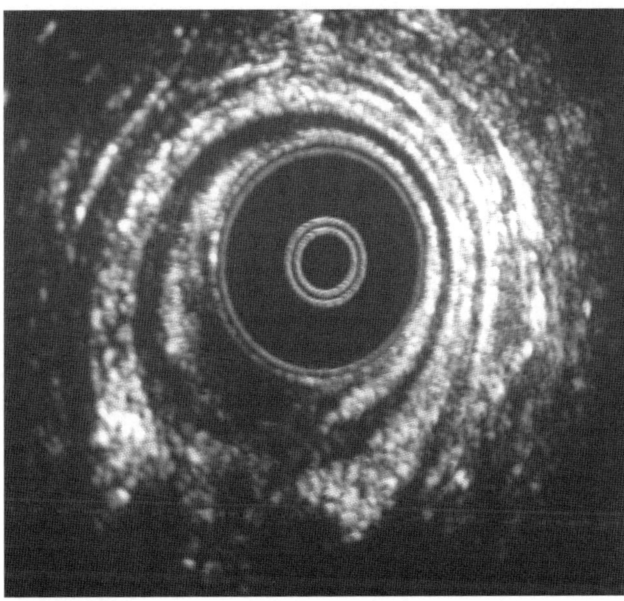

Figure 40.2

Endorectal Ultrasound Report

Transanal ultrasound shows involvement of external and internal sphincters with intact mucosa.

◼ Approach

Larger tumors staged as T2–4 and smaller tumors close to the anal verge should be treated with combined modality therapy. Abdominoperineal resection is reserved for recurrent disease after failed chemoradiation. Standard chemoradiation consists of continuous infusion 5-fluorouracil (5-FU) at 1,000 mg/m^2 on days 1 to 4 and 29 to 33 with mitomycin C at 10 mg/m^2 on days 1 and 29. The mitomycin C was given IV push and the 5-FU was given through a continuous-infusion pump on an outpatient basis along with concurrent radiotherapy. A total of 50.4 Gy in 18-Gy/day fractions over 55 days was delivered in three phases. An initial large pelvic field of 30.6 Gy to the whole pelvis and inguinal lymph nodes utilizing 6- and 18-MV photons using three fields with custom blocking was delivered. A reduced pelvic field of 3.60 Gy was delivered to the bottom of the sacroiliac joints and inguinal nodes.

Discussion

Small superficial carcinomas (T1) have a small chance of lymph node involvement and can be treated with local excision with 1-cm margins or with radiotherapy. Local recurrences, if small and away from the sphincter, may be treated with re-excision. In a series of 51 patients with epidermoid anal margin cancer treated by local excision alone, a 5-year, cancer-specific survival rate of 88% was achieved. Locoregional recurrence was seen in almost half the patients, and was managed with re-excision or inguinal lymphadenectomy. Results of these patients were similar to those of the 13 patients in the series who were treated with abdominoperineal resection. Local recurrences after excision may also be treated by radiation therapy. Local excision for tumors close to the anal verge may result in incontinence if a significant portion of sphincter muscle is resected.

In a recent study, there were no failures at 2-year follow-up in 10 patients with anal margin tumors staged as T2/T3 N0 and treated with radiotherapy alone or combined with concurrent chemotherapy. Thus, radiation therapy and local excision are reasonable treatments for T1 and perhaps T2 cancers. Chemoradiation therapy is suitable for more advanced lesions, with abdominoperineal resection reserved for patients with local recurrence after radiotherapy. Overall, radiation therapy seems to be a suitable alternative to surgery for anal margin tumors, and should be considered as part of a sphincter-sparing regimen for tumors close to the anal verge.

Case Continued

Due to the extensive nature of the tumor, the patient is treated with combined chemoradiation therapy, and the tumor has a greater than 80% regression at the completion of chemoradiation. He is seen 4 weeks after completion of therapy, and he is symptom free. There is some hair loss and mild hypopigmentation in the perianal area. Rectal examination shows nontender, healed mucosa with no masses.

At the 6-month follow-up visit, he presents again with recurrent pain and bleeding. Examination reveals an ulcerated firm mass at the anal verge, which is recurrent squamous cancer on biopsy. CT scans of the abdomen and pelvis show no metastasis.

Recommendation

Perform salvage abdominoperineal resection.

Case Continued

The patient undergoes an uneventful abdominoperineal resection and is discharged on postoperative day 4. The omentum was mobilized on the left gastroepiploic artery to fill the void in the pelvis. The perineum was left open to heal by secondary intention. The tumor was deeply ulcerated. Pathology evaluation showed poorly differentiated squamous carcinoma with perineural invasion in two areas of deep ulceration 2 cm in diameter. All proximal, distal, and radial margins were free of tumor, and eight lymph nodes were negative.

Discussion

The alternative approach for the patient, instead of the abdominoperineal approach, is to consider salvage chemoradiation therapy using cisplatin and perhaps adding an extra 10 Gy of radiation therapy, as tested for anal canal cancer. The role of cisplatin-based chemoradiation therapy following the Nigro regimen was reported in a phase II trial by the Radiation Therapy Oncology Group (RTOG), where an additional 50% of patients were salvaged.

Suggested Readings

Newlin HE, Zlotecki RA, Morris CG, et al. Squamous cell carcinoma of the anal margin. *J Surg Oncol* 2004;86:55–62.
Rousseau DL Jr, Petrelli NJ, Kahlenberg MS. Overview of anal cancer for the surgeon. *Surg Oncol Clin N Am* 2004;13:249–262.
Skibber J, Rodriguez-Bigas MA, Gordon PH. Surgical considerations in anal cancer. *Surg Oncol Clin N Am* 2004;13:321–338.

Presentation

A healthy 33-year-old man presents with a 2-month history of intermittent bright red blood with bowel movements associated with mild right-sided rectal pain. Otherwise, no change in bowel habits, such as constipation, diarrhea, or narrowed stool caliber, is reported. The patient denies experiencing similar symptoms in the past. A digital rectal examination reveals a small nodular mass at the anal verge.

Differential Diagnosis

In this young patient, the most likely diagnosis is a thrombosed hemorrhoid. A neoplastic process such as a polyp or a malignancy is also in the differential, but statistically is much less common. A presumed diagnosis of thrombosed hemorrhoid is made, and treated with conservative management including sitz baths, stool softeners, and suppositories.

Case Continued

Symptoms persist, however, and a proctoscopy is performed. With the patient in the prone jack-knife position, the presence of the mass at the 4 o'clock location is confirmed without obvious hemorrhoids. A polypoid mass is described with a small area of surrounding black mucosal pigmentation. A neoplastic process is entertained and a biopsy is performed.

Diagnosis and Recommendation

The histologic findings are consistent with a nodular melanoma in anal mucosa. The tumor thickness is at least 6 mm with a positive deep margin and some surrounding melanoma in situ. A careful physical examination fails to reveal palpable inguinal adenopathy. No pigmented lesions are identified around the perianal skin. A thorough rectal examination fails to reveal any other mucosal nodules or perirectal masses. A repeat proctoscopy reveals only some residual mucosal pigmentation around the biopsy site and no other areas of mucosal abnormalities. A complete imaging evaluation, including computed tomography (CT) scans of the chest, abdomen, and pelvis, reveals no evidence of distant visceral metastases and no pelvic, inguinal, or perirectal adenopathy. A rectal ultrasound confirms the absence of obvious suspicious perirectal lymph nodes. A sphincter-sparing transanal resection and a sentinel node biopsy (SNB) are offered to accomplish local and regional disease control and potential cure followed by adjuvant therapy.

Approach

Mucosal melanomas of the anorectum are extremely rare, and therefore standards of care are not well established because large single- or multi-institutional experiences are lacking. The management strategies are designed based on the stage at presentation, the predicted sites of recurrence, and the combining of principles learned from treating cutaneous melanoma with surgical techniques used for the more common histologic solid malignancies of the anus and rectum, while at the same time minimizing long-term morbidity. As in this patient, most present with clinically localized disease, but have a very high rate of regional lymph node failure and the development of distant disease and death, despite initial surgery with curative intent. No current data demonstrate that abdominoperineal resection (APR) improves survival or regional control compared with local excision with negative margins. Therefore, contemporary surgical approaches include sphincter-sparing resections, if technically feasible, and a selective approach to the regional nodes using lymphatic mapping and SNB. Adjuvant regional and systemic therapies are often recommended because of the potential for local recurrence and the high rate of systemic failure.

Surgical Approach

A careful digital and proctoscopic examination by the operating surgeon is critical to assess the local extent of disease and determine if a local excision is feasible. The digital examination can detect submucosal extent of disease and satellite nodules that will not be visible. Furthermore, a thorough digital evaluation may detect perirectal nodal enlargement as well as presacral adenopathy. Finally, endorectal ultrasound is a good adjunct in evaluating perirectal extent of disease, particularly in patients with pure rectal mucosal lesions. The proctoscopy not only identifies the exact location of the primary tumor, but also the presence of multifocal mucosal disease.

Preoperative lymphoscintigraphy can be accomplished accurately by peritumoral mucosal injections of radiolabeled colloids to assess if unilateral or bilateral inguinal drainage exists or if the primary regional drainage is directly to the rectal mesenteric nodes. On the morning of surgery, the injection is repeated to facilitate performing the SNB in the same operative setting as the formal excision. The transanal resection is performed with the patient in either the lithotomy or prone position, depending on the location of the tumor. The SNB can be performed before or after the excision of the primary, and therefore one position change is required if the primary tumor resection is facilitated by the prone position. It should be cautioned that peritumoral blue dye injections for SNBs might obscure the surgeon's ability to determine the mucosal extent of the tumor. Patients with positive sentinel nodes are offered completion node dissections.

Full-thickness resections of the primary tumor are advocated. Careful orientation of the specimen and direct communication with the pathologist are critical so additional margins can be removed from the correct locations.

Lymphoscintigrams

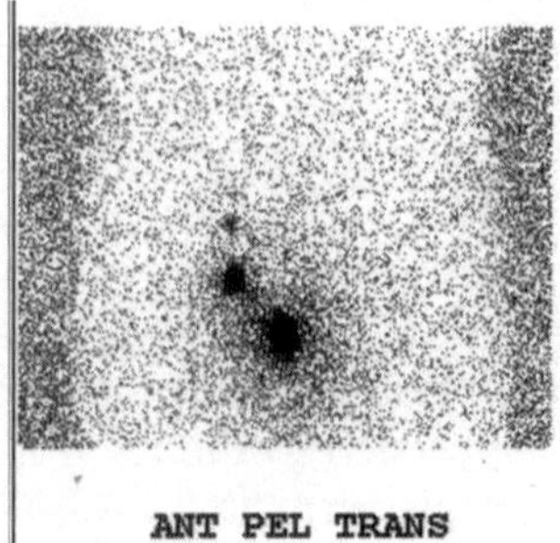

Figure 41.1A

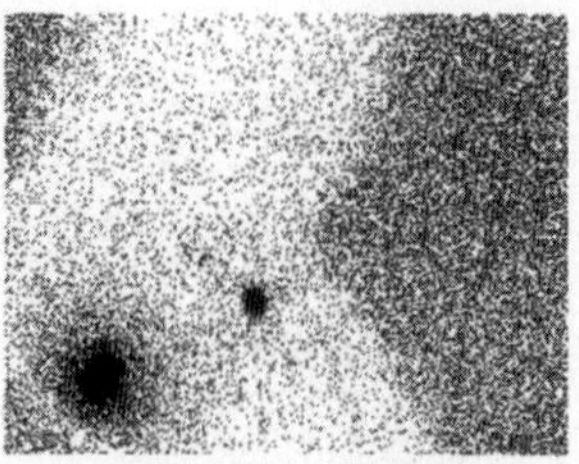

Figure 41.1B

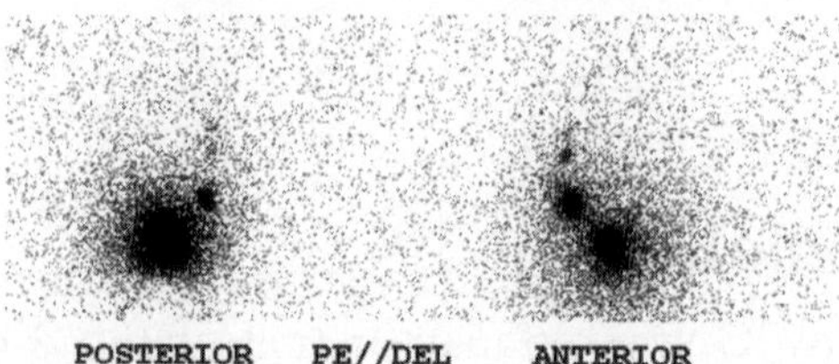

Figure 41.1C

Lymphoscintigraphy Report

Lymphoscintigraphy shows lymphatic drainage from the right lateral anal wall to the right inguinal nodes in preparation for SNB.

Case Continued

The SNB is performed first without difficulty. With the patient in the prone position, transanal resection is performed from the lateral anal canal at the 4 o'clock location. All formal resection margins are negative. The sentinel node is positive for metastatic melanoma, and the patient elects to receive adjuvant radiation therapy to the groin in addition to the anorectal region rather than completion inguinal dissection. He elects not to pursue any systemic therapy options. He is currently without any evidence of local/regional recurrence or distant metastases 2 years postoperatively. Follow-up includes digital and proctoscopic examinations at 3- to 6-month intervals.

Discussion

Primary anorectal mucosal melanoma is an uncommon aggressive malignancy characterized by early systemic dissemination, and therefore a poor prognosis. Presenting symptoms are rectal bleeding, rectal pain, or a palpable mass. The primary lesions are most often identified at the squamocolumnar junction where most of the melanocytes reside, but can develop purely in rectal (columnar) mucosa or anal (squamous) mucosa. Such information may be important when assessing and/or predicting lymphatic drainage patterns and likely sites of regional lymph node failure. Despite the fact that most patients present with clinically localized disease to the primary site, with or without regional lymph node disease but no demonstrable distant disease, the vast majority succumb to distant dissemination regardless of the extent of local/regional therapy. The poor overall prognosis is most likely explained by a delay in diagnosis until symptoms develop. The chance for early diagnosis in anorectal melanoma patients, and for almost all mucosal melanomas in general, is limited because these lesions develop in occult anatomic locations. Unlike cutaneous melanoma, where early change can be readily detected visually, mucosal lesions remain asymptomatic until they are locally advanced and ulcerated. Most of the mucosal primaries are comparable to stage IIC cutaneous lesions (larger than 4 mm in thickness, and ulcerated) and are likely to harbor micrometastatic disease at diagnosis. The only exception is when the diagnosis is made incidentally upon hemorrhoidectomy. Experience with mucosal melanomas further demonstrates the propensity for melanoma in general to develop metastases with relatively small primary tumor volumes compared with other solid tumors.

Because of its rarity, standards of care for anorectal mucosal melanoma have not been well established. Historically, APR with extensive elective pelvic and inguinal lymphadenectomy was promoted. Because survival rates were so poor (<25%), a more conservative and less morbid sphincter-preserving approach was selectively employed, with APR reserved for patients with unresectable local recurrences. Local/regional control rates after transanal excision were inferior to those reported after APR as the initial surgical procedure, but survival rates were not negatively affected. Recurrence patterns after local excision include either local tumor relapse and/or regional nodal failure (primarily inguinal) in up to 60% of patients. Borrowing the concept of margin-negative local excision and adjuvant radiation often used for rectal adenocarcinomas, combined with what we have learned about adjuvant radiation therapy regimens for high-risk cutaneous melanoma, a rational treatment strategy has been applied selectively to those patients with resectable anorectal melanoma in the hope of improving local/regional control and still providing sphincter preservation. Transanal excision and adjuvant postoperative radiation delivered in five 30-Gy fractions to the primary surgical site and potential regional nodal basins has been recently evaluated. Long-term results, for both local/regional control and overall survival, compare favorably with results achieved with APR but without the associated functional morbidity.

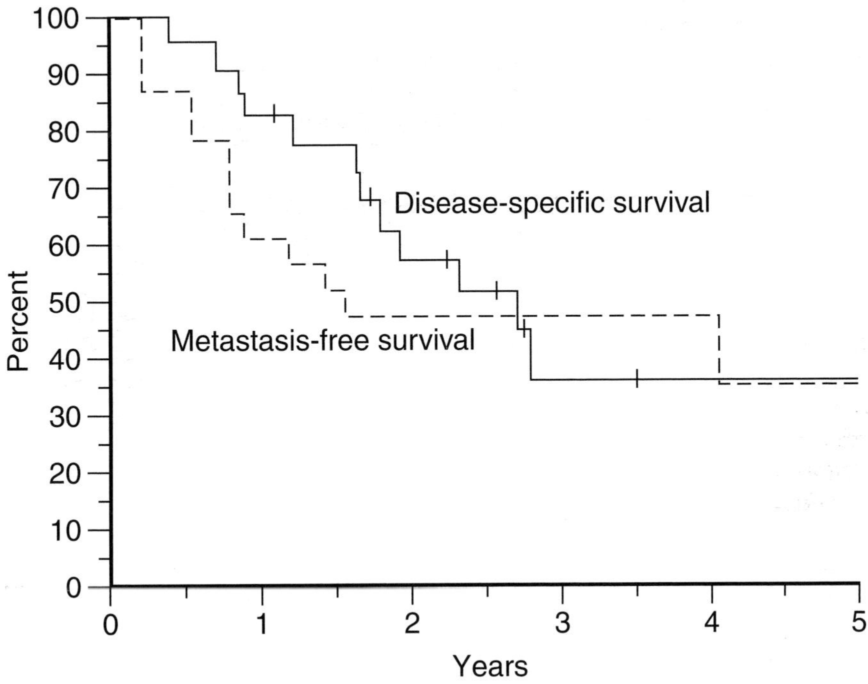

Figure 41.2A

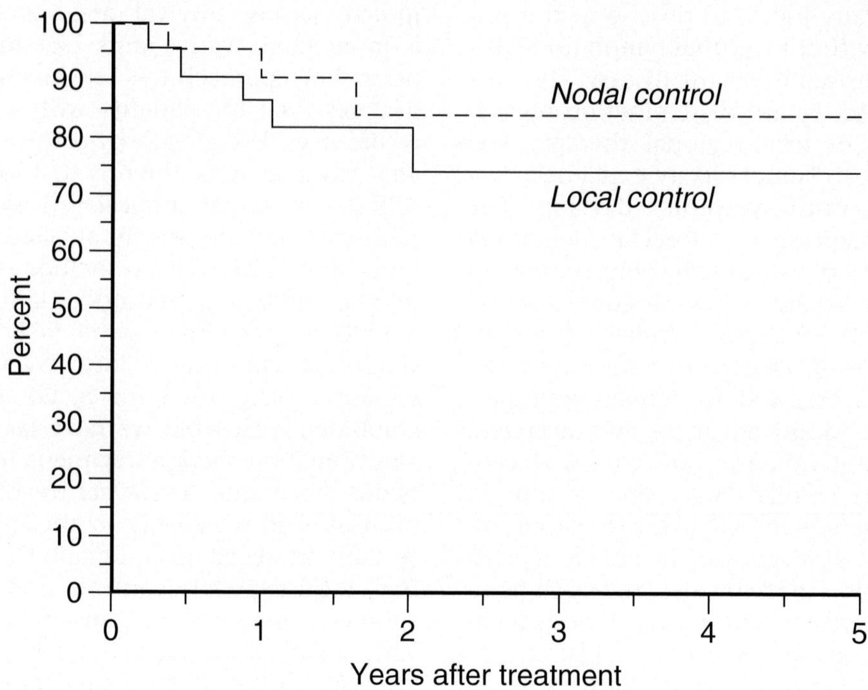

Figure 41.2B

Regional lymph node metastases are a common form of failure in anorectal melanoma patients. Extrapolating from a wealth of experience with lymphatic mapping and SNB in the management of primary cutaneous melanoma patients, such an approach has been applied to anorectal patients who present without clinically or radiographically identifiable nodal disease. While lesions arising at or below the squamocolumnar junction often drain primarily to one or both inguinal basins, lesions above this area are likely to spread through the rectal mesenteric nodes. Using lymphoscintigraphy, individual lymphatic drainage patterns can be defined and SNB can be performed if drainage to the inguinal nodes is demonstrated. In this way, a more selective approach to nodal treatment can be pursued, potentially reducing the morbidity associated with unnecessary lymphadenectomy or nodal irradiation.

The most difficult challenge to address in these patients is the development of distant metastases. The systemic metastatic patterns of relapse are not dissimilar to those of cutaneous melanoma. Again, extrapolating from experience with cutaneous melanoma, high-dose interferon alone or in combination with cisplatin-based chemotherapy and interleukin-2 (biochemotherapy) has been used anecdotally. On one hand, these patients are at such a high risk for relapse that an aggressive adjuvant approach has been routinely employed at some centers; on the other hand, an argument can be made that the toxicities of aggressive therapy may not be worth the small potential benefits in a patient population with a relatively short life expectancy. Recently, most of the cooperative groups have allowed anorectal melanoma patients to be eligible for adjuvant therapy programs that were designed for cutaneous melanoma patients. These trials include vaccine approaches as well as biochemotherapy regimens. Enrolling patients in one of these trials is probably the best option.

Neoadjuvant approaches are rational for those patients who present with locally advanced disease that would require an APR and for patients with measurable regional lymph node metastases. A preoperative response may facilitate a sphincter-preserving approach and/or identify a regimen that can be used in the adjuvant setting. Biochemotherapy may provide the best chance for a significant response.

Suggested Readings

Bentzen SM, Overgaard J, Thames HD, et al. Clinical radiobiology of malignant melanoma. *Radiother Oncol* 1989;16:169–182.

Brady MS, Kavolius JP, Quan SHQ. Anorectal melanoma: a 64-year experience at Memorial Sloan-Kettering Cancer Center. *Dis Colon Rectum* 1995;38:146–151.

Goldman S, Glimelium B, Pahlman L. Anorectal malignant melanoma in Sweden: report of 49 patients. *Dis Colon Rectum* 1990;33:874–877.

Kim KB, Sanuino AM, Hodges C, et al. Biochemotherapy in patients with metastatic anorectal mucosal melanoma. *Cancer* 2004;100:1478–1483.

Konstadoulakis MM, Ricaniadis N, Walsh D, et al. Malignant melanoma of the anorectal region. *J Surg Oncol* 1995;58: 118–120.

Ross M, Pezzi C, Pezzi T, et al. Patterns of failure in anorectal melanoma. *Arch Surg* 1990;125:313–316.

Roumen RMH. Anorectal melanoma in the Netherlands: a report of 63 patients. *Eur J Surg Cancer* 1996;22:598–601.

Siegel B, Cohen D, Jacob ET. Surgical treatment of anorectal melanomas. *Am J Surg* 1983;146:336–338.

case 42

Presentation

A 72-year-old woman with history of distal gastrectomy for early gastric cancer presents to your office after she was seen by her primary medical doctor with a suspected liver tumor detected by ultrasonography. She received a blood transfusion 30 years ago at the time of gastrectomy. She was diagnosed as having hepatitis C 10 years ago, and has been followed by her primary medical doctor. She denies history of alcohol abuse. On examination, liver and spleen are not palpable and she does not have ascites or jaundice.

Laboratory Tests

Laboratory values on admission were as follows: hepatitis B surface antigen (HBsAg) negative, hepatitis C virus antibody (HCV Ab) positive; platelet count: $8.1 \times 10^4/mm^3$; prothrombin time: 56.6% (international normalized ratio [INR] 1.48); serum total bilirubin: 1.0 mg/dL; alpha-fetoprotein (AFP): 240 ng/mL (normal range, <9); des-gamma-carboxy prothrombin (DCP): 100 mAU/mL (normal range, <40); 15-minute retention rate of indocyanine green (ICG): 24%; and plasma disappearance rate of ICG: 0.095 (min^{-1}).

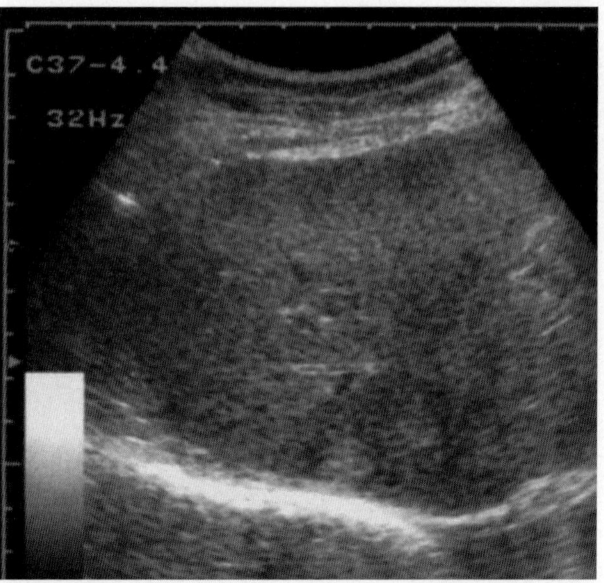
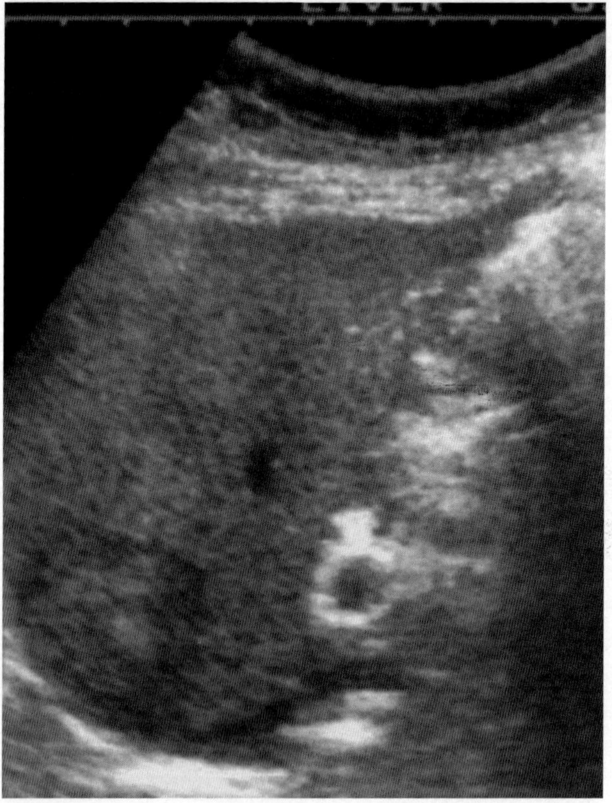

Figure 42.1

Ultrasonography Report

A round hypoechoic mass, 4 cm in diameter, is visualized in Couinaud segment VIII. The internal echo of the lesion shows a mosaic pattern and it is surrounded by a hypoechoic halo.

Differential Diagnosis

The differential diagnoses for a hypoechoic hepatic mass in the liver are hepatocellular carcinoma, cholangiocellular carcinoma, metastatic liver cancer, and cavernous hemangioma.

Discussion

Development of a liver mass in a hepatitis C-positive patient is usually highly suspicious for hepatocellular carcinoma. Ultrasound (US) findings and elevated serum levels of AFP and DCP are supportive of the diagnosis. Intrahepatic cholangiocellular carcinoma or a mixed type of hepatocellular-cholangiocellular carcinoma are relatively rare but cannot be excluded by US alone. To exclude metastatic liver tumor, common primary sites including the gastrointestinal tract (upper gastrointestinal study, colonoscopy), pancreas, breast, and genitourinary organs should be screened. Liver metastasis from early gastric cancer resected 30 years before is highly unlikely. A cavernous hemangioma is sometimes hypoechoic, but may be ruled out by computed tomography (CT) scan or angiography.

Laboratory data, including decreased platelet count and serum albumin and prolonged prothrombin time, suggest the presence of liver cirrhosis. To estimate the hepatic functional reserve precisely, ICG test is recommended.

Recommendation

A dynamic CT scan study, as well as hepatic angiography.

CT Scan

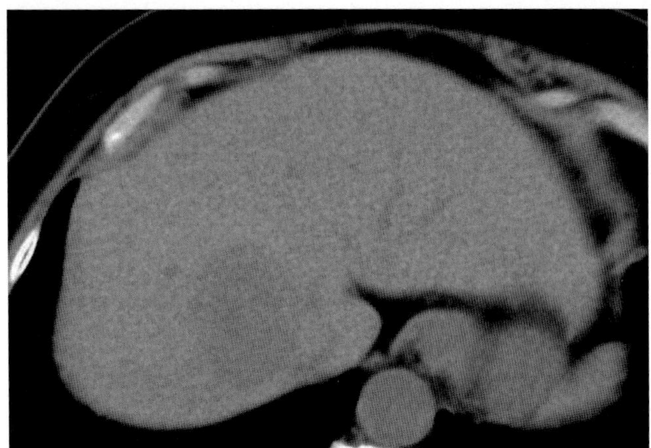

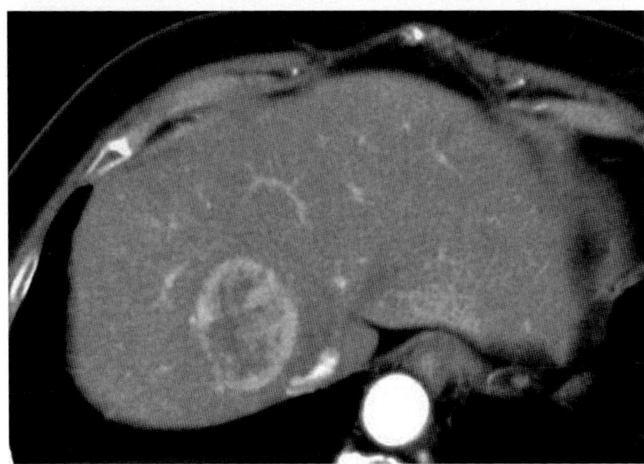

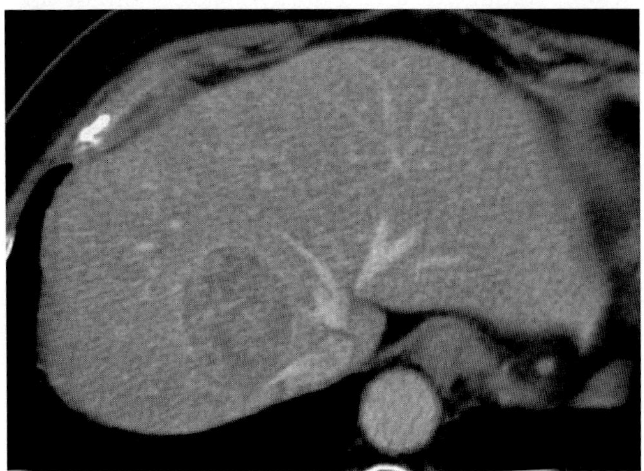

Figure 42.2

CT Scan Report

CT scan shows a 4 × 4-cm hypervascular mass in segment VIII of the liver. Compared to the density of the surrounding liver parenchyma, the density of the lesion is lower in plain CT, higher in early phase, and again lower in late phase.

Hepatic Angiogram

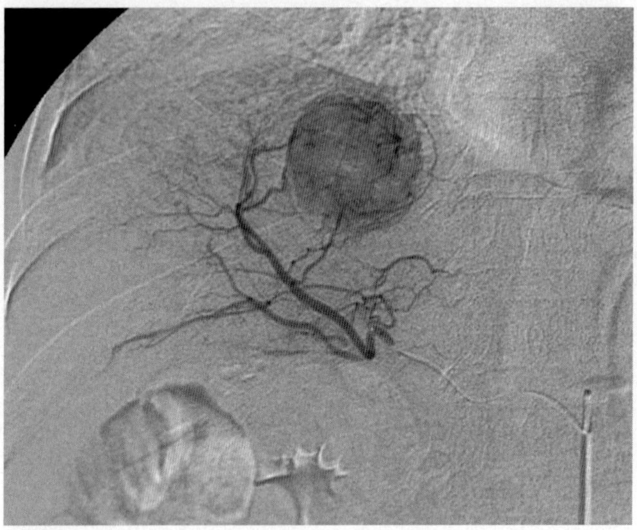

Figure 42.3

Hepatic Angiography Report

The 4 × 4-cm tumor is fed by the arterial branch for segment VIII. Tumor vessels are dense and irregular. In preparation for a lipiodol CT scan, 3 mL of lipiodol is injected via the right hepatic artery and 2 mL is injected via the left hepatic artery.

Lipiodol CT Scan of Liver

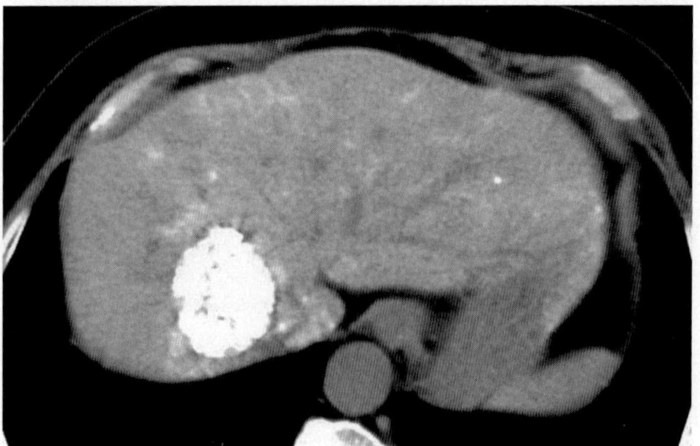

Figure 42.4

Lipiodol CT Scan Report

A noncontrast CT scan performed 2 weeks after lipiodol injection reveals a dense lipiodol accumulation in the hepatic tumor. There are no other lipiodol deposits inside the liver.

Diagnosis and Recommendation

Single hepatocellular carcinoma. ICG test to assess hepatic functional reserve.

Case Continued

Fifteen-minute retention rate of ICG was 24% and plasma disappearance rate of ICG was 0.095 (min^{-1}). The patient had no ascites, and serum total bilirubin level was normal.

Approach

This patient is offered an anatomical resection of segment VIII of the liver, which will be performed via a J-shaped thoracoabdominal approach. The patient is informed that her hepatic functional reserve is estimated to tolerate segmentectomy (up to one sixth resection of the liver) well according to the algorithm shown. The complications mentioned are bleeding, bile leakage, infection, pleural effusion, ascites, and death (<1%).

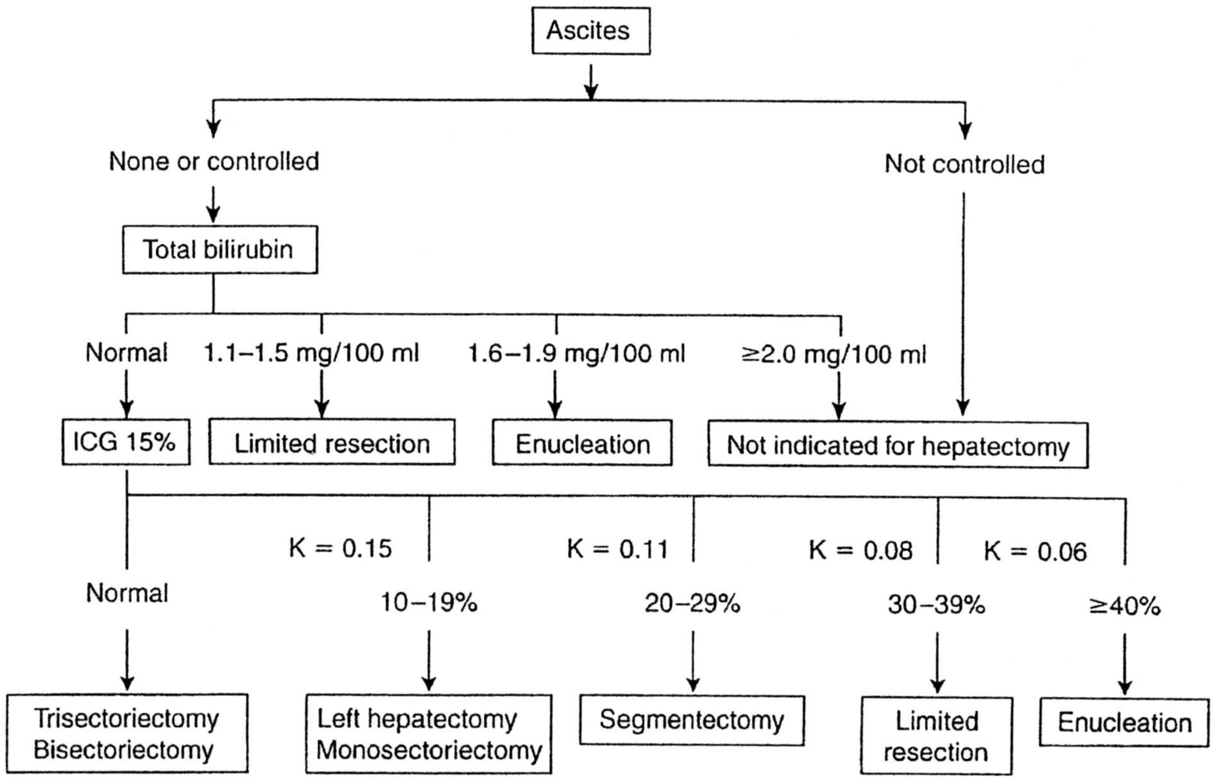

Figure 42.5

Intraoperative Image

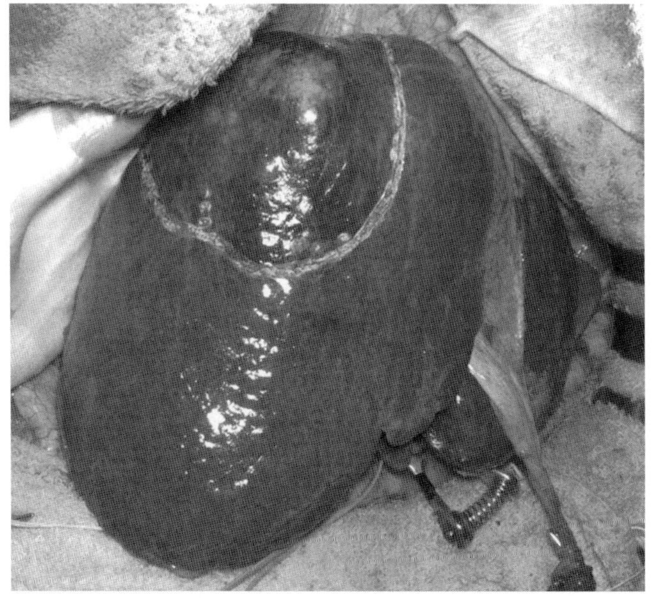

Figure 42.6

Surgical Approach

To remove possible intrahepatic metastases, anatomical resection of segment VIII is recommended. To identify the border of segment 8 on the liver surface, 5 to 10 mL of dye (indigo) is injected via the portal branch for segment VIII under US guidance. The border is marked with electrocautery, and hepatic parenchymal dissection is done using the so-called crush clamping method or ultrasonic surgical aspirator. To reduce the intraoperative blood loss, Pringle's maneuver (15-minute clamp and 5-minute release) is repeated during hepatic transection. Portal pedicles for segment VIII are ligated and divided, and the middle and the right hepatic vein are exposed on the cut surface. A 16F chest tube and a 24F silicone drain are placed at the conclusion of the operation, which are usually removed on the third and seventh to ninth postoperative day, respectively.

Discussion

Approximately 70% to 80% of patients with hepatoma are cirrhotic. To reduce the mortality and morbidity of liver resection in this setting, hepatic functional reserve should be precisely evaluated. The surgical decision tree for patient selection and surgical procedures was proposed by Makuuchi. This surgical algorithm is used extensively in Japan and has significantly improved operative mortality and morbidity in hepatoma patients. There are only three parameters: presence or absence of ascites, serum total bilirubin, and ICG retention rate at 15 minutes. Extent of liver resection is shown at the bottom.

Superiority of anatomical hepatic resection for hepatoma has been demonstrated by several centers. Precise identification of the segmental border using dye injection and exposure of landmarks, including hepatic veins and portal pedicles, are keys for curative resection.

Case Continued

Postoperative course is uneventful. The patient visits the hospital once a month to check serum AFP and DCP levels and to undergo US. CT scan is taken every 3 to 6 months.

Suggested Readings

Couinaud C. Lobes et segments hepatiques. Notes sur l'architecture anatomique et chirurgicale du foie. *Presse Med* 1954; 62:709–712.

Kokudo N, Vera DR, Tada K, et al. Predictors of successful hepatic resection: prognostic usefulness of hepatic asialoglycoprotein receptor analysis. *World J Surg* 2002;26:1342–1347.

Kokudo N, Vera DR, Makuuchi M. Clinical application of TcGSA. *Nucl Med Biol* 2003;30:845–849.

Makuuchi M, Kosuge T, Takayama T, et al. Surgery for small liver cancers. *Semin Surg Oncol* 1993;9:298–304.

Makuuchi M, Hasegawa H, Hirohashi S, et al. Strategy for the treatment of hepatocellular carcinoma accompanied with liver cirrhosis [in Japanese]. *Geka Shinryo* 1987;29:1530–1536.

Makuuchi M, Hasegewa H, Yamazaki S. Ultrasonically guided subsegmentectomy. *Surg Gynecol Obstet* 1985;161:346–350.

Presentation

A 39-year-old woman presents to her primary care physician. She has a history of intermittent upper abdominal pain but is otherwise healthy. There is no history of nausea, vomiting, or troublesome heartburn. Past medical history is essentially unremarkable except for migraines. Her medications include ibuprofen for her headaches and oral contraceptive pills for the past 5 years. The primary care physician orders an upper gastrointestinal (GI) endoscopy and right upper quadrant ultrasound. Upper GI endoscopy reveals antral gastritis with biopsy positive for *Helicobacter pylori*. She is started on an anti-*H. pylori* regimen. Ultrasound shows no evidence of gallstones but an incidental finding of a 1.5-cm solid hypoechoic mass. The patient's symptoms resolve with the anti-*H. pylori* regimen, and she is referred for further evaluation of the solid hepatic mass.

◼ Ultrasound Image

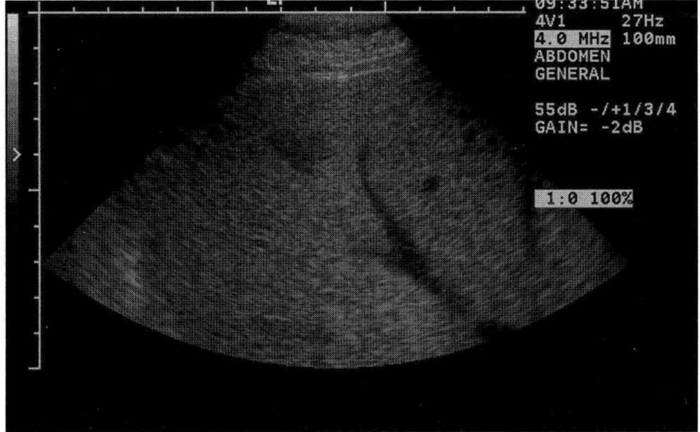

Figure 43.1

Ultrasonography Report

Presence of a well-circumscribed 1.5-cm hypoechoic mass.

Differential Diagnosis

Disease processes that may present as a hepatic mass can be broadly categorized into benign and malignant conditions. A variety of benign liver tumors have been described, but the common lesions include hemangiomas, hepatic adenomas, focal nodular hyperplasia, and bile duct hematomas. In the malignant category, primary malignancies include hepatocellular carcinoma, cholangiocarcinoma, and angiosarcoma. Malignancy can also include metastatic disease from an extrahepatic primary tumor.

Discussion

Solid hepatic lesions often create a diagnostic challenge, and management should incorporate a cost-effective diagnostic and therapeutic approach. The first step involves a careful history and physical examination with attention given to constitutional and gastrointestinal symptoms, with particular attention to prior exposure to hepatitis, carcinogens, or oral contraceptives. Physical examination should be directed at outlining any stigmata of chronic liver disease. Careful examination of the skin, eyes, and breast, as well as a pelvic and rectal examination should be performed to identify sources of primary tumor that may have metastasized to the liver. Laboratory tests include a complete blood cell count, coagulation profile, liver function tests, hepatitis A, B, and C screen, and measurement of serum tumor markers such as alpha-fetoprotein (AFP), carcinoembryonic antigen (CEA), and cancer antigen 19-9 (CA 19-9).

Many hepatic lesions can have overlapping radiographic features, causing a diagnostic dilemma. The ultrasound findings of focal liver lesions are frequently nonspecific, making differentiation between benign and malignant liver lesions problematic. The limitations of ultrasound scan include its dependence on the operator and patient limitations such as obesity and biliary tree distention. Prior to the development of magnetic resonance imaging (MRI), the diagnostic algorithm included obtaining nuclear medicine examinations, such as tagged red blood cell (RBC) scan to detect liver hemangiomas, and Tc-sulfur colloid scan (which enhances Kupffer cells) to distinguish focal nodular hyperplasia, which contains Kupffer cells, from hepatic adenoma, which contains hepatocytes. Spiral computed tomography (CT) scans with three-phase (arterial, portal, and parenchymal) images are obtained to categorize the vascularity of the various lesions according to the timing of the contrast bolus. With experience gained in bolus injection techniques, characteristic patterns of enhancements can be used to suggest a particular diagnosis, though no specific CT criteria can distinguish benign from malignant liver masses with absolute certainty. Many investigators have demonstrated that the sensitivity and accuracy of MRI in the detection and categorization of liver lesions exceed those of ultrasound scan and spiral CT. Unenhanced MRI helps the diagnosis of focal liver lesions because of the excellent information on morphology provided by T2-weighted and T1-weighted sequences. A variety of contrast media, including gadolinium, hepatobiliary, and tissue-specific MR contrast agents, have been investigated to improve the differential diagnostic potential of this modality. Fluorodeoxyglucose positron emission tomography (FDG-PET) has become an important tool in the staging of malignancies, but its role in evaluating solid hepatic lesions remains to be defined.

Recommendations

Perform liver function tests, hepatitis profile, and measurements of tumor markers including AFP, CEA, and CA 19-9, followed by a contrast-enhanced MRI of the liver.

Case Continued

The liver function tests are normal and the hepatitis profile was nonreactive. None of the tumor markers were elevated.

MRI

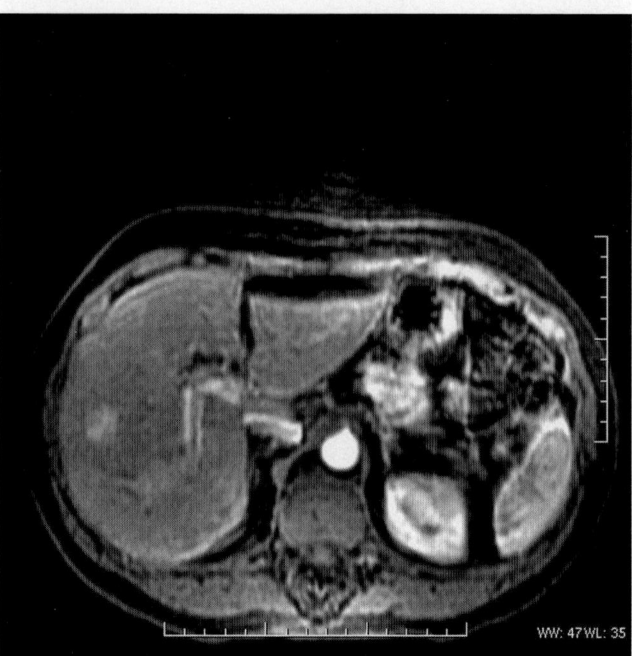

Figure 43.2

MRI Report

There is a well-demarcated hypervascular hepatic lesion with indistinct hypodense areas suggestive of a focal nodular hyperplasia (FNH), though a hepatic adenoma cannot be excluded.

Approach

In the case of solid hepatic tumors without clinical evidence of malignancy or serum elevation of tumor markers, a benign lesion must be considered during the differential diagnosis, most frequently hemangioma, FNH, or hepatic adenoma. Although not specific, findings of an avascular central scar or a feeding artery to the mass are highly supportive of FNH, and the presence of intralesional hemorrhage with necrosis is similarly supportive of hepatic adenoma. The possible presence of fibrolamellar hepatoma should be kept in the differential diagnosis because the clinical and biochemical characteristics of this carcinoma are nonspecific and the appearance of tumor on imaging may mimic FNH.

The strategy for management of benign hepatic tumors can range from surveillance to routine resection. The indications for surgery include the presence of symptoms, and if the histologic nature of the tumor is uncertain. Surveillance is an appropriate option for FNH because there is no evidence that these tumors can bleed or undergo malignant transformation. Similarly, cavernous hemangiomas have a low potential for complications such as rupture, growth, or mass effects, and thus do not justify surgery. In contrast to FNH and hemangioma, resection of hepatic adenoma is advocated regardless of symptoms, particularly for those larger than 5 cm, because these lesions carry the risk of malignancy and potential for rupture. A conservative approach may be justified with smaller hepatic adenomas, but female patients have to be advised to stop steroid use and avoid pregnancy. However, surgery should be strongly considered when any benign liver tumor causes sustained symptoms or when there is uncertainty regarding the diagnosis.

The value of percutaneous liver biopsy remains controversial. The lesion itself or an area of malignant transformation in an adenoma can be missed, leading to a false-negative result. With hemangioma, aspiration of blood without adequate cell yield may preclude the correct diagnosis; furthermore, there is a considerable risk of biopsy-induced bleeding in hypovascularized tumors. Needle biopsy of hepatic tumors is associated with the known hazard of hemorrhage, sampling error, misdiagnosis, and needle-track tumor seeding. Focal nodular hyperplasia may resemble cirrhosis, and needle samples of hepatic adenoma may be interpreted as normal tissue. In cases where the location of the tumor makes resection hazardous, a percutaneous liver biopsy with ultrasonographic or CT guidance may be valuable.

An asymptomatic patient with a diagnosis of hemangioma or FNH can be observed with imaging examinations at 6-month intervals. Surgical resection should be reserved for patients with symptomatic or enlarging lesions. Withdrawal from contraceptive steroids should be recommended in any case of observed hepatic adenoma, which can regress although the potential for rupture and hemorrhage persist. Therefore, the current recommendation for hepatic adenoma is to perform resection to eliminate the risk of rupture and bleeding that occur in 22% to 25% of patients and to avoid the potential for malignant transformation.

After a complete workup, including a fine-needle aspiration if uncertainty is still present regarding potential malignancy, surgical resection should be the first line of treatment when feasible. Patients who are selected for nonoperative management must be observed closely for the development of symptoms or a change in the radiographic size or characteristics of the lesion.

Case Continued

Due to the diagnostic uncertainty, the patient is advised to undergo exploration and resection of the hepatic mass. The risks, benefits, advantages, and disadvantages of the alternative option of observation are discussed. Due to the upcoming final examination for her master's in business administration program, the patient elects to proceed with observation, but requests a biopsy for her peace of mind. After the risks associated with percutaneous liver biopsy are explained, she undergoes this procedure. Pathology examination reveals a mixture of hepatocytes and fibrotic tissue, and is interpreted as inconclusive but suggestive of FNH. The patient is asked to stop the oral contraceptive pill, and a repeat ultrasound scan of the liver is obtained in 6 months. The ultrasound shows that the mass has increased in size to 3 cm. The patient wishes to continue surveillance, but misses her next ultrasound appointment. Another ultrasound obtained 1 year later shows that the mass measures 5 cm in size.

Recommendation

Surgical resection of the solitary hepatic lesion.

Surgical Approach

The risks, benefits, and complications of hepatic resection are explained to the patient and a full consent is obtained. The patient is placed in the supine position and the anesthesiologist is requested to provide a low central venous pressure (CVP) anesthesia.

A right subcostal incision is made, and a thorough exploration is performed to evaluate for evidence of distant metastatic disease. A vessel loop is placed around the porta hepatis for subsequent Pringle maneuver. The liver is mobilized by dividing the falciform ligament and the right triangular ligament. The right lobe of the liver is dissected from the inferior vena cava by dividing and ligating the small venous tributaries. The right hepatic vein is then carefully dissected and a vessel loop is placed around it. An intraoperative liver ultrasound scan is performed to delineate the relation of the tumor to the major blood vessels, exclude any other liver lesions, and confirm the surgical margin. Using the Glissonian technique, the right hepatic pedicle is isolated and then transected with the linear endogastrointestinal anastomosis (GIA) stapler. Next, the hepatic vein is also divided in a similar fashion. Transection of the liver parenchyma can be achieved using a variety of methods. Hemostasis is secured along the transected surface, and any biliary radicals are controlled with suture ligature. The incision is then closed in the standard fashion.

Case Continued

The patient undergoes a right hepatectomy without any complication. Pathology examination reveals a hepatic adenoma with a small focus of hepatocellular carcinoma. The margins of resections are negative.

Discussion

For optimal evaluation and management of solitary liver lesions, a multidisciplinary approach involving the surgeon, radiologist, and internist is necessary. Some of the clinically common benign hepatic tumors are discussed here.

Hemangioma

Hemangioma is the most common benign hepatic tumor of mesenchymal origin with a worldwide incidence of approximately 15%. Cavernous hemangiomas occur in all age groups, but are more frequently encountered in the 30- to 50-year-old age group. They occur primarily in women with a male:female ratio of 1:5. Hemangiomas appear to develop in women at an earlier age than in men, and in women they are more likely to be symptomatic. Nevertheless, most hemangiomas are asymptomatic until they reach a size greater than 10 cm. On contrast-enhanced spiral CT scan, hemangiomas are well-demarcated lesions that develop a peripheral zone of enhancement with a delayed centripetal flow of the contrast medium during the arterial phase. The RBC nuclear scan will show a typical blood pooling, and on MRI these are hyperintense on T1-weighted and on T2-weighted images. False-positive diagnosis of hemangiomas with MRI is uncommon and usually results from metastatic lesions of endocrine tumors. As a general rule, needle biopsies of hemangiomas should not be performed. When surgical treatment is necessary, it can be undertaken either as an enucleation or an anatomic resection.

Focal Nodular Hyperplasia

FNH is the second most common benign solid hepatic tumor, and is increasingly being diagnosed due to routine use of abdominal CT scan. Typically, FNH is seen more commonly in adult women (80%). Classically, these lesions are spherical with a central stellate scar. Histologically, there is a large central vessel without portal veins surrounded by nodules of hyperplastic liver plates. Like hemangiomas, the majority of these are asymptomatic. Unlike hepatic adenoma, the relation of FNH to oral contraceptive use is less apparent. On CT scan, FNH tends to be well demarcated, and these tumors are typically hypervascular on arterial phase examination with subsequent isodensity and hypodensity on portal venous phase. Nuclear scan using a hepatobiliary agent demonstrates hypoperfusion during the early phase with trapping during the late phase. MRI is thought to be superior for characterization of FNH, particularly the detection of the central scar. Unlike adenomas, FNH rarely has a higher signal intensity than the liver on T1-weighted images. The central scar appears hypodense on T1-weighted images and mostly hyperintense on T2-weighted images. Because FNH shows no malignant potential or serious risk of spontaneous hemorrhage, these are primarily managed with surveillance.

Hepatic Adenoma

There is a close association between the incidence of hepatic adenomas and the use of oral contraceptives. Hepatic adenomas are also seen in patients with rare metabolic diseases, such as glycogen storage disease type 1A (GSD type 1). These lesions usually tend to be solitary, although multiple tumors are characteristic in patients with anabolic steroid use and GSD type 1. Compared with FNH, incidental detection is much less common and studies have demonstrated that two thirds of hepatic adenomas cause symptoms, with 52% experiencing abdominal pain and approximately one third demonstrating an acute onset of symptoms secondary to intratumoral bleeding or rupture. Typically, on CT scan, these lesions show areas of hemorrhage and necrosis with a significant enhancement on the arterial phase, due in part to the presence of subcapsular feeding vessels and early draining veins. On T1-weighted MRI images, hepatocellular adenoma has increased signal intensity due to the high glycogen content of the cells, which enhances on the fat suppression images. Areas of recent internal hemorrhages are easily recognizable as marked hyperintense areas on both T1-weighted and T2-weighted images. No contrast pooling is noticed on delayed imaging due to arterial venous shunting. Because of the considerable risk of rupture, intraperitoneal hemorrhage, and malignant transformation, hepatic adenomas are treated with resection.

Suggested Readings

Alobaidi M, Shirkhoda A. Benign focal liver lesions: discrimination from malignant mimickers. *Curr Probl Diagn Radiol* 2004; 33:239–253.

Belghiti J, Pateron D, Panis Y, et al. Resection of presumed benign liver tumors. *Br J Surg* 1993;80:380–383.

Charny CK, Jarnagin WR, Schwartz LH, et al. Management of 155 patients with benign liver tumors. *Br J Surg* 2001;88:808–813.

Horton KM, Bluemke DA, Hruban RH, et al. CT and MR imaging of benign hepatic and biliary tumors. *Radiographics* 1999;19:431–451.

Kammula US, Buell JF, Labow DM, et al. Surgical management of benign tumors of the liver. *Int J Gastrointest Cancer* 2001;30:141–146.

Laurent C, Trillaud H, Lepreux S, et al. Association of adenoma and focal nodular hyperplasia: experience of a single French academic center. *Comp Hepatol* 2003;2:6.

Lepreux S, Laurent C, Balabaud C, et al. FNH-like nodules: possible precursor lesions in patients with focal nodular hyperplasia (FNH). *Comp Hepatol* 2003;2:7.

Mortele KJ, Ros PR. Benign liver neoplasms. *Clin Liver Dis* 2002;6:119–145.

Nakanuma Y. Non-neoplastic nodular lesions in the liver. *Pathol Int* 1995;45:703–714.

Paradis V, Laurent A, Flejou JF, et al. Evidence for the polyclonal nature of focal nodular hyperplasia of the liver by the study of X-chromosome inactivation. *Hepatology* 1997;26:891–895.

Reddy KR, Kligerman S, Levi J, et al. Benign and solid tumors of the liver: relationship to sex, age, size of tumors, and outcome. *Am Surg* 2001;67:173–178.

case 44

Presentation

A 56-year-old man is referred to your office by his primary care physician for evaluation of a rising carcinoembryonic antigen (CEA) level. Two years previously, the patient underwent a sigmoid colectomy for a T3 N1 (American Joint Committee on Cancer [AJCC] stage III) colon cancer, followed by adjuvant chemotherapy consisting of 5-fluorouracil (5-FU) and leucovorin. At that time, he had no evidence of metastatic disease. Recently, he has been found on routine follow-up to have an elevated CEA level (19.2 mg/dL).

CT Scan

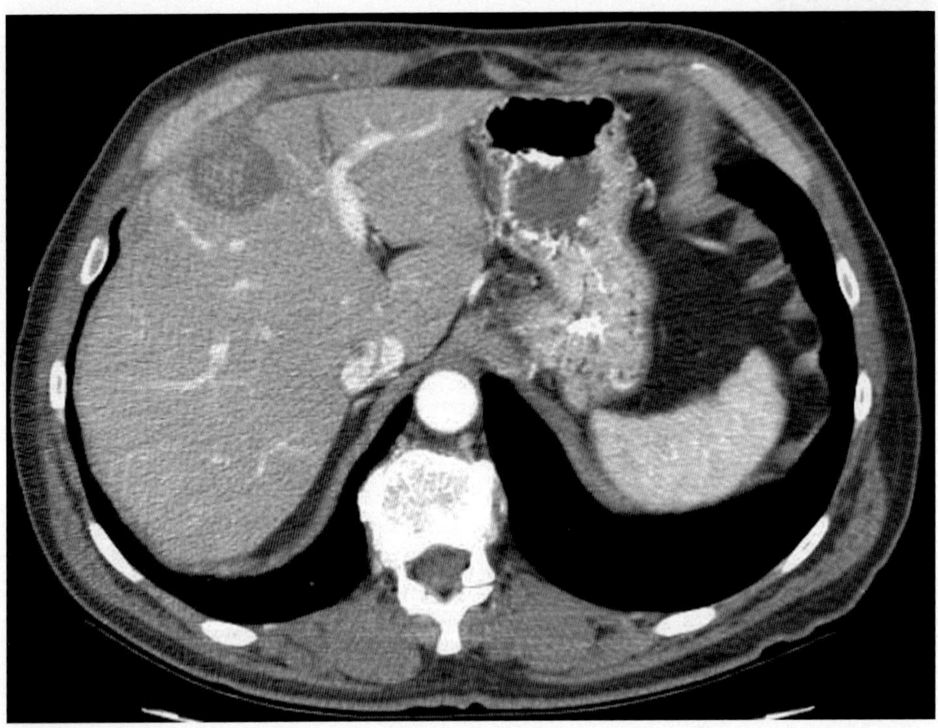

Figure 44.1

CT Scan Report

There is a solitary lesion in segment IV of the liver.

Differential Diagnosis

The differential diagnosis for liver lesions commonly includes hepatocellular carcinoma, cholangiocarcinoma, hepatic adenoma, metastatic tumor, hemangioma, focal nodular hyperplasia (FNH), and a benign cyst.

Discussion

A computed tomography (CT) scan using a quadphase liver protocol is currently the study of choice to evaluate liver tumors at most institutions. In a patient with a history of colorectal cancer with an elevated CEA level, and with CT findings consistent with metastatic colon cancer (low-attenuation irregular lesion with punctate calcifications), the diagnosis is all but certain. Fine-needle aspiration (FNA) is not routinely indicated for a tissue diagnosis if surgical exploration is contemplated. A negative biopsy will not alter management if there is no evidence of metastatic carcinoma elsewhere.

Case Continued

The CT scan demonstrates a single tumor in the medial segment of the left lobe (segment IV). A chest x-ray shows no evidence of metastatic lesions, and a colonoscopy demonstrates no recurrence or new primary.

PET Scans

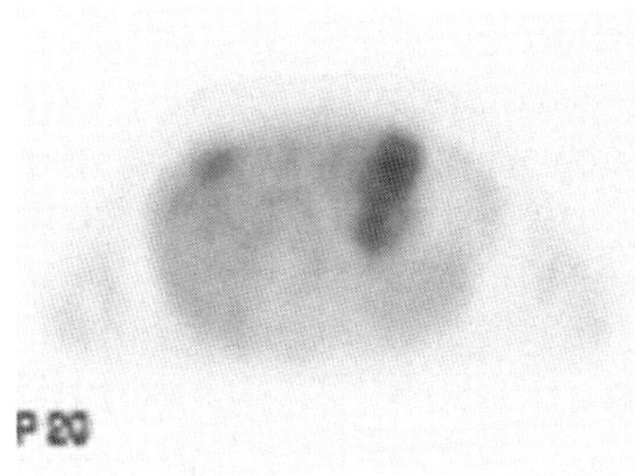

Figure 44.2A

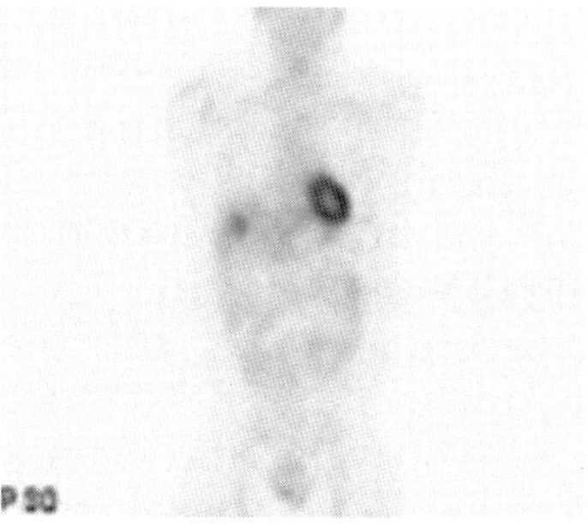

Figure 44.2B

PET Scan Report

A full-body positron emission tomography (PET) scan confirms focal high uptake in the liver consistent with the known lesion, but no evidence of extrahepatic tumors.

Case Continued

The patient has no other significant medical problems, takes no medications, and reports good exercise tolerance. Laboratory studies, including platelet count, total bilirubin, and prothrombin time, are normal.

Diagnosis and Recommendation

The patient has metastatic colorectal cancer, which appears to be confined to the liver. He is a good operative candidate, and should be offered exploratory laparotomy. If there is no evidence of disease outside the liver upon surgical exploration, he will undergo resection and/or ablation of the metastatic tumor.

Approach

Hepatic resection remains the only potentially curative intervention for these patients as long as R0 resection can be achieved while preserving adequate functional residual liver volume. If additional lesions are discovered during resection, these can either be resected or destroyed with radiofrequency ablation. The role of postresection adjuvant hepatic intra-arterial chemotherapy is uncertain, particularly given the recent availability of new systemic chemotherapeutic and biologic agents that appear to yield significantly improved response rates compared to traditional agents (e.g., 5-FU). Hepatic intra-arterial chemotherapy, at this time, should not be routinely used outside of clinical trials.

Discussion

The American Cancer Society estimated that approximately 150,000 cases of colorectal cancer would be diagnosed in 2004 in the United States. One fourth of these were expected to have hepatic metastases at presentation (synchronous metastases), and another quarter were expected to develop hepatic metastases during the course of their disease (metachronous metastases). The median survival time for patients with untreated (but potentially resectable) hepatic metastases is on the order of 14 to 18 months, with essentially no survivors beyond 3 years.

Initially, metastasectomy for colorectal liver metastases was met with some skepticism, given the morbidity of liver resection historically and the perception that liver metastases were a harbinger of widespread disease. However, since the initial reports in the early 1980s, mounting data have supported an aggressive approach. Specialized centers consistently report 5-year survival rates after metastasectomy of 30% to 50% with a perioperative mortality of less than 5%. Similar to other complex surgical procedures, outcome closely correlates with the case volume performed at a given medical center. Therefore, evaluation and treatment of these patients should be performed at centers where the staff—surgical, anesthesia, interventional radiology, oncology, intensive care unit, and nursing—routinely care for patients who undergo major hepatic resections.

The curative resection of metachronous colorectal liver metastases is generally predicated on the absence of metastases outside the liver. Routine evaluation therefore includes plain radiographs of the chest to identify possible pulmonary metastases. Chest CT scan only minimally improves detection of metastatic lesions in a patient with negative chest radiographs and has a high false-positive rate, and is therefore not routinely utilized. Either colonoscopy or barium enema is essential to rule out recurrence at the anastomosis or metachronous primary colonic tumors. A CT scan of the abdomen and pelvis (quadphase liver protocol) allows careful evaluation of the liver, as well as the remainder of the abdomen, for nodal disease or evidence of carcinomatosis. Helical CT scan also allows three-dimensional volumetry, which assists in operative planning to ensure adequate hepatic reserve after resection. Magnetic resonance imaging (MRI) is sometimes used as an alternative to delineate hepatic tumors and provide detailed information about the relation of a tumor to vascular and biliary structures. However, MRI is less useful for evaluating the remainder of the abdomen and is more expensive than CT. Whole-body PET, though not mandatory, is used with increasing frequency. PET is the most specific imaging modality in cases of uncertain hepatic lesions, and is especially useful for detecting extrahepatic disease, although its sensitivity is probably not greater than that of CT for liver lesions. Bone scans are not indicated in the absence of bony symptoms.

Preoperative evaluation includes a thorough assessment of comorbid conditions, particularly cardiac and pulmonary, that might preclude major surgery. Hepatic function is appraised simply by routine liver function tests, albumin, platelet count, and prothrombin time. More specialized estimation of functional hepatic reserve (e.g., indocyanine green clearance and 99m-Tc-galactosyl serum albumin scintigraphy) are not widely available and are not routinely utilized at our institution.

Metastasectomy is feasible in approximately 20% to 25% of patients with metachronous colorectal hepatic metastases. Unresectable extrahepatic disease (e.g., peritoneal carcinomatosis) or incompletely resectable hepatic tumors preclude curative resection. A tumor may be deemed unresectable because of proximity to hilar vasculature or biliary structures obviating adequate resection margins, because of multifocal liver involvement, or because of inadequate functional hepatic reserve. There is no absolute number of metastatic lesions that preclude curative resection, so long as all tumors can be resected with adequate margins. Though somewhat controversial, there is some evidence that, in selected patients with both liver metastases and *limited and resectable* extrahepatic disease (e.g., anastomotic recurrence, isolated portal node metastasis, limited lung metastasis), resection of all disease (hepatic and extrahepatic) may prolong survival. Similarly, disease that is contiguous with the liver, such as invasion into the diaphragm, bowel, kidney, or adrenal, may be resected en bloc with the liver and results in outcomes similar to those for patients with isolated hepatic disease. This represents relatively few patients, however, and remains a point of dispute.

Ablation serves as an important adjunct to resection. Cryotherapy was the first ablative technology that was widely available. Cryotherapy uses a liquid nitrogen cryoprobe to destroy tumors by creating intracellular and extracellular ice crystals, resulting in a hyperosmolar environment, membrane damage, and protein denaturation. A number of uncontrolled studies published in the early 1990s established the efficacy of cryoablation. However, cryotherapy has largely been abandoned. This is due partly to practical considerations (the freezing of each tumor takes 30 to 40 minutes, making the procedure quite lengthy), and partly to concern about the rate of complications (particularly myoglobinuria and renal injury in cases of aggressive ablation, as well as cracking of the liver). Radiofrequency ablation (RFA) has largely replaced cryotherapy. RFA utilizes an alternating-current probe to create thermal coagulation necrosis. The cost of the instrumentation is lower than cryoablation, and the ablation time is significantly shorter. Intraoperatively, the RFA probe is introduced into the liver with the aid of intraoperative ultrasound (IOUS). Previously, size was a limitation of the technology, because the electrodes allowed only small (3 cm) lesions to be ablated. However, newer probes that use a continuous saline infusion allow a 7-cm sphere to be ablated. Uncontrolled series with short follow-up report outcomes that are similar to those of cryoablation. Retrospective comparison suggests that RFA is inferior to resection, though no controlled trials have been conducted to date. At present, RFA should be considered an adjunct to resection rather than an alternative for resectable tumors.

Another investigational therapy for colorectal hepatic metastases is hepatic intra-arterial chemotherapy (HIAC). The logic behind regional chemotherapy is that anticancer drugs may be delivered directly to the tumor at high concentrations, while minimizing systemic toxicity. Perfusion studies have demonstrated that two thirds or more of the blood supply to hepatic metastases is from the hepatic artery, thus HIAC is preferentially delivered to the tumors. HIAC has been investigated in cases of unresectable colorectal metastases and as an adjunctive therapy after liver resection. Briefly, HIAC is delivered via a catheter directly into the hepatic artery (positioned at the takeoff of the gastroduodenal artery) attached to an implantable continuous-infusion pump placed in a subcutaneous pocket in the abdominal wall. Fluorodeoxyuridine (FUdR), a pyrimidine analog, and 5-FU are the agents most frequently employed. In the most widely publicized trial of HIAC after metastasectomy, published in the *New England Journal of Medicine* in 1999, Kemeny et al. reported a modest improvement in survival over resection and systemic chemotherapy (86% vs. 72% 2-year survival rate). However, other trials have not achieved as promising results, and meta-analysis suggests that the survival benefit of HIAC with conventional agents is, at best, quite small.

Surgical Approach

The abdomen is explored via a limited right subcostal incision. If carcinomatosis is encountered, the operation is terminated before proceeding further. In the absence of palpable disease outside the liver, the incision is extended to a bilateral subcostal incision with a vertical extension in the midline to the sternum (chevron incision). The liver is widely mobilized and the caudate lobe is exposed. The hepatogastric and hepatoduodenal ligaments are inspected for the presence of accessory/replaced left or right hepatic arteries. IOUS using a 5- or 7.5-MHz linear array probe is performed. The IOUS allows evaluation of the entire liver from anterior and interior surfaces to assess lesions seen on preoperative imaging, to identify any lesions (typically <14 cm) not seen on CT scan, and to define the relation of metastatic tumors to the hepatic vasculature. IOUS adds approximately 20 minutes to the operative time, but alters the surgical plan in approximately one fourth of cases. It therefore serves a critical role in liver resection for metastatic disease.

Laparoscopy in conjunction with laparoscopic ultrasound offers an alternative to open exploration. In some cases, laparoscopic staging may be limited by adhesions or less complete access to the liver. However, given the much-reduced morbidity, laparoscopy is an attractive alternative in patients with questionably resectable disease or who are poor operative candidates.

Surgical management proceeds according to the findings of the preoperative CT, the IOUS, and the findings on palpation and visual inspection. As a general rule, 70% of the liver parenchyma can be removed for an otherwise normal liver, although caution must be exercised in the elderly or diabetic patient or the patient with extensive fatty infiltration of the liver. Anatomic resection has been shown to provide superior oncologic outcomes to wedge resection, and resection appears superior to RFA. All surgical strategies, whether resection or RFA or a combination, aim toward achieving a 10-mm margin. In cases where (typically for technical reasons) the margin after resection is less than 10 mm, RFA of the cut edge is occasionally useful to increase the functional margin. Close or positive margins are associated with high local recurrence. In this setting, RFA should generally be reserved for smaller lesions (3 cm or less) that are not amenable to resection. It is difficult to ensure adequate ablation, even with multiple passes, for larger lesions.

Postoperatively, liver function tests and prothrombin time are monitored for evidence of hepatic insufficiency. Phosphorous repletion is commonly required. Median hospital stay is typically about 7 to 9 days.

Case Continued

The patient undergoes exploration via a subcostal chevron incision. There is no evidence of carcinomatosis.

Intraoperative Ultrasonograms

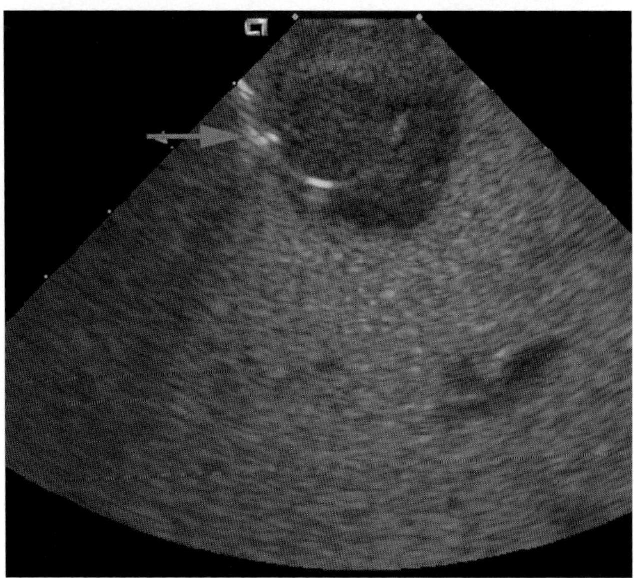

Figure 44.3A

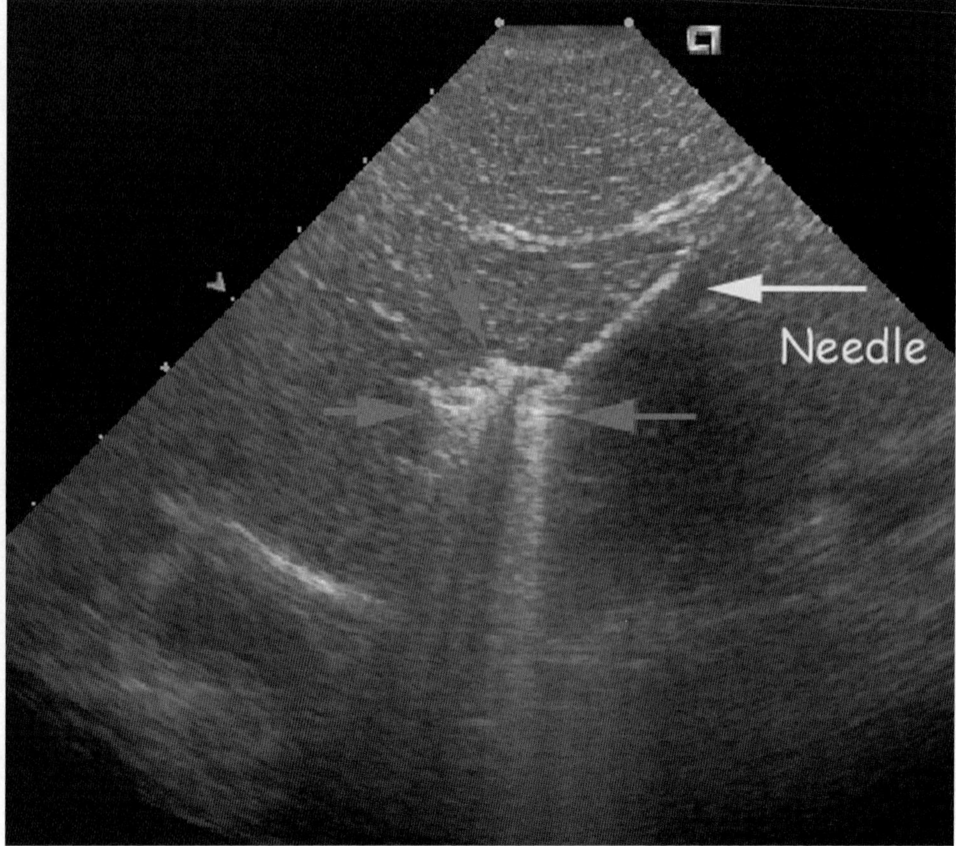

Figure 44.3B

Intraoperative Ultrasonography Report

The known lesion in segment IV is found to abut the middle hepatic vein. An 8-mm lesion is seen in the posterior-inferior right lobe (segment VI) that had not been seen on the preoperative CT (*left*). This was felt to be consistent with another metastatic deposit. The patient undergoes an extended left hepatectomy (segments II, III, IV, as well as portions of V and VIII) and RFA of the lesion in segment VI using a 2-cm probe (*right*).

Discussion

Recent series of metastasectomy for hepatic liver metastases report 5-year survival rates of 30% to 50%. Several investigators have sought to define prognostic indicators that would allow selection of patients who are most likely to benefit from resection. The most powerful clinical predictors of outcome are consistently found to be the number of metastases and the presence of a positive surgical margin. Additional factors predictive of recurrence are the presence of extrahepatic disease, a node-positive primary tumor, a short (<12 months) interval between the primary tumor and the metastasis, preoperative elevated CEA level, and the size of the largest hepatic metastasis (>5 cm). Promising research is ongoing into molecular markers that predict outcome (e.g., loss of heterozygosity at the specific gene MTSP2 or array bases analysis of the total fraction of the genome altered in a tumor).

The mortality associated with liver resection is now consistently less than 5% and often less than 2% at referral centers, with complications occurring in 20% to 50% of cases. Hepatic insufficiency, the most ominous complication, occurs in 1% to 5% of cases. Other serious complications include hemorrhage (1% to 3%), biliary leak or fistula (3% to 4%), and perihepatic abscess (1% to 9%). Cardiopulmonary complications, including myocardial infarction, pleural effusion requiring thoracostomy, pneumonia, and pulmonary embolism, occur in 5% to 10% of cases.

Unfortunately, cancer recurs in approximately 50% to 75% of patients after liver resection. Half of those recurrences are in the liver. Highly selected patients may be candidates for repeat hepatectomy following recurrence. The clinical evaluation and eligibility for re-resection are essentially the same as for initial hepatectomy. Several centers have reported

5-year survival following re-resection that approximates survival after the initial liver resection.

Follow-up after metastasectomy is therefore dependent on whether the patient is potentially a candidate for re-resection. If so, liver function tests, CEA level, and helical CT scan are obtained at 4- to 6-month intervals for at least 3 years. Patients who are not candidates for further surgery undergo further radiologic evaluation only as symptoms arise.

In the last 5 years, medical therapy for advanced colorectal cancer has changed dramatically. Treatment protocols that include new chemotherapeutic agents (e.g., irinotecan, oxaliplatin) and biologics (e.g., bevacizumab [Avastin], gefitinib [Iressa]) have considerably improved response rates (approaching 50%) over traditional 5-FU-based regimens. This progress in medical therapy may increase the number of patients who benefit from aggressive surgical intervention. As clinicians are armed with more effective weapons against microscopic disease, more patients may ultimately benefit from resection of hepatic metastases.

Suggested Readings

Abdalla EK, Vauthey JN, Ellis LM, et al. Recurrence and outcomes following hepatic resection, radiofrequency ablation, and combined resection/ablation for colorectal liver metastases. *Ann Surg* 2004;239:818–825; discussion 825–827.

DeMatteo RP, Palese C, Jarnagin WR, et al. Anatomic segmental hepatic resection is superior to wedge resection as an oncologic operation for colorectal liver metastases. *J Gastrointest Surg* 2000;4:178–184.

Fong Y, Fortner J, Sun RL, et al. Clinical score for predicting recurrence after hepatic resection for metastatic colorectal cancer: analysis of 1001 consecutive cases. *Ann Surg* 1999;230:309–318; discussion 318–321.

Kemeny N, Huang Y, Cohen AM, et al. Hepatic arterial infusion of chemotherapy after resection of hepatic metastases from colorectal cancer. *N Engl J Med* 1999;341:2039–2048.

Kinkel K, Lu Y, Both M, et al. Detection of hepatic metastases from cancers of the gastrointestinal tract by using noninvasive imaging methods (US, CT, MR imaging, PET): a meta-analysis. *Radiology* 2002;224:748–756.

Nelson RL, Freels S. A systematic review of hepatic artery chemotherapy after hepatic resection of colorectal cancer metastatic to the liver. *Dis Colon Rectum* 2004;47:739–745. Epub 2004 Mar 25.

Weber SM, Jarnagin WR, DeMatteo RP, et al. Survival after resection of multiple hepatic colorectal metastases. *Ann Surg Oncol* 2000;7:643–650.

case 45

A 40-year-old man with no past medical history is admitted for long-standing pain in the left upper quadrant. He is not a smoker or a drinker. Physical examination is unremarkable; the patient was in a good condition with normal blood pressure and stools. There is no sign of portal hypertension. Abdominal ultrasound shows hepatomegaly with several hypoechoic nodules.

CT Scans

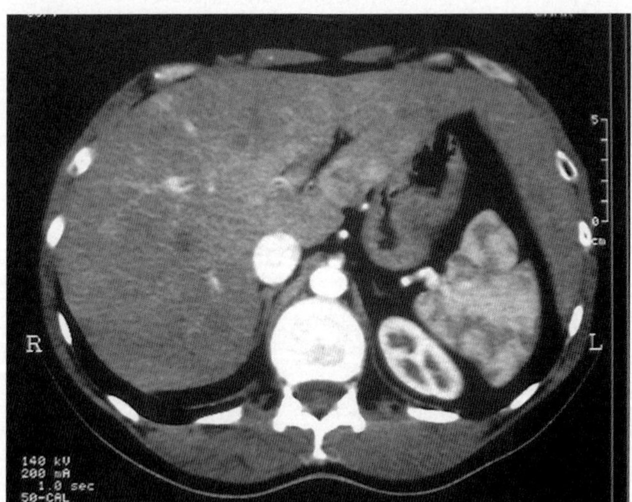

Figure 45.1A

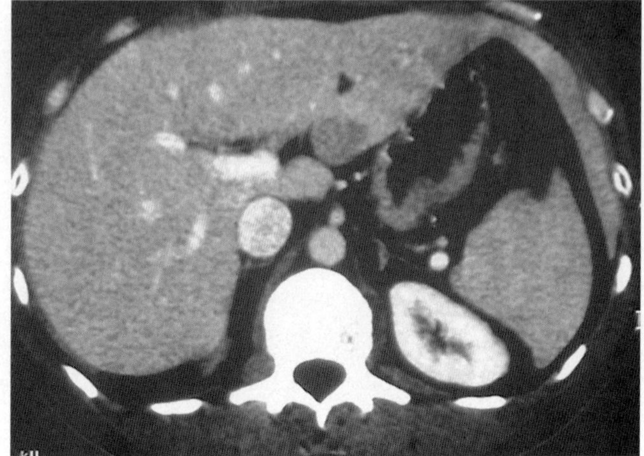

Figure 45.1B

CT Scan Report

Abdominal computed tomography (CT) scan shows four hypervascularized nodules during the arterial phase, favoring intrahepatic benign tumors. The lesions are hypodense in portal phase.

Differential Diagnosis

Differential diagnoses for intrahepatic tumors include hemangiomas, hepatocarcinomas, metastases of thyroid and kidney cancers, multiple nodular hyperplasias, and polyadenomas, even when there is no washout.

Case Continued

Esophagogastric endoscopy and colonoscopy are normal. Similarly, plasma levels of gastric vasoactive intestinal peptide (VIP) and calcitonin are normal. Levels of plasma serotonin and urinary 5-hydroxyindoleacetic acid (5-HIAA) are one and a half and two times normal, respectively, on two successive assays. Levels of carcinoembryonic antigen (CEA) and cancer antigen (CA) 19-9 are normal.

At this stage, we suspect the diagnosis of liver metastases of a carcinoid tumor located in the appendicular region (suspicion of a positive lymph node in the right inferior quadrant).

A CT-scan-guided biopsy leads to the diagnosis of well-differentiated endocrine (carcinoid) tumor.

MRI

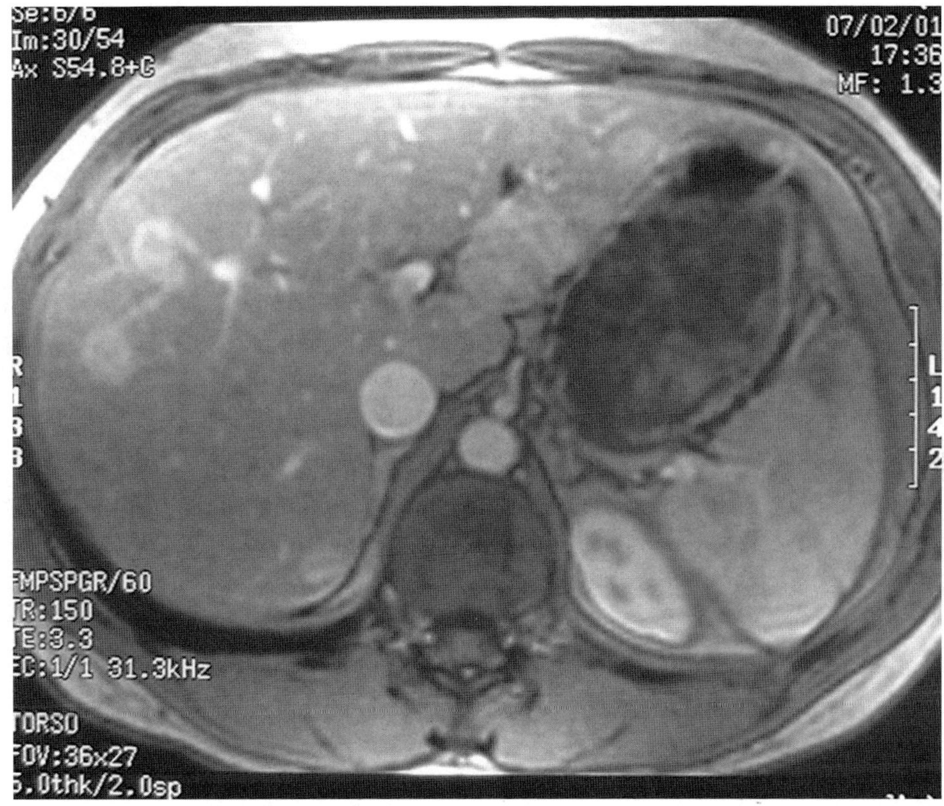

Figure 45.2

MRI Report

Magnetic resonance imaging (MRI) of the liver did not show the classic bulb sign, which would favor hemangioma, but disclosed more intrahepatic lesions in the right lobe.

Octreotide Scintigram

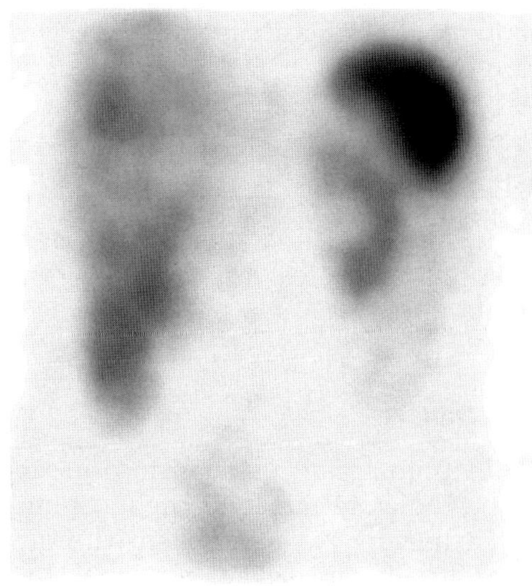

Figure 45.3

Octreotide Scintigraphy Report

There is increased uptake of radionucleotide by the terminal ileum in the location of the primary tumor, and uptake is revealed in other areas. There are several ileal and lymphatic foci in the right iliac region; multiple foci are identified in the liver.

CT Scan

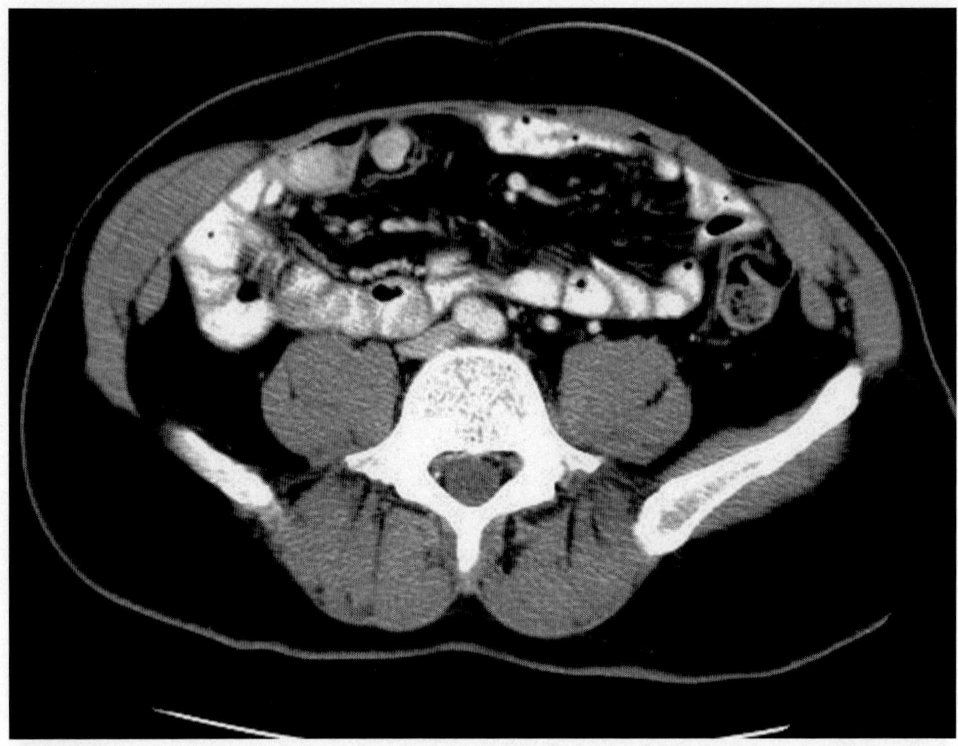

Figure 45.4

CT Scan Report

A CT scan reveals the presence of a 15-mm diameter hypervascularized tumor located in the ileocecoappendicular region. In addition, there are several intra-abdominal nodules suggestive of lymphatic metastases.

Diagnosis

The diagnosis is carcinoid tumor with lymphatic metastases in the ileocecal region and liver carcinoid tumor metastases.

Approach

Carcinoid tumors are notable for an indolent course, and therefore surgery is the most important aspect in achieving palliation even with advanced and metastatic disease where there is no hope for cure. If the patient presents with synchronous metastatic disease, the primary tumor is resected with the draining lymphatic basin. Carcinoid syndrome can be suspected by the presence of diarrhea, facial flushing, bronchospasm, and crampy abdominal pain. Carcinoid syndrome is confirmed by demonstrating elevation in 24-hour 5-HIAA and serotonin levels. Borderline cases can be diagnosed with serum chromogranin A, substance P, serotonin, and urinary 5-HIAA. Carcinoid syndrome can be treated with somatostatin, which can be effective in 50% to 80% of cases and may also stabilize the disease. Pretreatment with somatostatin is also effective in avoiding carcinoid crisis that can be induced by stress such as surgery, anesthetic induction, and chemotherapy.

Generally, the goal of treatment in patients with metastatic carcinoid syndrome is palliation. For healthy patients, an aggressive surgical approach that includes resection or ablation of the hepatic metastases is appropriate. Palliation can also be achieved with hepatic artery chemoembolization.

Recommendation

Surgical resection of the primary lesions and the hepatic metastases is proposed.

Surgical Approach

A bisubcostal incision is mandatory for complete exploration of the liver. The first step of the procedure is to remove the tumor located at the ileocecal junction with the adjacent mesentry to eliminate the lymph node metastases. The second step is to evaluate the liver with ultrasound, which also guides the resection and ablative therapy.

The primary tumor is resected, and 25 carcinoid liver metastases are treated (14 lesions are removed surgically and 11 nodules are treated by radiofrequency ablation). Ultrasound guidance is used for all resections. Pathological examination confirms that the primary tumor and all the metastases were well-differentiated tumors according to the World Health Organization's (WHO) 2000 classification. The primary tumor was located in the deep layer of the mucosa and submucosa. The other macroscopic lesions exhibited characteristic features of metastases.

CT Scan

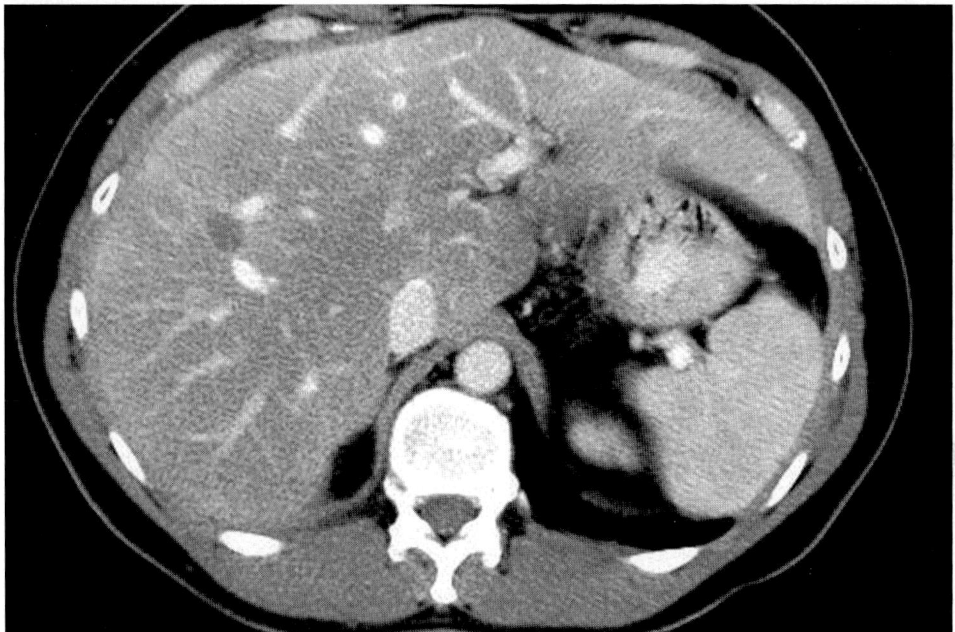

Figure 45.5

CT Scan Report

Aftereffects of radiofrequency ablation.

Discussion

Carcinoid tumors arise from enterochromaffin cells found throughout the body. The incidence is 3 to 15 cases per million. Thus, it is one of the most common neuroendocrine tumors of the gut. Foregut primary carcinoid tumors arise in the stomach, lung, and proximal duodenum, midgut tumors arise from the remainder of the small intestine and colon to the midtransverse colon, and hindgut tumors arise from the distal colon and rectum. The tumors are said to be distinct in their hormone production. Midgut tumors produce large amounts of serotonin.

The majority of midgut carcinoid tumors found outside the appendix arise in the ileum or cecum, and remain clinically silent until the development of carcinoid syndrome and/or hepatic metastases.

Most carcinoid tumors are malignant. The overall 5-year survival rate of those with liver metastases from midgut tumors is between 25% and 38%, though in those with one to four hepatic metastases it is 79%, falling with increasing numbers of metastases. Poor prognostic factors include a high level of circulating tumor markers and urinary 5-HIAA. A combination of anatomic imaging studies (CT, MRI, and ultrasonography) and radionuclide investigations (octreotide scan) can usually locate the primary tumor and metastatic dissemination.

Chemotherapy has been disappointing in the control of carcinoid tumors, even with combined streptozocin, 5-FU, and cyclophosphamide. Surgical treatment includes resection of the primary tumor and resection of the liver metastases. There are two types of liver resection. If there is no other tumor left, liver transplantation can be proposed for multiple liver metastases. This is the only indication for liver transplantation for neuroendocrine tumors. One of our patients, a 28-year-old woman with liver metastases of a midgut carcinoid tumor, received a transplant in 1989; she is alive and well. In this patient, however, there was some suspicion about other intra-abdominal lesions. We preferred to use multiple metastases resection. With so many atypical resections, there is a real risk of postoperative liver insufficiency. Radiofrequency can be combined with surgical resection to spare more functional liver tissue than surgical resection alone.

Suggested Readings

Fenwick SW, Wyatt JI, Toogood GJ, et al. Hepatic resection and transplantation for primary carcinoid tumors of the liver. *Ann Surg* 2004;239:210–219.

Fenwick SW, Wyatt JI, Toogood GJ, et al. Hepatic resection and transplantation for primary carcinoid tumors of the liver. *Ann Surg* 2004;239:210–219.

Moertel CG. Chemotherapy of gastrointestinal cancer. *N Engl J Med* 1978;299:1049–1052.

Schillaci O, Spanu A, Scopinaro F, et al. Somatostatin receptor scintigraphy in liver metastasis detection from gastroenteropancreatic neuroendocrine tumors. *J Nucl Med* 2003;44: 359–368.

Stanley SA, Bloom R. Endocrine aspect of liver tumors. In: Blumgart LH, Fory Y, eds. *Surgery of the Liver and Biliary Tract.* London: WB Saunders; 2000.

Sutcliffe R, Maguire D, Ramage J, et al. Management of neuroendocrine liver metastases. *Am J Surg* 2004;187:39–46.

Presentation

A 66-year-old woman with no significant past medical history presents with a 3-day history of right upper quadrant pain. She is referred by her primary medical doctor. Physical examination reveals no jaundice, anemia, lymphadenopathy, or specific abdominal findings.

Ultrasonogram

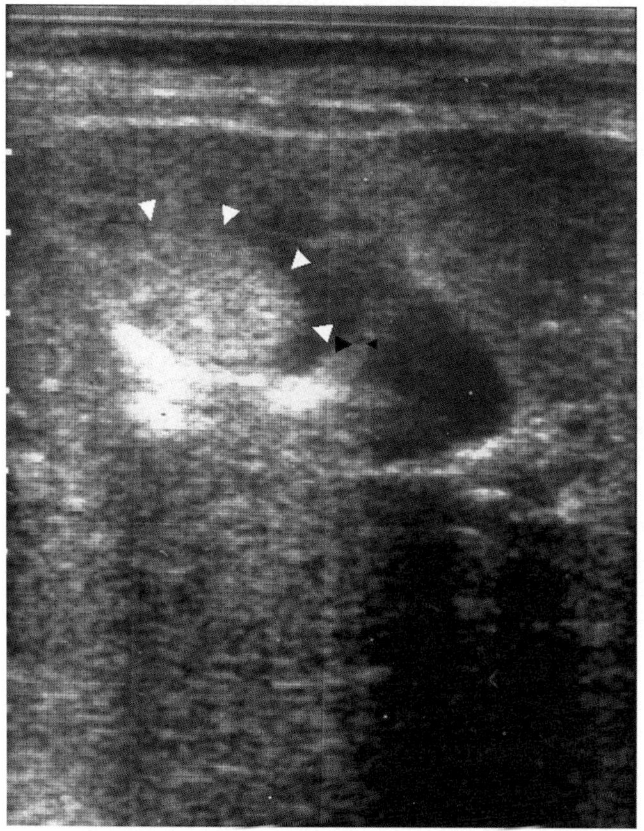

Figure 46.1

Ultrasonography Report

Ultrasonography shows a sessile protruding mass *(arrowheads)*, measuring 3.5 × 3.0 cm, in the fundus

of the gallbladder, which does not involve the liver. A gallstone is present in the gallbladder lumen *(not shown).*

Endoscopic Retrograde Cholangiogram

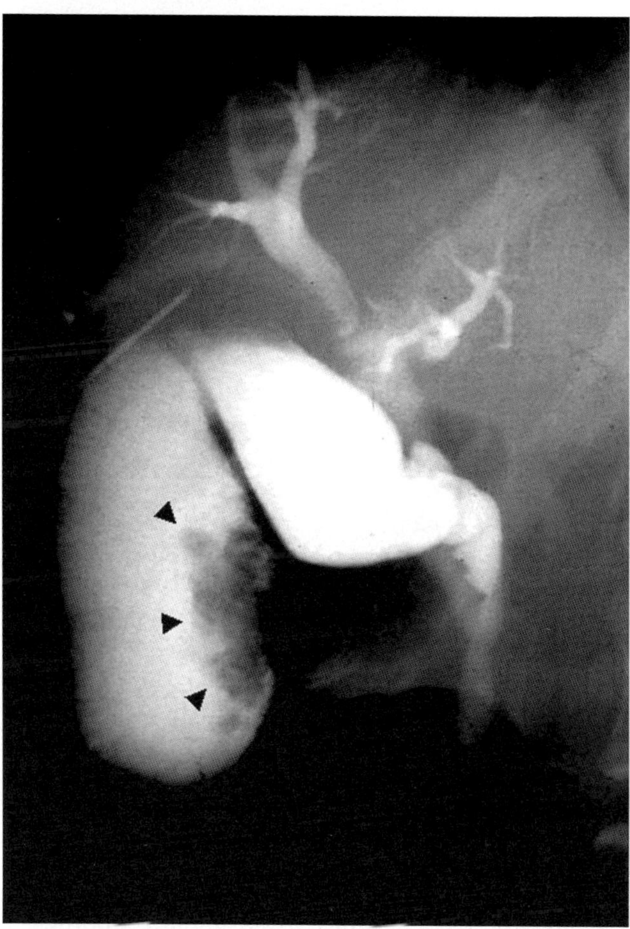

Figure 46.2

Endoscopic Retrograde Cholangiography Report

A 3.5-cm mass with granular appearance *(arrowheads)* is depicted as a filling defect in the fundus of the gallbladder. It does not involve the extrahepatic bile ducts.

Differential Diagnosis

There are a variety of tumors or tumor-like lesions arising in the gallbladder, which often present as protruded (polypoid) lesions. Epithelial tumors include carcinoma, dysplasia, and adenoma, whereas tumor-like lesions comprise hyperplasia, adenomyomatosis, polyps, and others. Among protruded lesions of the gallbladder, the cholesterol polyp is the most common. Once protruded lesions are detected on imaging, the discrimination between benign and malignant is clinically important, and it mainly depends on the size of the lesion. Most protruded lesions smaller than 1 cm in maximum diameter are benign. In contrast, many cancers appear as large polypoid lesions, and those exceeding 1.5 cm in maximum diameter are very likely to be malignant. The shape of the lesion is another useful hint when discriminating benign from malignant lesions. Carcinoma is usually sessile (with the exception of carcinoma in pedunculated adenoma), while most benign lesions are pedunculated.

In this patient, with a sessile protruded lesion far exceeding 1.5 cm in the gallbladder, one must consider gallbladder carcinoma as the primary diagnosis. The irregular (granular) contour of the lesion on cholangiography (Fig. 46.2) also supports this diagnosis.

Diagnosis and Recommendation

Gallbladder carcinoma. A computed tomography (CT) scan of the abdomen is recommended for staging of the tumor.

CT Scan

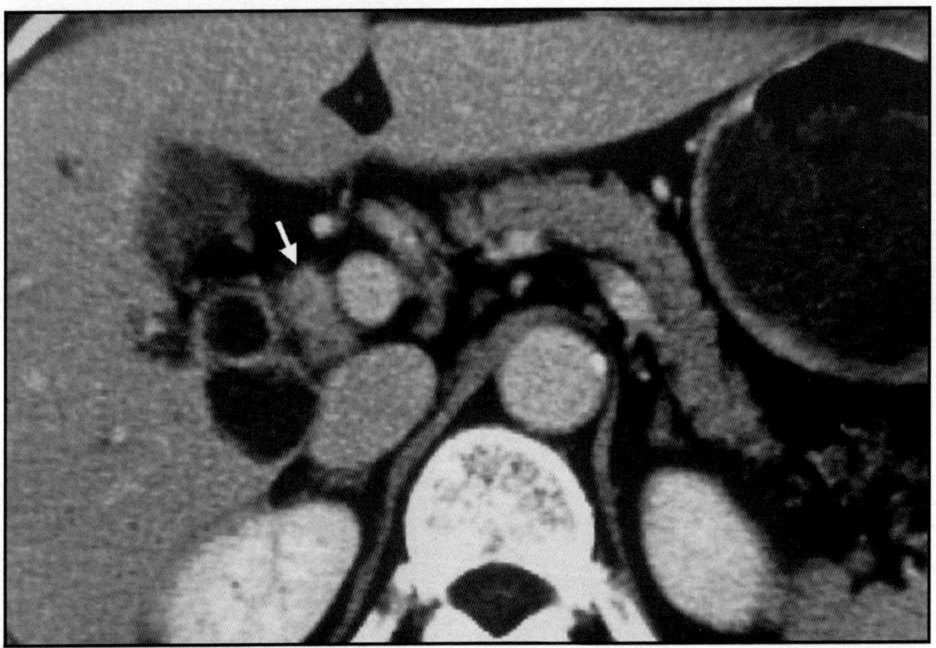

Figure 46.3

CT Scan Report

A 3-cm mass with contrast enhancement is depicted in the fundus of the gallbladder *(not shown)*. It does not involve the adjacent organs, including the liver. There are neither liver metastases nor peritoneal seeding. A 2 × 1-cm soft tissue mass with heterogeneous contrast enhancement *(arrow)*, suggestive of a positive lymph node, is located on the right side of the main portal vein.

Approach

Although gallbladder carcinoma has been considered to be a highly lethal disease, resection provides the only chance for a cure. The outcome of resection depends on the extent of the primary tumor. The Tis or T1 tumor is designated as *early* carcinoma and bears a favorable prognosis after resection (cumulative 5-year survival rate >90%). The outcome of radical resection of a T2 tumor is better (cumulative 5-year survival rate >50%) than the poorer resection outcomes of T3 or more advanced tumors.

In 1954, Glenn and Hays first proposed a radical cholecystectomy procedure (the Glenn operation) for gallbladder carcinoma, which consists of en bloc resection of the gallbladder, gallbladder bed, and regional lymph nodes within the hepatoduodenal ligament and lesser omentum. Since 1982, we have been using a modified Glenn operation for this disease, in which the suprapancreatic segment of the extrahepatic bile duct is excised and the regional lymph nodes adjacent to the posterosuperior aspect of the head of the pancreas are dissected, in addition to the original Glenn operation. The bile duct is usually divided at the upper border of the pancreas and then just below the confluence of the right and left hepatic ducts. The application of bile duct resection to gallbladder carcinoma is controversial; the rationale for bile duct resection is to accomplish en bloc resection including the pericholedochal/cystic duct lymph nodes (first echelon nodes), to facilitate regional lymphadenectomy, to eliminate possible bile duct involvement, and to prevent ischemic stricture of skeletonized bile ducts. Because the objective of hepatic resection for gallbladder carcinoma is to eliminate possible hepatic involvement, the extent of hepatectomy during radical cholecystectomy should be weighed against the degree of such involvement. Although a non-anatomic resection of the gallbladder bed, an integral part of the Glenn operation, is sufficient for minor liver involvement, marked hepatic involvement and/or invasion of the pedicle of the right lobe requires a more extensive hepatectomy procedure, such as an extended right hepatectomy.

The choice of resectional procedure for each patient depends on the extent of the tumor. The Tis or T1 tumor is usually not accompanied by any regional spread, and cholecystectomy alone is appropriate for this stage of tumor. T2 or more advanced tumor bear a greater than 50% incidence of nodal involvement, for which regional lymphadenectomy is indicated. For T2 tumors, radical cholecystectomy (the Glenn, or modified Glenn operation) is appropriate. Radical resections for T3 or T4 tumors depend on the organs or structures involved. Major hepatic involvement requires extensive hepatectomy; involvement of the duodenum and/or pancreas usually requires pancreaticoduodenectomy (Whipple or pylorus-preserving); gastric or colonic involvement requires partial resection of the viscus. Combined hepatectomy and pancreaticoduodenectomy is indicated for selected patients with both hepatic and pancreaticoduodenal involvement. As bile duct involvement usually indicates extensive involvement of the hepatoduodenal ligament, malignant biliary obstruction is a sign of local irresectability in gallbladder carcinoma, with the exception of selected patients with localized ductal involvement. Although radical resection for locally advanced gallbladder carcinoma has been accepted by many surgeons, further investigation is warranted to refine the indications and specific details.

When a radical resection is planned for gallbladder carcinoma, the preoperative staging of the tumor with the help of plain and contrast-enhanced CT scanning or other imaging techniques is essential. The presence of distant metastases is a contraindication for radical resection. The CT scan depicts a positive lymph node as a soft tissue mass with an anteroposterior dimension of at least 10 mm and ringlike or heterogeneous contrast enhancement. Laparoscopic staging prior to definitive surgery may be useful to avoid unnecessary laparotomies in selected patients with advanced disease. Finally, intraoperative staging by the surgeon is indispensable, because it is more accurate and reliable than preoperative staging. The presence or absence of liver metastases and/or peritoneal seeding and local resectability of the tumor should be assessed carefully before starting resectional procedures.

Recommendation

After confirming the absence of lung metastases on chest radiograph (not shown), the diagnosis of gallbladder carcinoma with metastasis to a pericholedochal lymph node, categorized as stage IIB (cT2 N1 M0), is made. This patient is offered radical resection of the gallbladder tumor (en bloc resection of the gallbladder, gallbladder bed, bile duct, and regional lymph nodes).

It is also explained to the patient that more than half of the patients with stage II tumors will survive for 5 years after the resection, provided that the resection is potentially curative. The complications mentioned are bleeding, biliary fistula, infection, lymphorrhea, and death.

Surgical Approach

A laparotomy reveals a tumor in the fundus of the gallbladder, which grossly has no extension beyond the serosa or into the liver. The tumor is considered resectable because of limited nodal disease and the absence of both liver metastases and peritoneal seeding.

Initially a careful exploration is performed to exclude evidence of peritoneal seeding, liver metastases, and extensive nodal disease. The gallbladder is inspected to determine if it is resectable. In the absence of distant metastases and if the tumor is considered resectable, the radical cholecystectomy begins. After an extensive Kocher maneuver, the posterosuperior pancreaticoduodenal lymph node group is dissected from the head of the pancreas, and then the common bile duct is secured and divided at the upper border of the pancreas. The common hepatic artery and the portal vein are secured, together with the dissection of the hepatic artery nodes, right celiac nodes, and retroportal nodes. The regional lymphadenectomy procedure continues toward the hepatic hilum within the hepatoduodenal ligament in an en bloc fashion, during which the right hepatic artery is secured and the cystic artery is divided at its origin. The gallbladder bed (a rim of liver tissue around the gallbladder) is resected with a 2-cm margin of liver tissue together with the gallbladder. The right hepatic pedicle is exposed as the division of the liver is completed. The cystic plate is divided at its base, and the adipose tissue in Calot's triangle is dissected caudad along the right hepatic pedicle. The common hepatic duct is secured and divided just below the confluence of the hepatic ducts. The gallbladder, gallbladder bed, bile duct, and node-bearing adipose tissue are retrieved en bloc. Bilioenteric anastomosis is constructed using a Roux-en-Y jejunal limb. Drains are placed into the foramen of Winslow. The abdomen is closed primarily.

Case Continued

Histologic examination of the resected specimen reveals a well-differentiated adenocarcinoma of the gallbladder with two pericholedochal lymph nodes involved, categorized as stage IIB (pT2 N1 M0). The resection margins are negative. The patient shows uneventful recovery with the exception of delayed gastric emptying persisting for a week, and is then discharged on the 16th postoperative day. Because a potentially curative resection was done, no adjuvant treatment is given. The patient remains well, with no evidence of recurrence 6 years and 7 months after resection.

Discussion

Adjuvant treatment after resection is a matter of debate in the management of gallbladder carcinoma.

There have been no standardized chemotherapeutic regimens in adjuvant settings. Recently, the use of gemcitabine, alone or in combination with 5-fluorouracil or other agents, has been investigated. Adjuvant treatment after resection for gallbladder carcinoma is at the discretion of the individual surgeon in Japan, where some patients receive oral administration of 5-fluorouracil or its derivatives for 6 to 12 months after the resection, while others do not.

Gallbladder carcinoma first discovered after cholecystectomy for presumed benign disease, designated *inapparent* carcinoma, poses another critical problem in the surgical management of gallbladder carcinoma. Because the extent of the primary tumor affects the surgical strategy for the inapparent tumor, the depth of invasion should be determined histologically for each tumor-bearing cholecystectomized specimen prior to definitive treatment. A radical second resection improves the unfavorable outcome after cholecystectomy alone for the pathologic T2 or more advanced inapparent tumors, whereas the pathologic T1 inapparent tumor bears a favorable outcome after cholecystectomy alone, provided that the resection margins are negative. A radical second resection should be offered to patients with a pathologic T2 or more advanced inapparent carcinoma of the gallbladder whenever appropriate. Follow-up without a second resection is the treatment of choice for the pathologic T1 tumor with free margins.

Suggested Readings

Fahim RB, McDonald JR, Richards JC, et al. Carcinoma of the gallbladder: a study of its modes of spread. *Ann Surg* 1962;156: 114–124.

Glenn F, Hays DM. The scope of radical surgery in the treatment of malignant tumors of the extrahepatic biliary tract. *Surg Gynecol Obstet* 1954;99:529–541.

Ohtani T, Shirai Y, Tsukada K, et al. Carcinoma of the gallbladder: CT evaluation of lymphatic spread. *Radiology* 1993;189: 875–880.

Shirai Y, Ohtani T, Hatakeyama K. Is laparoscopic cholecystectomy recommended for large polypoid lesions of the gallbladder? *Surg Laparosc Endosc* 1997;7:435–436.

Shirai Y, Ohtani T, Tsukada K, et al. Combined pancreaticoduodenectomy and hepatectomy for patients with locally advanced gallbladder carcinoma: long term results. *Cancer* 1997;80:1904–1909.

Shirai Y, Yoshida K, Tsukada K, et al. Inapparent carcinoma of the gallbladder: an appraisal of a radical second operation after simple cholecystectomy. *Ann Surg* 1992;215:326–331.

Shoup M, Fong Y. Surgical indications and extent of resection in gallbladder cancer. *Surg Oncol Clin N Am* 2002;11:985–994.

Presentation

A 52-year-old white woman is referred to your office with a 4-week history of pruritus, jaundice, and dark urine. The patient denies abdominal pain but noted intermittent nausea without vomiting. She has mild anorexia with a 10-pound weight loss over the past 4 weeks. She denies any change in bowel habit or hematochezia but reports pale stools. There is no prior history of these symptoms. Patient had previously undergone laparoscopic cholecystectomy. On physical examination, the patient has icteric sclera, but does not appear cachectic or in any acute distress. There are scratch marks on her extremities and trunks from the pruritus. Her abdomen is soft, nontender, and nondistended with no evidence of intra-abdominal masses or hepatosplenomegaly.

Differential Diagnosis

The presence of progressive painless jaundice with associated constitutional symptoms points toward a malignant neoplasm of the extrahepatic biliary tree, head of the pancreas, or ampulla of Vater. Given the prior history of laparoscopic cholecystectomy, benign biliary stricture or choledocholithiasis should also be considered. Injury resulting from the laparoscopic cholecystectomy would have presented soon after the operative procedure period. Although only about 10% of patients with postoperative strictures are actually suspected within the first week after cholecystectomy, nearly 70% of patients are diagnosed within the first 6 months, and over 80% within 1 year of surgery. In the remaining patients, presentation may be delayed for many years after the initial operative procedure. However, patients with postoperative bile duct strictures who present months to years after the initial operation frequently have evidence of repeated episodes of cholangitis. Less commonly, patients may present with painless jaundice and no evidence of sepsis.

Recommendation

Obtain liver function tests, complete blood count, and coagulation studies. The first imaging test recommended is abdominal ultrasonography, which can be subsequently complemented with computed tomography (CT) scan of the abdomen and pelvis for further anatomical definition of the hepatobiliary and pancreatic system.

◼ Ultrasonogram

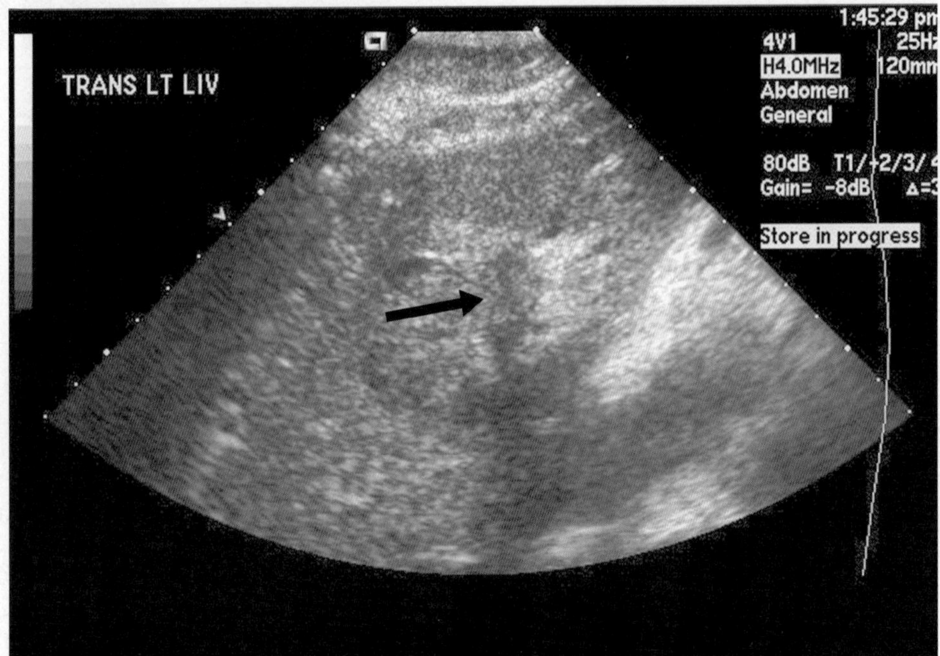

Figure 47.1

Ultrasonography Report

There is a dilated bile duct extending throughout the right and left hepatic lobe emanating from the porta hepatis. There is a hypoechoic mass at the portal bifurcation and extending toward the left hepatic duct. The common bile duct is of normal caliber and does not contain any stones. The gallbladder is not distended and does not show evidence of wall thickening.

Case Continued

Liver function test results are total bilirubin 24.9, alkaline phosphatase 336, ASD 82, albumin 2.7, and cancer antigen (CA) 19.9: 64,154. CT scan of the abdomen and pelvis reveals the presence of a hepatic duct confluence mass, which is confirmed with associated dilated intrahepatic biliary tree. There is no evidence of suspicious lymphadenopathy.

Diagnosis and Recommendation

The clinical, laboratory, and radiologic studies strongly indicate the presence of a hilar cholangiocarcinoma with possible extension to the left hepatic duct. To further delineate the extent of local disease, percutaneous transhepatic cholangiography (PTC) is traditionally obtained. However, recent developments in magnetic resonance (MR) technology allow detailed noninvasive imaging of the biliary tree, that is, magnetic resonance cholangiopancreaticography (MRCP). It also provides additional valuable information regarding parenchymal involvement by tumor, nodal metastasis, and vascular invasion. On the other hand, PTC has the advantage of allowing concurrent placement of a biliary stent for relief of jaundice and also obtaining brushings to establish a tissue diagnosis. However, it should be stated that if the magnetic resonance imaging (MRI) indicates that the presumed hilar cholangiocarcinoma is judged to be resectable, then a percutaneous cholangiogram or tissue diagnosis is not necessary, because it does not influence the choice of resection.

The presence on ultrasound scan and MRI of a 4.5-cm mass in the patient with a history of jaundice supports the diagnosis of cholangiocarcinoma that may have initially arisen in the left or the right biliary tree before extending to the confluence, at which time jaundice appears. When the tumor arises in the confluence of the common hepatic duct (type 1 and 2), the mass is much smaller at the time of presentation with jaundice. The greatly dilated intrahepatic branches on the left and some degree of atrophy of the left lobe (segment II and III) are in favor of the initial location of this tumor to be on the left side with subsequent extension to the confluence. This pattern of progression provides orientation to the treatment approach: no drainage of the left duct is necessary because it is not functional, and the appropriate option is to manage with resection by means of a left hemihepatectomy (segment II, III, IV, and segment I).

Discussion

Bile duct cancers are very uncommon tumors. In autopsy series, the incidence ranges from 0.01% to 0.2%. The frequency of proximal bile duct carcinomas ranges from 1 in 40,000 to 4 in 100,000. In the United States, approximately 4,500 tumors of the extrahepatic bile duct occur each year, and of these, 2,500 are limited to the confluence of the hepatic duct. Cholangiocarcinomas located at the hepatic duct bifurcation are known as Klatskin tumors, named after Dr. Klatskin who described this condition in 1965. Bile duct cancers have a slight male predominance and occur primarily in older individuals, with a median age of 70 years at diagnosis. The risk of developing bile duct cancer is distinctly elevated in patients with ulcerative colitis. Patients with ulcerative colitis have an incidence 9 to 22 times higher than that of the general population, and predisposition is independent of whether patients have had adequate therapy of their inflammatory colonic disease. Although there is an association between bile duct cancers and gallstones, no clear causal relationship has been demonstrated. Chronic infections, such as *Clonorchis sinensis* infection, have been shown to increase the risk of developing bile duct cancer. Other risk factors include sclerosing cholangitis, choledochal cysts, and congenital hepatic fibrosis.

About 90% of malignant bile duct tumors are adenocarcinomas. These tend to grow very slowly, and the pattern of spread is most frequently by local extension, though 30% may develop nodal metastasis. Distal metastases are seen less frequently than in other cancers. Morphologically, these tumors are described as nodular, papillary, sclerosing, or diffusely infiltrating with the nodular variant being the most frequent variety. Longmire proposed a classification according to location, with 60% occurring in the upper third of the ductal system, which includes the confluence of the hepatic ducts. The middle third is located between the cystic duct and the upper part of the duodenum. Finally, the lower third is located between the upper border of the duodenum and up to, but not including, the ampulla of Vater. The hilar cholangiocarcinomas are further classified into four types according to Bismuth: type 1, common hepatic duct to the level of the confluence; type 2, extension to the confluence of the hepatic duct up to the communication between the two branches; type 3, extension into either the right or left hepatic duct; and type 4, extension into both

the right and left hepatic ducts. The distinct morphologic varieties also show a pattern of occurrence; the nodular variety commonly occurs in the upper duct and presents as a small localized mass. The papillary lesions seldom present in the hilar region, but are commonly seen in and near the ampulla and may be multifocal. The diffusely infiltrating variant presents as a thickening or an extensive area of the extrahepatic biliary tree, and can be difficult to distinguish from sclerosing cholangitis.

Clinically these tumors most commonly present with jaundice (90%), but initial findings may include abdominal pain (30% to 50%) and cholangitis (10% to 30%). The presence of weight loss and anorexia usually indicates locally advanced disease. Certain patients may present solely with an elevated alkaline phosphatase level. Evaluation of patients presenting with obstructive jaundice often begins with abdominal ultrasonography, but the imaging studies that are most valuable in cholangiocarcinoma include CT scan of the abdomen, or better still, magnetic resonance imaging with MRCP and MR-angiography to delineate the biliary anatomy and assess involvement of the adjacent portal vein and the hepatic artery. Percutaneous transhepatic cholangiogram allows visualization of the proximal portion of the biliary tree, placement of biliary stents, and performance of brushings for cytologic diagnosis. However, it has to be noted that there is no evidence that placement of preoperative biliary drainage stents improves outcome but, in fact, may increase mortality and morbidity secondary to postoperative septic complication. Operative intervention may also become difficult due to the extensive inflammatory action resulting from placement of stents.

MRI

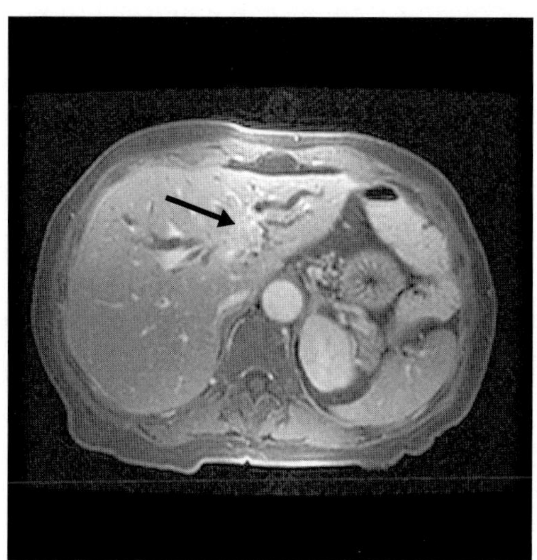

Figure 47.2A

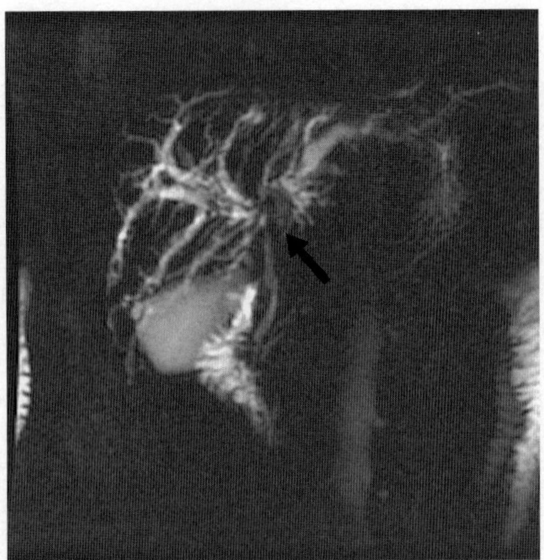

Figure 47.2B

MRI Report

MRI scan with MRCP reveals a 4.5-cm mass involving the confluence of the hepatic duct and extending into the left hepatic lobe along the hepatic duct. It causes diffuse intrahepatic biliary ductal dilatation that is particularly marked on the left side. The mass abuts the left portal vein, which may be compressed but there is no evidence of thrombosis.

Approach

Evaluation of a hilar cholangiocarcinoma should focus on the decision of whether to pursue a curative surgical resection. First, the clinician should maintain a high index of suspicion for the presence of malignant hilar biliary obstruction in the presence of progressive jaundice and imaging studies demonstrating dilated intrahepatic ducts with a relatively nondilated distal common bile duct. Alkaline phosphatase level is abnormal in virtually all patients, with variable increases in serum bilirubin and transaminase levels. CA 19.9 level is often elevated and is associated with a sensitivity of 75% and specificity of 80%. The preoperative imaging modalities are central not only to establish a diagnosis but also to facilitate surgical planning. MRI and MRCP have rapidly been established as the imaging modalities of choice for evaluation of hilar biliary obstruction because they provide invaluable information about the tumor itself, vascular involvement, and the presence of segmental ductal obstruction. MRI and MRCP with gadolinium enhancement and magnetic resonance angiography yield information similar to that of CT scan, invasive cholangiography, and angiography combined. Endoscopic ultrasonography can be valuable in the visualization of hilar lesions as well as allowing fine-needle aspiration of the malignant lesion and the adjacent enlarged lymph nodes, but this technique requires expertise and the availability of the technology. Imaging modalities can, to a certain degree, also assist the surgeon in determining whether the patient has any contraindication to resection such as (a) main portal vein thrombosis; (b) insufficient hepatic remnant volume in case en bloc hepatic resection is necessary; and (c) presence of N_2 lymphadenopathy (celiac, superior mesentery, periduodenal, and pancreatic) and presence of distant disease (liver, peritoneum). In the absence of these contraindications, as long as the patient is medically fit, all patients whose tumors are thought to be potentially resectable should undergo exploration. However, despite recent improvements in radiologic imaging, the resolution capacity of currently available technology still fails to detect subcentimeter metastases, and almost 25% of patients during exploration are found to harbor advance nodal, peritoneal, or hepatic metastasis that precludes curative resection. Two techniques are available to enhance the existing limitation of anatomic imaging studies: positron emission tomography (PET) scan and diagnostic staging laparoscopy. PET scan has been used for staging in a variety of solid organ malignancies, but its resolution is limited, where metastatic disease less than 7 to 10 mm in size may not be detected, and the presence of a false-positive results for distant metastases may deny the patient the only chance of a cure, that is, surgical exploration and resection. Diagnostic-staging laparoscopy has the advantages of a minimally invasive inspection of the peritoneal surface to exclude carcinomatosis and allowing intraoperative ultrasonography of the liver to exclude previously undetected liver metastasis. Studies have demonstrated that 25% of patients will have evidence of unresectability with this approach, which thus obviates the need for a nontherapeutic laparotomy.

Case Continued

Given the findings on imaging studies, the patient is advised to undergo surgical resection. The risks, benefits, and complications are discussed and informed consent is obtained. The patient is notified that resection will not be performed at the time of surgery if there is evidence of the following: (a) metastatic disease, (b) extensive vascular invasion (i.e., invasion of the main portal vein or involvement of the both right and left portal vein or hepatic artery), and (c) tumor extension into secondary biliary radicals of both hepatic lobes.

Surgical Approach

After induction of anesthesia, the patient first undergoes an exploratory staging laparoscopy, where the peritoneum is carefully examined for carcinomatosis, followed by careful examination of the liver with a laparoscopic linear ultrasound. Once the patient is deemed to be potentially curable, a right subcostal incision is made. The porta hepatis is then encircled and a vessel loop placed. Cholecystectomy is performed, which facilitates the subsequent conduct of the operation. After dividing the cystic duct, the common bile duct is identified, encircled with the vessel loop, and dissected and divided just above the first portion of the duodenum. A sliver of distal ductal tissue is sent for frozen section to exclude microscopic tumor involvement. The hepatic artery and its branches are dissected and encircled with vessel loops. The divided common bile duct is then dissected proximally and a plane is developed between the tumor and the anterior wall of the portal vein. After the confluence is mobilized, dissection proceeds along the right and left hepatic duct to evaluate the extent of ductal involvement proximal to the hilum. In this case, a left lobectomy (segments II and III) is mandatory and segment IV and the caudate lobe must be resected to remove the hilar plate and the extent of the tumor to the small ducts of segment IV and I. The specimen is then labeled and sent for frozen section of the proximal margin. Following this, a Roux-en-Y limb is prepared and hepaticojejunostomy is performed on the two sectoral branches of the right biliary system with an end-to-side anastomosis using a single layer of interrupted monofilament suture. Closed suction drains are placed in the subhepatic space.

Case Continued

During diagnostic laparoscopy, there are a few peritoneal nodules seen, and biopsy of these confirms metastatic adenocarcinoma. Given this finding, the patient is determined to have incurable disease and is scheduled for percutaneous drain placement by interventional radiology. Interventional radiology places internal and external drains through the right ductal system. Two weeks later, the drains are internalized by placement of a metallic stent and the external biliary drains are capped and left in place. The patient is then returned to have the external drains removed after confirmations of patency of the internal stent. The patient is subsequently referred to medical oncology to consider palliative chemotherapy or enrollment in a clinical trial.

KUB Image

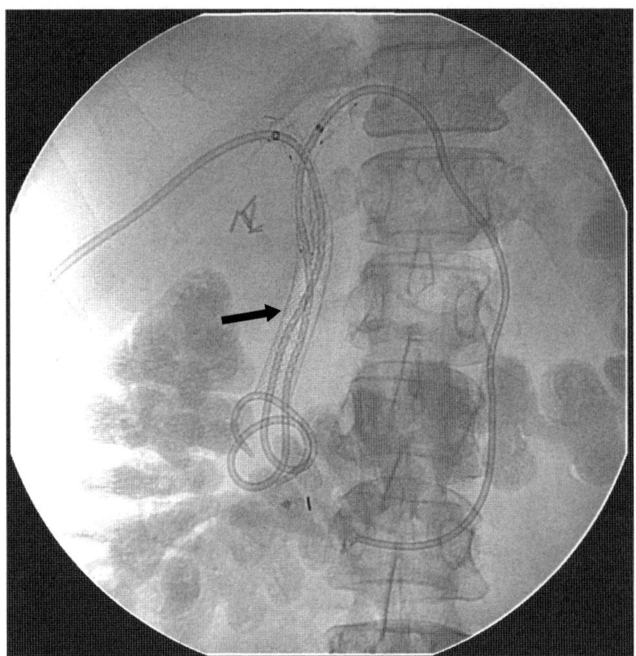

Figure 47.3

KUB Report

The permanent metallic stent can be seen along with the external biliary drains.

Discussion

The extent of surgical resection for hilar cholangiocarcinoma is based on the Bismuth classification of the disease. For type 1 disease, tumor resection of the extrahepatic bile duct, gallbladder, and regional lymphadenectomy is performed. For type 2, as the roof of the confluence is invaded, resection of the hilar plate is mandatory: if the tumor is small without extension to the left or right branches as confirmed by frozen section, a central liver resection (segment IV and I) is advocated. For type 3, either a left or right hepatectomy is added to the above resection. If the estimated liver remnant is thought to be small, then preoperative portal vein embolization of the diseased lobe has to be performed. For type 4 lesions that extend to both ductal systems, the patient is best treated with palliative stent placement. Results of studies of surgical resection for hilar cholangiocarcinoma performed in the 1990s report a 30% to 40% resection rate, achieved with mortality of 2% to 10 % with a 5-year survival rate of 15% to 40%.

Hepatic transplantation has been performed for these tumors, but it is followed by a high rate of recurrence and therefore is not a recommended modality of treatment. The role of adjuvant or therapeutic radiation therapy is unclear. Use of either systemic or regional 5-FU-based combination chemotherapy has resulted in a collective response rate of 29% to 39% without any impact on survival. When curative resection cannot be performed, the patient can be palliated most commonly with biliary stents. Usually, a transhepatic plastic internal/external stent is placed initially. Once the transhepatic tract has developed, an expandable internal wall stent is inserted. Once the jaundice is resolved, the external stents can be removed. The median survival time of patients with unresectable hilar cholangiocarcinoma is 9 to 12 months; interestingly, the mean patency duration of the internal expandable stent is approximately 9 months. Durable palliation can also be achieved with a bilioenteric bypass if unresectable disease is identified at exploration.

Suggested Readings

Bismuth H, Nakache R, Diamond T. Management strategies in resection for hilar cholangiocarcinoma. *Ann Surg* 1992;215:31–38.

Chamberlain RS, Blumgart LH. Hilar cholangiocarcinoma: a review and commentary. *Ann Surg Oncol* 2000;7:55–66.

D'Angelica MI, Jarnagin WR, Blumgart LH. Resectable hilar cholangiocarcinoma: surgical treatment and long-term outcome. *Surg Today* 2004;34:885–890.

Jarnagin WR, Fong Y, DeMatteo RP, et al. Staging, resectability, and outcome in 225 patients with hilar cholangiocarcinoma. *Ann Surg* 2001;234:507–517; discussion 517–519.

Nimura Y. Extended surgery in bilio-pancreatic cancer: the Japanese experience. *Semin Oncol* 2002;29:17–22.

Saldinger PF, Blumgart LH. Resection of hilar cholangiocarcinoma—a European and United States experience. *J Hepatobiliary Pancreat Surg* 2000;7:111–114.

Presentation

The patient is a 60-year-old white woman who presents with abdominal pain. The computed tomography (CT) scan shows a tumor of the anatomical left lobe that extends to segment IV. The left branch of the portal vein is not seen and the right branch of the portal vein is well visualized, suggesting an arteriovenous fistula. There are no retroperitoneal or intraperitoneal lymph nodes, with no evidence of a gastric or colonic primary tumor. Serum transaminases and gamma glutamyl transpeptidase are normal. The other liver tests are normal. Percutaneous transhepatic biopsy reveals a strongly mucosecretory adenocarcinoma of the liver.

CT Scan

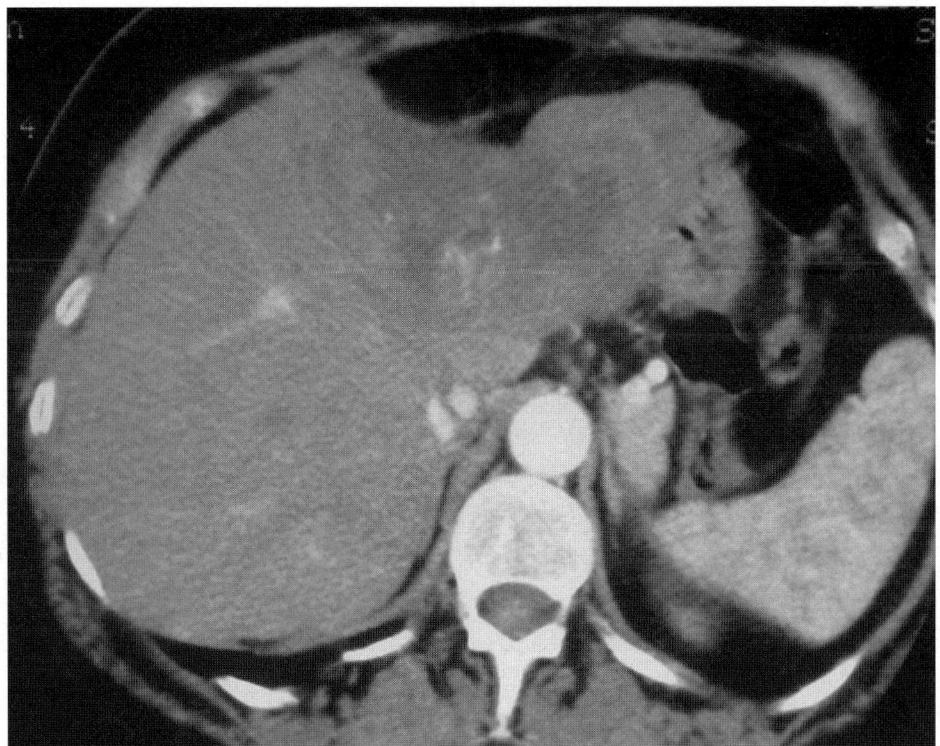

Figure 48.1

CT Scan Report

CT scan shows cholangiocarcinoma of the left liver before chemotherapy.

Differential Diagnosis

Various primary or secondary liver tumors constitute the differential diagnosis of cholangiocarcinoma (see Chapter 43), but endoscopic examinations are normal.

Case Continued

Immunohistochemistry is in favor of intrahepatic cholangiocarcinoma, because of positive cytokeratin 7 and negative cytokeratin 20 and carcinoembryonic antigen (CEA).

Diagnosis and Recommendation

The diagnosis is intrahepatic cholangiocarcinoma. The patient has no major comorbid conditions and therefore is judged to be suitable for surgery.

Approach

Cholangiocarcinoma is known to have a poor prognosis. Though some may treat these tumors with chemotherapy alone, the mainstay of ensuring cure is surgical resection. In high-risk patients, such as those with large tumors, consideration can be given to treating the patient initially with neoadjuvant chemotherapy.

Case Continued

The patient received preoperative chemotherapy with six cycles of 5-fluorouracil (5-FU) and cisplatin with good tolerance.

CT Scan

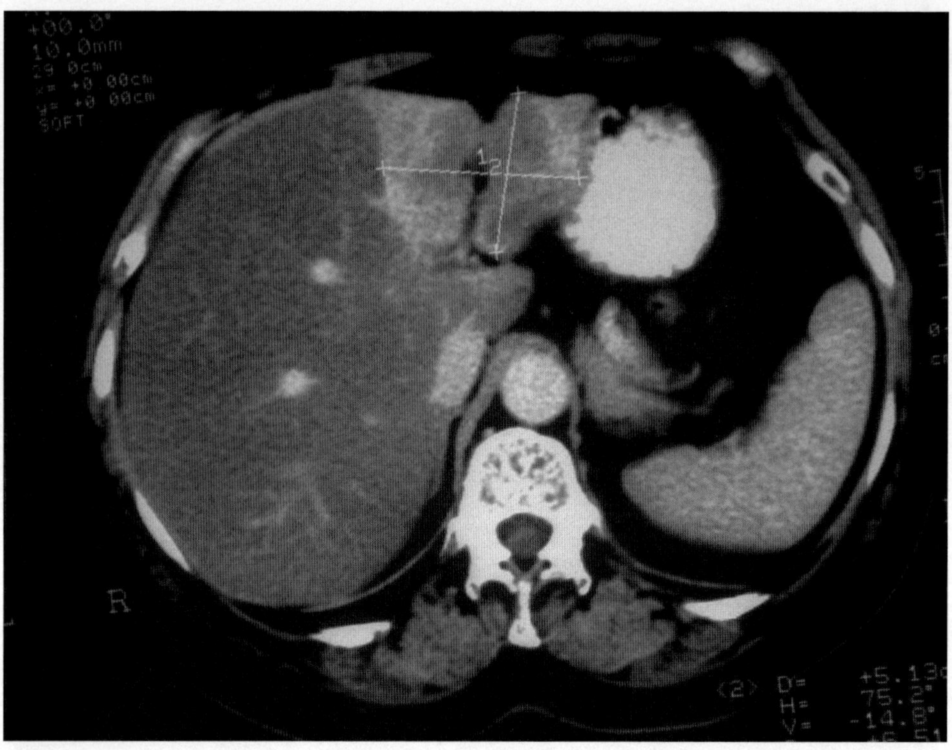

Figure 48.2

CT Scan Report

The postchemotherapy CT scan performed showed tumor regression. The tumor measures 8 × 6 cm; by comparison, on the previous scan it measured 12 × 7 cm. Liver retraction in front of the tumor is noted, a good sign of downstaging. The right liver is hypotrophic with the same steatosis as on the left, probably related to chemotherapy.

Surgical Approach

The abdomen is explored through a bilateral subcostal incision, and careful exploration is performed to exclude peritoneal and lymph node metastases. The extent of the tumor is assessed by palpation and confirmed with intraoperative liver ultrasonography. The lesser omentum is opened and a vessel loop is placed around the porta hepatis in preparation for a subsequent Pringle maneuver. The liver is mobilized by division of the falciform and the left triangular ligament while avoiding injury to the phrenic vein. The confluence of the middle and left hepatic vein with the suprahepatic vena cava is exposed, and a vessel loop is secured around the left hepatic vein. The portal triad is clamped and a hepatotomy is made at the hilum in segment IV and caudate lobe, allowing isolation of the left hepatic pedicle, which is transected with a linear stapler. The liver parenchyma is transected and the left hepatic vein is divided when encountered.

Case Continued

Abdominal exploration shows no peritoneal deposit or lymph node metastases. The tumor is located in segments II and III with segment IV involvement, and a left hepatectomy is performed. Pathologic examination of the surgical specimen reveals complete resection with a negative surgical margin.

CT Scan

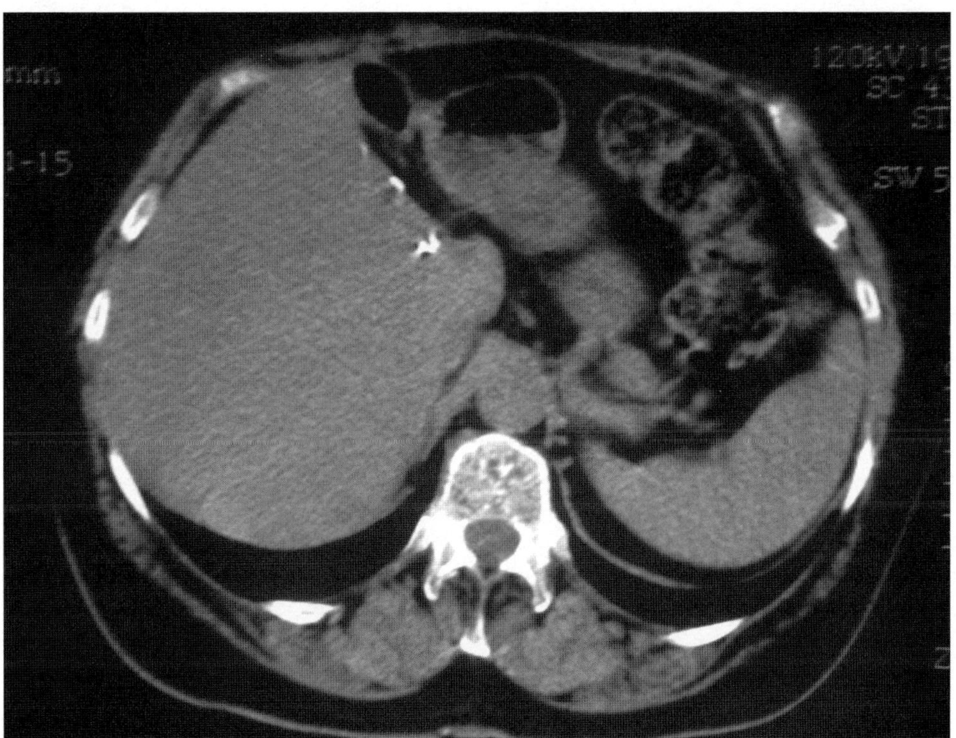

Figure 48.3

CT Scan Report

There is no evidence of recurrent tumor in the liver on a surveillance CT scan 6 months after the left hepatectomy.

Case Continued

Two years later, the patient presents with recurrent disease and undergoes re-exploration. Intraoperative ultrasound shows recurrent tumor located in segments VIII and V. Three other superficial nodules are located in segments VI and VIII. The last one is located at the limit between segments V and VIII. A bisegmentectomy V and VIII is performed (anterior segmentectomy) with resection of the three superficial nodules. Radiofrequency ablation is used for the deepest nodule. The postoperative course is uneventful.

CT Scan

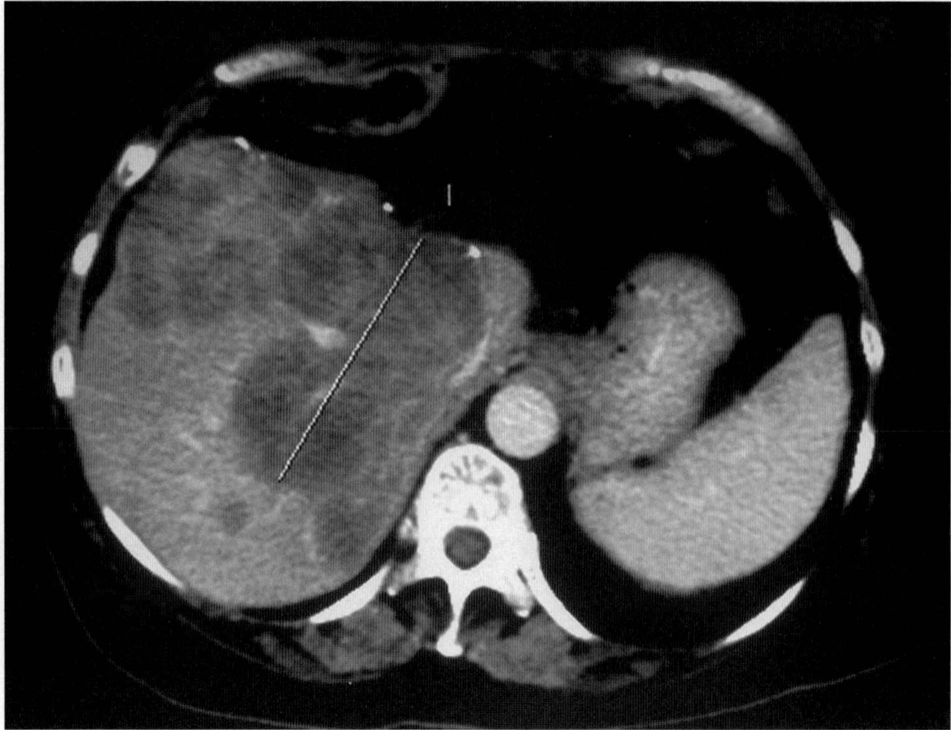

Figure 48.4

CT Scan Report

The CT scan shows massive liver recurrence involving the entire right liver 1 year later.

Case Continued

The patient is noted to have recurrence again and is treated with systemic chemotherapy using 5-FU and cisplatin, but eventually dies from progressive disease.

Discussion

Two types of tumor are classified as cholangiocarcinoma. The first type is called *bile duct* or *proximal cholangiocarcinoma,* when the tumor is located high in the extrahepatic biliary tree. The terms *hilar cholangiocarcinoma at the confluence of the bile duct* and *Klatskin tumo*r are also used, and the location and the extension of the tumor have led to a treatment-oriented classification. The second type is an *extrahepatic peripheral cholangiocarcinoma,* sometimes called *cholangiocellular carcinoma.* This is a primary tumor of the liver, occurring less frequently than the other types of primary hepatocellular cancer.

Outcomes of treatment are different for the two types of tumor. Indeed, the term *cholangiocarcinoma*

should be avoided for the first type, that is, bile duct cholangiocarcinoma. Intrahepatic cholangiocarcinoma is a primary liver tumor arising from intrahepatic bile duct canaliculi. The tumor presents as a firm white liver mass, sometimes with satellite tumors. It is histologically similar to, but clinically different from, extrahepatic cholangiocarcinoma.

Because of risk factors such as *Clonorchis fluke* or hepatolithiasis, primary cholangiocarcinoma of the liver occurs more commonly in Asian countries than in Europe and the United States. In Europe, an adenocarcinoma of the liver is more likely a metastasis than a primary tumor. If no primary tumor from a site outside the liver can be identified, the mass may be presumed to be a primary cholangiocarcinoma rather than a metastasis to the liver from another site. Cholangiocarcinoma may be suspected clinically if the patient has hepatitis, cirrhosis, or an increased alpha-fetoprotein level.

Imaging studies can frequently establish the benign nature of a mass in the liver. If a liver tumor is probably malignant, because of the clinical presentation, laboratory results, and imaging studies, and is considered to be resectable by anatomical criteria in a patient with normal hepatic reserve, then it should be resected. In our opinion, because of the risk of cell seeding, most resectable liver tumors should not be biopsied before surgery. Liver biopsy, however, may be indicated in two situations: (1) to establish the indication for preoperative chemotherapy to achieve tumor reduction and (2) to establish the diagnosis of benign tumor and rule out possible malignancy.

Histologically, it is usually difficult to differentiate cholangiocarcinoma from metastatic adenocarcinoma. In our patient, immunohistochemistry staining for specific markers is useful. Primary risk factors for cholangiocarcinoma are previous exposure to Thorotrast, biliary tract infection with *C. fluke*, hepatolithiasis, congenital biliary dilatation, and sclerosing cholangitis. Median survival of patients with untreated intrahepatic cholangiocarcinoma is less than 1 year. With chemotherapy, radiotherapy, or both, mean survival ranges from 1.8 to 12 months. Survival after palliative resection has also been found to be poor. Resection plays a primary role in the treatment of cholangiocarcinoma because there is no known effective chemotherapy or radiotherapy. Hepatic resection remains the mainstay of treatment. Liver transplantation may be a viable treatment for the patient whose disease is limited to the liver and when resection is not technically possible. Large tumor size alone and close adhesion of the tumor to major vessels or biliary strictures that need to be preserved are not contraindications for resection. On

the contrary, the uniformly poor survival in Huang's study of patients who had metastases to lymph nodes suggests a limited role for aggressive resection in these circumstances. There is no consensus concerning the role of lymph node dissection. Hepatic recurrence remains problematic. In Huang's series, recurrent cancer was identified in 58% of patients, and 89% of those cancers were in the liver. The presence of multicentric disease and a high rate of liver recurrence are arguments favoring an underlying abnormal epithelial proliferation of the biliary canaliculi, which could precede the development of carcinoma.

Suggested Readings

Aishima S. Intrahepatic cholangiocarcinoma: its mode of spreading and therapeutic modalities. *Surgery* 2002;131(1 suppl): S159–S164.

Chen MF. Peripheral cholangiocarcinoma (cholangiocellular carcinoma): clinical features, diagnosis and treatment. *J Gastroenterol Hepatol* 1999;14:1144–1149.

Huang JL, Biehl TR, Lee FT, et al. Outcomes after resection of cholangiocellular carcinoma. *Am J Surg* 2004;187(5):612–617.

Okuda K, Nakanuma Y, Miyazaki M. Cholangiocarcinoma: recent progress. Part 2: molecular pathology and treatment. *J Gastroenterol Hepatol* 2002;17:1056–1063.

Shirabe K, Shimada M, Harimoto N, et al. Histologic factors affecting prognosis following hepatectomy for intrahepatic cholangiocarcinoma. *World J Surg* 2001;25(7):865–869. Erratum in *World J Surg* 2002;26:283.

case 49

Presentation

A 67-year-old woman with no relevant past history has experienced vague epigastric discomfort and anorexia for the last several weeks. She now presents with jaundice, acholic stools, and dark urine. A 15-pound weight loss is documented. Physical examination shows scleral icterus. There is no palpable abdominal mass or evidence of ascites. Total bilirubin is elevated at 9 mg/dL.

Abdominal X-Ray

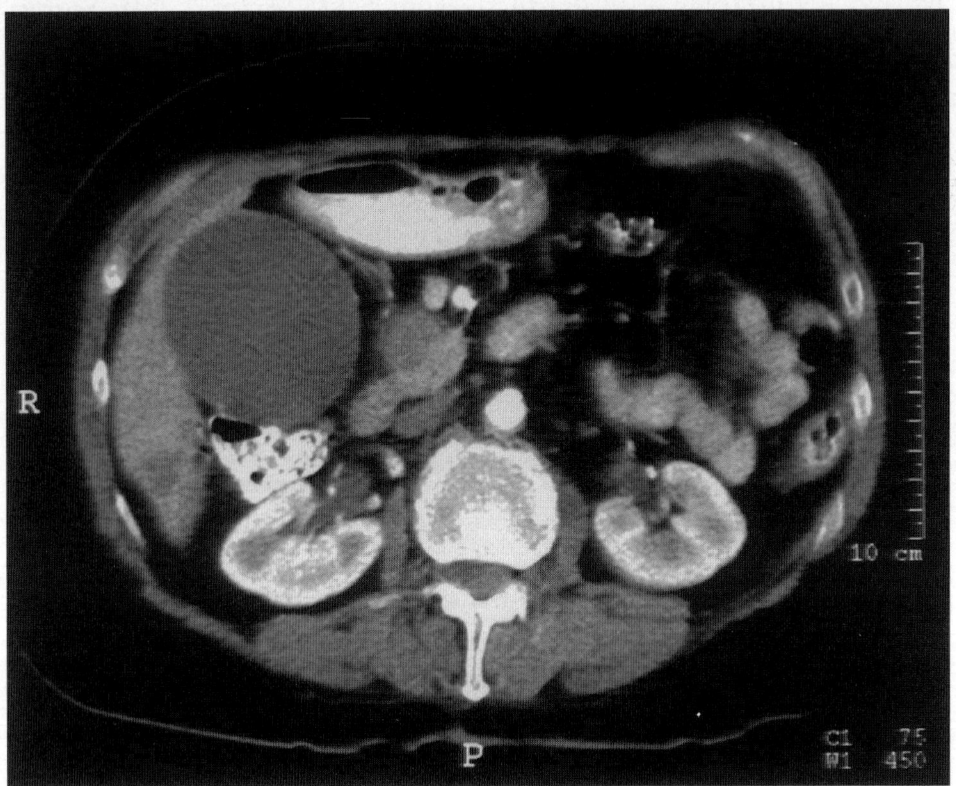

Figure 49.1

Abdominal X-Ray Report

The gallbladder is markedly dilated, representing distal bile duct obstruction. A 3-cm mass is seen in the head of the pancreas. There is no evidence of liver metastases, and the major visceral vessels (superior mesenteric vein, portal vein, superior mesenteric artery, and hepatic artery) are not involved.

Differential Diagnosis

The diagnosis for obstructive jaundice (as diagnosed by the obstructed biliary tree on computed tomography [CT]) includes periampullary cancer (pancreatic, distal bile duct, ampullary, or duodenal carcinoma), common bile duct stone, and benign distal bile duct stricture, usually due to chronic pancreatitis. Other pancreatic neoplasms, such as cystic neoplasms or islet cell tumors, may also uncommonly present with jaundice. The clinical scenario presented is classic for cancer of the head of the pancreas.

Discussion

The extent of further workup necessary at this time is variable. Many surgeons would proceed with an operation to potentially resect the tumor without further evaluation, based on a high-quality contrast-enhanced spiral CT scan. Endoscopic retrograde cholangiopancreaticography (ERCP) with or without endostent placement may be advisable if the level of jaundice is high or if a delay in definitive surgery is anticipated. Endoscopic ultrasound can be used to further assess the local extent of disease (vascular invasion, lymph node involvement) and can successfully obtain a cytologic diagnosis by fine-needle aspiration in a high percentage of patients. A preoperative tissue diagnosis is not required prior to surgery, although it can be useful, especially if neoadjuvant chemoradiation is planned. Finally, many surgeons will perform a prelaparotomy diagnostic laparoscopy because of a 10% to 15% incidence of detecting unsuspected small liver or peritoneal metastases.

Diagnosis and Recommendation

This patient has potentially resectable pancreatic carcinoma. She should undergo appropriate preoperative medical evaluation in preparation for pancreaticoduodenectomy.

Surgical Approach

If thorough exploration at laparotomy (or laparoscopy) reveals that the tumor is curable, the next step is to determine whether the primary tumor is resectable. After a wide Kocher maneuver, the right gastroepiploic vein and the gastroduodenal artery are divided, and if necessary, the common hepatic duct can also be transected to achieve access to the anterior surface of the portal vein. The surgeon should perform careful digital examination to exclude encroachment of the tumor to the major regional vessels (portal vein, superior mesenteric vein, and artery). In the absence of such regional invasion, a pancreaticoduodenectomy should be performed. Either the classic procedure or the pylorus-preserving modification is a suitable option. There is no evidence to support extended lymphadenectomy. After resection is complete, frozen sections of the margins of the bile duct, pancreatic body, and uncinate process should be obtained. A jejunal limb is prepared, and to restore gastrointestinal continuity, pancreaticojejunostomy is performed, followed by choledochojejunostomy 10 cm distally. Approximately 15 cm distal to the choledochojejunostomy, the gastrojejunostomy or duodenojejunostomy is performed. Drains are placed adjacent to the pancreaticojejunostomy and choledochojejunostomy to drain potential anastomotic leaks.

The perioperative mortality following pancreaticoduodenectomy has been consistently reported in high-volume centers at <5%. Complications occur in 30% to 45% of patients and most commonly include pancreatic anastomotic leak, delayed gastric emptying, and wound infection.

Discussion

The survival following pancreaticoduodenectomy for periampullary carcinoma is highly dependent on the site of origin of the primary tumor. Survival is highest for duodenal carcinoma (5-year survival rate, 50% to 70%) followed by ampullary carcinoma (30% to 50%), distal bile duct carcinoma (20% to 35%), and pancreatic carcinoma (15% to 25%). Other factors influencing survival include tumor differentiation, node status, and margin status. The role of adjuvant therapy following resection for pancreatic carcinoma is somewhat controversial. In the United States, most centers employ postoperative chemoradiation, although recent European results question the benefit of radiation. Novel therapies, including immunotherapy, may be available in the future.

Case Continued

At laparotomy, the tumor is found to be unresectable due to local invasion of the superior mesenteric vein.

Surgical Approach

Patients found to be unresectable at laparotomy should undergo operative palliation, which includes hepaticojejunostomy, gastrojejunostomy, and chemical splanchnicectomy.

Discussion

Patients with periampullary carcinoma that is found to be unresectable during preoperative evaluation generally should be palliated by nonoperative techniques. However, if a patient is found to be unresectable at the time of laparotomy, surgical palliation should be considered. Operative palliation should include bypass of the biliary tree, usually by hepaticojejunostomy. An exception is in selected patients with advanced disease, such as peritoneal carcino-mastosis, who have already undergone endoscopic biliary stenting. Level I published evidence has shown the performance of a prophylactic gastroje-junostomy prevents the development of late duode-nal obstruction with increasing perioperative compl-ications. Similarly, chemical splanchnicectomy with 50% alcohol can improve and/or prevent cancer-related pain due to unresectable pancreatic cancer.

Suggested Readings

Billingsley KG, Hur K, Henderson WG, et al. Outcome after pan-creaticoduodenectomy for periampullary cancer: an analysis from the Veterans Affairs National Surgical Quality Improve-ment Program. *J Gastrointest Surg* 2003;4:484–491.

Li D, Xie K, Wolff R, et al. Pancreatic cancer. *Lancet* 2004;363: 1049–1057.

Lillemoe KL, Cameron JL, Hardacre JM, et al. Is prophylactic gas-trojejunostomy indicated for unresectable periampullary can-cer? A prospective randomized trial. *Ann Surg* 1999;230: 322.

Neoptolemos JP, Dunn JA, Stocken DD, et al. Adjuvant chemora-diotherapy and chemotherapy in resectable pancreatic cancer: a randomized controlled trial. *Lancet* 2001;358:1576–1585.

Sohn TA, Lillemoe DK, Cameron JL, et al. Surgical palliation of un-resectable periampullary adenocarcinoma in the 1990s. *J Am Coll Surg* 1999;176:1–10.

Stojadinovic A, Brooks A, Hoos A, et al. An evidence-based ap-proach to the surgical management of resectable pancreatic adenocarcinoma. *J Am Coll Surg* 2003;196:954–964.

Yeo CJ, Cameron JL, Sohn TA, et al. Six hundred fifty consecutive pancreaticoduodenectomies in the 1990's: pathology, compli-cations, outcomes. *Ann Surg* 1997;226:248–260.

Yeo CJ, Sohn TA, Cameron JL, et al. Periampullary adenocarci-noma: analysis of 5-year survivors. *Ann Surg* 1998;227: 821–831.

Presentation

A 63-year-old woman with a past medical history significant for type 2 diabetes mellitus, cerebrovascular disease, hypertension, psoriasis, hysterectomy with oophorectomy (for uterine fibroids), and alcohol abuse presents to your office after she was seen by her primary medical doctor 1 month previously with right upper quadrant tenderness secondary to trauma. She denies any prior gastrointestinal or constitutional symptoms such as abdominal pain, nausea, vomiting, early satiety, diarrhea, constipation, anorexia, or weight loss. On abdominal examination, no organomegaly, masses, tenderness, or ascites are noted. Previous abdominal ultrasound shows a 5.5-cm cystic mass in the tail of the pancreas.

CT Scan

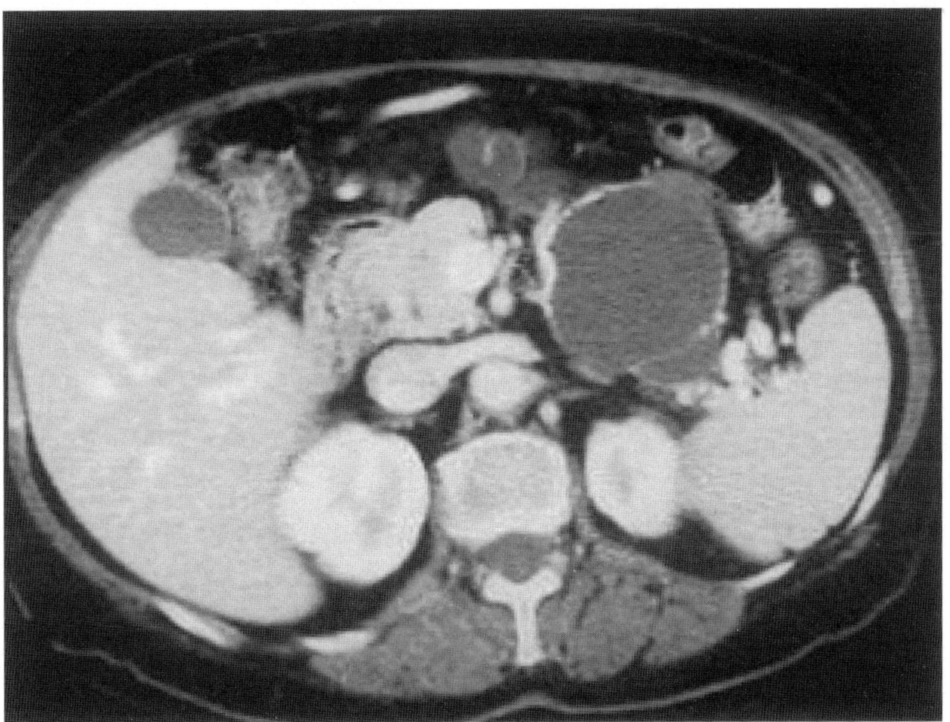

Figure 50.1A

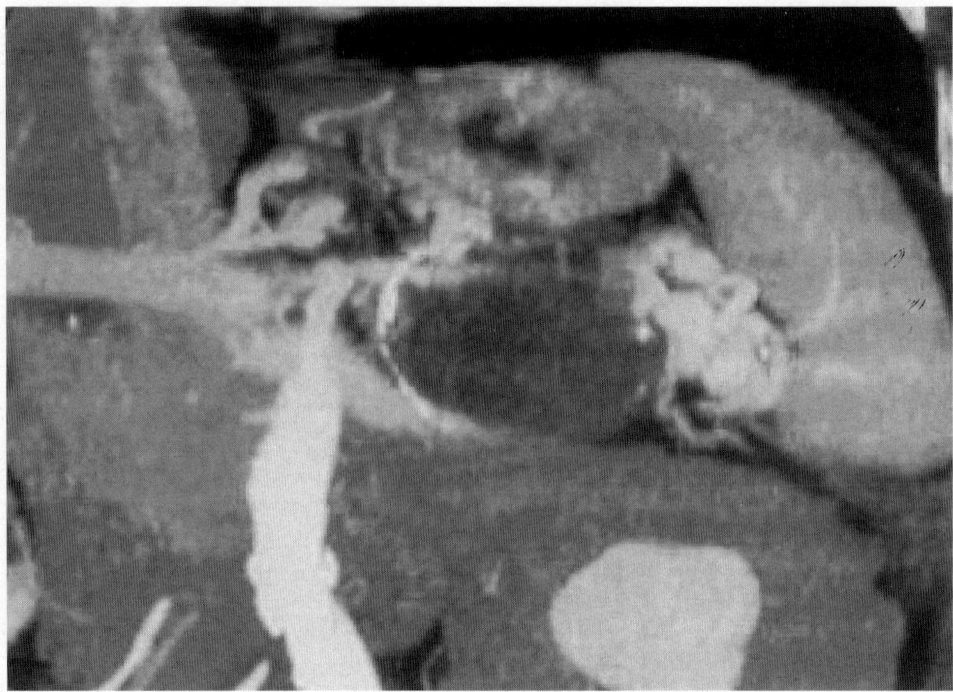

Figure 50.1B

CT Scan Report

A 7-cm multiloculated, septated fluid collection with dense calcifications in the tail of the pancreas is identified on computed tomography (CT) scan. Three-dimensional reconstruction CT-pancreatography demonstrates splenic vein compression and multiple venous collaterals.

Differential Diagnosis

The differential diagnosis of a patient with a cystic pancreatic lesion includes pseudocyst, serous cystadenoma, mucinous cystic neoplasm, intraductal papillary mucinous neoplasm, cystic islet cell tumor, solid and cystic papillary (Hamoudi) tumor, and mucinous cystadenocarcinoma.

Discussion

Cystic pancreatic neoplasms are rare and account for only 1% of primary pancreatic malignancies and 50% to 60% of cystic lesions of the pancreas. The most common cystic lesions of the pancreas are pseudocysts, which usually are the result of gallstone-induced or alcohol-induced pancreatitis or trauma. Cystic pancreatic neoplasms occur at a median age of 50 to 60 years and with a female:male predominance of 9:1. Symptoms commonly encountered are vague, nonspecific abdominal pain, early satiety, nausea, and vomiting. In many patients no symptoms are evident, and lesions are initially identified as an incidental finding, as in the case being presented.

In the absence of pancreatitis, which otherwise might suggest a pseudocyst, benign lesions include serous cystadenoma and solid and cystic papillary (Hamoudi) tumors. Mucinous cystic neoplasms, intraductal papillary mucinous neoplasms, and cystic islet cell tumors are premalignant or malignant, whereas mucinous cystadenocarcinomas are malignant. A recent analysis from our institution (Medical College of Wisconsin) has shown that symptoms and age are predictors of neoplasia. The absence of gallstones on ultrasound, no prior history of alcoholic pancreatitis, and the calcifications make a pseudocyst unlikely. Although this patient is asymptomatic, her age (63 years) raises concerns about a premalignant or malignant cystic tumor.

Recommendation

Endoscopic ultrasound (EUS) with fine-needle aspiration is recommended for this patient.

Case Continued

Possible further workup could include EUS with fine-needle aspiration (FNA), which may yield further information not only about the type of cyst, but also about the relationship of the pancreatic duct to the cystic lesion. In this patient, EUS shows a complex cystic mass in the tail of the pancreas with multiple irregular septations. The rest of the pancreas is sonographically normal with no pancreatic duct dilatation. FNA shows hypocellular smears with monolayered groups of benign duct epithelium, rare histiocytes, and mucus/debris consistent with a mucinous cystic neoplasm.

Discussion

Noninvasive imaging techniques such as CT and magnetic resonance imaging (MRI) are unreliable to accurately distinguish among the different pancreatic cysts. As a result, many authorities recommend surgical removal, especially in patients who are younger and otherwise fit. Others have recommended percutaneous aspiration with fluid analysis. More recently, EUS with FNA has been suggested as a method to differentiate among benign, premalignant, and malignant lesions. However, percutaneous or endoscopic aspiration has the potential to spill malignant cells into the peritoneum with subsequent seeding and reduced survival. For this reason, as well as concerns about diagnostic accuracy, we do not recommend preoperative aspiration. Nevertheless, EUS was performed prior to referral in this patient. Endoscopic retrograde cholangiopancreatography (ERCP) and magnetic resonance cholangiopancreatography (MRCP) may be helpful in defining cyst and pancreatic duct anatomy. However, CT pancreatography and intraoperative ultrasound may be just as useful, less invasive, and potentially less expensive than ERCP.

In the absence of a good radiologic or pathologic test to determine the diagnosis preoperatively, clinical characteristics such as age, gender, and the presence of symptoms may be helpful in the decision to operate. Cyst size and location do not predict premalignant or malignant pathology.

Diagnosis and Recommendation

The preoperative diagnosis is mucinous cystic neoplasm. The patient is offered distal pancreatectomy that will be performed by laparotomy. She is told that splenic preservation may be possible. The common complications mentioned are bleeding, infection, and pancreatic fistula.

Surgical Approach

A complete resection of the cystic lesion is crucial to prevent recurrence or subsequent manifestation of malignant disease. A midline laparotomy is performed; after examination of the abdominal contents, the lesser sac is entered, and the pancreas is inspected. The body and tail of the pancreas are mobilized from the retroperitoneum. The splenic artery is ligated near its origin as well as in the splenic hilum. The venous collaterals in the splenic hilum are suture ligated after dissection of the pancreatic tail. The splenic vein is ligated at the point of pancreatic transection 2 cm from the lesion, preserving the inferior mesenteric vein. A Jackson-Pratt drain is placed adjacent to the resected pancreas. A large multiloculated cystic structure measuring 7.5 cm in greatest diameter is identified. The cyst wall is hyalinized and focally calcified, and the cavity contains abundant mucin, consistent with a diagnosis of benign mucinous cystic neoplasm.

Histopathology Slide

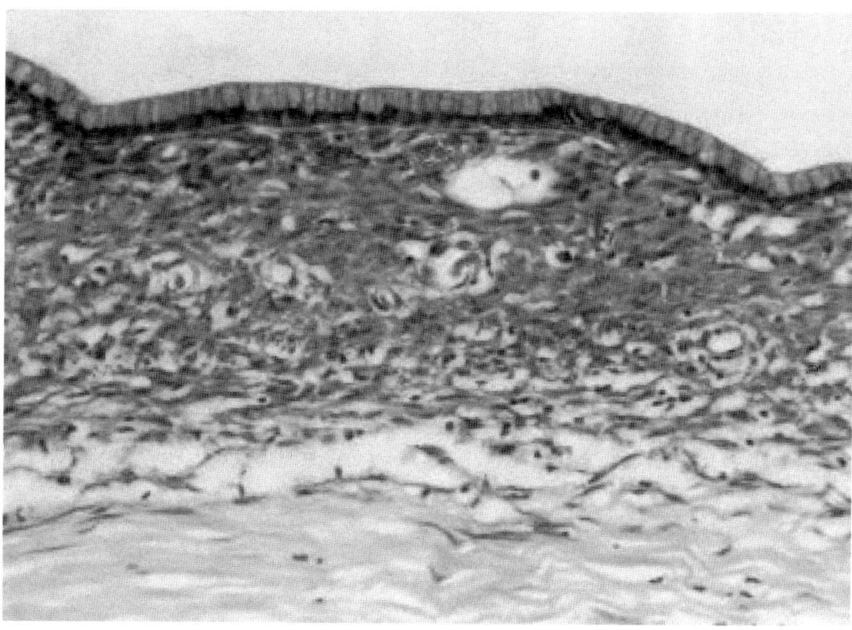

Figure 50.2

Histopathology Report

The microscopic histologic examination demonstrates a columnar epithelial lining above a matrix of typical ovarian stroma, the classic histology of a benign mucinous cystic neoplasm.

Case Continued

The patient has minimal elevation of her serum amylase on the first postoperative day. She continues to make good progress and advances to full liquids by postoperative day 4 and a low-fat diet by postoperative day 5. The drain amylase is checked on postoperative days 5 and 6 and found to be 3,355 and 13,310 u/dL, respectively. Despite this increase in drain amylase, the drain output is low and averages 60 mL per day. She continues to improve, is ambulating by postoperative day 9, and is discharged home with the drain in situ. The drain output continues to decrease gradually, and at follow-up in clinic 3 weeks later, the drain is removed with no further problems.

Approach

Pancreatic fistula is defined as drainage of >50 mL of amylase-rich fluid through operatively placed drains on or after postoperative day 7. In this instance, the patient is tolerating the fistula well, and a bag without suction can be connected to drain residual fluid with nursing advice before discharge home.

Discussion

The morbidity of a "pure" pancreatic fistula is less than that of a fistula from a pancreatic-enteric anastomosis. A low-output fistula from the resected pancreatic margin after a distal pancreatectomy is rarely of clinical consequence if the remainder of the pancreas is normal with no pancreatic duct obstruction. In this setting, octreotide is usually not necessary, and stenting of the pancreatic duct may cause more trouble by introducing bacteria from the duodenum and causing a stricture.

Case Continued

The initial 3-month postoperative CT scan shows no recurrent mass or fluid within the operative bed.

CT Scans

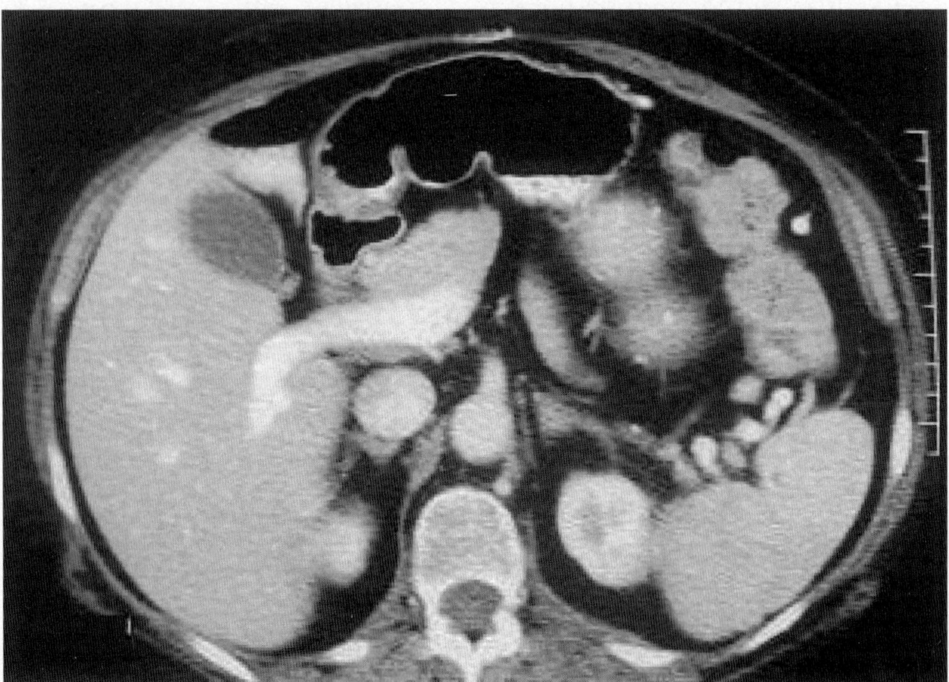

Figure 50.3A

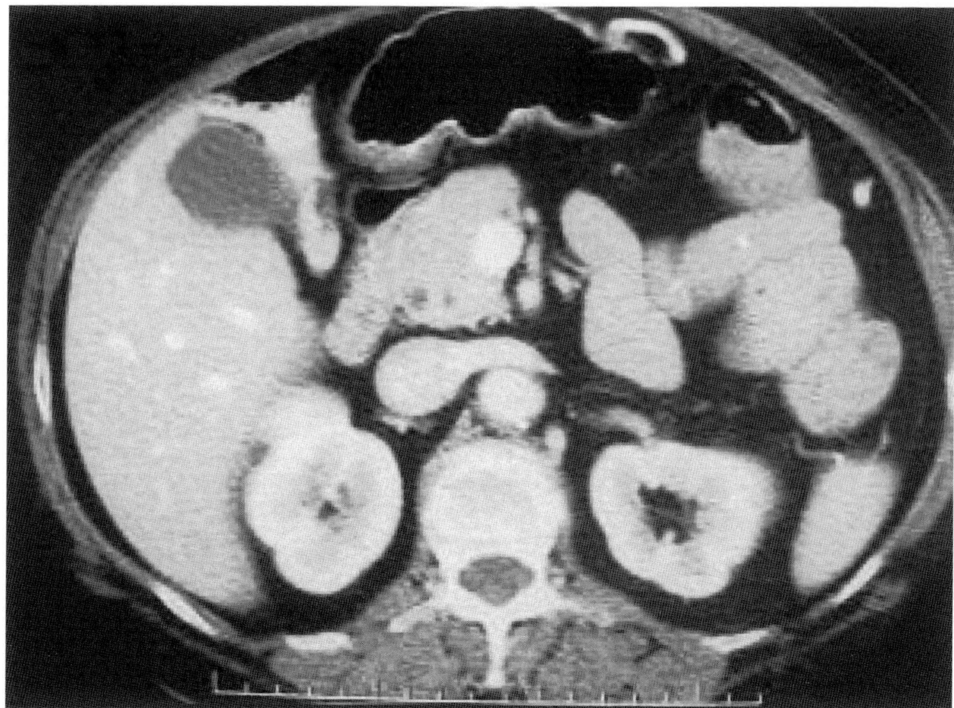

Figure 50.3B

CT Scan Report

A subsequent follow-up CT scan at 3 years again demonstrates no tumor recurrence. Pancreatic neck and preserved spleen are evident. Lower cut of same scan demonstrates normal head of pancreas.

Case Continued

At present, 4 years postsurgery, the patient is doing well and is symptom free.

Discussion

The majority of benign cystic neoplasms of the pancreas are serous cystadenomas, whereas solid and cystic papillary (Hamoudi) tumors are quite rare. These benign lesions frequently can become quite large and symptomatic, eventually requiring a major pancreatic resection, whereas early intervention might allow enucleation or limited resection. In patients with mucinous cystic neoplasms, cystic neuroendocrine tumors, and benign intraductal papillary mucinous neoplasms, early surgery will prevent malignant degeneration and is likely to be more cost-effective than observation. Moreover, even small lesions in older patients, especially if they are symptomatic or present with jaundice or pancreatitis, are likely to be malignant and deserve exploration in fit patients. Thus, surgical excision is recommended for pancreatic cysts that increase under observation, are symptomatic, and are discovered in healthy older patients.

For cystic tumors in the tail of the pancreas, resection remains the operation of choice. Splenic preservation should be strongly considered in patients suspected to have a benign or premalignant lesion in the pancreatic tail. For small cystic tumors in the uncinate, head, neck, and body of the pancreas, enucleation may have advantages over pancreatic resection with respect to operative time, blood loss, and preservation of pancreatic parenchyma. Because the pancreas is otherwise normal in these patients, the risk of pancreatic fistula is high. However, the morbidity of a "pure" pancreatic fistula that may occur after an enucleation is generally less than that of a fistula from a pancreatic-enteric anastomosis after a pancreatoduodenectomy.

Suggested Readings

Ahrendt SA, Komorocki RA, Demure MJ, et al. Cystic pancreatic neuroendocrine tumors: is preoperative diagnosis possible? *J Gastrointest Surg* 2002;6:66–74.

Alles AJ, Warshaw AL, Southern JF, et al. Expression of CA 72-4 (TAG-72) in the fluid contents of pancreatic cysts: a new marker to distinguish malignant pancreatic cystic tumors from benign neoplasm and pseudocysts. *Ann Surg* 1994;219: 131–134.

Kiely JM, Nakeeb A, Komorowski RA, et al. Cystic pancreatic neoplasms: enucleate or resect? *J Gastrointest Surg* 2003;7:890–897.

Moesinger RC, Talamini MA, Hruban RH, et al. Large cystic pancreatic neoplasms: pathology, resectability, and outcome. *Ann Surg Oncol* 1999;6:682–691.

Sand JA, Hyoty MK, Mattila J, et al. Clinical assessment compared with cyst fluid analysis in the differential diagnosis of cystic lesions in the pancreas. *Surgery* 1996;119:275–280.

Spinelli KS, Fromwiller TE, Daniel RA, et al. Cystic pancreatic neoplasms: observe or operate? *Ann Surg* 2004;239:651–659.

Talamini MA, Moesinger R, Yeo CJ, et al. Cystadenomas of the pancreas: is enucleation an adequate operation? *Ann Surg* 1998;227:896–903.

Walsh RM, Henderson JM, Vogt DP, et al. Prospective preoperative determination of mucinous pancreatic cystic neoplasms. *Surgery* 2002;132:628–634.

Presentation

A 45-year-old woman with no significant past medical history was found to have an abnormality in the right breast on routine bilateral screening mammogram. She presents to your office for evaluation and further treatment recommendations. The patient is without any complaints, including nipple discharge, skin changes, tenderness, or palpable mass. There is a family history of breast carcinoma in her paternal aunt at age 70. The patient's age of menarche was 12 years. Her last menstrual cycle was 2 weeks prior to presentation. The patient is gravida 2, para 1, abortion 1, with her first childbirth at age 35. She has been on birth control pills in the past but currently takes no hormones. On examination, the skin, nipples, and areolas appear normal. There is no skin dimpling with movement of the pectoralis. There is no nipple retraction. No nipple discharge can be elicited. There are no dominant masses in either breast. The axillary tails are normal. The supraclavicular, axillary, and cervical regions are free of significant lymphadenopathy bilaterally.

Mammograms

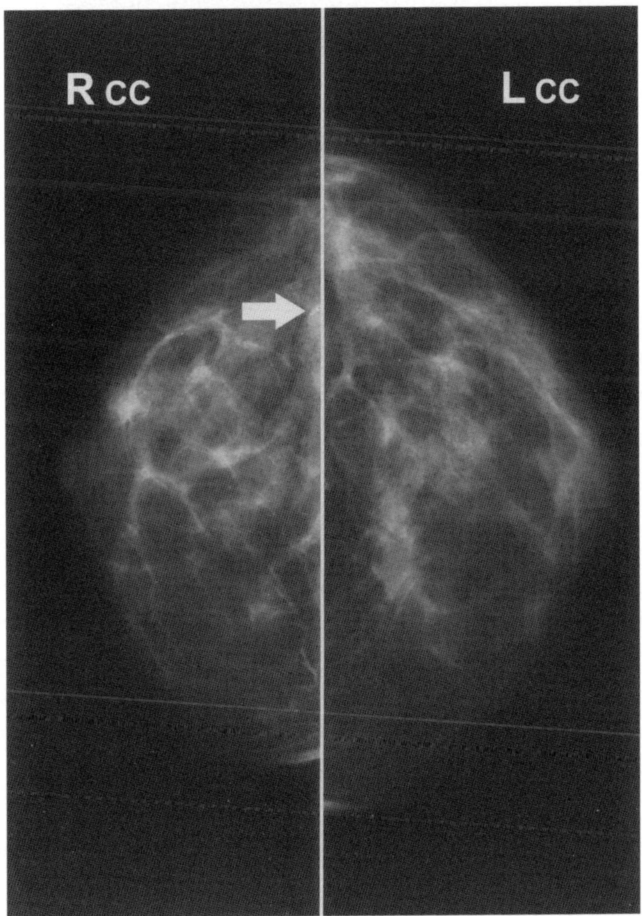

Figure 51.1A

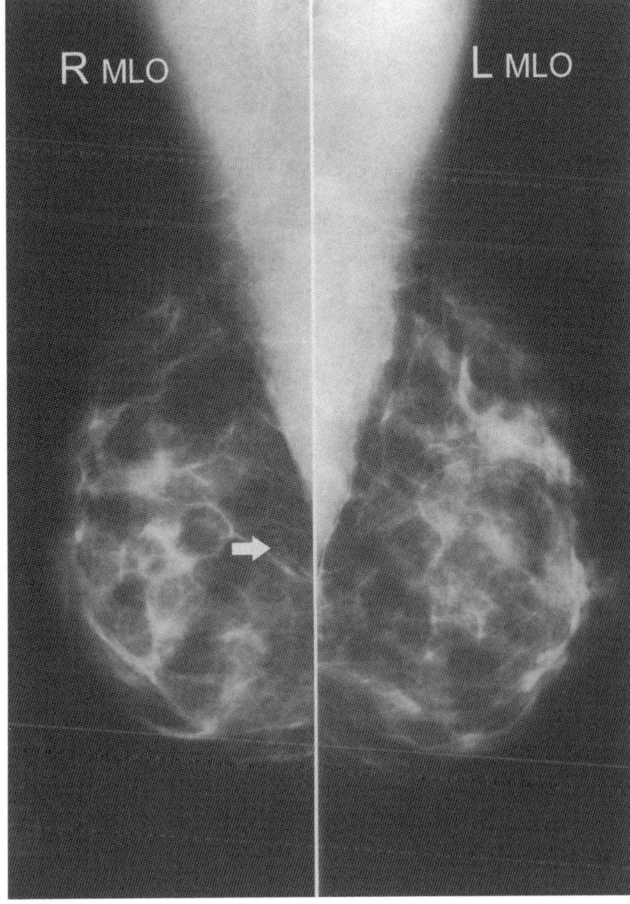

Figure 51.1B

Mammography Report

On screening mammography of the bilateral breasts in **(A)** craniocaudal (CC) and **(B)** mediolateral oblique (MLO) views, *white arrows* on the right breast mammogram demonstrate fine, linear, heterogeneous calcifications. A new group of clustered fine, linear, heterogeneous, and punctuate calcifications is seen in the lower outer quadrant of the right breast.

Differential Diagnosis

The differential diagnosis for mammographic calcifications includes fibrocystic diseases, true mineral deposits, milk of calcium (calcium within the fluid of a noncancerous cyst), inflammation (mastitis), fibroadenomas, and cancer. In this patient with clustered fine, linear, heterogeneous, and punctuate calcifications, a further diagnostic mammogram of the right breast is needed, including magnified views.

Discussion

Mammography remains the best method of detection for early breast cancer. Calcifications in the breast are common, and most breast calcifications are benign. However, certain patterns or appearances of calcifications can be associated with cancer and further workup is needed to rule out malignancy. There are different types of breast calcifications, such as: microcalcifications, which are very fine calcifications that may be scattered or clustered and can be associated with either benign or malignant lesions; "popcorn" calcifications, which appear fluffy and are benign; macrocalcifications, which are large calcifications that are usually benign; and spiculated calcifications, which appear as spider webs and are associated with cancer.

Recommendation

Additional diagnostic views of the breast are needed to differentiate the microcalcifications in mammography. Magnified views best delineate the shape and extent of calcifications. If calcifications are suspicious (i.e., clustered, pleomorphic, or branched), then biopsy is required to rule out malignancy.

Mammograms

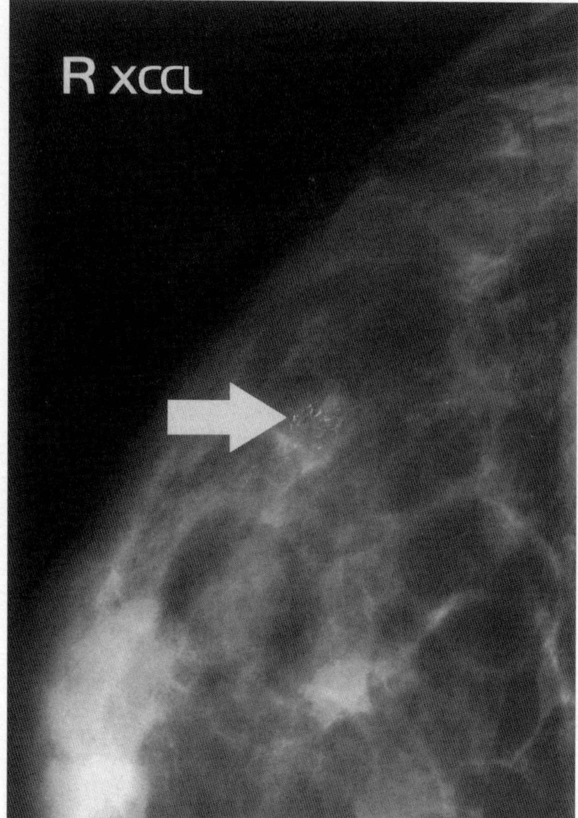

Figure 51.2A

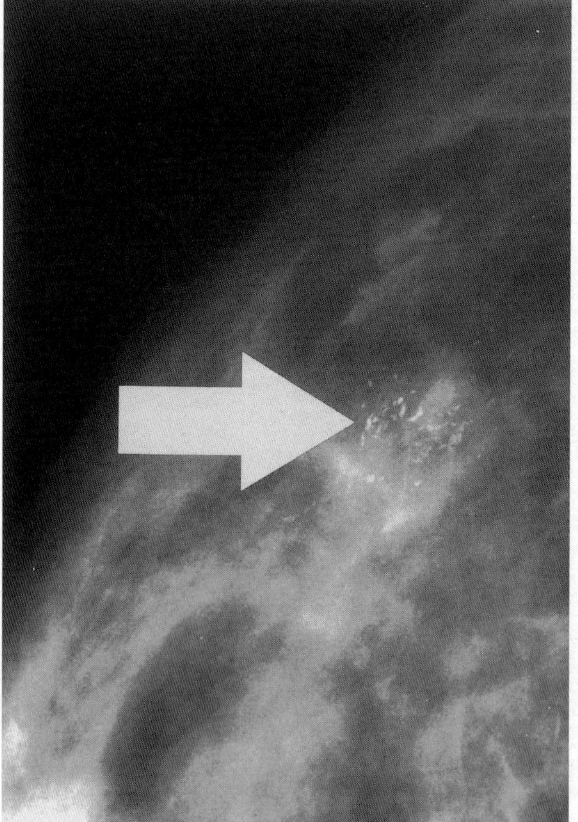

Figure 51.2B

Mammography Report

Additional diagnostic views of the right breast demonstrate 15 × 20-mm clustered fine linear branching and pleomorphic calcifications in the right lower outer quadrant *(white arrows)*—**(A)** exacerated craniocaudal lateral (XCCL) view, **(B)** magnified XCCL view. Core biopsy is the procedure of choice for the biopsy of a nonpalpable mammographic abnormality.

Specimen Photograph

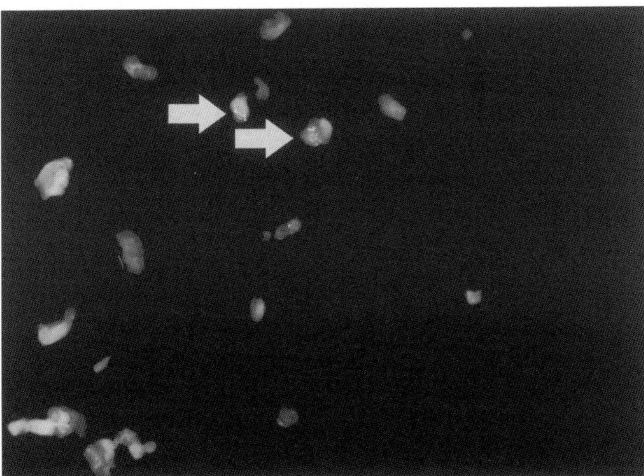

Figure 51.3

Pathology Report

A stereotactic core biopsy of the calcifications demonstrates a well-differentiated invasive ductal carcinoma with associated ductal carcinoma in situ (DCIS).

Diagnosis and Recommendation

The diagnosis is invasive ductal carcinoma. The patient needs a basic staging workup, including complete blood cell (CBC) count, liver function test (LFT), and chest x-ray. Any abnormality on chest x-ray can be evaluated with computed tomography scan of the chest.

Case Continued

CBC, LFT, and chest x-ray are normal.

Approach

Surgical options are discussed, including breast-conserving therapy consisting of segmental mastectomy with axillary lymph node dissection (ALND) or modified radical mastectomy. The patient desires breast conservation and does not wish routine ALND. Thus, the recommendation of right segmental mastectomy with sentinel lymph node biopsy with preoperative mammographic localization is made to the patient. ALND will be performed if the sentinel node contains metastasis. The risks and complications of the operation, including breast edema, scar, breast deformity, retained tumor, paresthesias, lymphedema, weakness, bleeding, infection, hematoma, discoloration of skin from isosulfan blue dye, allergy to the dye, and even (rarely) more serious complications, are discussed with the patient.

Surgical Approach

The patient has a nonpalpable cancer in the right lower outer quadrant and requires preoperative mammographic localization, which is performed by a mammographer. It is critical to review the films prior to starting the surgical procedure to decide on the location of the incision and relation of the tumor to the localizing needle. After induction of general anesthesia, 5 mL of isosulfan blue dye is injected around the primary tumor site in the right lower outer quadrant. After 5 minutes of gentle massage to distribute the dye, a transverse incision is made in the axilla. A blue lymphatic is identified and traced to a blue sentinel node. All blue-stained nodes and any suspicious nodes are excised. A curvilinear incision is then made in the right lower outer quadrant. The entire segment of the breast containing the cancer is resected with a rim of 1 to 2 cm of normal tissue. Specimen mammography is obtained to confirm the retrieval of the calcification and clip. The margins of resection are sampled and are marked with clips.

Discussion

Breast cancer accounts for approximately 31% of all new cancer cases in women and is second only to lung cancer as the leading cause of death in women. In the United States, the overall lifetime risk for the development of breast cancer in women is one in eight. The malignancy arises either in the small or terminal ducts. The most common histologic type of breast cancer is infiltrating ductal carcinoma; this accounts for 70% of breast cancer cases in the United States. Infiltrating lobular carcinoma accounts for about 15% to 20%. After the diagnosis of breast cancer, the clinical stage of the disease should be determined. For patients with small tumors, no palpable lymph nodes, and no symptoms of metastases, the preoperative workup should include bilateral mammograms, chest radiograph, CBC, and blood chemistry tests. More extensive staging procedures (computed tomography, bone scan) are useful only if the tumor is larger than 2 cm, there are palpable lymph nodes, the patient has symptoms, or results of blood tests are abnormal. Breast cancer is staged based on the size of the primary tumor, the status of lymph nodes, and the presence of metastases. The most updated staging for breast cancer is available from the American Joint Committee on Cancer (AJCC).

During the 20th century, the treatment of breast cancer was modified to improve functional and cosmetic results. The National Surgical Adjuvant Breast and Bowel Project (NSABP) conducted a randomized trial comparing Halsted radical mastectomy with total mastectomy with or without radiation therapy. After a 25-year follow-up, there was no significant difference among the three groups of women with negative nodes or between the two groups of women with positive nodes with respect to disease-free survival, relapse-free survival, distant-disease-free survival, or overall survival. Veronesi et al. reported the first major, prospective, randomized trial comparing standard Halsted radical mastectomy with a combination of quadrantectomy, ALND, and adjuvant radiotherapy (XRT). Patients with stage I disease were considered for this trial. After a 20-year follow-up, there were no statistically significant differences between the two groups in contralateral breast cancer, distant metastases, second primary cancer, or overall survival. The NSABP conducted a

trial that extended these observations to tumors as large as 4 cm, and showed that segmental mastectomy (or lumpectomy), ALND, and postoperative XRT were as effective as modified radical mastectomy for the management of patients with stage I and II breast cancer. Thus, adjuvant radiation after breast-conserving therapy is essential for obtaining local recurrence rates equivalent to those obtained by mastectomy.

Similarly, the removal of level I and II axillary nodes has been routine for staging of early breast cancer for many years. However, with increased screening by mammography, the size of breast cancers and concomitant nodal involvement have been decreasing. This has led to questioning the value of routine axillary dissection in patients with early invasive breast cancer, because most women have tumor-free nodes and derive no benefit from their removal. Sentinel lymphadenectomy is a minimally invasive procedure that accurately stages patients by removing the one or two sentinel nodes that are most likely to contain tumor if metastasis has occurred. It has been shown that if the sentinel node is free of tumor, then this predicts with great accuracy that the rest of the axillary nodes are likely to be free of tumor. A complete ALND may not be needed. If the sentinel node contains metastatic disease, then the standard treatment has been complete axillary dissection, although radiation and/or systemic therapy may be reasonable options.

Histopathology Slides

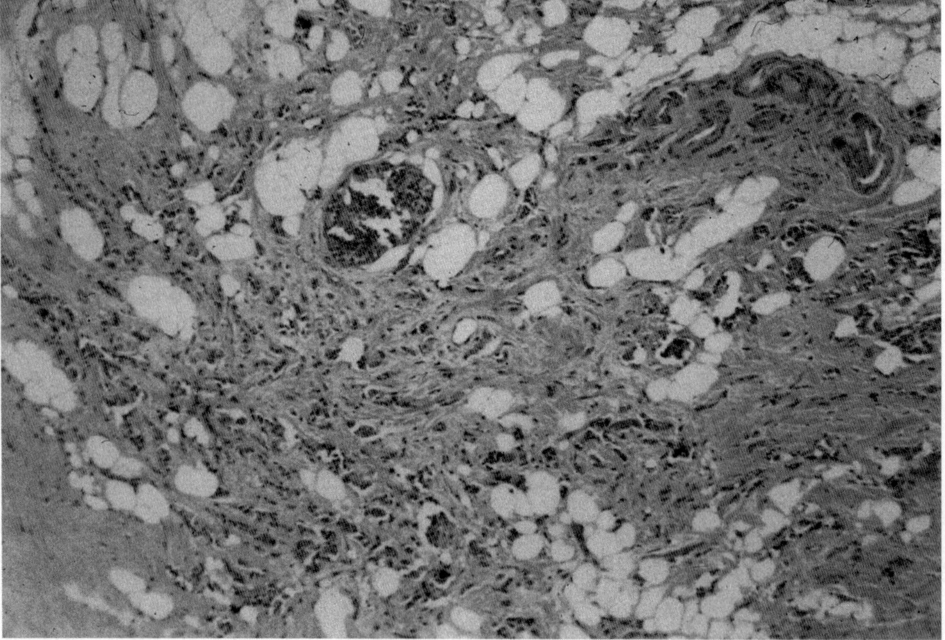

Figure 51.4A

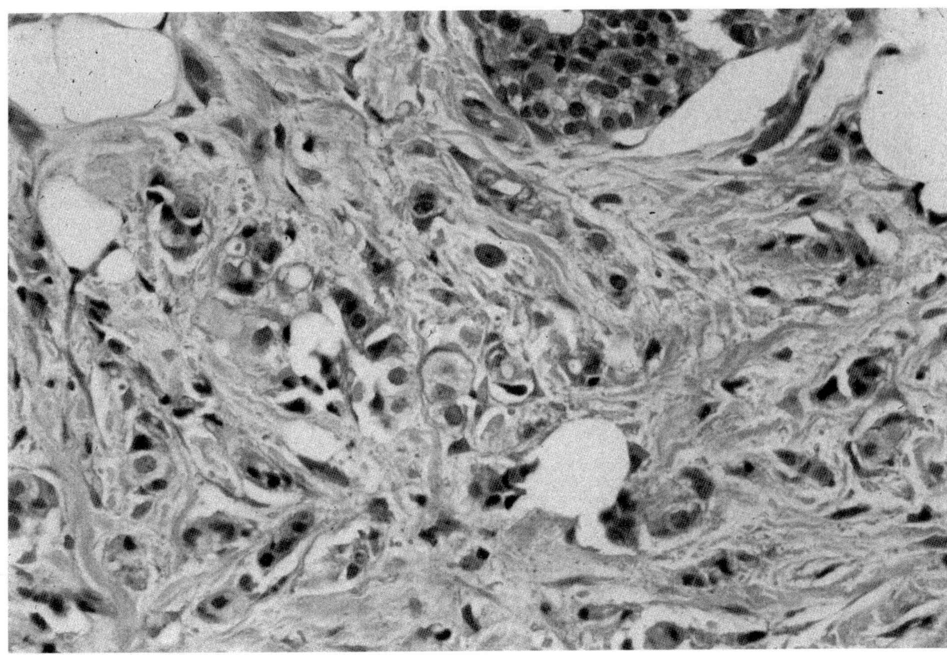

Figure 51.4B

Histopathology Report

Final histopathologic examination demonstrates a 0.2-cm infiltrating ductal carcinoma, the usual type associated with DCIS. All three sentinel nodes are negative for metastatic disease. Estrogen and progesterone receptor assays are both positive.

Case Continued

The patient will receive radiation therapy and will consider tamoxifen.

Acknowledgments

Supported by funding from the Ben B. and Joyce E. Eisenberg Foundation (Los Angeles, CA), the Fashion Footwear Association of New York Charitable Foundation (New York, NY), the Leslie and Susan Gonda (Goldschmied) Foundation (Los Angeles, CA), the John Wayne Cancer Institute Auxiliary (Santa Monica, CA), the Rabinovitch Foundation (Beverly Hills, CA), the Witherbee Foundation (Santa Monica, CA), and Mr. and Mrs. Fernando Diez-Barroso (Beverly Hills, CA).

Suggested Readings

Bassett LW, Giuliano AE, Gold RH. Staging for breast carcinoma. *Am J Surg* 1989;157:250–255.

Feuer EJ, Wun L-M, Boring CC, et al. The lifetime risk of developing breast cancer. *J Natl Cancer Inst* 1993;85:892–897.

Fisher B, Anderson S, Bryant J, et al. Twenty-year follow-up of a randomized trial comparing total mastectomy, lumpectomy, and lumpectomy plus irradiation for the treatment of invasive breast cancer. *N Engl J Med* 2002;347:1233–1241

Fisher B, Jeong JH, Anderson S, et al. Twenty-five year follow-up of a randomized trial comparing radial mastectomy, total mastectomy, and total mastectomy followed by irradiation. *N Engl J Med* 2002;347:567–575.

Giuliano AE, Haigh PI, Brennan MB, et al. Prospective observational study of sentinel lymphadenectomy without further axillary dissection in patients with sentinel node-negative breast cancer. *J Clin Oncol* 2000;18:2553–2559.

Giuliano AE, Jones RC, Brennan M, et al. Sentinel lymphadenectomy in breast cancer. *J Clin Oncol* 1997;15:2345–2350.

Giuliano AE, Kirgan DM, Guenther JM, et al. Lymphatic mapping and sentinel lymphadenectomy for breast cancer. *Ann Surg* 1994;220:391–401.

Green FL, Page DL, Fleming ID, eds. *AJCC cancer staging manual.* 6th ed. New York: Springer-Verlag; 2002.

McDivitt RW, Stewart FW, Berg JW. *Atlas of tumor pathology: tumors of the breast.* Fascicle 2, second series. Washington, DC: Armed Forces Institute of Pathology; 1968.

Veronesi U, Cascinelli N, Mariani L, et al. Twenty-year follow-up of a randomized study comparing breast-conserving surgery with radical mastectomy for early breast cancer. *N Engl J Med* 2002;347:1227–1232.

case 52

Presentation

A 46-year-old woman presents to your office with a large palpable mass in her right breast, which she first noted 7 months earlier. Physical examination reveals thin shiny skin over the central portion of the right breast around the nipple-areolar complex. There is distortion of the nipple-areolar complex. The right breast is larger than the left, and contains a mass measuring 15×10 cm, which occupies the entire outer and central portion of the breast. The mass is not fixed to the chest wall and does not invade the skin. There are no palpable right supraclavicular nodes. There is a firm, nonfixed, 1.5-cm node in the right axilla that is clinically suspicious for metastatic disease. Examination of the left breast and axilla is normal.

Clinical Photograph

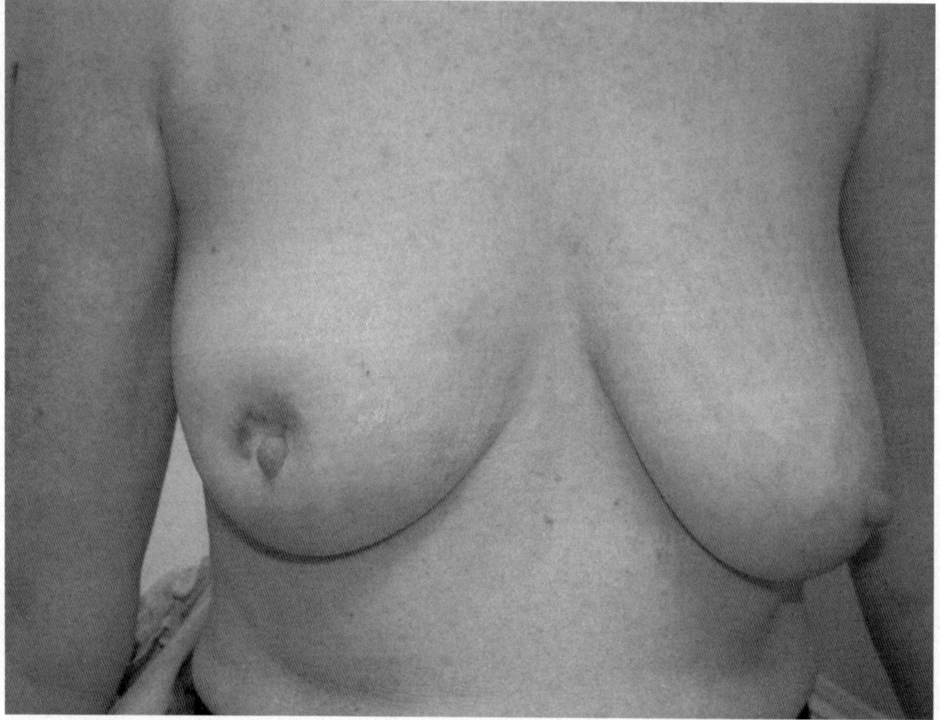

Figure 52.1

The distortion of the nipple-areolar complex due to the underlying large mass is seen.

Differential Diagnosis

The differential diagnosis of a large breast mass such as the one in this case is primarily between breast carcinoma and phyllodes tumor, either benign or malignant.

Discussion

Nonepithelial breast malignancies are rare. A review of 363,801 malignant breast tumors reported to 26 population-based registries between 1994 and 1998 identified only 0.4% (1,401) as nonepithelial in origin. The median age of women with nonepithelial cancer was 53 years, 10 years younger than that of women with epithelial cancer. Clinical characteristics suggestive of adenocarcinoma of the breast rather than phyllodes tumor include skin invasion, ulceration, or *peau d'orange*. Shiny thin skin is a characteristic of phyllodes tumors, but this is due to pressure necrosis rather than actual skin invasion. On mammography, phyllodes tumors are often smooth or lobulated, with well-defined margins. Ultrasound will occasionally demonstrate fluid-filled, elongated clefts within a solid mass, a classic sign of phyllodes tumors. Although many of these are present in the patient in this case, one aspect of her presentation that was not suggestive of phyllodes tumor was the presence of clinically positive axillary lymph nodes. The malignant component of a phyllodes tumor is sarcomatous, so metastases to axillary nodes are rare. Although clinical and imaging characteristics may suggest phyllodes tumor or epithelial malignancy, a histologic diagnosis is the only method of reliably distinguishing between these entities.

Recommendation

A diagnostic mammogram, ultrasound if necessary, and a core biopsy to establish tissue diagnosis are recommended for this patient.

Case Continued

The mammogram reveals an abnormal large suspicious mass in the right breast. By ultrasound, the mass measured 8.8 cm in diameter and was hypoechoic with heterogeneous internal echoes. A core needle biopsy revealed grade III infiltrating ductal carcinoma with negative hormone receptors and no overexpression of HER-2.

Mammogram

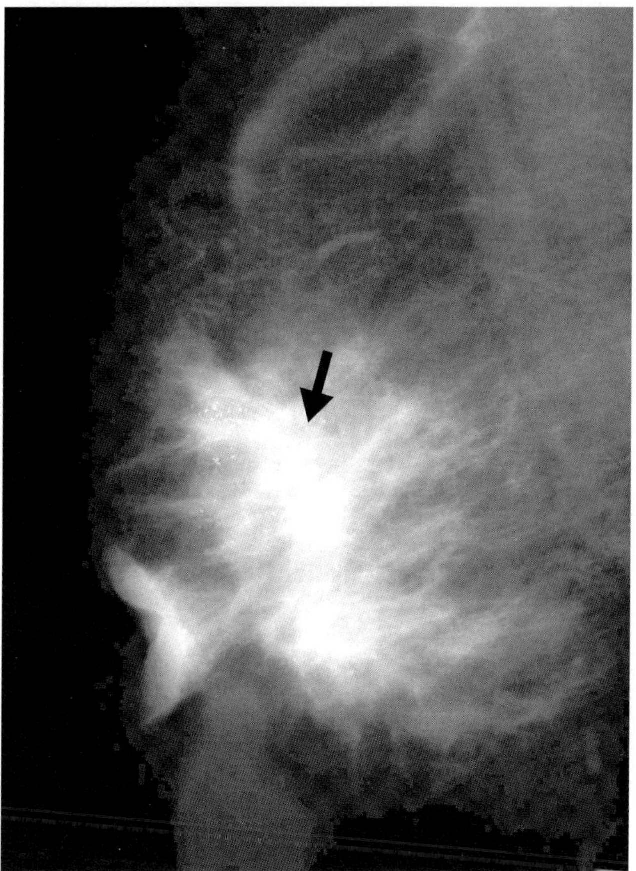

Figure 52.2

On pretherapy mammogram, a large mass occupying the entire lower half of the breast is present. The mass was bilobulated with a poorly defined posterior border.

Diagnosis and Recommendation

Locally advanced breast carcinoma. After the diagnosis of carcinoma is established, a metastatic workup consisting of chest and abdominal computed tomography (CT) scans and a bone scan should be completed.

Case Continued

There was no evidence of visceral or bony metastases. The chest CT scan reveals enlarged lymph nodes in the right axilla.

Approach

The patient's disease is assigned as T3 N1 M0, stage IIIA, and she is referred for induction chemotherapy. Current recommendations for the treatment of locally advanced breast carcinoma are multimodal and include combinations of induction chemotherapy, surgery, and radiation therapy. Although patients with inoperable disease (T4, N2, or N3) require neoadjuvant chemotherapy or hormone therapy prior to local treatments, even those with operable disease at the time of diagnosis can benefit from induction chemotherapy if tumor shrinkage will not allow them to undergo breast-conserving surgery. This patient had a large unicentric tumor, and wished to preserve her breast if possible.

Discussion

A clinical response to initial anthracycline-based chemotherapy occurs in about 72% to 97% of cases. The majority of these are partial responses, with complete pathologic response seen in fewer than 15% of patients in most series. Characteristics predictive of a good response to induction chemotherapy include high histologic grade, estrogen receptor negativity, and ductal rather than lobular histology, all of which were present in this patient. In studies of neoadjuvant therapy for large operable breast cancers, breast conservation is reported in 63% to 90% of cases.

A prospective, randomized trial performed by the National Surgical Adjuvant Breast and Bowel project (NSABP B27) demonstrated that the addition of four cycles of preoperative docetaxel to preoperative doxorubicin and cyclophosphamide increased the pathologic complete response rate from 13.7% to 26.1% (p <0.001) and the proportion of node-negative patients from 50.8% to 58.2% (p >0.001).

Case Continued

The patient has a repeat clinical evaluation 3 weeks after completion of four cycles of doxorubicin and cyclophosphamide therapy. Physical examination is remarkable for a significant decrease in the size of the right breast mass and resolution of the enlarged right axillary lymph node. Residual nodularity measuring 2 cm in size is palpable in the lower outer quadrant of the breast. However, repeat imaging reveals that a residual mass measuring 4.6 cm in its greatest dimension is present. For this reason, it was elected to give four cycles of taxane therapy prior to surgery.

At repeat evaluation 3 weeks after her fourth cycle of docetaxel, only a vague thickening is palpable in the lower outer quadrant of the breast. By ultrasound, a residual mass measuring 2.5 × 2.0 cm is seen.

Mammogram

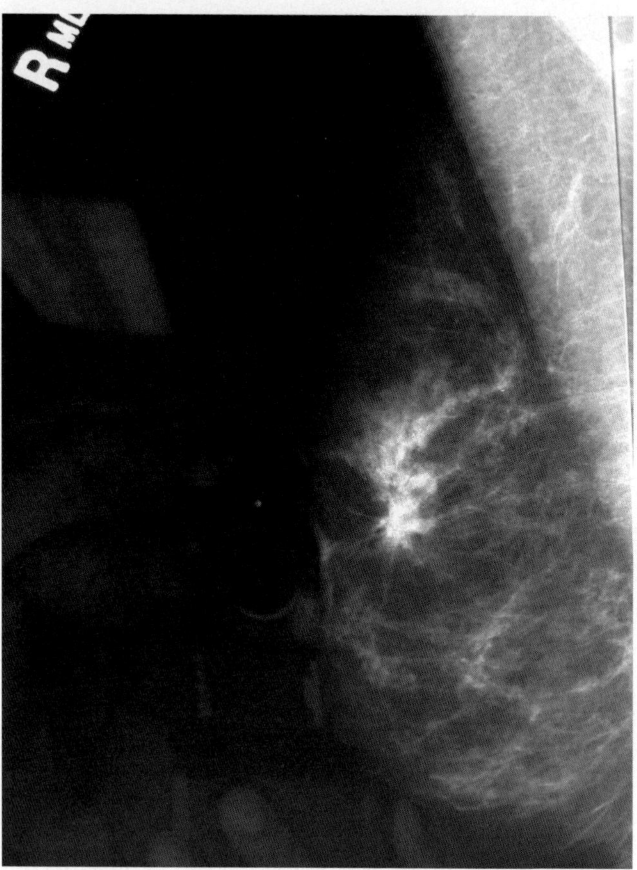

Figure 52.3

Mammography Report

On postchemotherapy mammogram, there is a persistent density present in the right breast.

Surgical Approach

The patient was believed to be an appropriate candidate for breast-conserving surgery and underwent lumpectomy and axillary dissection. Although the entire area encompassed by the tumor initially was not resected, a generous 10 × 10-cm specimen was excised. Final pathology demonstrated fibrosis, but no residual tumor was found in the 10-cm specimen, and 19 lymph nodes were negative for disease.

Case Continued

The cosmetic outcome was excellent in the early postoperative period.

Discussion

The appropriate extent of resection after induction chemotherapy is poorly defined. It is clearly not feasible to resect the entire area initially involved by tumor. Any residual clinical or image-detected abnormalities should be removed along with a sample of apparently normal breast tissue. If viable residual tumor is present scattered throughout the specimen, consideration should be given to the resection of additional breast tissue, even if the margins are negative. The use of sentinel node biopsy in patients with clinically positive nodes at presentation is also controversial. Mamounas reported a 14% false-negative rate in a series of over 400 patients undergoing sentinel node biopsy after neoadjuvant chemotherapy. This patient will receive breast irradiation postoperatively. Reported rates of local recurrence after breast preservation following neoadjuvant therapy vary widely, ranging from 6% to 28%. This undoubtedly reflects variation in response rates and extent of surgical resection. No further systemic therapy is indicated at this time.

Suggested Readings

Bear HD, Anderson S, Broron A, et al. The effect on tumor response of adding sequential preoperative docetaxel to preoperative doxorubicin and cyclophosphamide: preliminary results from National Surgical Adjuvant Breast and Bowel Project Protocol B27. *J Clin Oncol* 2003;21:4165–4174.

Buchberger W, Strasser K, Heim K, et al. Phyllodes tumor: findings on mammography, sonography, and aspiration cytology in 10 cases. *Am J Roentgenol* 1991;157:715–719.

Gajdos C, Tartter PI, Estabrook A, et al. Relationship of clinical and pathologic response to neoadjuvant chemotherapy and outcome of locally advanced breast cancer. *J Surg Oncol* 2002;80:4–11.

Giordano S. Update on locally advanced breast cancer. *Oncologist* 2003;8:521–530.

Hortobagyi GN, Singletary SE, Strom EA. Treatment of locally advanced breast cancer. In: Harris JR, Lippman ME, Morrow M, et al., eds. *Diseases of the breast.* 3rd ed. Philadelphia, PA: Lippincott Williams & Wilkins; 2004.

Kuerer HM, Hunt KK, Newman LA, et al. Neoadjuvant chemotherapy in women with invasive breast carcinoma: conceptual basis and fundamental surgical issues. *J Am Coll Surg* 2000;3:350–363.

Mamounas EP. Sentinel lymph node biopsy after neoadjuvant systemic therapy. *Surg Clin North Am* 2003;83:931–942.

Mauriac L, MacGragen G, Avril A, et al. Neoadjuvant chemotherapy for operable breast carcinoma larger than 3 cm: a unicentric randomized trial with 124-month median follow-up. Institut Bergone Bordeaux Group Sein (IBBGS). *Ann Oncol* 1999;10:47–52.

Norris HJ, Taylor HB. Relationship of histologic features to behavior of cystosarcoma phyllodes, analysis of 94 cases. *Cancer* 1967;20:2090–2099.

Petrek JA. Phyllodes tumor in diseases of the breast. In: Harris JR, Lippman ME, Morrow M, et al., eds. *Diseases of the breast.* 2nd ed. Philadelphia, PA: Lippincott Williams & Wilkins; 2000:669–676.

Veronesi U, Bonadonna G, Zurrida S, et al. Conservation surgery after primary chemotherapy in large carcinomas of the breast. *Ann Surg* 1995;222:612–618.

Young JL Jr, Ward KC, Wingo PA, et al. The incidence of malignant non-carcinomas of the female breast. *Cancer Causes Control* 2004;15:313–319.

case 53

Presentation

A 55-year-old woman presents with a change in the shape of her left breast and the appearance of her nipple for approximately 2 months. In the 2 weeks prior to her appointment, she noted a pink discoloration of the central portion of her breast. She denies fever, chills, weight loss, or systemic symptoms. On physical examination, the left breast is erythematous with *peau d'orange* of the central third. There is loss of projection of the nipple and distortion of the inferolateral contour of the breast. There are no palpable axillary, supraclavicular, or infraclavicular lymph nodes. The central portion of the left breast is firm and diffusely thickened throughout the inferior half of the gland. Examination of the left breast is normal.

Clinical Photograph

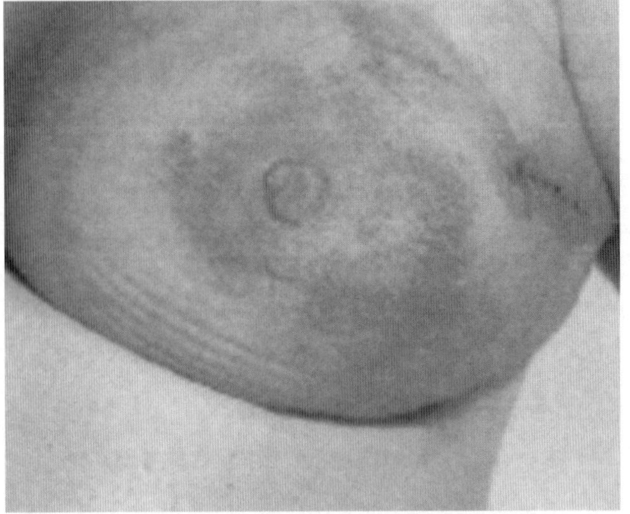

Figure 53.1 (From Moore KL, Dalley AF II. *Clinical oriented anatomy.* 4th ed. Baltimore, MD: Lippincott Williams & Wilkins; 1999.)

Clinical Examination Report

The erythema surrounding the nipple-areolar complex can be seen.

Differential Diagnosis

The differential diagnosis in this case includes inflammatory breast cancer, breast infection, and fat necrosis.

Discussion

Although inflammatory breast cancer (IBC) is included in the group designated as locally advanced breast cancer (LABC), it has some distinguishing characteristics, which are important both for treatment selection and prognosis. Inflammatory breast cancer represents only 1% to 5% of newly diagnosed breast cancers. This case illustrates the classic clinical signs of inflammatory cancer: an ill-defined mass, due to diffuse infiltration of the breast tissue with tumor, and skin erythema and edema (the classic *peau d'orange*), caused by obstruction of the dermal lymphatics with tumor cells. The extent of disease is often underestimated mammographically, with nonspecific signs of asymmetric density and skin thickening, as in this case. These features, coupled with the absence of an obvious breast mass, often result in confusion with breast infection. Patients with IBC are often initially prescribed antibiotics for a suspected breast infection, which does not resolve with treatment. There are several other infectious processes with similar clinical signs and symptoms, which must be distinguished from IBC. Periductal mastitis can occur in a single duct or in multiple ducts, and can present with erythema and tenderness in the skin overlying the involved duct. Breast abscess may have clinical findings that are very similar to the clinical features of IBC. In general, IBC is distinguished from infection by the absence of pain and fever. If abscess is suspected, it can be diagnosed by ultrasound examination and aspiration of purulent fluid from the mass. In patients suspected of having mastitis, a 1-week trial of antibiotics can be considered, but unless the clinical examination reverts to normal, a biopsy is indicated.

Trauma to the breast can produce fat necrosis or hematoma with surrounding inflammation, which occasionally is difficult to distinguish from inflammatory cancer. Patients who have had a previous breast or thoracic cancer and have received radiation therapy can have persistent erythema and skin edema lasting several years. This diagnosis should be easily made on the basis of the history. Edema of the breast can occur in patients with congestive heart failure or nephrotic syndrome who have generalized edema, but inflammatory changes and thickening of the breast parenchyma are not usually present. These conditions can usually be distinguished by a thorough history and physical examination. Definitive diagnosis may require a tissue biopsy, particularly in the case of fat necrosis.

Histologically, IBC is most commonly high-grade, poorly differentiated, estrogen-receptor (ER) and progesterone-receptor (PR) negative, infiltrating ductal carcinoma without a propensity for any particular subtype. Mutations of p53 and epidermal growth factor receptor are often present. The presence of tumor cells in the dermal lymphatics provides pathologic confirmation of the diagnosis of IBC, but the diagnosis can also be made on the basis of clinical signs of diffuse erythema and edema in the presence of a tumor in the breast parenchyma.

Recommendation

Bilateral mammogram, ultrasound scan, and full-thickness skin biopsy in the edematous/erythematous region.

Case Continued

The patient is unable to tolerate breast compression; therefore, a magnetic resonance imaging (MRI) study of the breast is obtained.

MRI

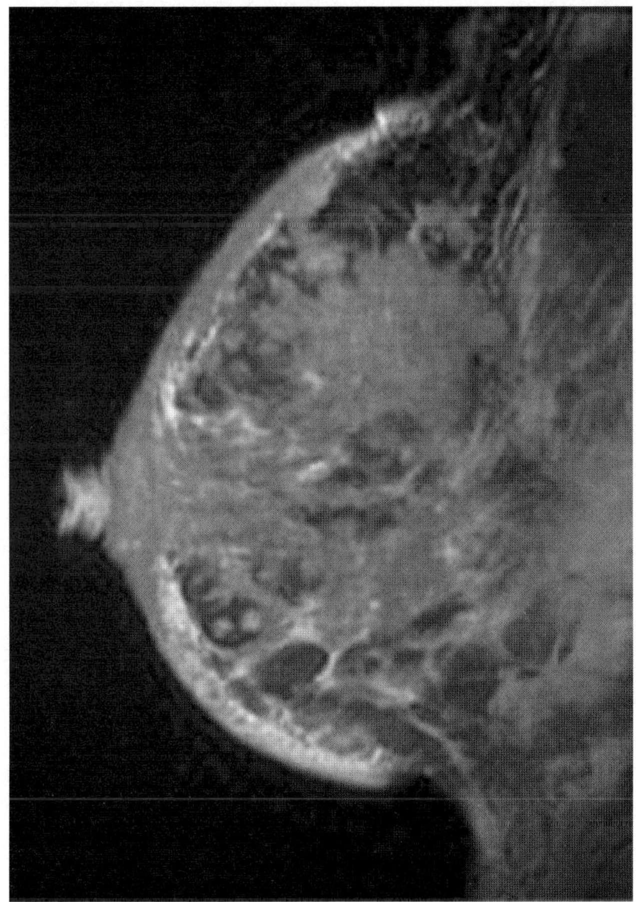

Figure 53.2A

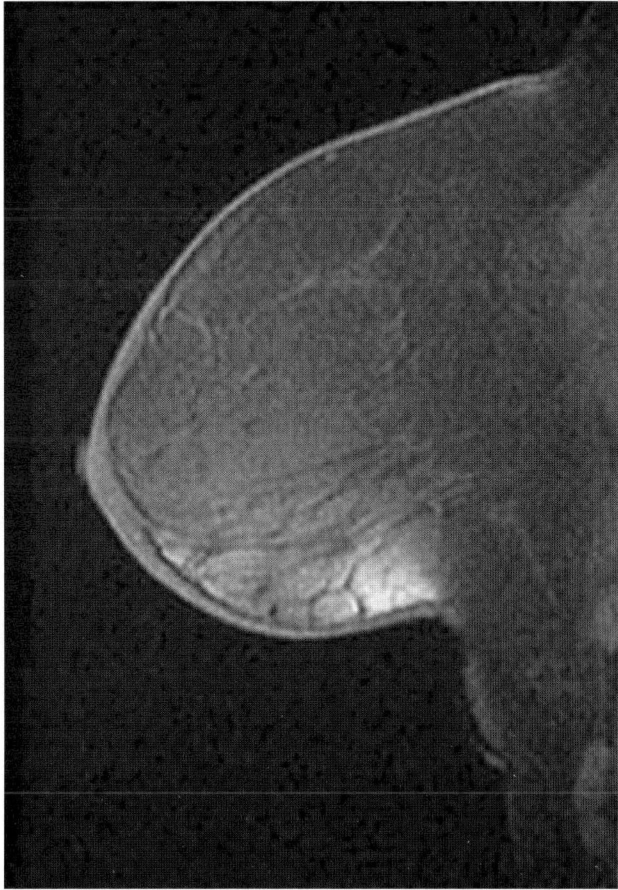

Figure 53.2B

MRI Report

There is diffuse, extensive skin thickening and enhancement of the left breast *(left)* in comparison to the normal contralateral breast *(right)*.

Case Continued

Ultrasound scans of the left breast show three irregular hypoechoic lesions in the superior hemisphere of the breast at 9 o'clock, 11–12 o'clock, and 2 o'clock.

A core needle biopsy of the central thickening in the breast shows grade 3 infiltrating ductal carcinoma that was ER and PR negative and HER-2 positive. A punch biopsy of the skin shows dermal lymphatic invasion.

Diagnosis and Recommendation

After the clinical and pathologic diagnosis of IBC is established, a metastatic workup consisting of chest and abdominal computed tomography (CT) scans and a bone scan is completed.

Case Continued

CT and bone scans reveal no evidence of metastases. The patient's cancer is assigned as T4 N0 M0 stage IIIb. She is referred for induction chemotherapy.

▨ Approach

Current recommendations for the treatment of IBC are multimodal and include combinations of induction chemotherapy, surgery, and radiation therapy. However, the diagnosis of IBC is an absolute contraindication to surgery prior to chemotherapy. Initial surgery or surgery and radiation are associated with local failure rates of 50% to 80% and 5-year survival rates approaching zero. Radiation is routinely employed because of the high risk of local recurrence when chemotherapy and surgery alone are used.

Discussion

Dramatic improvements in disease-free and overall survival rates were observed in the 1970s with the addition of systemic treatment to surgery and radiotherapy. A clinical response to initial chemotherapy occurs in about 80% of cases. Local recurrence rates for those receiving chemotherapy, radiation, and mastectomy are less than half of those receiving chemotherapy and radiation only. Radiation can be administered preoperatively or postoperatively, and the sequence of delivering these methods does not appear to affect disease-free or overall survival. Pathologic response determines the need for postoperative chemotherapy, and the regimen given will depend on the agents used preoperatively. Various anthracycline-based regimens have yielded at least partial pathologic responses (>50% reduction in tumor diameter) in up to 70% of patients and complete responses in 7% to 15%. Minimal response (25% to 50% reduction in tumor size) is seen in 15% to 35% of patients, and up to 14% have stable or progressive disease.

Case Continued

After the patient completes four cycles of doxorubicin and cyclophosphamide therapy, clinical evaluation demonstrates decreased but persistent skin erythema and softening of the breast. Due to the persisting erythema, four cycles of docetaxel are administered. Physical examination 3 weeks after the fourth cycle of docetaxel suggested a complete clinical response with resolution of the erythema and the skin and breast tissue thickening.

▨ Surgical Approach

Following completion of induction chemotherapy, a modified radical mastectomy should be performed. This involves designing an elliptical incision that encompasses the prior biopsy site and the nipple-areolar complex. Superior and inferior flaps are created to the level of the clavicle and the rectus sheath, respectively. The breast tissue, along with the underlying pectoralis major fascia, is resected. After identifying the lateral border of the pectoralis major muscle, the interpectoral (Rotter) nodes are removed and the axilla is entered by incising the axillary fascia along the lateral border of the pectoralis minor. The level I and II lymph node package is removed while preserving the long thoracic, thoracodorsal, and intercostobrachial nerves.

Pathology Report

Complete pathologic response is confirmed by absence of residual tumor in the breast. The breast parenchyma showed scarring, foreign body giant cell reaction, and fat necrosis, but no residual tumor. Two lymph nodes of the 17 that were removed contained small tumor cell intralymphatic emboli; however, the viability of these cells was questionable due to the appearance of therapy effect.

Case Continued

No further systemic therapy is administered because the patient experienced complete or near complete response to the original treatment. Radiation is delivered to the chest wall and supraclavicular nodal fields to a dose of 50.40 Gy and 45 Gy, respectively. The patient will be monitored with clinical breast examinations every 3 to 4 months for the first 2 postoperative years, and annual mammograms. Subsequent clinical examinations will occur twice yearly. Screening for metastatic disease will be performed on the basis of clinical symptoms.

Discussion

The criterion for operability is complete resolution of the inflammatory skin changes. Initial evaluation can occur after four cycles of chemotherapy, historically an anthracycline. If complete resolution of the inflammatory changes has not occurred, four cycles of another agent, usually a taxane, are administered. If resolution of skin erythema still has not occurred, chemoresistant disease is most likely present, and radiotherapy should be the next therapeutic modality. Surgery should be avoided prior to resolution of all inflammatory changes because local recurrence often occurs prior to complete wound healing if tumor in the dermal lymphatics is not controlled prior to mastectomy. When the inflammatory changes have resolved, modified radical mastectomy (MRM) remains the procedure of choice due to the diffuse tumor involvement characteristic of IBC. Breast conservation in this setting is treacherous, because discerning the amount of remaining disease is extremely difficult. In a small study of 13 patients treated with breast-conserving therapy, seven experienced local recurrence. The limited experience with sentinel node biopsy in IBC suggests an unacceptably high false-negative rate for the procedure. Axillary dissection remains the standard procedure for nodal staging.

After a complete pathologic response to induction therapy, 5- and 10-year survival rates of 65% and 46%, respectively, and disease-free survival rates of 59% and 50%, respectively, are reported. Overall 5-year survival rates for women with inflammatory cancer treated with a multimodal approach range from 10% to 75%, reflecting all levels of response, the small size of many of these studies, and the variety of chemotherapeutic agents used.

Suggested Readings

Anderson WF, Chu KC, Chang S. Inflammatory breast carcinoma and noninflammatory locally advanced breast carcinoma: distinct clinicopathologic entities? *J Clin Oncol* 2003;21: 2254–2259.

Greene FL, Page DL, Fleming ID, et al., eds. *Breast: AJCC cancer staging manual.* 6th ed. New York, NY: Springer; 2002: 221–240.

Brun B, Otamezguine Y, Feuilhade F, et al. Treatment of inflammatory breast cancer with combination chemotherapy and mastectomy versus breast conservation. *Cancer* 1988;61: 1096–1103.

Harris ER, Schula D, Bertsch H, et al. Ten-year outcome after combined modality therapy for inflammatory breast cancer. *Int J Radiat Oncol Biol Phys* 2003;55:1200–1208.

Hortobagyi GN, Singletary SE, Strom EA. Treatment of locally advanced and inflammatory breast cancer. In: Harris JR, Lippman ME, Morrow M, et al., eds. *Diseases of the breast.* 2nd ed. Philadelphia, PA: Lippincott Williams & Wilkins; 2000: 645–667.

Ozmen V, Cabioglu N, Igci A, et al. Inflammatory breast cancer: results of anthracycline-based neoadjuvant chemotherapy. *Breast J* 2003;9:79–85.

Riou G, Le MG, Travagli JP, et al. Poor prognosis of p53 gene mutation and nuclear overexpression of p53 protein in inflammatory cancer. *J Natl Cancer Inst* 1993;85:1765–1767.

Stearns V, Ewing CA, Slack R, et al. Sentinel lymphadenectomy after neoadjuvant chemotherapy for breast cancer may reliably represent the axilla except for inflammatory breast cancer. *Ann Surg Oncol* 2002;9:235–242.

Presentation

A 52-year-old woman presents for routine follow-up 3 years after right breast-conserving surgery and radiation therapy for a 2.5-cm invasive ductal carcinoma. Original pathology included an intermediate-grade tumor, all surgical margins were clear, estrogen and progesterone receptors were positive, and all lymph nodes were negative for metastatic disease.

Clinical Photograph

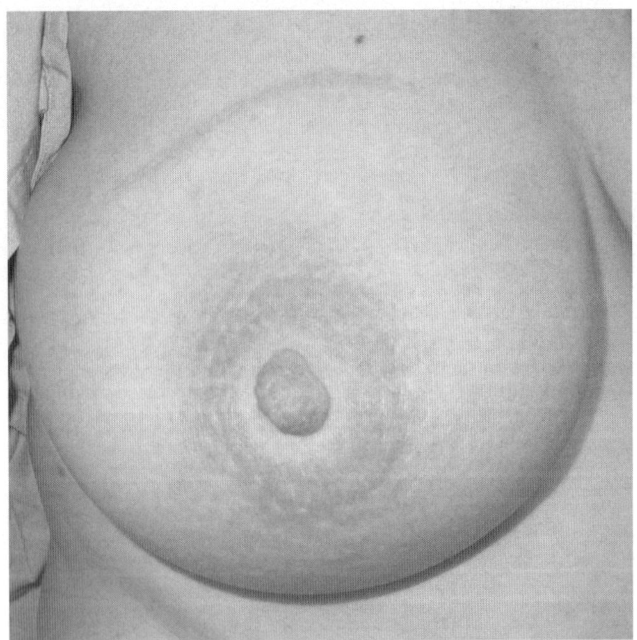

Figure 54.1

Physical Examination Report

Physical examination reveals mild thickening of the breast and slight retraction in the area of wide local excision. There is no palpable mass. There is no lymphadenopathy in the axilla or supraclavicular area, and no other concerning features are found on physical examination. A diagnostic mammogram is obtained.

Mammogram

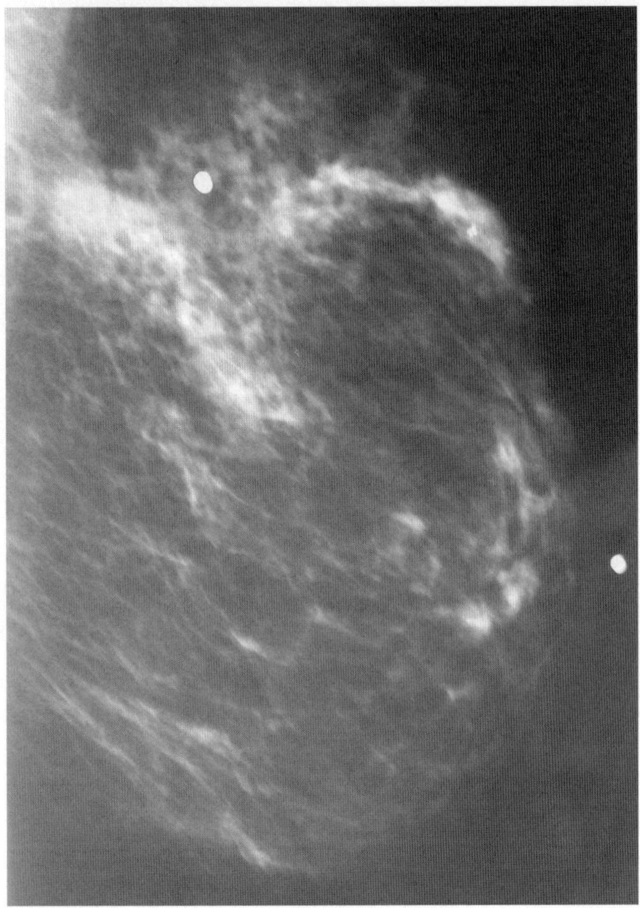

Figure 54.2

Mammography Report

The skin marker is placed over the prior skin incision. On the mediolateral oblique (MLO) view, a density is demonstrated within the posterior third of the upper breast. The density is worrisome for recurrent breast carcinoma.

Differential Diagnosis

In general, mild thickening without a mass may be related to initial surgery and radiation therapy. Also, scar tissue and radiation-associated fibrosis may present as mass-like regions that are difficult to distinguish from local recurrence. Fat necrosis from surgical trauma may present as a hard mass with skin dimpling and may occur under flaps following mastectomy and reconstruction. Changes in the physical examination occurring 1 to 2 years after initial surgical and radiation therapy must be viewed with suspicion.

Local recurrence, defined as any recurrence of cancer in the ipsilateral breast, chest wall, or skin, may present with minimal thickening or retraction at the site of prior surgery. Local recurrence should be distinguished from regional recurrence (i.e., axillary, internal mammary, or supraclavicular lymphadenopathy). Approximately one third of recurrent breast cancers are diagnosed by mammography alone. Physical examination may detect a suspicious mass, asymptomatic nodule, skin dimpling, or retraction, similar to the presentation of primary breast cancer in approximately two thirds of patients. Less commonly, diffuse breast thickening and increasing induration may be indicative of local recurrence and is easily confused with radiation-induced changes. Rarely, local recurrence may present as an area of nipple excoriation or Paget disease.

Mammography may note features similar to the original primary tumor including irregular or clustered microcalcifications, a spiculated mass, increased density, or distorted architecture. Fat necrosis and scarring may mimic a primary or recurrent breast cancer. Rarely, areas of well-circumscribed sclerosis can occur following radiation therapy. Certain histologies, such as infiltrative lobular breast cancer, can be mammographically occult.

Discussion

Because it is often difficult to interpret the physical examination and mammogram, suspicious findings should be histologically evaluated. Fine-needle aspiration and core biopsies have up to a 15% false-negative rate in this setting. Mammography-guided or ultrasound-guided and mammotome biopsies produce more accurate and larger specimens, respectively. However, it still may be difficult to distinguish radiation-induced atypia from malignancy. An open surgical biopsy may be required. An expert breast pathologist is very helpful in equivocal tissue diagnoses.

The National Cancer Institute (NCI) randomized control trial (RCT) comparing breast-conserving surgery (BCS) with mastectomy noted a 22% risk of local recurrence following BCS, axillary dissection, and adjuvant radiation therapy at a median follow-up of 18 years. Most patients with local recurrence were salvaged by mastectomy, and disease-free and overall survival were comparable in the two groups. The National Surgical Adjuvant Breast Project (NSABP) B-06 trial comparing modified radical mastectomy, lumpectomy, and lumpectomy plus radiation for breast cancer (4 cm or less) noted a 14.3% local recurrence rate following BCS and radiation at 20 years of follow-up. Local recurrence occurred in 39.2% of patients treated by lumpectomy alone. A similarly designed RCT from Europe in early-stage breast cancer (2 cm or less) noted an 8.8% local recurrence rate at 20 years following BCS and adjuvant radiation.

An overview of these RCTs confirms the risk of local recurrence is three times lower when radiation therapy is utilized in addition to BCS. Although radiotherapy is associated with a slightly lower breast cancer-specific death rate, overall survival is unchanged when comparing surgery with surgery plus radiation therapy.

Risk factors for local recurrence in various studies include multicentricity, increasing primary tumor size and grade, close or positive margins, an extensive intraductal carcinoma component, vascular or lymphatic invasion, increasing number of metastatic axillary lymph nodes, hormone receptor-negative tumors, younger patients (<45 years of age), and absence of adjuvant radiation therapy.

Case Continued

Mammogram-guided core biopsy confirms invasive breast cancer. Histology is the same as the primary breast cancer.

Diagnosis and Recommendation

Recurrent breast carcinoma. The patient should be restaged, which includes history and physical examination, chest x-ray, liver imaging, ultrasonography, and bone scan. There is no evidence of metastatic disease.

Approach

Staging tests, including chest x-ray, liver ultrasound, and bone scan, have a low yield in stage I and II primary breast cancer. However, full staging is generally warranted in patients with locally recurrent breast cancer following BCS even though most will not have clinically detectable distant metastases at the time of diagnosis.

Locally recurrent breast cancer may have a devastating psychological impact. The recurrence is a visible reminder of failure to respond to therapy and has significant implications for prognosis. A holistic approach is paramount. It is important to inform the patient adequately regarding optimal treatment and prognosis but also to maintain hope.

In most series, locally recurrent breast cancer after BCS and radiation appears to have a better prognosis than local recurrence following mastectomy. Individual patients with locally recurrent breast cancer have a worse prognosis as a reflection of a more aggressive biology; however, as a group, overall survival is similar in RCTs comparing BCS with mastectomy despite differences in local control. A provisional explanation of these data includes the idea that local recurrence following BCS may be secondary to residual cancer, a new primary breast cancer, or secondary to circulating tumor cells from distant metastases recurring in the wound. The first two scenarios will have a much better prognosis than the latter.

Surgical Approach

With no evidence of regional or distant disease, the patient undergoes salvage right mastectomy. An elliptical incision is made, and after creating superior and inferior flaps, the breast tissue is resected with the underlying pectoralis fascia. The skin is approximated carefully after placement of closed suction drains.

Discussion

The most common treatment following local recurrence is salvage mastectomy with no further treatment of the previously dissected axilla. However, up to 30% of cases are managed by further wide local excision in some series. Although overall survival is likely unaffected, a local re-recurrence is more common in patients managed in this manner. Patients and physicians are often reluctant to consider a second attempt at BCS due to this reason, unless radiotherapy was not utilized initially. Furthermore, the final cosmetic results are unlikely to be satisfactory with a second wide excision.

Most authors consider prior axillary surgery a contraindication to sentinel lymph node biopsy. However, a few small reports describe this technique in locally recurrent breast cancer. Reoperative sentinel node biopsy is technically successful in up to 75% of cases; it is most successful when less than ten or an inadequate number of lymph nodes were removed at the initial dissection. Because most patients with locally recurrent breast cancer will be offered adjuvant therapies, repeat sentinel lymph node assessment has limited value in directing further therapy.

Many patients consider prophylactic surgery for the contralateral breast following the diagnosis of a locally recurrent breast cancer. The unfortunate reality, however, is that the primary breast cancer, now locally recurrent, will determine the patient's long-term outcome rather than the attempt to avoid a new primary breast cancer of the opposite breast.

Case Continued

The patient remains disease free several years following salvage mastectomy.

Discussion

A different, yet equally important, issue is the risk of locally recurrent breast cancer following mastectomy.

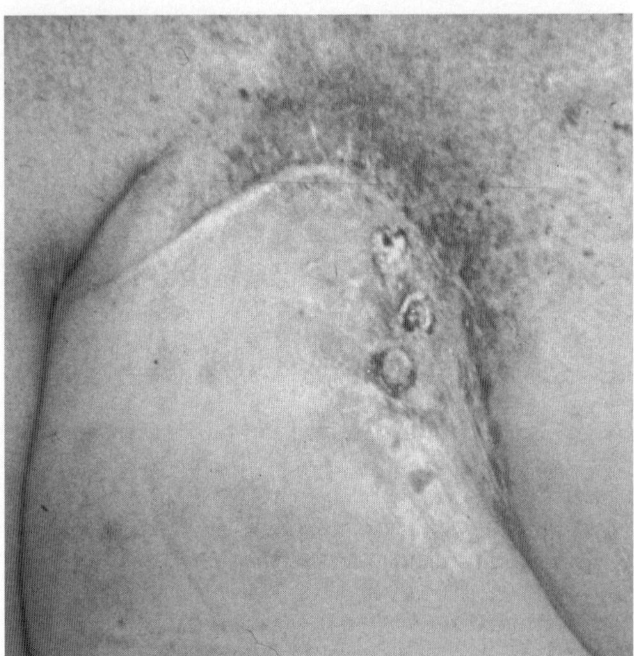

Figure 54.3 Chest wall recurrence following mastectomy.

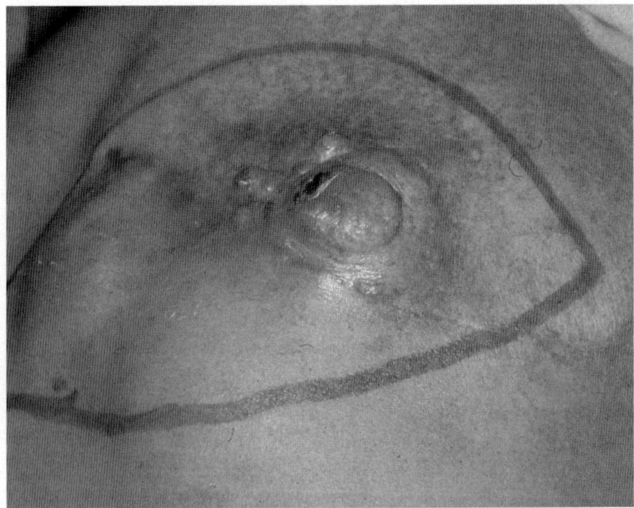

Figure 54.4 Local recurrence requiring bony chest wall excision.

Twenty-five-year follow-up data for the NSABP-04 trial note a 5% overall local recurrence rate in 1,665 patients following radical mastectomy, total mastectomy, or total mastectomy with radiation therapy. Patients with positive axillary nodes had a 3% to 8% risk of local recurrence, depending on treatment modality, and those with negative nodes had a 1% to 7% risk. An absolute improvement from 13% to 5% in *locoregional* recurrence rates was noted comparing total mastectomy with total mastectomy plus radiation therapy, respectively. Six percent of all women had regional nodal recurrences, and 34% had distant recurrences. There were no significant disease-free or overall survival differences between treatment modalities. At the 20-year follow-up, local recurrence rates of 2.3% and 10.2% occurred in the mastectomy treatment arms of the World Health Organization and NSABP-06 RCTs, respectively. All of the preceding trials dealt with early-stage (T1 or T2) breast cancer, and local recurrence rates following mastectomy can be considerably higher in more advanced cancers.

An increasing number of patients receive postmastectomy radiation of the chest wall in primary treatment of cancers with four or more positive lymph nodes. Level I evidence confirms a reduced locoregional recurrence rate with this approach. Extended nodal field radiation is controversial and currently is being investigated in an RCT. In addition, increasing numbers of patients receive adjuvant systemic therapies that decrease the incidence of locoregional recurrence as the first site of relapse.

As noted previously, local recurrence following BCS is usually secondary to residual or recurrent tumor cells growing in the breast and is not a marker of distant disease. However, local recurrence following mastectomy is found in the previous incision, dermal lymphatics, or subcutaneous nodules on the chest wall. It may also result from migration of circulating tumor cells from a distant metastatic site back to the surgical field.

Most reports confirm local recurrence following mastectomy is a harbinger of distant disease and eventual fatality. Most patients develop detectable distant metastases within 2 years. However, some recent reports challenge this concept. In two European RCTs, 133 patients had isolated locoregional recurrences; most occurred on the chest wall (69%) or in the breast (72%) after mastectomy or wide local excision, respectively. Subsequent 5-year actuarial local recurrence rates and overall survival were no different after salvage treatment (excision plus radiation compared with salvage mastectomy). Similarly, a series of 105 patients with locally recurrent breast cancer noted no significant difference in prognosis based on initial surgical therapy (55 breast conservation; 50 mastectomy) and an overall 10-year survival rate of 56%.

There is a subgroup of postmastectomy patients with locally recurrent breast cancer and long-term survival. More favorable outcomes are seen in patients with a solitary chest wall nodule, a relatively long disease-free interval (more than 1 year), and a primary node-negative tumor smaller than 5 cm, and in cases where the local recurrence can be controlled.

Patients should undergo complete restaging of their disease, which includes physical examination, chest x-ray, bone scan, liver imaging, and additional investigations if suggested by history or physical evaluation. A number of treatment modalities have been employed, including surgical excision, irradiation therapy, systemic hormonal therapy, and chemotherapy, as well as other investigational methods such as combined hyperthermia and irradiation and topical chemotherapeutics.

The most common treatment strategy for local recurrence not invading the underlying bony chest wall is wide local excision (with margins of 1 to 3 cm) and subsequent irradiation if the individual did not have radiation therapy following mastectomy. Wide local excision plus complete chest wall irradiation maintains local control in 80% to 90% of patients at 5 years. Focused or limited irradiation following wide local excision has a higher local recurrence rate of 35% to 40%. Wide local excision alone has a significant risk (50% to 75%) of further local relapse, with most occurring within 24 months. Radiation therapy alone has a high initial response rate, but nearly one third of patients will develop further local recurrence at a median interval of 11 to 12 months.

If distant metastatic disease is present or if the recurrence occurs rapidly following primary treatment, most clinicians will offer palliative chemotherapy (generally anthracycline-based) or hormonal therapy (tamoxifen or an aromatase inhibitor). Estrogen-receptor-positive tumors will respond in approximately 40% to 50% of cases or more. An RCT compared tamoxifen with placebo in postmastectomy patients following excision and radiation therapy for locoregional recurrence of breast cancer. To be eligible for the trial, all tumors were estrogen-receptor positive or occurred in patients with a disease-free interval longer than 12 months. All had fewer than four recurrent tumor nodules and all were <3 cm in size. An isolated local recurrence with skin or chest wall involvement was seen in 91% of cases. At an 11-year median follow-up, 5-year disease-free survival rates were 61% and 40% in the tamoxifen and observation arms, respectively. This was primarily due to a reduction in further local recurrence in the tamoxifen arm. Improved disease-free survival rate in the tamoxifen arm did not translate into an overall survival benefit.

Combined short-term complete and partial response rates to chemotherapy alone are reported in

25% to 80% of cases. Five-year disease-free recurrence rates of 30% are quoted for some chemotherapy regimens in patients with isolated local recurrence, following local surgical excision. Critical evidence is lacking, with no RCTs comparing chemotherapy with placebo or different chemotherapy regimens in this setting. Multidisciplinary consultation is paramount, even in the setting of metastatic disease, because surgery (wide local excision) or radiation therapy remains an excellent option for local control in patients expected to survive more than 6 months.

Limited residual soft tissue overlying the ribs following mastectomy may result in local recurrence invading the bony chest wall. This type of local recurrence is often treated with radiation therapy and the addition of chemotherapy or hormonal therapy. At times, the local recurrence is resistant to treatment and progresses into painful, ulcerating lesions. Chest wall resection including bony resection (ribs or sternum) should be considered when other treatment measures have failed. Morbidity and mortality rates following aggressive surgical procedures are generally low. Ideally, the local recurrence should be limited to a single location without evidence of systemic disease. However, there is often a role for palliative resection in cases where a relatively prolonged survival time is expected. Reconstruction generally involves permanent mesh and soft tissue coverage with myocutaneous flaps. The primary goal is local control, although some have reported a prolonged disease-free interval and possible cure following chest wall resection.

Combined hyperthermia and irradiation has been used in some centers. Five underpowered RCTs combined into one meta-analysis examined the role of irradiation alone versus combined hyperthermia and irradiation. A heterogeneous group was eligible, including patients with primary advanced cancers that were deemed inoperable, and patients with locally recurrent disease, with or without previous irradiation. All patients had superficial lesions and surgery was not feasible. Patients received 28 Gy or >40 Gy depending on whether they had previously been irradiated. Local complete response rates of 41% and 59% were obtained comparing radiation alone with combined radiation and hyperthermia, respectively. Primary or recurrent lesions occurring in an area not previously irradiated had a higher rate of complete response. Time to complete response ranged from 70 to 149 days. Among complete responders, 30% in the radiation arm and 17% in the combined treatment arm developed further local recurrence found at follow-up (2-year actuarial relapse-free survival rate).

Topical chemotherapy agents (miltefosine, ceramides) are currently being explored for the palliative treatment of postmastectomy local recurrence or cutaneous metastases. Thus far, combined complete and partial responses appear limited to one third of patients, and median time to treatment failure is <2 months.

Suggested Readings

Early Breast Cancer Trialists' Collaborative Group. Effects of radiotherapy and surgery in early breast cancer: an overview of the randomized trials. *N Engl J Med* 1995;333:1444–1455.

Faneyte IF, Rutgers EJT, Zoetmulder FAN. Chest wall resection in the treatment of locally recurrent breast cancer: indications and outcome for 44 patients. *Cancer* 1997;80:886–891.

Fisher B, Jeong J, Anderson S, et al. Twenty-five-year follow-up of a randomized trial comparing radical mastectomy, total mastectomy, and total mastectomy followed by irradiation. *N Engl J Med* 2002;347:567–575.

International Collaborative Hyperthermia Group. Radiotherapy with or without hyperthermia in the treatment of superficial localized breast cancer: results from five randomized controlled trials. *Int J Radiat Oncol Biol Phys* 1996;35:731–744.

Leonard R, Hardy J, van Tienhoven G, et al. Randomized, double-blind, placebo-controlled, multicenter trial of 6% miltefosine solution, a topical chemotherapy in cutaneous metastases from breast cancer. *J Clin Oncol* 2001;19:4150–4159.

Waeber M, Castiglione-Gertsch M, Dietrich D, et al. Adjuvant therapy after excision and radiation of isolated postmastectomy locoregional breast cancer recurrence: definitive results of a phase III randomized trial (SAKK 23/82) comparing tamoxifen with observation. *Ann Oncol* 2003;14:1215–1221.

Willner J, Kiricuta IC, Kolbl O. Locoregional recurrence of breast cancer following mastectomy: always a fatal event? Results of univariate and multivariate analysis. *Int J Radiat Oncol Biol Phys* 1997;37:853–863.

Presentation

A 36-year-old multiparous Hispanic woman, 20-weeks pregnant, presents in clinic with a complaint of a persistent, tender left breast mass of 3 weeks' duration. She is otherwise healthy, has no past history of breast problems and no family history of breast or ovarian cancer, and she previously successfully breast-fed her other children. Physical examination discloses a firm but not hard, slightly tender, mostly discrete 2.5 × 2-cm mass beginning 3 cm above the areolar margin without any overlying skin changes. The patient came with a recent bilateral mammogram, which showed only dense breast tissue without any obvious abnormalities, read as BIRADS 1. A targeted left breast ultrasound is obtained.

Breast Ultrasonogram

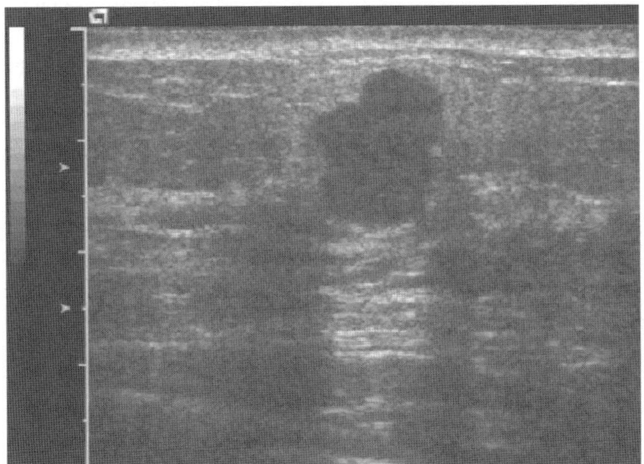

Figure 55.1

Breast Ultrasonography Report

Ultrasound of the left breast reveals an 11 × 12 × 14-mm macrolobulated hypoechoic mass, taller than wide, with good through transmission but some increased blood flow at the edges, read as BIRADS 4.

Discussion

Mammography is both safe and useful in the evaluation of the breast in pregnant women. The radiation dose to the properly shielded fetus is only 0.01 rad, well below the accepted 5-rad limit. However, owing to the increased density of breast tissue in younger and pregnant women, mammography has a high false-negative rate in these settings, with reported sensitivities of only 64% or less in pregnant women. Conversely, ultrasound is 93% accurate for the evaluation of masses in pregnant women, and should be used in most cases, especially when the mammogram is normal during the evaluation of a suspicious mass. The safety of magnetic resonance imaging (MRI) of the breast is still being established in pregnant women; some radiologists recommend it not be used in the first trimester, but there are no consistent data for this.

Differential Diagnosis

The differential diagnosis includes cancer, fibroadenoma, lobular hyperplasia, lipoma, and (rarely) leukemia, lymphoma, sarcoma, neuroma, and tuberculosis. A cyst, including galactocele, seems less likely given the ultrasound result. Because the mass has persisted longer than 2 weeks, it requires further evaluation by completion of a modified triple test (addition of a needle biopsy to the clinical breast examination and ultrasound).

Case Continued

Fine-needle aspiration done in the clinic immediately following the ultrasound shows malignant cells (modified triple test score of 7). Alkaline phosphatase level is elevated, but a chest x-ray and low-dose bone scan are normal. A subsequent core biopsy shows a high-grade invasive ductal cancer, estrogen-receptor and progesterone-receptor positive, and HER-2/neu negative.

Discussion

Because of the tendency for delayed diagnosis of pregnancy-associated breast cancer, a high index of suspicion and an easy, rapid, "one-stop" method of evaluating suspicious masses in the pregnant patient are required. The modified triple test (MTT) is accurate (scores of 6 or more indicate cancer) and allows the clinician to move ahead quickly with a metastatic workup and treatment planning. Malignancies diagnosed by fine-needle aspiration as part of the MTT should be confirmed by core needle biopsy (which caries a small risk of milk fistula in lactating patients) or intraoperative frozen section.

As in nonpregnant patients, a primary metastatic workup (chest x-ray, alkaline phosphatase, and liver function tests) is usually sufficient for early stage breast cancer (stages I and IIA). Chest x-rays are safe throughout pregnancy, but alkaline phosphatase levels may be falsely elevated, so that a low-dose bone scan may be needed. Low-dose bone scans reduce the fetal radiation exposure by half (from 0.19 to 0.08 rad). For higher stage or symptomatic patients, MRI of the liver and/or brain should be added to the workup; MRI is superior to ultrasound for evaluation of the liver in pregnant patients. Gadolinium crosses the placenta and is a class C drug in pregnancy, meaning that it can potentially cause fetal abnormalities, and should be used only if the benefit justifies risk.

Diagnosis and Recommendation

Pregnancy-associated invasive breast cancer. Because this patient was already in her second trimester and was likely to be a candidate for chemotherapy, she is offered either mastectomy or lumpectomy and radiation. She chose the latter.

Approach

Once thought to be rare, pregnancy-associated breast cancer (breast cancer during, or within a year after, a pregnancy) is expected to increase in frequency as women delay childbearing until later in life, when the general risk of breast cancer begins to rise. At present, breast cancer is the second most common malignancy in pregnancy (after cervical cancer), occurring in 1 in 5,000 deliveries. At least 10% of women younger than 40 with breast cancer are pregnant at diagnosis. Although women with a genetic predisposition to breast cancer may be over-represented among pregnant patients with cancer, the majority of cases are considered sporadic. Breast cancers in pregnant women are histologically similar to those in nonpregnant women, with 75% to 90% being ductal cancers in either group. Many studies have shown decreased estrogen-receptor positivity in pregnancy-associated cancers, possibly due to receptor downregulation in pregnancy. Some recent studies suggest that HER-2/neu overexpression may be as high as 36% to 58% in these tumors.

Nevertheless, older notions of pregnancy-associated breast cancer being more aggressive have been replaced by data suggesting a similar stage-for-stage prognosis as breast cancer in nonpregnant women (with perhaps a worse prognosis in later stages), although stage at presentation tends to be later due to the difficulty of assessing the breast in pregnant and lactating women. Thus, it is generally felt that pregnant patients should be treated with the same principles used for nonpregnant patients, that is, aggressively for cure in most cases.

Accordingly, surgery is an important part of the treatment for pregnancy-associated cancers, and the choice of operation is based not only on the same factors as for nonpregnant women (technical issues, patient choice), but also on gestational dates. Standard therapeutic radiation courses expose the fetus, even with shielding, to 15 to 200 rad, depending on the size of the fetus (i.e., proximity to the diaphragm), which is higher than the 5 to 10 rad felt to be safe. These doses expose the fetus to risks of both teratogenicity and childhood cancers or hematologic disorders. Thus, breast radiation during pregnancy is contraindicated, and lumpectomy and radiation should be offered only if the radiation can be given postpartum (i.e., if the patient is in the latter stages of the pregnancy), or if the radiation will be delayed by prior chemotherapy. Otherwise, a mastectomy is typically chosen. Reconstruction after mastectomy should be delayed until after delivery and cessation of lactation when the remaining breast has returned to normal size, to maximize the chance of attaining a balanced reconstruction.

With either approach, the standard axillary evaluation for invasive cancer is still two-level axillary dissection. The accuracy and safety of sentinel node biopsy in pregnancy is unknown, and pregnant patients are excluded from pending national trials of this technique. Further, while technetium does not cross the placenta and the standard dose of 1 mCi (or less) may give a very low dose to the fetus, isosulfan blue dye is a class C drug, and has not been tested in pregnant animals or humans.

Surgical Approach

General anesthesia and breast operations are generally safe throughout pregnancy. Nevertheless, for pregnancies more advanced than 32 weeks, consideration should be given to induction or cesarean section prior to the breast operation. Otherwise, the general principles of operation during pregnancy apply; the surgical team should be aware of the physiologic changes of pregnancy that can complicate sedation and surgery (hypercoagulability, delayed gastric emptying, increased blood volume and cardiac output, decreased pulmonary functional residual capacity, and decreased serum cholinesterase activity). The pregnant patient should be given preoxygenation, antacids or acid-decreasing medications, fetal monitoring, rapid-sequence induction with cricoid pressure, and elevation of the right hip (to decrease vena caval compression).

If the patient is lactating, this should be stopped preoperatively with ice packs, breast binding, or bromocriptine (2.5 mg po bid or tid).

Patients undergoing lumpectomy should be advised that milk production after chemotherapy will be decreased, and that lactation after radiation is often difficult due to changes in the nipple and milk ducts.

Case Continued

Pathologic examination of material from the lumpectomy and axillary dissection reveals a 1.7-cm high-grade infiltrating cancer, negative surgical margins, with one of 18 lymph nodes positive for metastatic disease (no extracapsular extension). The patient recovers well and is seen in consultation by a medical oncologist who advises four cycles of chemotherapy with doxorubicin (Adriamycin) and cyclophosphamide, followed by a taxane. The patient accepts the recommendation.

Discussion

Although all chemotherapy drugs are category D (teratogenic), these risks have generally been seen only in the first trimester; later in pregnancy they are surprisingly safe, with only a 1.3% risk. In the only prospective trial of chemotherapy in pregnancy to date, Berry, at the M.D. Anderson Cancer Center, utilized the cyclophosphamide, doxorubicin, fluorouracil (CAF) regimen to treat 24 pregnant patients after the first trimester, and saw no birth defects. Complications were few, but did include preterm delivery (three cases), transient newborn tachypnea (two cases), low birth weight, hyaline membrane disease, and transient leukopenia (one case each). The long-

term health of these children is being evaluated. No data exist to compare patient outcomes after chemotherapy in patients who received it during pregnancy with patient outcomes for those in whom systemic treatment was delayed until after delivery.

Almost all chemotherapeutic agents cross the placenta. Anthracyclines are considered safer than alkylating agents in pregnancy. Taxane use was found safe in one case report. Recent studies of dose-dense schedules excluded pregnant patients. Methotrexate, an abortifacient and the leading cause of birth defects due to chemotherapy, is strongly contraindicated in pregnancy

Physiologic changes during pregnancy, including increased plasma volume, decreased albumin concentration, increased liver and kidney function, and decreased gastric motility, may affect chemotherapy dosing. Because the newborn's kidneys and liver excrete drugs slowly, it is generally recommended to decrease or hold chemotherapy for approximately 3 weeks prior to delivery. Cyclophosphamide, doxorubicin, and methotrexate all enter breast milk, and breast-feeding is therefore usually contraindicated during chemotherapy. Many drugs typically used to treat chemotherapy side effects are safe in pregnancy, including ondansetron, haloperidol, selective serotonin reuptake inhibitors (SSRIs), methylphenidate hydrochloride, metoclopramide, acetaminophen, and morphine sulfate; in neonates, morphine sulfate may cause a withdrawal syndrome that can be treated with paregoric.

Case Continued

The patient begins chemotherapy at 24 weeks' gestation. She receives two cycles, and then, following a rest period, delivers a healthy 7-pound baby girl by cesarean section at 34 weeks' gestation. Lactation is stopped, and she continues chemotherapy. After completion of chemotherapy, she is started on tamoxifen. The patient expresses an interest in possibly having another child in the future.

Discussion

There is no evidence that therapeutic abortion improves the outcome in pregnancy-associated breast cancer. One exception may be in patients with advanced breast cancer diagnosed in the first trimester, in whom immediate chemotherapy is planned. A large meta-analysis recently showed no link between previous abortion and subsequent increased risk of breast cancer.

Tamoxifen has been associated with fetal abnormalities, is not recommended during pregnancy, and is usually stopped if a breast cancer patient subsequently becomes pregnant. Oophorectomy has not been shown to improve the prognosis in pregnancy-associated breast cancer. Similarly, future pregnancies do not appear to increase the likelihood of progressive or recurrent disease, as long as the first cancer is in remission. In fact, some data suggest that breast cancer survivors who subsequently become pregnant have a better 5-year survival than controls matched for age and stage. Further, the standard advice to avoid pregnancy for at least 2 years after treatment for a breast cancer seems arbitrary, given that the risk of relapse goes on for years, and that follow-up in any breast cancer survivor should be long term.

Suggested Readings

Beral V, Bull D, Doll R, et al. Breast cancer and abortion: collaborative reanalysis of data from 53 epidemiological studies, including 83,000 women with breast cancer from 16 countries. *Lancet* 2004;363:1007–1016.

Berry D, Theriault R, Holmes F, et al. Management of breast cancer during pregnancy using a standardized protocol. *J Clin Oncol* 1999;17:855–861.

Melnick DM, Wahl WL, Dalton VK. Management of general surgical problems in the pregnant patient. *Am J Surg* 2004;187:170–180.

Morris KT, Vetto JT, Petty JK, et al. A new score for the evaluation of palpable breast masses in women under age 40. *Am J Surg* 2002;184:346–347.

Petrek J. Breast cancer during pregnancy. *Cancer* 1994;74(suppl 1):518–527.

Woo JC, Yu T, Hurd TC. Breast cancer in pregnancy: a literature review. *Arch Surg* 2003;138:91–98.

Presentation

A 45-year-old asymptomatic woman with no significant past medical history undergoes annual screening mammography and presents to your office with an abnormal mammogram report. She has no family history of breast or ovarian cancer. No abnormalities are detected upon physical examination. A review of her current mammogram, with magnification views, demonstrates indeterminate microcalcifications in the upper outer quadrant of the right breast.

Mammograms

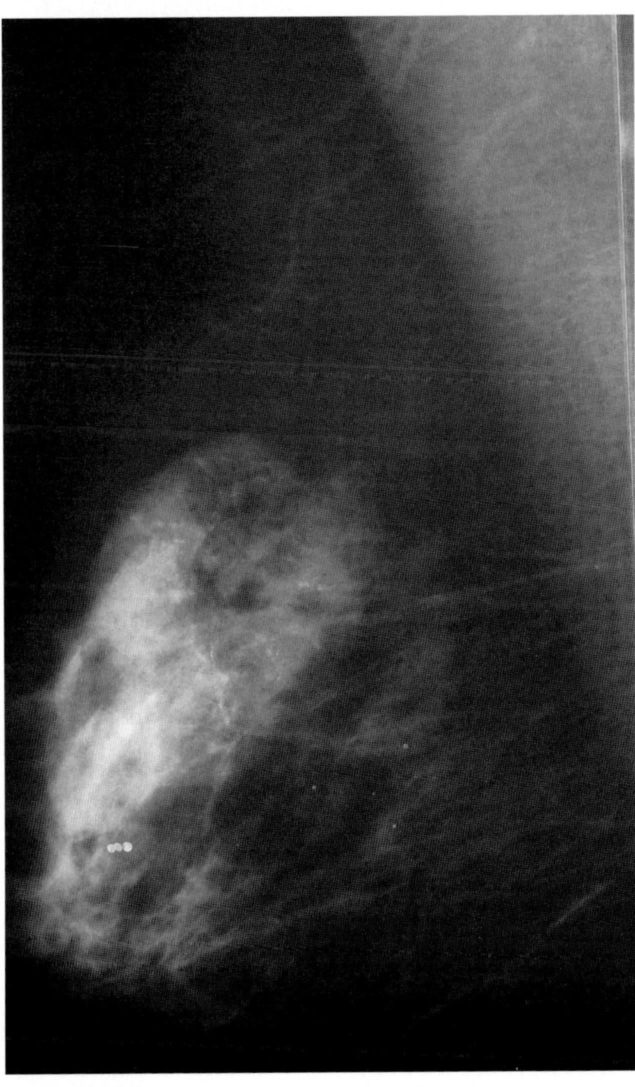

Figure 56.1A

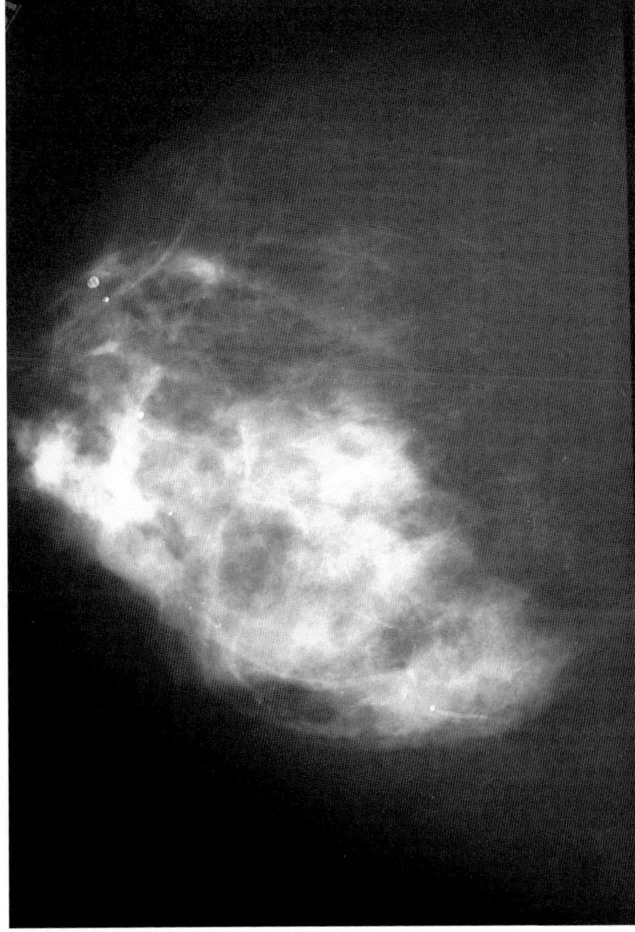

Figure 56.1B

Figure 56.2

Mammography Report

Standard two-view screening mammography demonstrates indeterminate calcifications in the upper outer quadrant of the right breast. Magnification view demonstrates amorphous calcifications in a grouped distribution.

Differential Diagnosis

Indeterminate microcalcification may be benign, though the likelihood of malignancy (noninvasive or invasive) needs to be kept in mind. Pathologic diagnosis may include fibrocystic disease, atypical ductal/lobular hyperplasia, lobular carcinoma in situ (LCIS), or ductal carcinoma in situ (DCIS)

Discussion

Calcification can occur both in carcinoma and in adjacent benign breast lesions and may be present in adjacent epitheliosis. The origin and distribution of microcalcification appears to be the same in epithelial hyperplasia, noninvasive carcinoma, and invasive carcinoma, and there may be a relationship between the amount of calcification and the activity of the epithelial cells. Microcalcification is not specific to breast cancer, but is a product of increased cellular activity in the lobuloductal complex and may be extruded into the surrounding interstitial tissue. This implies that microcalcification on the mammogram, particularly if sparse, demonstrates a high-risk area of breast rather than a certainty of the presence of carcinoma.

A retrospective review of 859 cases conducted at the Mayo Clinic analyzed 11 morphologic categories that were encountered in a mammogram and correlated to pathological findings. Within these categories, the percentages of cases with a surgical pathologic diagnosis of malignant involvement were as follows: benign calcification (0% malignant); indeterminate calcification (22%); malignant calcification (92%); smooth mass (1%); irregular mass (40%); architectural distortion (47%); asymmetric breast tissue (3%); smooth mass with calcification (0%); irregular mass with calcification (66%); architectural distortion with calcification (57%); and asymmetric breast tissue with calcification (29%). The overall rate of malignant involvement for the 859 cases was 34%.

Recommendation

Compare with previous mammogram to determine if the microcalcifications are a new finding. If they are a new finding, then stereotactic needle core biopsy (SNCB) should be considered to establish tissue diagnosis. If this procedure is not available, then a needle-localized excisional biopsy should be performed.

Case Continued

You recommend that a stereotactic core biopsy be performed. The pathology demonstrates lobular carcinoma in situ and fibrocystic changes including sclerosing adenosis. Calcifications are seen in association with benign fibrocystic changes.

Discussion

LCIS, also known as lobular neoplasia, is a marker of abnormal proliferative activity of both breasts, increasing the risk for subsequent breast cancer. Typically, LCIS is an incidental pathologic finding in breast tissue that has been removed for some mammographic or physical examination finding. There are no gross or mammographic findings specifically associated with LCIS. It does not form a mass, produce nipple discharge, or routinely produce mammographic findings such as calcifications or architectural distortion. In retrospective reviews of benign breast biopsies, LCIS occurs 0.5% to 4.3% of the time. An increasing incidence of LCIS has been noted in recent years, with most LCIS being detected in the fifth decade of life, as is most invasive breast cancer.

Patients diagnosed with LCIS have an increased probability of developing invasive breast cancer, with a relative risk ranging from 6.9 to 12. In the longest follow-up series, the probability of developing an invasive breast cancer by 10 years after a diagnosis of LCIS was 13%; it was 26% after 20 years and 35% by

35 years, or approximately 1% per year. Stated another way, 87% of patients at 10 years and 74% of patients at 20 years will remain free of invasive disease during the 15 years subsequent to diagnosis. The disease-related mortality rate is about 2.8% in patients treated with observation. It is important to note that this risk is equal for both breasts, regardless of the side on which the original biopsy was performed. The most common histology of invasive breast cancer occurring following the diagnosis of LCIS is invasive ductal carcinoma, not invasive lobular carcinoma, as many would expect to be evident.

As depicted in the case presentation, most LCIS is diagnosed as an incidental finding in a biopsy for another cause. It is not necessary to attempt wide local excision for margin control when LCIS is detected. In all situations, however, one must review the reason for recommending the original biopsy: if the microscopic pathologic findings *in addition* to the LCIS finding are not concordant with prebiopsy imaging findings, then a repeat core biopsy or open surgical biopsy is necessary to completely rule out malignancy because LCIS alone would not account for any physical or mammographic/ultrasonographic abnormalities. If the microscopic findings *in addition* to the finding of LCIS are concordant with the prebiopsy imaging findings, then open surgical biopsy may be omitted. If there are equivocal findings on core biopsy, then an open surgical biopsy is mandated. The pleomorphic variety of LCIS is sometimes difficult to distinguish from DCIS microscopically. E-cadherin staining may assist with the diagnosis; however, if a definitive diagnosis of LCIS or DCIS cannot be made, surgical biopsy is warranted, as the management of DCIS is quite different from the management of LCIS.

When LCIS is found in association with invasive cancer, lumpectomy margins should be free of invasive cancer and DCIS, but margin control of the LCIS component is not necessary. Several studies have shown that patients with primary invasive cancer associated with LCIS have equivalent locoregional recurrence and survival to those without an LCIS component.

Approach

For those patients with LCIS, there are three management strategies: surveillance, chemoprevention, and prophylactic surgery. A thorough discussion with the patient should ensue so that she may participate in the decision-making process regarding management of her risk.

As stated previously, patients diagnosed with LCIS have a low likelihood of developing subsequent breast cancer, albeit a higher rate than the general population. Observation with mammography and history and physical examination is an acceptable management strategy for most of these women. Patients should be seen every 6 to 12 months for a complete history and physical examination, in addition to breast self-examination and awareness. Annual mammography is also recommended.

Tamoxifen, a selective estrogen-receptor modulator, is the only medication approved by the Food and Drug Administration for chemoprevention in breast cancer. Data from the National Surgical Adjuvant Breast and Bowel Project (NSABP) Breast Cancer Prevention Trial show that tamoxifen is effective in reducing risk associated with LCIS. In this prospective randomized study of tamoxifen versus placebo in more than 13,000 women at increased risk for breast cancer, tamoxifen decreased the incidence of breast cancer by 49%. A subset analysis revealed that 826 women in the study had an increased risk for breast cancer secondary to LCIS. For the 415 women in the tamoxifen arm, tamoxifen decreased the risk of breast cancer by 56%, as reported by Fisher et al. The decision to recommend tamoxifen must be made in the context of the risk versus benefit. In addition to breast cancer risk reduction, tamoxifen improves bone density in postmenopausal women; further, its use reduces the risk of osteoporosis-induced fractures. Adverse side effects of tamoxifen include hot flashes and vaginal dryness. Rarely, endometrial cancer, thromboembolic events, and cataracts are observed in the postmenopausal patient population taking tamoxifen.

Prophylactic mastectomy is usually only considered in those patients who prefer mastectomy because of their anxiety or who have a strong family history of breast cancer. In patients who have a strong family history of breast cancer, prophylactic mastectomy can decrease the incidence of subsequent breast cancer by 90%. Bilateral mastectomy is indicated in these patients because the breast cancer risk conferred by LCIS is bilateral in nature. The mastectomy can be done with or without immediate reconstruction, as the patient prefers.

Follow-up of patients with LCIS includes interval history and physical examinations every 6 to 12 months for 5 years, and then annually. For patients treated without bilateral prophylactic mastectomy, annual mammography is recommended.

Case Continued

After the options have been explained, the patient elects to pursue chemoprevention with tamoxifen. She understands that tamoxifen is very well tolerated, with few adverse side effects seen in premenopausal women. She will continue with breast self-examination, yearly mammography, and biannual clinician breast examination.

Suggested Readings

Bland KI, Copeland EM III, eds. *The breast: comprehensive management of benign and malignant disorders*. 3rd ed. St. Louis, MO: WB Saunders; 2004.

Fisher B, Costantino JP, Wickerham DL, et al. Tamoxifen for prevention of breast cancer: report of the National Surgical Adjuvant Breast and Bowel Project P-1 Study. *J Natl Cancer Inst* 1998;90:1371–1388.

Frykberg ER. Lobular carcinoma of the breast. *Breast J* 1999;5:296–303.

Harris JR, Lippman ME, Morrow M, et al, eds. *Diseases of the breast*. 3rd ed. Philadelphia, PA: Lippincott Williams & Wilkins; 2004.

Hartmann LC, Schaid DJ, Woods JE, et al. Efficacy of bilateral prophylactic mastectomy in women with a family history of breast cancer. *N Engl J Med* 1999;340:77–84.

Knutzen AM, Gisvold JJ. Likelihood of malignant disease for various categories of mammographically detected, nonpalpable breast lesions. *Mayo Clin Proc* 1993 8:454–460.

Singletary SE. Lobular carcinoma of the breast: a 31-year experience at the University of Texas M.D. Anderson Cancer Center. *Breast Dis* 1994;7:157–163.

Presentation

A 39-year-old woman underwent a routine screening mammogram and is found to have clustered microcalcifications in the upper outer quadrant of the left breast. The patient's mother had undergone a mastectomy for "breast cancer" at age 47 and is alive and free of disease. There is no other family history of breast or ovarian cancer. Review of systems and physical examination are normal. There is no palpable breast mass or axillary/supraclavicular lymphadenopathy.

Differential Diagnosis

The analysis of microcalcifications can be challenging. If they are scattered, the most important determination is whether or not there are casting calcifications present. If so, malignancy cannot be excluded. If clustered, then analysis of their form becomes critical. Teacup or pearl-type calcifications are benign. Granular or casting calcifications are malignant. Clustered calcifications that appear obviously malignant or highly suspicious for malignancy warrant a biopsy whether or not an associated mass is clinically palpable. Some of the pathological entities that can cause calcifications include ductal ectasia, fat necrosis, atypical ductal hyperplasia, ductal carcinoma in situ (DCIS), and invasive carcinoma with extensive intraductal component (EIC). If calcifications are obviously benign, then routine follow-up at 4- to 6-month intervals is recommended if there is a high probability that they are benign. Otherwise, biopsy should be performed at the discretion of the clinician.

Discussion

Cancer cells are classified as in situ or invasive depending on whether or not they invade through the basement membrane. Broder's original description of in situ breast cancer stressed the absence of invasion of cancer cells into the surrounding stroma and their confinement within natural ductal and alveolar boundaries. Because areas of invasion may be minute, the accurate diagnosis of in situ cancer necessitates the analysis of multiple microscopy sections to exclude invasion. In 1941, Foote and Stewart published a landmark manuscript, which distinguished lobular carcinoma in situ (LCIS) from DCIS. In the late 1960s, Gallagher and Martin published a descriptive study of whole breast sections and described a stepwise progression from benign breast tissue to in situ cancer and subsequently to invasive cancer. They coined the term *minimal breast cancer* (LCIS, DCIS, and invasive cancers smaller than 0.5 cm in size) and stressed the importance of early detection.

DCIS accounts for 20% of all breast cancers in women and up to 5% of breast cancers in men. It occurs most commonly in the fifth decade of life. The term *intraductal carcinoma* is frequently applied to DCIS, which carries a high risk for progression to an invasive cancer. DCIS is suspected when clustered microcalcifications are detected on screening mammogram. These clusters demonstrate pleomorphic or fine, linear, and branching microcalcifications. Palpable DCIS tumors have been described, but these are uncommon. DCIS presents as a single lesion (unifocal DCIS) or as multiple lesions, which may be limited to one quadrant of the breast (multifocal DCIS) or may involve two or more quadrants (multicentric DCIS).

Before the widespread use of mammography, diagnosis of breast cancer was by physical examination. At that time, in situ cancers constituted approximately 5% of all breast cancers and, by a ratio of more than 2:1, LCIS was diagnosed more frequently than DCIS. However, now that screening mammography is widely utilized, a 10-fold increase in the incidence of in situ cancer (50%) has been seen and, by a ratio of more than 2:1, DCIS is more frequently diagnosed than LCIS.

Tissue for histological diagnosis can be obtained by percutaneous stereotactic core biopsy. However, negative core biopsy of a suspicious mammography lesion should be followed by confirmatory needle-localization excisional biopsy to avoid diagnostic failure secondary to sampling error. Similarly, a stereotactic core biopsy diagnosis of atypical ductal hyperplasia should result in a confirmatory needle-localization excisional biopsy to avoid missing associated DCIS.

Specific classification of DCIS is problematic because of tumor heterogeneity and interobserver variation in histological classification. However, two broad categories for DCIS are agreed upon: comedo and noncomedo types. DCIS is classified as comedo type based on the presence of necrotic cellular debris within the ducts, the presence of numerous mitoses and large pleomorphic nuclei, and the absence of specific architectural changes.

Recommendation

Compression mammography is recommended for this patient to further characterize the microcalcifications. Stereotactic core biopsy is recommended to establish tissue diagnosis. However, if this is not available, then a needle-localized excisional breast biopsy should be performed.

Mammograms

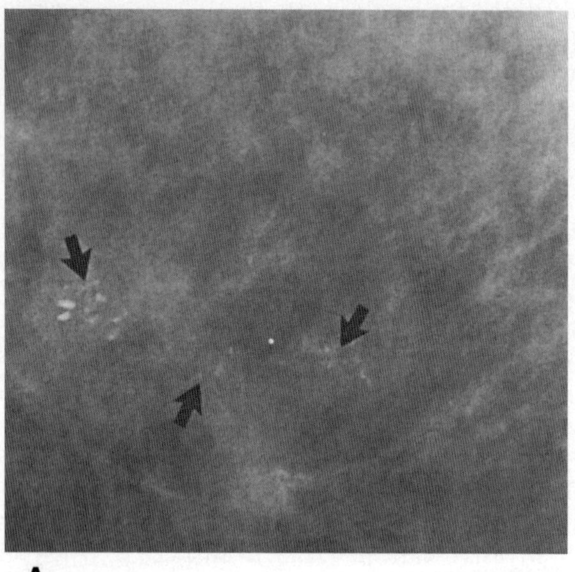

A

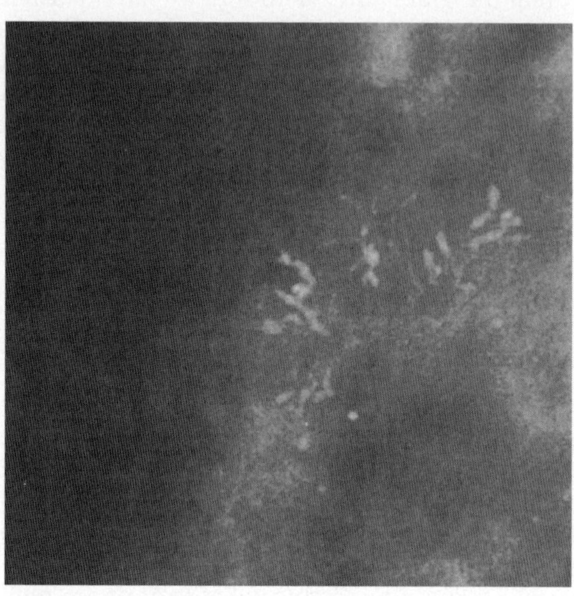

B

Figure 57.1

Mammography Report

Compression mammography demonstrates two foci of calcifications in the upper outer quadrant of the left breast, each measuring <2.0 cm in size and separated by 1.0 cm of apparently uninvolved breast tissue. Clusters of pleomorphic microcalcifications **(A)** and fine, linear, and branching microcalcifications **(B)** are present.

Case Continued

Stereotactic core biopsy is performed. Histological examination of the submitted specimen reveals noncomedo DCIS. Follow-up mammography reveals that most, but not all, of the microcalcifications had been removed with the core biopsy.

Approach

The two general options for management of DCIS are either a total mastectomy or breast conservation that involves a wide local excision with or without adjuvant radiation therapy. The role of sentinel node biopsy in the treatment algorithm for DCIS is controversial and is still evolving. Skin-sparing mastectomy with immediate reconstruction is generally performed only for multicentric DCIS or for multifocal DCIS that is not amenable to lumpectomy. When DCIS is large (>4 cm) and high grade, there is an increased chance of an invasive component, and if the patient has elected mastectomy, then sentinel lymph node biopsy is indicated. If a patient elects to undergo a lumpectomy, then sentinel lymph node biopsy is not performed at the initial operation because approximately 70% may not have an associated invasive component, and thus they can avoid an unnecessary procedure even though it is minimally invasive.

Most frequently, needle-localization lumpectomy is performed, which implies complete removal of the DCIS with a margin of normal appearing breast tissue. This requires a preoperative visit to the mammography suite for placement of a localization wire. Using the wire as a guide, the surgeon subsequently excises the DCIS along with a 1.0-cm margin of normal-appearing breast tissue. After excision of the DCIS, the lumpectomy tissue specimen is orientated for the pathologist using sutures, surgical clips, or dyes. Histological evaluation of the lumpectomy specimen determines whether there is a 0.5-cm or larger surgical margin of normal-appearing tissue. If this is not the case, re-excision is performed. A margin of 1.0 cm is required for unifocal DCIS larger than 2.5 cm, for multifocal DCIS, or for DCIS with microinvasion.

For subareolar and centrally located DCIS, circumareolar incisions provide adequate exposure and result in acceptable scars. For DCIS located elsewhere, incisions that parallel Langer lines (lines of tension in the skin that are generally concentric with the nipple-areola complex) result in acceptable scars. It is important to maintain lumpectomy incisions within the boundaries of the skin excision that may be required as part of a subsequent mastectomy. Radial incisions in the upper half of the breast are not recommended because of possible scar contracture resulting in displacement of the nipple-areola complex.

After lumpectomy (and re-excision for adequate margins if necessary), patients are stratified into three groups for subsequent therapy: (a) those with unifocal DCIS measuring <0.5 cm and favorable histology (low grade, noncomedo) may forego adjuvant radiation therapy; (b) those with unifocal DCIS measuring 0.5 to 2.5 cm require external beam radiotherapy to the ipsilateral breast or accrual to a prospective clinical trial; and (c) those with unifocal DCIS measuring >2.5 cm, multifocal DCIS, or DCIS with microinvasion require external beam radiotherapy.

Case Continued

Management options were discussed with the patient. These included (a) needle-localization lumpectomy followed by external beam radiotherapy to the ipsilateral breast and (b) skin-sparing mastectomy (with or without sentinel node biopsy) with immediate reconstruction. After thorough discussion, the patient opted for needle-localization lumpectomy followed by radiation therapy.

■ Surgical Approach

The patient undergoes placement of a localizing wire adjacent to the mammographic abnormality. In the operating room, the patient is placed in the supine position with the ipsilateral arm in 90 degrees abduction. The breast and the localizing wire are prepped and draped in a sterile fashion. Using the two views (mediolateral and craniocaudal) of the mammograms with the wire in situ, the surgeon needs to develop a three-dimensional relationship of the abnormal microcalcification to the localizing wire. Often the area of concern is a considerable distance from the skin entry site of the wire, and therefore its location needs to be assessed to allow correct placement of the incision.

A curvilinear skin crease incision is made (avoid radial incisions), after which the depth of the lesion from the skin is assessed to determine the thickness of the flaps. Circumferential dissection is performed, and the wire is carefully brought out through the main incision. Usually the hook portion of the wire is distal to the lesion. Therefore, as long as the hook is not encountered during the distal dissection, the surgeon can be confident of being beyond the target lesion. Once resected, the specimen is oriented for the pathologists with sutures, and is first sent to radiology for a specimen radiograph to confirm complete resection of the lesion. If there is doubt regarding any of the margins, then shave biopsies of the appropriate area can be taken. Some surgeons routinely take shave biopsies from all four quadrants of the cavity as well as a deep margin. Small titanium surgical clips are then placed in the lumpectomy site to delineate the area for subsequent radiotherapy.

Case Continued

The patient undergoes needle-localized wide local excision of the DCIS. Specimen mammography reveals that all clustered microcalcifications have been removed. Histological examination of the submitted specimen shows multifocal involvement of the surgical margins by DCIS. There is no invasive carcinoma.

Recommendations

The options at this juncture include undergoing a re-excision, although with widely positive margin the success of breast conservation is unlikely. The other alternative is to perform either a standard total or a skin-sparing mastectomy, with or without reconstruction, depending on the wishes for the patient. The various options for reconstruction necessitate a preoperative consultation with a plastic surgeon, and this may include tissue transfer (pedicle or free transverse rectus abdominis muscle [TRAM] flap) or using implants. To allow symmetry, additional interventions are often required on the contralateral breast. The patient therefore needs to be aware that choosing reconstruction usually involves undergoing additional surgical procedures. If the wide local excision had shown evidence of an invasive component, then a sentinel node biopsy would be offered. However, even in the absence of an invasive component, a sentinel biopsy would be appropriate when total mastectomy is being considered for DCIS only. If pathology subsequently shows an invasive carcinoma, the patient would have avoided an axillary lymph node dissection and its attendant potential complications.

Case Continued

The patient undergoes skin-sparing mastectomy and reconstruction utilizing a free TRAM flap. The internal mammary vessels are used for arterial/venous anastomosis.

Suggested Readings

Cady B, Chung M. Surgical management of "early" breast cancer. In: Bland KI, Copeland EM III, eds. *The breast.* 3rd ed. St. Louis, MO: Saunders; 2004:1103–1128.

Deawr M. Legal issues in breast disease. In: Bland KI, Copeland EM III, eds. *The breast.* 3rd ed. St. Louis, MO: Saunders; 2004: 1585–1596.

Page DL, Simpson JF. In situ carcinomas of the breast: ductal carcinoma in situ, Paget's disease, lobular carcinoma in situ. In: Bland KI, Copeland EM III, eds. *The breast.* 3rd ed. St. Louis, MO: Saunders; 2004:255–278.

Robinson DS, Sundaram M. Stereotactic imaging and breast biopsy. In: Bland KI, Copeland EM III, eds. *The breast.* 3rd ed. St. Louis, MO: Saunders; 2004:685–696.

Silverstein MJ, Woo C. Ductal carcinoma in situ: diagnostic and therapeutic controversies. In: Bland KI, Copeland EM III, eds. *The breast.* 3rd ed. St. Louis, MO: Saunders; 2004:985–1018.

Vicini FA, Kestin L, Martinez A. Radiotherapy and ductal carcinoma in situ. In: Bland KI, Copeland EM III, eds. *The breast.* 3rd ed. St. Louis, MO: Saunders; 2004:1151–1158.

Presentation

A 60-year-old woman presented with an itching right nipple, with some crust, redness, and occasional bloody discharge. This abnormality has developed gradually over the past 5 months. An ointment containing corticosteroids, prescribed by the family practitioner about 2 months before, did not improve the symptoms. The family practitioner referred the patient to your breast clinic for further evaluation.

History reveals no specific breast complaints or symptoms, previous surgery, or mammographic screening. There is no family history of breast cancer. The patient has had psoriasis for many years, but is otherwise healthy.

Clinical Photographs

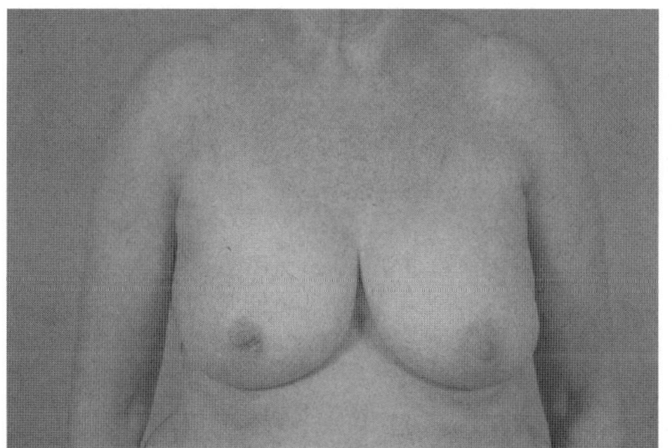

Figure 58.1A

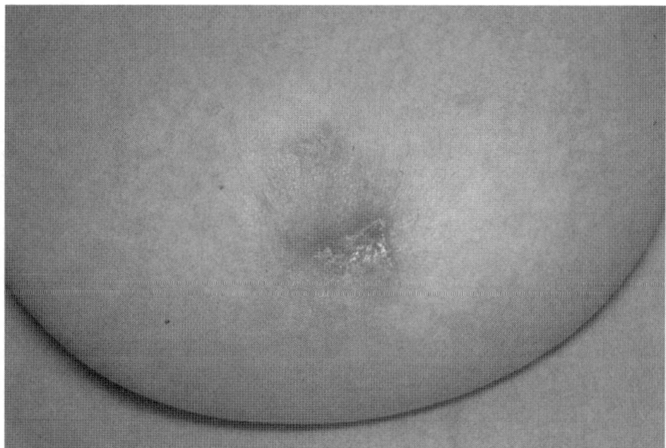

Figure 58.1B

Physical Examination Report

On physical examination, the right nipple shows a crusted, eczematous, elevated redness over an area of about 2 cm. The areola feels somewhat indurated without any lumps or firm tissues in the retroareolar region. The remaining breast tissue is unremarkable without suspicious enlarged axillary lymph nodes.

Differential Diagnosis

Paget disease of the nipple is suspected. Nipple adenoma, papillomatosis, invasive ductal carcinoma, squamous cell carcinoma, eczema of the nipple, and chronic infection or fistulae by duct ectasia cannot be excluded on clinical grounds.

Discussion

Paget disease of the nipple is an uncommon manifestation of breast carcinoma, representing approximately 1% to 3% of all cases. Patients present clinically with eczematous changes of the nipple occasionally associated with itching, ulceration, and bleeding. Histologically, Paget disease is characterized by intraepidermal spread of large round or ovoid tumor cells with abundant pale cytoplasms and large pleomorphic and hyperchromatic nuclei with prominent nucleoli. Regarding the exact origin of these Paget cells, currently most authors postulate the epidermotropic theory, which assumes that Paget cells are ductal carcinoma cells that have migrated from the underlying mammary ducts to the epidermis of the nipple. This theory is supported by the presence of underlying ductal carcinoma in situ (DCIS) or invasive breast carcinoma in nearly all patients (97%).

Paget disease can only be diagnosed with a punch (2 to 3 mm) biopsy. Punch biopsy is advised when any abnormality of the nipple is encountered. Further, a two-view mammography should be performed to evaluate for any abnormality within the breast parenchyma, such as microcalcifcations that could be associated with DCIS, or invasive cancer. Spot magnification view of the retroareolar region may be helpful for improved definition of the extent of microcalcifications. Ultrasound of the breast may show signs of invasive cancer. If this is encountered, ultrasound-directed core biopsies should be taken to confirm this suspicion. The role of magnetic resonance imaging (MRI) of the breast is not completely clear, but if further extension of the disease in the retroareolar area or further in the breast is suspected, MRI may be helpful to exclude the possibility of invasive cancer.

Case Continued

The following tests are performed: two-view mammography of both breasts and retroareolar spot compression view of the right breast; ultrasound of the retroareolar area of the right breast; and a punch biopsy (3 mm) of the right nipple in the abnormal area.

▣ Mammogram

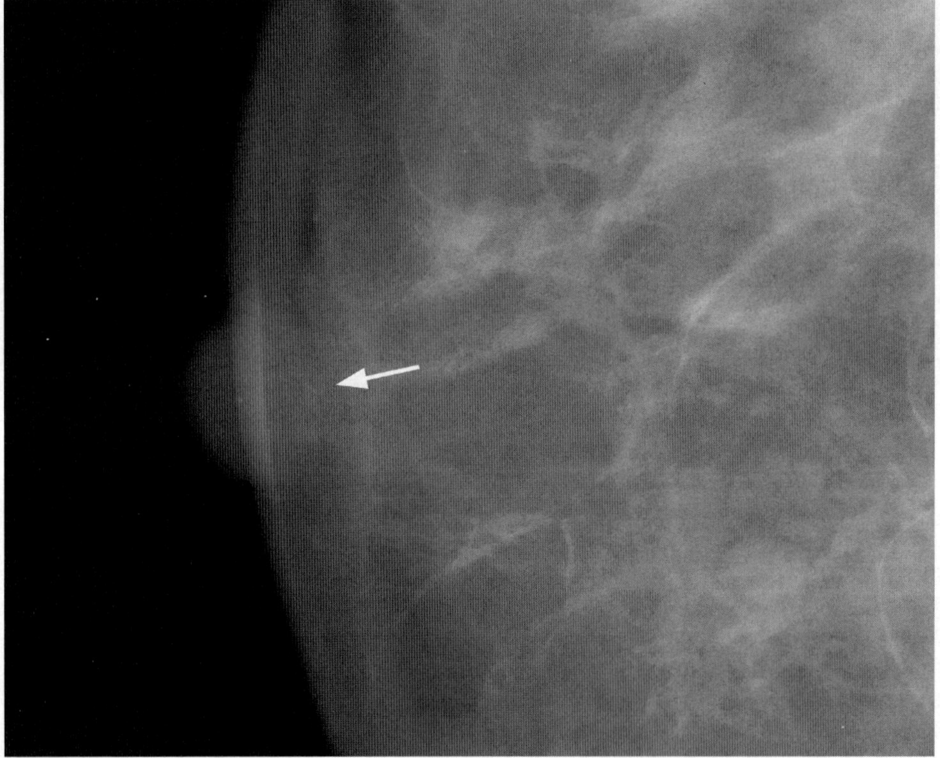

Figure 58.2

Mammography Report

On mammography, the left breast is without abnormalities; in the right breast, a few microcalcifications are found in the immediate retroareolar region, but no other abnormalities are seen. A magnification view of the retroareolar region confirms the three or four microcalcifications without signs of further extension.

Case Continued

On ultrasound, there is some duct ectasia but no further abnormality or suspicious reflections and no enlarged or suspicious lymph nodes in the axilla.

Histopathology Slide

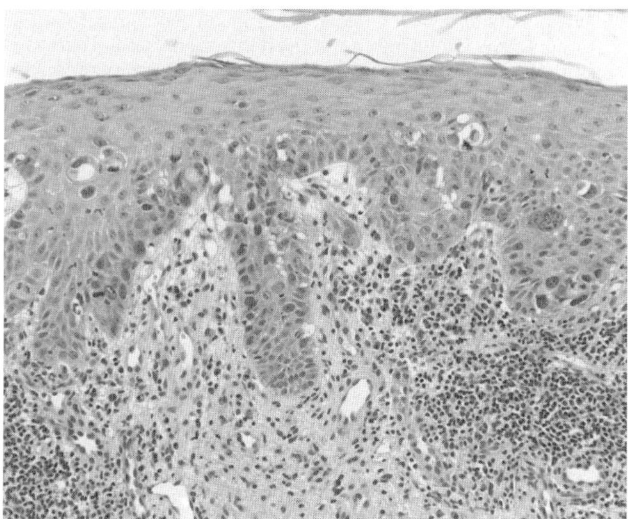

Figure 58.3

Histopathology Report

The punch biopsy showed the typical, large, pale-staining Paget cells, including the round or oval nuclei and large nucleoli in the epidermis. In the retroareolar area, one duct was seen with poorly differentiated DCIS.

Diagnosis

The diagnosis of Paget disease of the nipple is established, with probably associated retroareolar DCIS. There are no signs of invasive cancer in the breast or presence of lymph node metastasis.

Recommendation

Different options are discussed with the patient: simple mastectomy; modified radical mastectomy; excision of the nipple areolar complex, including a cone-shaped part of the central breast (as the first step of breast conservation, followed by radiation therapy); and definitive radiation therapy of the breast with a boost to the nipple.

In the absence of signs of invasive cancer and the associated retroareolar DCIS, we advised breast-conserving central cone excision followed by radiation therapy as the preferred option. The patient consents to this recommendation.

Surgical Approach

The resection can be performed with general anesthesia or with local anesthesia and sedation. The nipple-areolar complex (NAC) is excised with a 1-cm margin using an elliptical incision oriented in a horizontal direction, and the underlying subcutaneous and breast tissue directly under the NAC is resected over an area about 4 cm deep and 4 cm in diameter. The specimen should be marked with a stitch at the cranial side (at the 12 o'clock position) and sent immediately to the pathology lab. After hemostasis is achieved, the skin is closed intracutaneously with absorbable material. The postoperative course is uneventful and the patient is discharged home the same day.

Case Continued

The final diagnosis of Paget disease is confirmed, and this is associated with poorly differentiated DCIS over about 1 cm. All resection margins are free of tumor, with a minimal margin of 7 mm. No invasive cancer is seen.

Recommendation

For treatment of DCIS, the patient is advised to undergo whole breast irradiation. Axillary treatment is not necessary, because no invasive cancer is encountered.

Case Continued

The patient receives radiation therapy to the breast in two tangential fields, in 25 fractions of 2 Gy delivered in 5 weeks, for a total dose of 50 Gy. Apart from some redness of the skin at the end of the radiotherapy course, the treatment is uneventful. Four years later, the patient is free of disease and without abnormality on physical examination and mammography.

Discussion

Paget disease of the nipple is associated with DCIS in the majority of cases (77%) and with invasive cancer in 20%; Paget cells alone are seen only rarely (3%). Once invasive cancer is suspected or proven, the invasive lesion may be much more extensive, and axillary lymph node involvement is seen in over half of the patients. In patients with Paget disease associated with invasive cancer, a modified radical mastectomy is still considered standard treatment. Alternatively, a total mastectomy with a sentinel node biopsy for axillary staging can be performed. If the lesion is not associated with any abnormality on imaging or with only a limited extension of micro-calcifications without density, the lesion can be approached as poorly differentiated DCIS. The role of lymphatic mapping by sentinel node biopsy in DCIS is unclear, as it is in DCIS associated with Paget disease of the nipple. Breast-conserving therapy can be considered, including a central wide local exci-sion with free margins. If radiation therapy is pro-vided, local control is comparable to that of breast-conserving therapy in DCIS: 95% in 5 years. Some authors report from small series that radiation ther-apy of the breast and a boost dose on the nipple may suffice and lead to comparable results.

In conclusion, Paget disease of the nipple can only be diagnosed histologically with punch biopsy. If no apparent invasive cancer is suspected or proven, breast-conserving therapy with a central cone excision, including the NAC and followed by radiotherapy, may be the preferred option. If inva-sive cancer is suspected or proven, more extensive spread is likely and a modified radical mastectomy or a total mastectomy with sentinel node biopsy is advised. If an invasive component is present, adju-vant systemic treatments should be considered.

Suggested Readings

Bijker N, Rutgers EJ, Duchateau L, et al. EORTC Breast Cancer Cooperative Group. Breast-conserving therapy for Paget dis-ease of the nipple: a prospective European Organization for Research and Treatment of Cancer study of 61 patients. *Cancer* 2001;91:472–477.

Kaelin CM. Paget's disease. In: Harris JR, Lippman ME, Morrow M, et al., eds. *Diseases of the breast*. 3rd ed. Philadelphia, PA: Lippincott Williams & Wilkins; 2004:1007–1013.

Kothari AS, Beechey-Newman N, Hamed H, et al. Paget disease of the nipple: a multifocal manifestation of higher-risk disease. *Cancer* 2002;95:1–7.

Marcus E. The management of Paget's disease of the breast. *Curr Treat Options Oncol* 2004;5:153–160.

Marshall JK, Griffith KA, Haffty BG, et al. Conservative manage-ment of Paget disease of the breast with radiotherapy: 10- and 15-year results. *Cancer* 2003;97:2142–2149.

Schelfhout VR, Coene ED, Delaey B, et al. Pathogenesis of Paget's disease: epidermal heregulin-alpha, motility factor, and the HER receptor family. *J Natl Cancer Inst* 2000;92:622–628.

Presentation

A 39-year-old woman with a family history of breast cancer presents to your office with pain in the left arm after physical activity and a tender nodule in her left axilla of 10 days' duration. Her family history is positive for breast cancer with her mother and a paternal aunt diagnosed at a postmenopausal age. There is no family history of ovarian cancer. On examination, two left axillary masses, one measuring 1 cm and the other high in the axilla measuring 2.5 cm, are palpated. There are no breast abnormalities. Prior to her presenting to your office, she had undergone a bilateral diagnostic mammogram, an ultrasound of the left axilla, a core biopsy of the axillary mass, and a metastatic workup. Bilateral mammogram showed dense breast parenchyma with no mammographic evidence of malignancy and the ultrasound findings are shown below.

Ultrasound

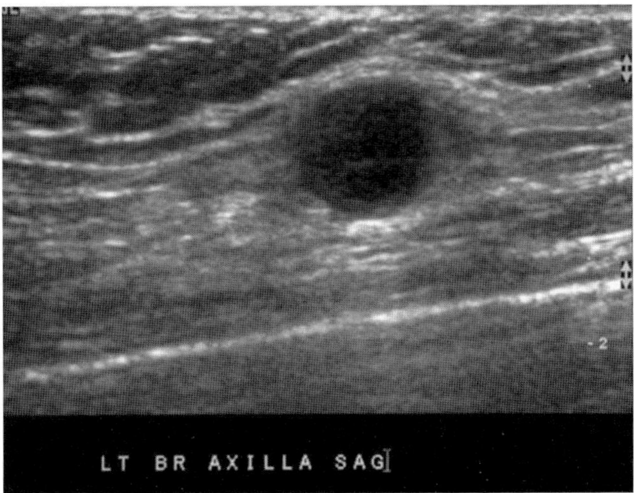

Figure 59.1

Ultrasonography Report

Ultrasound of the left axilla reveals two lesions in the axilla: a 3.3-cm ovoid hypoechoic lesion, highly vascular and with a shallow fatty cleft, and an additional adjacent 1.3-cm hypoechoic lesion. Both lesions are interpreted as lymph nodes. The impression is that these lymph nodes are most consistent with reactive adenopathy; however, malignancy cannot be excluded.

Case Continued

Biopsy of the lymph node revealed metastatic adenocarcinoma.

Differential Diagnosis

The most likely primary tumor site for metastatic adenocarcinoma to the axilla in a woman is the breast. Other potential primary tumor sites include the gastrointestinal and genital tracts and, in a smoker, the lung. A metastatic workup targeting these areas should be based on clinical findings. Serum tumor markers may be helpful in elucidating the primary tumor site.

Discussion

Occult breast cancer presenting with axillary adenopathy is infrequent and constitutes 1% of all breast cancers. In the woman presenting with axillary metastasis from an adenocarcinoma, the most likely primary site is the breast. The breasts should be evaluated by mammography as the initial diagnostic test. Other imaging modalities, such as ultrasound and magnetic resonance imaging (MRI), are also potentially useful for finding the primary breast lesion. MRI with a dedicated breast coil can identify the primary breast cancer in 75% to 80% of patients presenting with axillary adenopathy without mammographic findings, and is most useful in the patient with dense breast parenchyma. Ultrasound can also be helpful in identifying the primary breast tumor; like MRI, it is most useful in patients with dense breast parenchyma. However, breast ultrasound can be operator dependent. If a primary tumor cannot be identified in the breast, then an appropriate metastatic workup can be performed to identify the primary lesion and may include a colonoscopy, gastroscopy, and computed tomography (CT) scans of the chest, abdomen, and pelvis.

Tissue to document the etiology of the adenopathy can be obtained easily with fine-needle aspiration cytology (FNAC) or core needle biopsy. FNAC is the easier technique to perform and can be done with or without sonographic guidance. In addition to verifying the presence of metastatic adenocarcinoma, immunohistochemical evaluation of the biopsy specimen for hormone-receptor status or markers associated with certain primary tumor sites may also be requested. Serum tumor markers may be obtained for these patients, but are not sufficiently specific for any particular organ site.

Recommendation

MRI of the breast and whole breast ultrasound.

Case Continued

The breast MRI did not reveal any specific abnormality.

Ultrasonogram

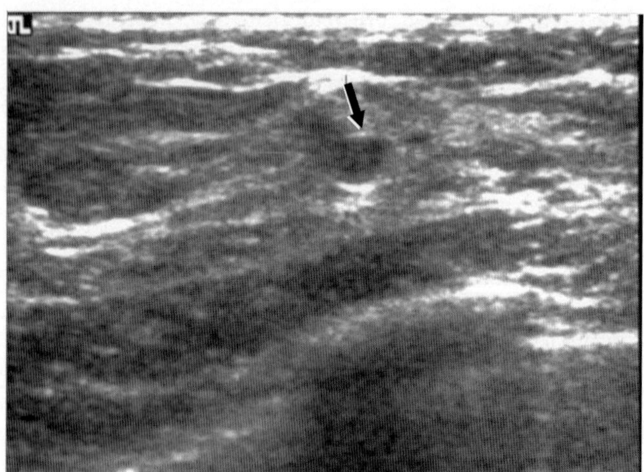

Figure 59.2

Ultrasonography Report

Ultrasound evaluation of the left breast reveals a small irregular density in the breast parenchyma measuring 7 × 4 × 3 mm in the 2 to 3 o'clock position *(arrow)*. The lesion is suspicious for malignancy, and an ultrasound-guided core biopsy of this mass is performed.

Histopathology Slide

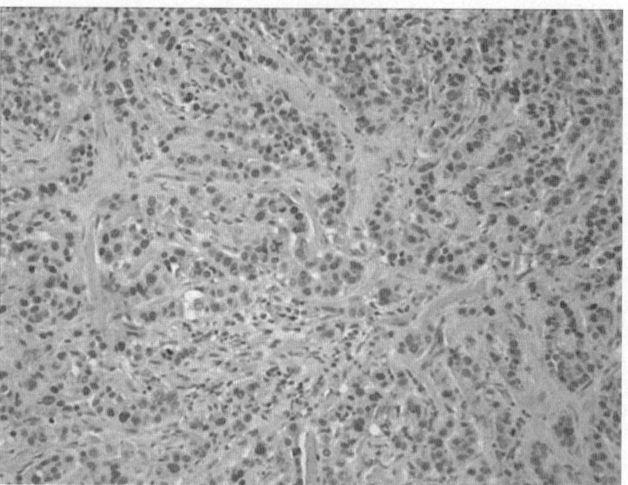

Figure 59.3

Histopathology Report

Positive for infiltrating ductal carcinoma.

Diagnosis and Recommendation

The patient is diagnosed with a primary breast cancer with metastasis to the axilla. Prior to any therapy, she needs a staging workup including CT scan of the chest, abdomen, and pelvis as well as a bone scan.

Case Continued

CT scan of the chest, abdomen, and pelvis and bone scans are all normal with no evidence of distant metastases.

Approach

In the absence of systemic disease, and if a primary lesion can be identified, patients should be treated according to current breast cancer treatment guidelines. Neoadjuvant chemotherapy should be considered in these patients because response to chemotherapy is the best prognostic indicator of outcome. However, if a primary breast tumor cannot be identified, these patients should undergo a level I and II axillary node dissection followed by systemic chemotherapy with or without hormonal therapy. Management of the breast is controversial. If a mastectomy is performed, the primary tumor is not identified in one third of patients. If the breast is observed without intervention until a lesion is identified, a primary tumor does develop in the vast majority of women. Some series have shown a significantly lower overall survival with this approach, compared with patients who received some treatment to the breast. Whole breast radiotherapy in addition to axillary radiotherapy after axillary node dissection and chemotherapy is another option. Based on current results, it appears that the latter would be the most appropriate management of patients who present with axillary metastases from an unknown breast primary. All patients are candidates for systemic cytotoxic chemotherapy, or hormonal treatment, or both.

Case Continued

The patient elects breast-conserving therapy, and appropriate consent is obtained.

■ Surgical Approach

To localize the tumor, first, ultrasonography of the breast is performed and a guide wire is placed, following which the partial mastectomy is performed.

■ Intraoperative Ultrasound

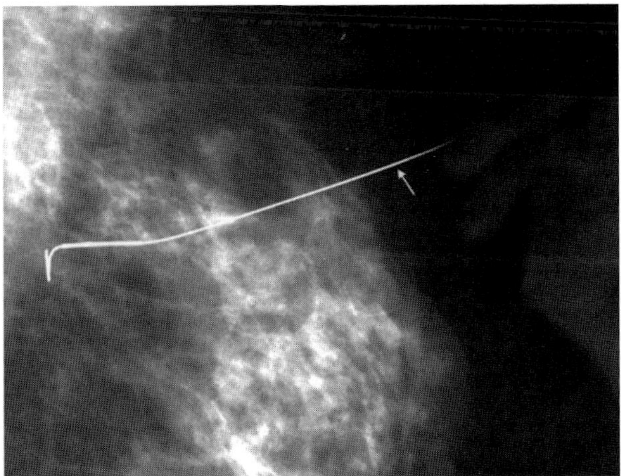

Figure 59.4

Intraoperative Ultrasonography Report

The primary breast tumor was localized using sonographic imaging and a guide wire was placed for localization *(right arrow)*. The lesion had been previously marked by a clip. The lesion cannot be visualized by mammography because of the dense breast parenchyma.

■ Surgical Approach (Continued)

A transverse incision is made in the axilla, and after creating flaps, the important structures should be identified. These include the axillary vein, long thoracic nerve, thoracodorsal nerve, and intercostobrachial nerve. If there is evidence of abnormal lymph nodes in level III, these should also be resected. Often, to improve access to level III, the pectoralis minor tendon needs to be transected. Particular care needs to be taken to avoid injury to the underlying axillary vein while dividing the pectoralis minor. Closed suction drains are placed after hemostasis is achieved.

Case Continued

After a lengthy discussion, the patient declines neoadjuvant chemotherapy. Breast-conserving surgery and axillary node dissection are performed, and the patient is found to have a 7-mm invasive ductal carcinoma. She has four axillary lymph nodes positive for metastasis after a level I/II dissection. She receives systemic adjuvant cytotoxic chemotherapy, followed by whole-breast radiotherapy and comprehensive axillary radiation therapy. She continues to have no evidence of disease approximately 2 years after her initial presentation.

Discussion

Most patients who present with axillary adenopathy from a breast primary have outcomes similar to those who present with nodal disease. A metastatic workup should be performed on these patients because they have a high risk of systemic disease. The breast should be evaluated with a mammogram and ultrasound, and when appropriate with breast MRI. If a primary breast tumor can be identified, these patients should be managed according to current breast cancer treatment guidelines. If a primary breast tumor cannot be found and there is no evidence of systemic disease, the patient should undergo an axillary node dissection, comprehensive whole-breast and axillary radiotherapy, and cytotoxic chemotherapy with or without hormonal therapy. Approximately 40% of the patients will develop systemic disease within 5 years.

Suggested Readings

Chen C, Orel SG, Schnall MD, et al. Breast conservation treatment for patients presenting with axillary lymphadenopathy from presumed primary breast cancer: the role of breast magnetic resonance imaging for staging. *Clin Breast Cancer* 2002;3:219–222.

Foroudi F, Tiver KW. Occult breast carcinoma presenting as axillary metastases. *Int J Radiat Oncol Biol Phys* 2000;47:143–147.

Jackson B, Scott-Conner C. Axillary metastasis from occult breast carcinoma: diagnosis and treatment. *Am Surg* 1995;61:431–435.

Leibman AJ, Kossoff MB. Mammography in women with axillary adenopathy and normal breasts on physical examination: value in detecting occult breast carcinoma. *AJR Am J Roentgenol* 1992;159:493–495.

Matsuoka K, Ohsumi S, Takashima S, et al. Occult breast carcinoma presenting with axillary lymph node metastases: follow-up of eleven patients. *Breast Cancer* 2003;10:330–334.

Medina-Franco H, Urist M. Occult breast carcinoma presenting with axillary lymph node metastases. *Rev Invest Clin* 2002;54:204–208.

Orel SG, Weinstein SP, Schnall MD, et al. Breast MR imaging in patients with axillary node metastases and unknown primary malignancy. *Radiology* 1999;212:543–549.

Rouzier R, Extra JM, Klijanienko J et al. Incidence and prognostic significance of complete axillary downstaging after primary chemotherapy in breast cancer patients with T1 to T3 tumors and cytologically proven axillary metastatic lymph nodes. *J Clin Oncol* 2002;20:1304–1310.

Scoggins CR, Vitola JV, Sandler MP, et al. Occult breast carcinoma presenting as an axillary mass. *Am Surg* 1999;65:1–5.

Presentation

A 64-year-old man presents to your office complaining of a 7-month history of a lump in the left breast, with a bloody discharge from the left nipple that occurs with mild pressure noted over the last 2 months. He has no significant past medical history. He is a nonsmoker and is not receiving hormone therapy for any disease. He has no family history of breast carcinoma. On physical examination, a retroareolar hard, irregular mass fixed to the thoracic wall is evident. No skin retraction can be detected. You observe a bloody discharge from the left nipple with mild pressure. No enlarged axillary nodes are palpable.

Differential Diagnosis

The differential diagnosis includes several conditions of breast mass; the most frequent is benign breast hypertrophy during adolescence. This condition develops around puberty or some years later than male breast carcinoma (mean age of male breast cancer, 64 years), and usually presents as a discoid mass under the areola. The young age of the patient and the well-delimited, mobile lump help to make the correct diagnosis.

Gynecomastia, which affects men in the second and third decades of life, is a diffuse enlargement of the breast gland of soft consistency, with characteristics similar to the small female breast. Male breast hypertrophy, which may be idiopathic or related to liver malfunction, can present as a round, mobile, sometimes painful breast mass under the areola.

Male breast carcinoma is so unusual under 30 years of age that there is no indication for biopsy in a clinically benign breast mass in this subgroup of men.

In patients older than 50 years, breast carcinoma should be differentiated from hypertrophy related to different clinical conditions or to medications, which interact with hormonal functions. Benign hypertrophy is usually an elastic, sharp, and regular mass under the areola.

Recommendation

Mammogram, breast ultrasound, and magnetic resonance imaging (MRI) for further characterization are recommended. Because the patient is older than 50 years, and the breast lump has suspicious clinical features, fine-needle aspiration biopsy (FNAB) is recommended to establish a tissue diagnosis.

Mammogram

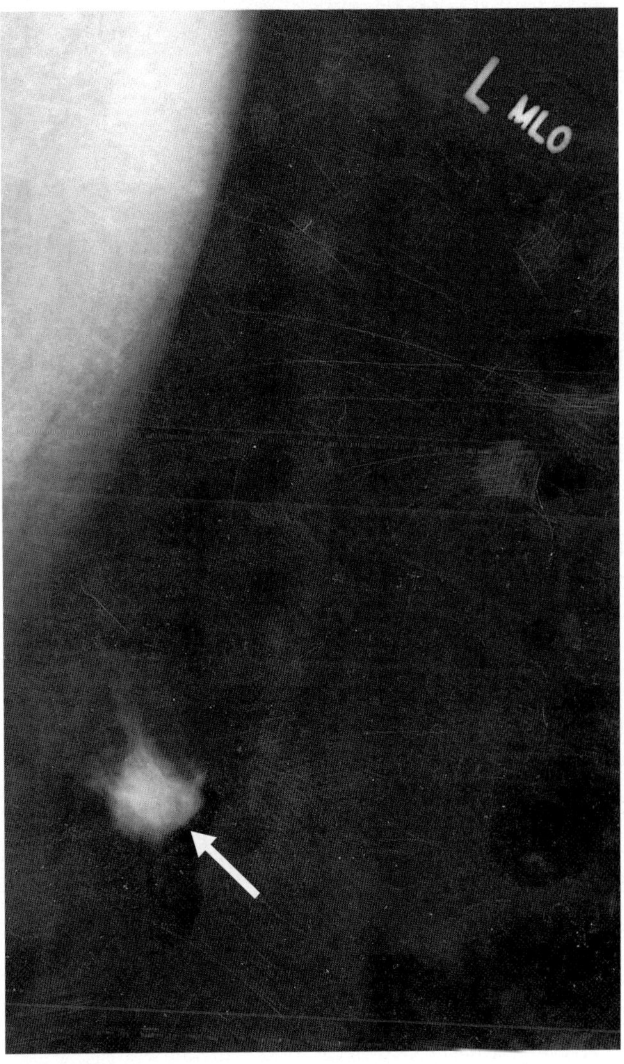

Figure 60.1

Mammography Report

A well-defined density *(arrow)* is seen in the retroareolar region of the left breast.

Ultrasound and Doppler Analysis

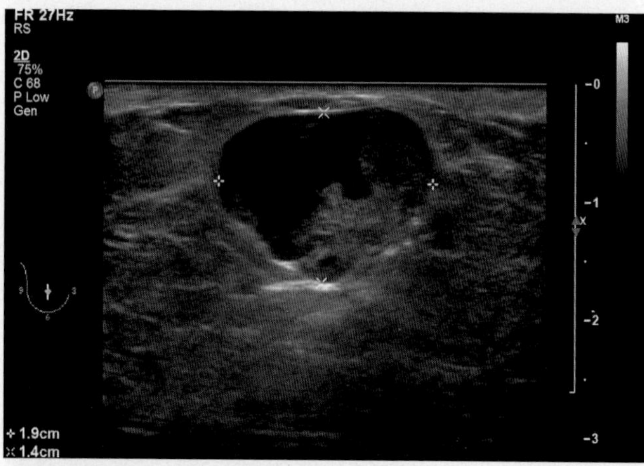

Figure 60.2A

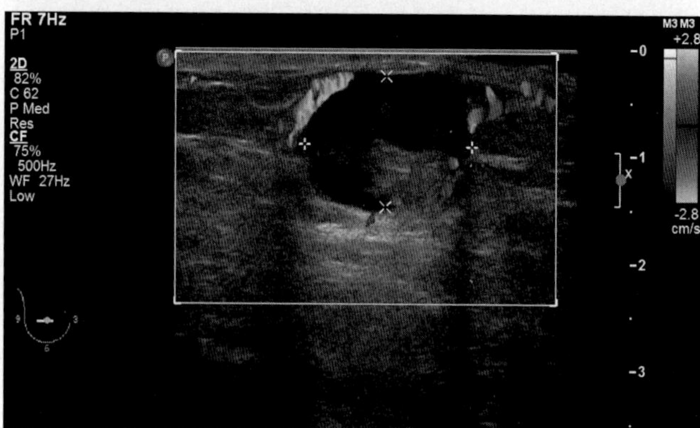

Figure 60.2B

Ultrasonography and Doppler Analysis Report

Ultrasound reveals a 1.9-cm complex lesion in the left breast with irregular margins. Enhanced vascular flow is noted on Doppler analysis.

MRI

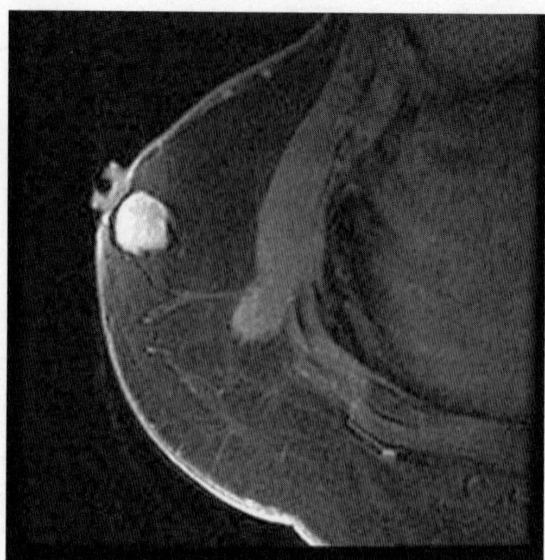

Figure 60.3

MRI Report

MRI demonstrates a 19 × 18 × 18-mm cystic mass with high T1 and T2 signals containing an irregular, 11- to 12-mm, enhancing intracystic solid component and septation. Kinetic assessment demonstrates rapid initial rise with washout of the solid intracystic component. The appearance is highly suspicious for a cystic malignancy.

FNAB Report

FNAB of the breast lesion reveals the presence of malignant tumor cells. Cytologic examination of the bloody nipple discharge reveals the presence of rare atypical cells.

Diagnosis and Recommendation

Male breast cancer. The next step is to perform a staging workup including chest x-ray, liver ultrasound, and bone scan.

Discussion

The diagnosis of breast carcinoma in men is usually done in the presence of symptoms or signs. Men are not screened for breast carcinoma and are not referred to the physician for early signs of breast disease. Risk factors are Klinefelter syndrome, a previous bilateral orchitis, or chronic exposure to high temperature in the work environment. There is evidence that liver damage of any origin, or toxic agents may contribute to a higher risk of developing this disease.

The most typical initial presentation is a breast lump, just as in women. There is no doubt that a man affected by breast carcinoma comes to the observation of the physician later than does a woman with similar symptoms, even if the information about breast cancer currently given to the male population is now more widespread.

The breast lump is hard, not painful, with less delimitation of clinical margins than in the female breast, and is usually proximal to the pectoralis major muscle. It is usually located under the nipple-areolar complex, with a frequent retraction of the nipple; the lump rapidly creates adherence with the skin. In more advanced stages, the neoplasm can infiltrate the skin and create ulceration. The possibility of Paget disease should be kept in mind: the first description of this pathological condition in men is from Treves (1954). The characteristics of Paget disease in men are exactly the same as in women.

A particular aspect of male breast cancer is the association of bloody nipple discharge with the breast lump: this sign is more frequent than in female breast carcinoma. Some authors consider bloody nipple discharge pathognomonic for carcinoma, even in the absence of a breast lump. The differential diagnosis should take into account three other conditions usually associated with bloody nipple discharge: estrogen-induced gynecomasty in prostate cancer; the use of high doses of androgens; and the extremely rare event of ductal papillomatosis.

Just as in women, a good clinical examination should not miss the regional lymph nodes (axilla and supraclavicular region), taking into account that the late diagnosis and the supposed aggressiveness of the disease make the likelihood of nodal involvement significantly high. Alternative lymphatic pathways have not been described in the literature.

Case Continued

Chest x-ray, bone scintigraphy, and liver ultrasound are negative. Due to the clinical negativity of axillary lymph nodes, the identification of the sentinel lymph node with radiotracer is performed the day before surgery.

Lymphoscintigraphy Report

Human serum albumin containing 5 to 10 MBq of technetium-labeled colloid particles ranging between 100 and 1,000 nm in diameter are injected around the tumor, in volumes ranging from 0.2 to 0.3 mL. Frontal and lateral view planar scintigraphy images of the breast and axilla are obtained with a gamma camera. The lymphatic basin at risk is identified, and the location of the highest radioisotope uptake is marked on the skin to facilitate intraoperative identification of the sentinel node.

Approach

Male breast carcinoma has been considered for years a disease with no possible surgical therapy; nowadays it is a neoplasm with a difficult surgical approach. The diagnosis is, in fact, usually late, and some technical problems are related to breast surgery in the male, such as the amount of skin to be removed to ensure a low rate of local recurrence (there is often the need to use a rotation skin flap to close the surgical breach). There is also the open question of whether or not pectoralis muscles should be sacrificed.

Our approach at the European Institute of Oncology in Milan is the Patey mastectomy, with the removal of a skin portion including the nipple, the areola, and a small portion of healthy skin, with the conservation of the pectoralis muscles, and with sentinel lymph node biopsy or axillary dissection in the same way as in women. Sentinel node biopsy can reliably predict the state of the axilla, so that when the sentinel node is negative for metastases, the entire axilla can be assumed to be clear, and axillary dissection can safely be avoided. This is important because the dissection removes immunocompetent tissue and may have complications, such as reduced mobility of the arm, numbness, pain, and lymphedema. Recent reports have shown that male breast cancer is similar to its female counterpart: this finding allowed us to propose similar therapeutic approaches.

When necessary, axillary dissection is performed completely with the removal of lymph nodes of Berg levels I and II.

We do not advocate adjuvant radiotherapy to the thoracic wall, even if some authors are in favor of it, except in cases of skin or pectoralis muscle infiltration.

The partial resection with sentinel node biopsy or axillary dissection and adjuvant radiotherapy, which is indicated in women affected by breast carcinoma of small size, could also offer the same results in men in terms of overall survival and local relapse. However, the frequent location of the tumor under the nipple makes partial surgery inapplicable.

Surgical Approach

General anesthesia is used to perform surgery. Sentinel node biopsy is first performed by making a transverse skin incision in the axilla and identifying the blue lymphatic channel leading to a lymph node that may be blue from 1% isosulfan blue (Lymphazurin) and/or "hot" due to entrapment of the technetium-labeled colloid. Next, a Patey mastectomy (modified radical mastectomy) should be performed. The sentinel node can be examined during surgery by frozen section, and if found to be positive, a complete axillary dissection (level I and II) is performed.

Case Continued

The sentinel node is positive for metastases; complete axillary dissection is performed. The final histology is ductal invasive carcinoma G3, with extension to the nipple. The sentinel node shows evidence of metastases with extracapsular spread. The remaining 33 axillary lymph nodes show no evidence of metastatic disease. The other markers are as follows: ER 90%, PgR 5%, ki-67 40%, c-erbB2, absent; peritumoral vascular invasion, absent.

Discussion

The presence of lymph node metastases, the dimension of the tumor, and the stage of disease influence the prognosis of patients who undergo radical surgery. Some authors consider the length of time that disease was present before diagnosis as a significant prognostic factor. Men affected by noninfiltrating neoplasms have an excellent prognosis with a very low incidence of local relapse; the same consideration is valid for particular histologies such as medullary carcinoma, colloid carcinoma, and papillary carcinoma. The most important prognostic factor is axillary involvement.

◼ Approach

At the European Institute of Oncology, the next step after breast surgery is the multidisciplinary meeting among breast surgeons, medical oncologists, radiation therapists, pathologists, radiologists, physicians from the chemoprevention unit, and plastic surgeons. During the meeting, all the patients treated surgically for breast carcinoma are discussed. The prognostic factors, together with personal and family history, are taken into account for a tailored prescription of adjuvant therapy.

Case Continued

The patient receives chemotherapy (doxorubicin and adriamycin cyclophosphamide [AC] for four cycles), which he tolerates well, followed by tamoxifen 20 mg/day, which is continued for 5 years. He remains free of disease 17 months after surgery.

Suggested Readings

Anelli M, Anelli A, et al. Tamoxifen is associated with high rate of treatment limiting symptoms in male breast cancer patients. *Cancer* 1994;74:74.

Borgen PI, Wong GY, Vlamis V, et al. Current management of male breast cancer, a review of 104 cases. *Ann Surg* 1994;215:451–459.

Donegan WL. Cancer of the male breast. In: Donegan WL, Spratt JS, eds. *Cancer of the breast.* 4th ed. Philadelphia, PA: WB Saunders; 1995.

Gennari R, Renne G, Travaini L, et al. Sentinel node biopsy in male breast cancer: future standard treatment? *Eur J Surg* 2001;167:461–462.

Guinee V, Olsson H, et al. The prognosis of breast cancer in males: a report of 335 cases. *Cancer* 1993;71:154.

Mabuchi K, Bross DS, Kessler, et al. Risk factors for male breast cancer. *J Natl Cancer Inst* 1985;74:371.

Presentation

A 53-year-old minister presents to your office with a 7- to 8-month history of swelling and bruising of the right posterior thigh. There was initial improvement in the ecchymosis, but the mass persisted and then recently increased in size. He denies any neurovascular symptoms in the right lower extremity. Examination of the right lower extremity reveals a 21 × 17-cm mass in the distal aspect of the right thigh. The distal aspect of the mass can be felt at the level of the popliteal fossa. The femoral and the dorsalis pedis pulses are palpable.

Differential Diagnosis

The differential diagnosis of a soft-tissue mass includes benign lesions such as lipomas, leiomyomas, neuromas, lymphangiomas, and soft-tissue sarcomas. Besides sarcomas, other malignant lesions (e.g., primary or metastatic carcinoma, melanoma, or lymphoma) should also be considered.

Discussion

Soft-tissue sarcomas represent a diverse histologic group of rare tumors, but they share a common embryonic origin, the mesoderm. Exceptions include neurosarcomas, Ewing sarcoma, and peripheral neuroectodermal tumors (PNETs) that arise from the ectoderm. Of particular note, although more than 75% of the human body weight consists of soft tissue skeleton, these tumors comprise only 1% of adult malignancies and 15% of all pediatric malignancies. In 2004, approximately 8,680 new cases were expected to have been diagnosed in the United States, with 3,660 deaths, thus underscoring the relatively high overall mortality associated with this malignancy. Soft-tissue sarcomas can occur anywhere in the body but most commonly originate in the extremities (upper extremity, 13%; lower extremity, 32%), the trunk (19%), the retroperitoneum (15%), or the head and neck (9%).

Case Continued

Given the antecedent history of local trauma, the primary care physician orders an ultrasound scan, which demonstrates a mass in the posterior thigh measuring 9 × 5 cm that was thought to be a hematoma. Subsequently, due to continued increase in size of the mass, a computed tomography (CT) scan is obtained, which reveals a 12 × 12-cm mass with areas of central necrosis. Prior to referral to the tertiary center, an incisional biopsy is performed, which reveals a high-grade leiomyosarcoma.

Clinical Photograph

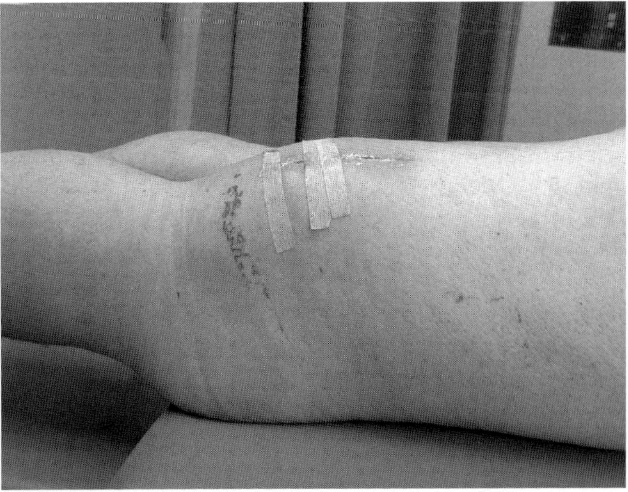

Figure 61.1

Physical Examination Report

View of the posterior thigh shows the mass and the recent incisional biopsy.

Diagnosis and Recommendation

Pretreatment radiologic imaging provides valuable information that aids in the diagnosis by defining the local extent of the tumor, which also assists in local staging of the disease and planning of the biopsy. Plain radiographs are useful for providing information on primary bone tumors, but are not as useful for evaluating soft-tissue tumors of the extremities, except for chronic hematomas for which they may reveal diagnostic calcification. Ultrasonography is also of limited value, except to guide percutaneous biopsies. The current imaging modalities of choice are either contrast-enhanced CT scan or magnetic resonance imaging (MRI), and the debate continues regarding which one is superior. A large multi-institutional trial by the Radiology Diagnostic Oncology Group compared these modalities, correlated their interpretations of the histologic and intraoperative findings, and found no statistical differences. Nevertheless, MRI is the preferred imaging modality for extremity sarcoma because it can provide multiplanar images with better spatial orientation. It also has the advantage of permitting concurrent MR angiography, which allows delineation of the tumor's relationship to adjacent vascular structures. Behavior of the primary tumor following administration of gadolinium contrast allows differentiation from lipomatous benign tumors. Dynamic postcontrast images may also facilitate differentiating viable tumor in adjacent muscle from tumor-associated edema. For low-grade sarcomas, chest radiography should be performed to look for lung metastases, while CT of the chest should be considered for patients with high-grade sarcomas or tumors larger than 5 cm.

To establish a histologic diagnosis, fine-needle aspiration biopsy (FNAB) may be used at centers where experienced cytopathologists are available. The diagnostic accuracy of FNAB in finding sarcomas ranges from 60% to 96%. If tumor grading is essential for treatment planning, then FNAB has limitations due to the small amount of material obtained. Office-based core needle biopsy has a diagnostic accuracy of about 95%, and its yield can be further enhanced by the use of ultrasonography to avoid sampling necrotic and cystic areas, and importantly avoiding neurovascular bundles that may have been displaced superficially. The core biopsy provides enough tissue to establish a histologic diagnosis and tumor grade, and in difficult cases allows additional diagnostic tests, such as electron microscopic examination and cytogenetic analysis. It also has an advantage over open biopsies, which can delay preoperative radiation therapy, and are particularly fraught with wound complications, particularly if the tumor is very large and primary closure can be under tension. If a core biopsy reveals nondiagnostic material, then an incisional biopsy can be performed, but should ideally be part of a well-planned treatment strategy. With a history of a rapidly growing soft-tissue mass, mass larger than 5 cm, and all the deep lesions (deep to the superficial fascia), the clinician should maintain a high degree of suspicion for the possibility of a sarcoma. When performing a biopsy, proper placement of the incision is vital, and it should be performed at a site that can be excised en bloc during the definitive surgery resection. Transverse incisions in the extremities are always contraindicated. The principles of incisional biopsy are as follows: (a) use a small longitudinal incision; (b) avoid flaps; (c) do not expose neurovascular structures; (d) sample the peripheral tumor, which is the most viable representative of the diagnostic portion; (e) avoid crushing the specimen with forceps; (f) obtain frozen section to determine adequacy of the sample; (g) achieve meticulous hemostasis; (h) avoid suction drains; (i) close the wound carefully to prevent necrosis or ulceration of the skin; and (j) biopsy tracks should not traverse normal anatomical muscular skeletal compartments.

Recommendation

Obtain an MRI scan with MR angiogram to determine proximity of the tumor to the neurovascular bundle, as well as determine vessel patency. Obtain CT scan of the chest to exclude metastatic disease.

MRI

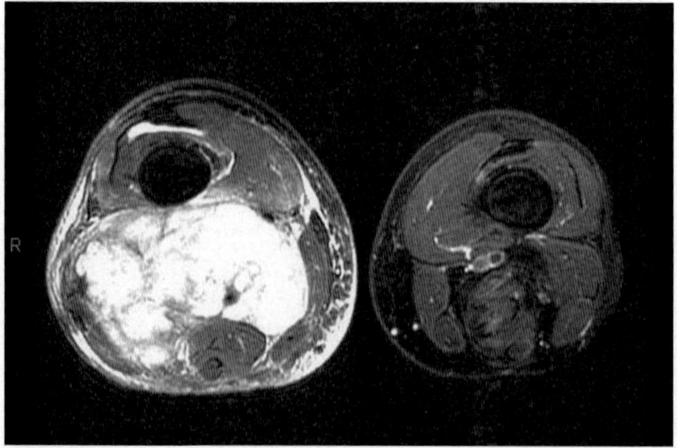

Figure 61.2A

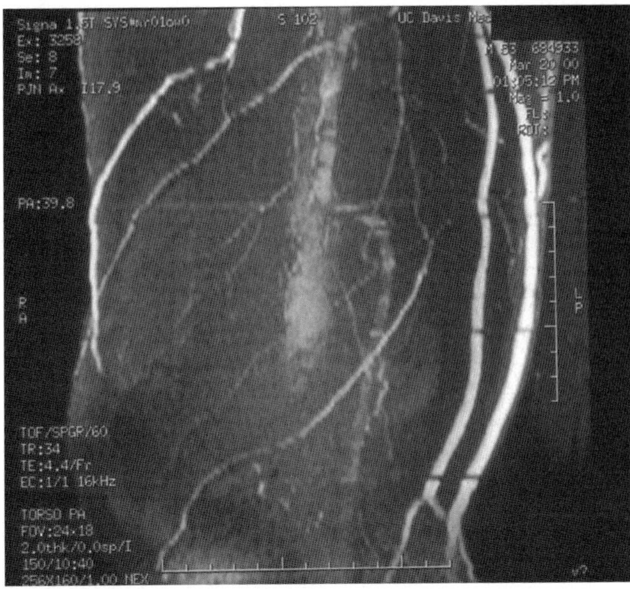

Figure 61.2D

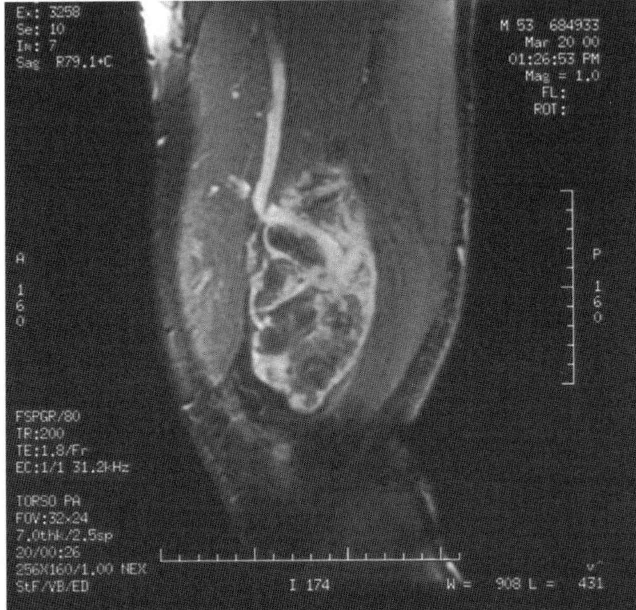

Figure 61.2B

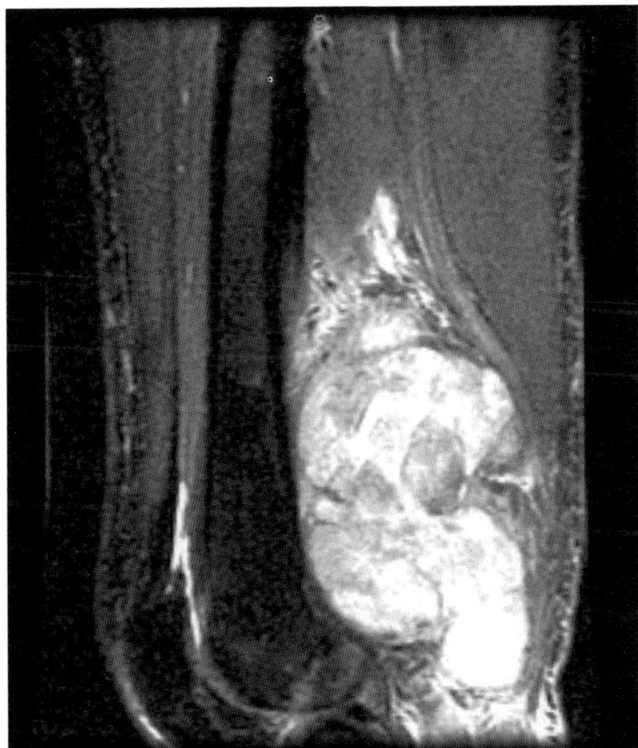

Figure 61.2C

MRI Report

MRI demonstrates a 10 × 14 × 14-cm heterogeneous enhancing mass in the right posterior thigh with complete encasement of the popliteal vessels. The sciatic nerve appears to be displaced posteriorly. The tumor abuts the posterior surface of the femur for at least 10 cm. Axial view **(A)** and sagittal view **(B)** show encasement of popliteal artery, and the sagittal view **(C)** shows abutment to femur. MR angiogram **(D)** reveals distortion of the popliteal artery.

Case Continued

No pulmonary metastases are seen.

Approach

Given the locally extensive nature of the sarcoma with encasement of the vessels, possible involvement of the sciatic nerve, and abutment to the femur, one of the options is an above-knee amputation. The alternative would be a limb-sparing approach that would combine wide local resection with radiation therapy. The principle of wide local excision involves achieving a goal of resecting the tumor with a 2-cm margin of surrounding normal soft tissue. Considerable debate exists regarding the optimal mode (external beam radiation therapy or brachytherapy) and timing (preoperative, intraoperative, or postoperative) of adjunctive radiation therapy. Theoretical advantages are proposed for each modality. The only randomized study comparing preoperative with postoperative radiation therapy, conducted by the National Cancer Institute of Canada Clinical Trials Group, reported similar high rates of local control and progression-free survival at a median follow-up of 3.3 years. Nevertheless, for tumors with proximity to the neurovascular bundle, where, clearly, wide margins would not be achievable in every plane, perhaps preoperative radiation therapy can facilitate a negative surgical margin resection. The single-institutional experience from Massachusetts General Hospital reported that, following preoperative radiation therapy, the extent of negative margin (1 mm vs 10 mm) did not influence the local control rate. For high-grade extremity sarcomas, the randomized trial from the National Cancer Institute reported a 10-year local control rate of 98%, and the randomized trial conducted at Memorial Sloan-Kettering observed a 5-year local control rate of 89% with the use of brachytherapy.

There is no role for adjuvant chemotherapy, and the Sarcoma Meta-analysis Group reported that combination chemotherapy did not influence overall survival, though it did enhance disease-free survival. Phase II trials have been reported for the preoperative use of the MAID regimen (mesna, Adriamycin, ifosfamide, DTIC) in combination with radiation therapy for large (>10 cm), high-grade tumors.

Case Continued

The patient receives preoperative radiation to a dose of 50 Gy given in 25 fractions. Six weeks following completion of radiation therapy, the patient is scheduled to undergo wide local resection.

Intraoperative Photographs

Surgical Approach

The MRI scan of the extremity is carefully reviewed to allow the development and conceptualization of a three-dimensional approach to wide resection. An elliptical incision that encompasses any prior biopsy is designed with a width that will balance the goal of achieving primary closure, but also to leave viable skin flaps and avoid inadvertent entry into the tumor, particularly if it is fairly superficial. Flaps are then created beyond the confines of the tumor. The thickness of the flaps can be judged by the depth of the tumor as assessed from the preoperative imaging study. Once the outer perimeter of the tumor is reached, the investing fascia can be incised to expose the underlying muscle. If the tumor is in close proximity to vascular structures, these should be isolated proximally and distally and vessel loops placed. If the neurovascular structures are displaced as well in very close proximity to the tumor, dissection can proceed beneath the adventitia of the vessels and beneath the perineurium of the nerve to facilitate negative surgical margins. The sarcoma is then resected en bloc with the adjacent muscles with a margin of 2 to 5 cm of normal tissue to encompass any unappreciated microscopic disease. If the compartmental vessels are encased, these are resected and reconstructed appropriately. The surgeon needs to be constantly cognizant of the regional normal anatomy, which, in fact, is often distorted by the sarcoma. Following resection, any exposed vascular structures should be covered with adequate local muscle tissue and, to avoid seroma formation, suction drains should be placed with the exit site close to the wound. The skin flaps are then meticulously approximated.

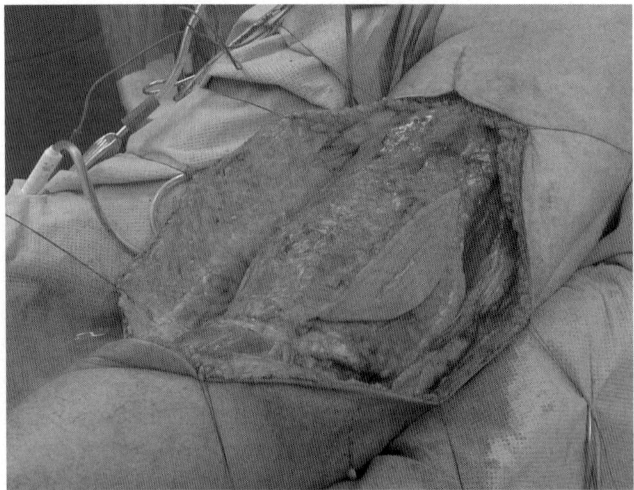

Figure 61.3A

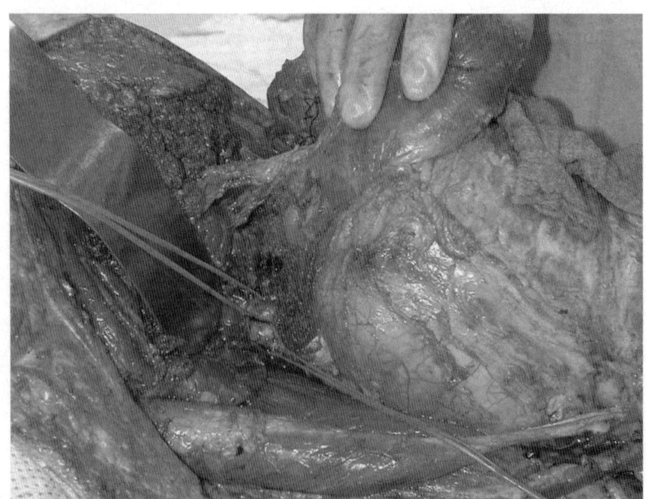

Figure 61.3B

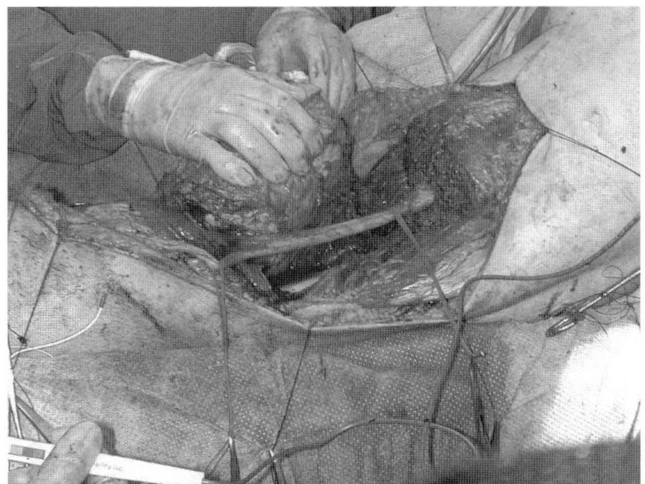

Figure 61.3C

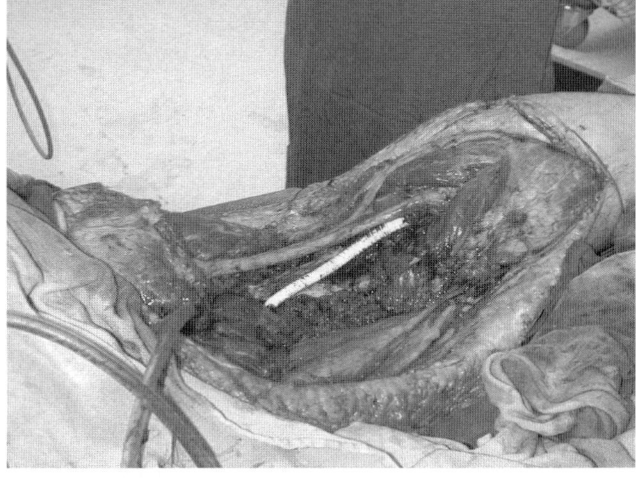

Figure 61.3D

Case Continued

The patient undergoes radical resection of right posterior thigh sarcoma with en bloc resection of hamstring muscles and popliteal vessels with preservation of the sciatic nerve. Flaps are created **(A)**, vessels isolated **(B)**, and the sciatic nerve preserved **(C).** The resected segment of the vessel is reconstructed with a polytetrafluoroethylene graft **(D).** Coverage of the popliteal graft and the sciatic nerve is achieved with a gastrocnemius, gracilis, and adductor longus muscle flap with primary closure of the overlying skin flaps. After a 6-week period of wound healing, the patient recovered well. Eight months later, during surveillance chest x-ray, the patient was noted to have an abnormal right-sided pulmonary nodule. CT scan of the chest demonstrated two nodules in the right lung.

Chest X-Ray and CT Scan

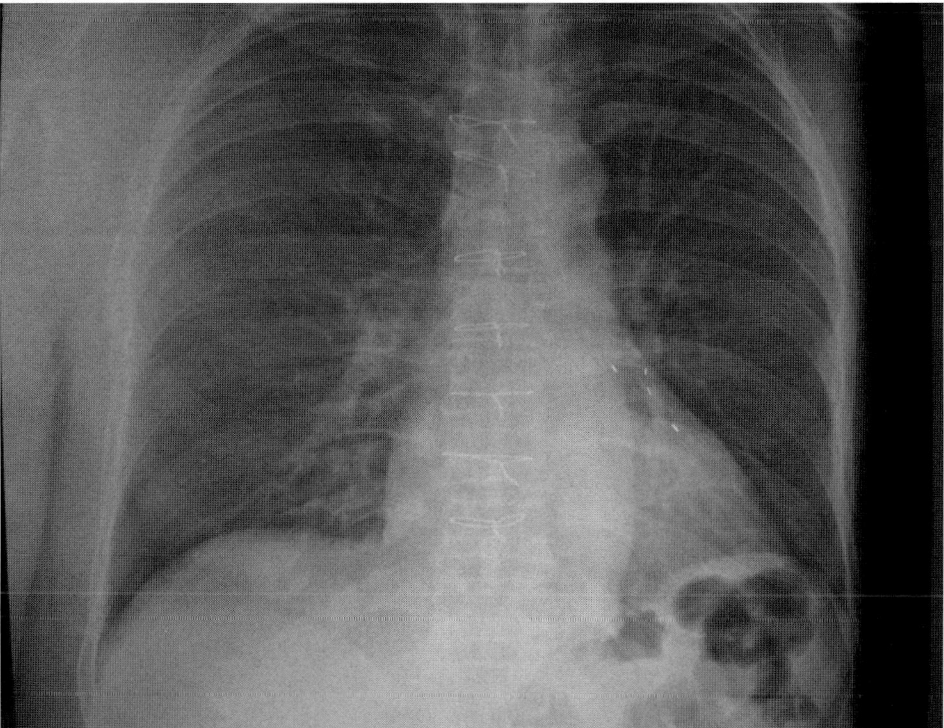

Figure 61.4A

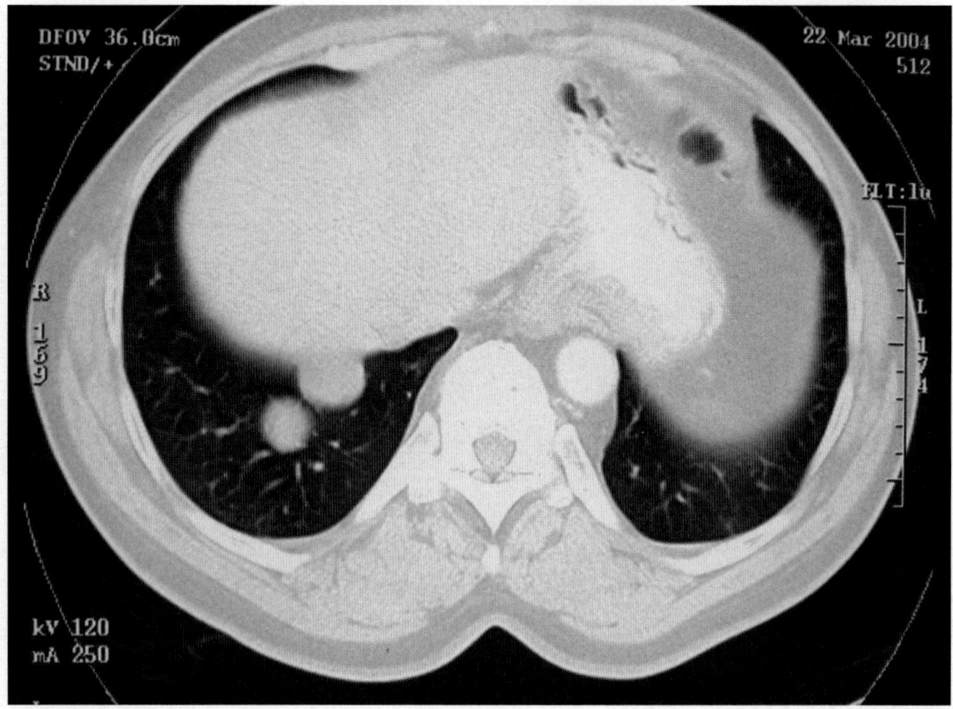

Figure 61.4B

Chest X-Ray and CT Scan Report

X-ray reveals the presence of an abnormal round density in the right lower lung field. On CT, two solitary nodules are present in the right lower lobe, one measuring about 2 cm and the other 1.5 cm, consistent with pulmonary metastases.

Recommendation

Pulmonary metastasectomy.

Intraoperative and Specimen Photographs

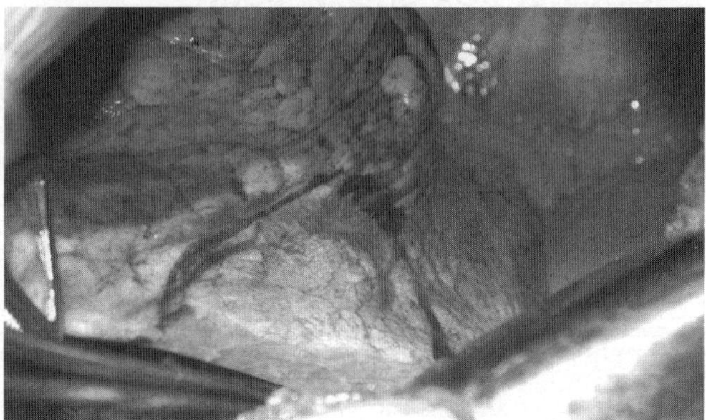

Figure 61.5A

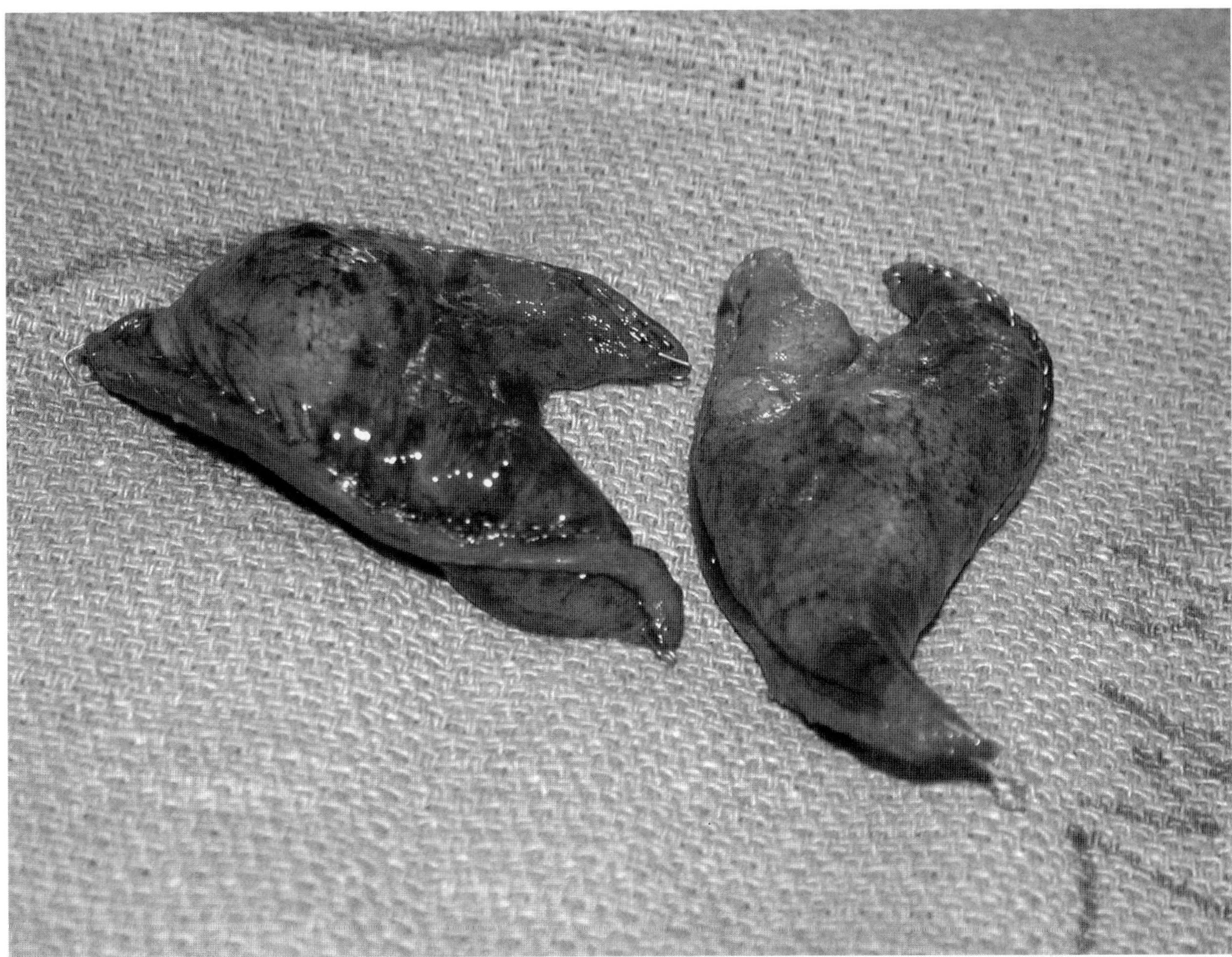

Figure 61.5B

Case Continued

The patient underwent a muscle-sparing right thoracotomy with wedge resections of the pulmonary metastases. Currently, the patient is without evidence of disease.

Discussion

The metastatic potential for soft tissue sarcoma is dependent on the grade and size of the sarcoma. The metastatic potential of soft-tissue sarcoma by grade is as follows: 5% to 10% for low-grade lesions, 25% to 30% for intermediate-grade lesions, and 50% to 60% for high-grade tumors. If achievable, a complete pulmonary resection should be offered, because it can offer long-term survival in 15% to 40% of patients with lung metastases. Wedge resection with negative margins is the procedure of choice. For bilateral metastases, a median sternotomy, staged thoracotomy, or video-assisted thoracoscopic surgery (VATS) can be used.

For those in whom a complete resection is achieved, a median survival of 19 months is noted, compared to 10 months for patients with incomplete resections and 8 months for those who do not undergo an operation. For patients who present with recurrent pulmonary metastases, a National Cancer Institute study demonstrated that 72% were able to undergo resection at second thoracotomy, which provided a median survival of 25 months. The most important prognostic factor influencing survival was the ability to achieve complete resection. Adverse prognostic factors include a shorter disease-free interval, presence of multiple (more than three) pulmonary metastases, and incomplete pulmonary resection.

Suggested Readings

Brennan MF, Hilaris B, Shiu MH, et al. Local recurrence in adult soft-tissue sarcoma. A randomized trial of brachytherapy. *Arch Surg* 1987;122:1289–1293.

Demas BE, Heelan RT, Lane J, et al. Soft-tissue sarcomas of the extremities: comparison of MR and CT in determining the extent of disease. *AJR Am J Roentgenol* 1988;150:615–620.

O'Sullivan B, Davis A, Turcotte R, et al. Preoperative versus postoperative radiotherapy in soft-tissue sarcoma of the limbs: a randomized trial. *Lancet* 2002;359:2235–2241.

Pisters PW, Leung DH, Woodruff J, et al. Analysis of prognostic factors in 1,041 patients with localized soft tissue sarcomas of the extremities. *J Clin Oncol* 1996;14:1679–1689.

Rosenberg SA, Tepper J, Glatstein E, et al. The treatment of soft-tissue sarcomas of the extremities: prospective randomized evaluations of (1) limb-sparing surgery plus radiation therapy compared with amputation and (2) the role of adjuvant chemotherapy. *Ann Surg* 1982;196:305–315.

Yang JC, Chang AE, Baker AR, et al. Randomized prospective study of the benefit of adjuvant radiation therapy in the treatment of soft tissue sarcomas of the extremity. *J Clin Oncol* 1998;16:197–203.

Presentation

A 69-year-old white man presents with a 6-month history of fatigue, early satiety, and an abdominal mass. On examination, there is a large, hard mass to the left of the midline. The inferior border of the mass is somewhat indistinct, suggesting that it extends into the pelvis. The primary physician performs an ultrasound scan, which demonstrates a large intra-abdominal mass occupying the left half of the abdomen and surrounding the kidney and the body and tail of the pancreas.

Clinical Photograph

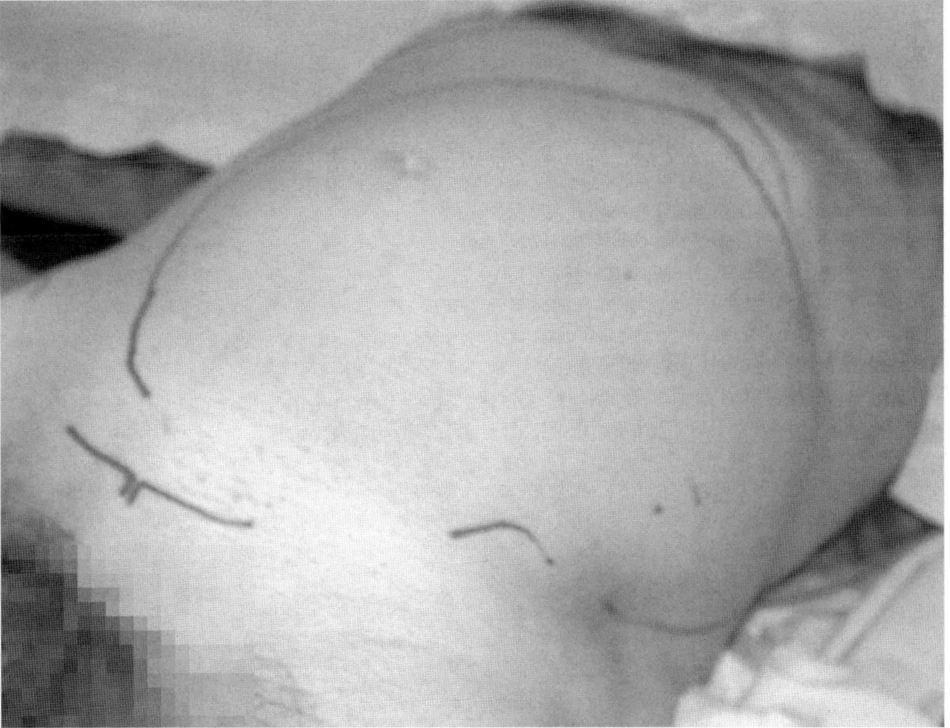

Figure 62.1

Physical Examination Report

View of the abdomen shows visible distension due to the mass.

Differential Diagnosis

The clinical features and the ultrasound scan findings are highly suggestive of a retroperitoneal sarcoma. The differential diagnosis of a retroperitoneal tumor includes lymphoma, germ cell tumors, and undifferentiated carcinomas.

Discussion

Most tumors of the retroperitoneum are malignant. About one third are soft-tissue sarcomas. Soft-tissue sarcomas are rare tumors, with an annual incidence around 2 to 3 per 100,000. Overall, soft-tissue sarcomas comprise <1% of all malignant tumors, and they account for 2% of the total cancer-related mortality. About 15% of all patients with soft-tissue sarcomas present with disease arising in the retroperitoneum. Retroperitoneal sarcomas have a peak incidence in the fifth decade of life. In patients with retroperitoneal neoplasms, 82% are malignant, 18% are benign. Of those with malignancies, 40% are lymphomas or a variety of urogenital cancer, and 55% are sarcomas. Stated another way, nearly one half of all retroperitoneal solid neoplasms will prove to be soft-tissue sarcomas. Patients most frequently present with a nontender palpable mass (80% to 90%). They may give a history of increasing abdominal girth and frequently (40% to 70%) describe vague, poorly localized discomfort due to stretching of the peritoneum. One third of patients have some distal neurologic signs and symptoms from the mass effect, stretching or compression of the lumbar or pelvic nerve plexuses. Gastrointestinal symptoms of a partially obstructive nature, due to displacement or direct invasion by the expanding mass, are found in 10% to 15% of the patients.

The rarity of retroperitoneal sarcomas and their location make it common for these tumors to be misdiagnosed preoperatively. Most often, retroperitoneal sarcomas are diagnosed as ovarian malignancies, but other diagnoses are possible, including genital, urinary, and gastrointestinal tumors, adrenal tumors, and metastatic tumors. History of fever and night sweats with findings of generalized lymphadenopathy and elevated lactate dehydrogenase levels suggest lymphoma. In men, a testicle mass or mass with elevated beta-human chorionic gonadotrophin or alpha-fetoprotein levels suggests a germcell tumor.

The most definitive radiographic study is a computed tomography (CT) scan of the abdomen and pelvis, because it will establish the retroperitoneal location of such tumors, and they are often heterogenous in appearance due to the presence of solid viable tumor intermixed with areas of necrosis and possible hemorrhage. The CT scan allows definition of the extent of the tumor and its relationships to the surrounding intra-abdominal organs, and particularly, the major vessels. Any discontinuous disease within the abdomen will also be revealed, and the liver can be assessed for the presence of metastases. A CT scan of the chest will disclose metastases that could influence future operative management. In situations where better definition of the tumor in relation to the spine and major vascular structures is necessary for operative planning, a magnetic resonance (MR) scan can be obtained. In addition, it has the advantage of providing an MR angiogram of the aorta and/or vena cava to evaluate displacement, encasement, thrombosis, and/or direct invasion. Any extension through this bowel perimeter can be determined for tumors in the paraspinal location.

Percutaneous CT or ultrasound-guided biopsy are most often unnecessary except for an unresectable tumor, or if the clinical presentation or CT scan findings do not support the diagnosis of a retroperitoneal sarcoma.

Recommendation

A CT scan of the chest, abdomen, and pelvis is recommended.

Case Continued

The patient undergoes a CT scan of the abdomen and pelvis. Prior to referral, a CT-guided biopsy requested by the primary physician establishes a diagnosis of a high-grade liposarcoma.

CT Scan

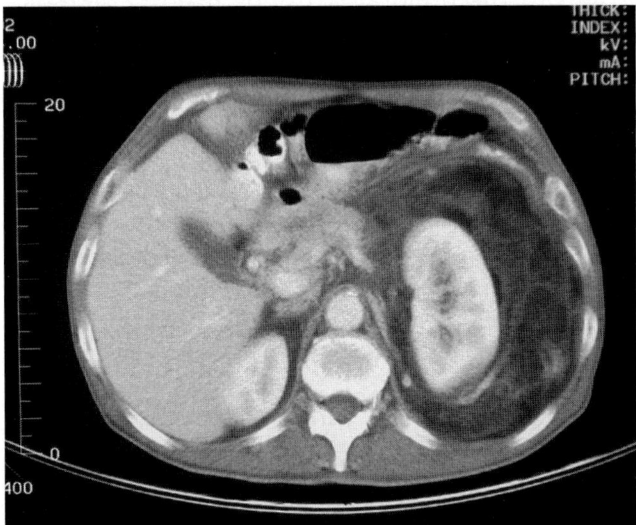

Figure 62.2A

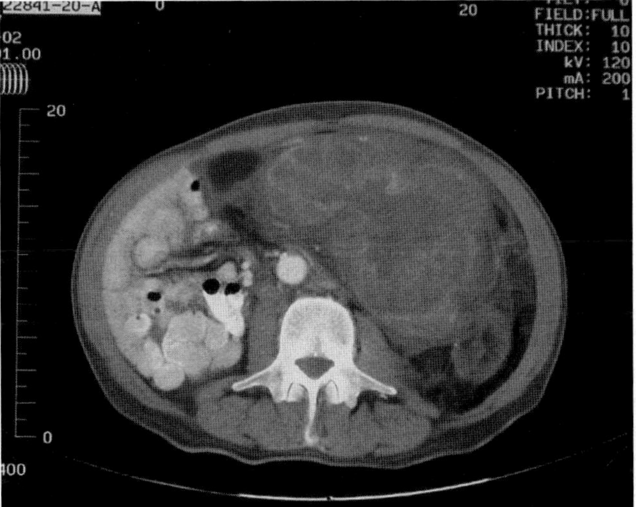

Figure 62.2B

CT Scan Report

There is a large retroperitoneal mass extending from the retrogastric area involving the spleen, surrounding the kidney and pancreas, and extending toward the pelvis. The tumor overlies the left-sided vena cava, but a plane exists with the intra-abdominal aorta.

Approach

The cornerstone of the treatment of retroperitoneal sarcoma involves complete surgical resection. Unlike extremity soft-tissue sarcomas, procuring a wide margin around the tumor is often difficult due to the presence of vital structures, though aggressive en bloc visceral resection of the intestine, kidney, pancreas, spleen, and retroperitoneal muscles may often be necessary. If preoperative imaging studies suggest doubtful resectability, exploratory laparotomy should still be strongly considered as the findings intraoperatively are often less worrying and microscopic clearance and complete resection can still be achieved. This is primarily due to the pushing nature of most retroperitoneal sarcomas.

To date, there has been little success with either adjuvant chemotherapy or radiation therapy in the local control of retroperitoneal sarcoma or in achieving improvement in overall survival. Chemotherapy in soft-tissue sarcoma has been reported to achieve only a 25% response rate with the best-known single-agent or multiagent regimens. Postoperative external beam radiation therapy has been limited primarily due to the associated toxicity to the adjacent intra-abdominal viscera. Though there have been studies demonstrating a delay in local recurrence after radiation therapy, this apparent benefit did not translate into an ultimate survival benefit.

Radiation therapy to the retroperitoneum is complex, owing to the frequent large field sizes and proximity of adjacent radiosensitive structures. Intraoperative radiation therapy or the use of adjuvant brachytherapy is an alternative approach, but these require special expertise; they are associated with late toxicity, but their effectiveness was not clearly demonstrated in a prospective clinical trial. For several reasons, preoperative radiation therapy may be appealing because the gross tumor volume is readily definable for accurate treatment planning, and the tumor displaces the radiosensitive viscera outside the treatment field to minimize dose-limiting toxicity. The University of Toronto group demonstrated Radiation Therapy Oncology Group (RTOG) toxicity of 2 or less for patients who have undergone 45 Gy of preoperative radiation therapy with a median radiation volume exceeding 7 liters.

Resectability rates for primary tumors range from 50% to 75%, but despite complete gross resection, there is a high propensity for local recurrence and tumor grade-specific risk for distant metastases. Therefore, in the absence of effective chemotherapy and radiation therapy, aggressive surgical re-exploration and resection for recurrence is appropriate. Evaluation of combined modality approaches should be evaluated with national cooperative group randomized trials.

Case Continued

Preoperative imaging studies suggest that the tumor is resectable with en bloc visceral resection that may require splenectomy, left nephrectomy, and distal pancreatectomy. Informed consent is obtained and vaccinations are provided in anticipation of a splenectomy.

Surgical Approach

The patient is generally placed in the supine position, although a Lloyd-Davies position is preferable if the tumor extends into the pelvis. A midline incision is commonly adequate, but depending on the extent of the tumor, extensions may be necessary for improved exposure. A thoracoabdominal incision for upper quadrant tumors, a lateral extension for flank tumors, and abdominoinguinal incision for lower quadrant tumors with iliac vessel involvement may facilitate resectability. Assessment of resectability is an ongoing intraoperative dynamic process that often is begun by determining if any of the hollow or solid viscera are densely adherent to the retroperitoneal tumor, and whether these structures can be spared while leaving an extra layer of tissue on the side of the tumor to achieve a narrow, yet negative, margin. If a plane of dissection does not exist between the tumor and the visceral structure, then the latter has to be sacrificed. A multidimensional dissection strategy is necessary, with continuous adjustment of the surgical plan in response to the operative findings and frequent changes to the location of dissection to exploit any obvious path of least resistance. The tumor is usually dissected from its lateral attachments, followed by its bed, and then in the subadventitial plane along the aorta and the vena cava.

Intraoperative Photographs

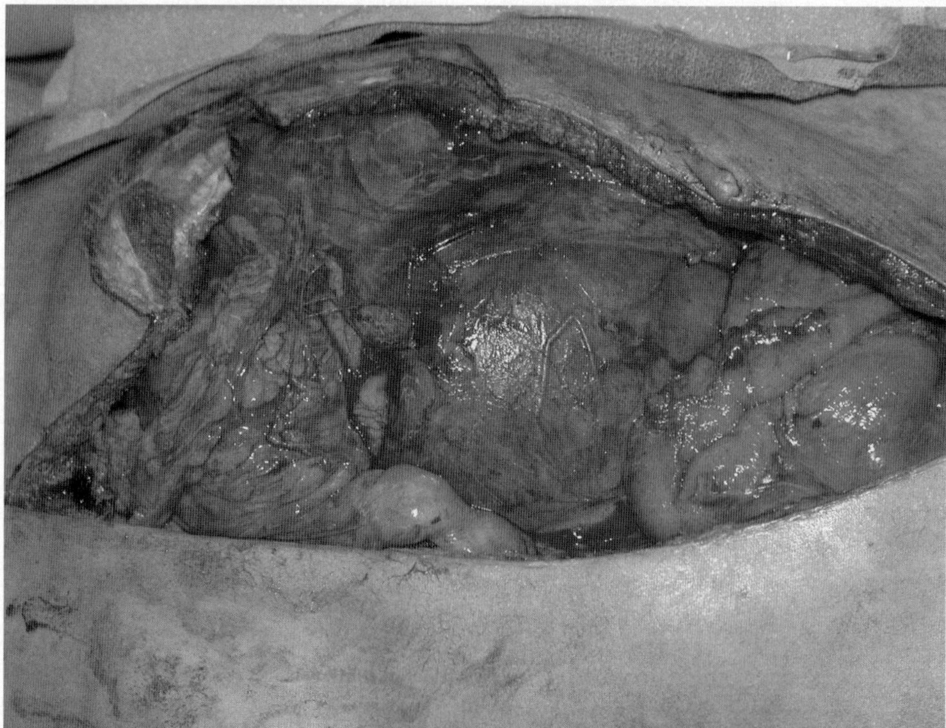

Figure 62.3A

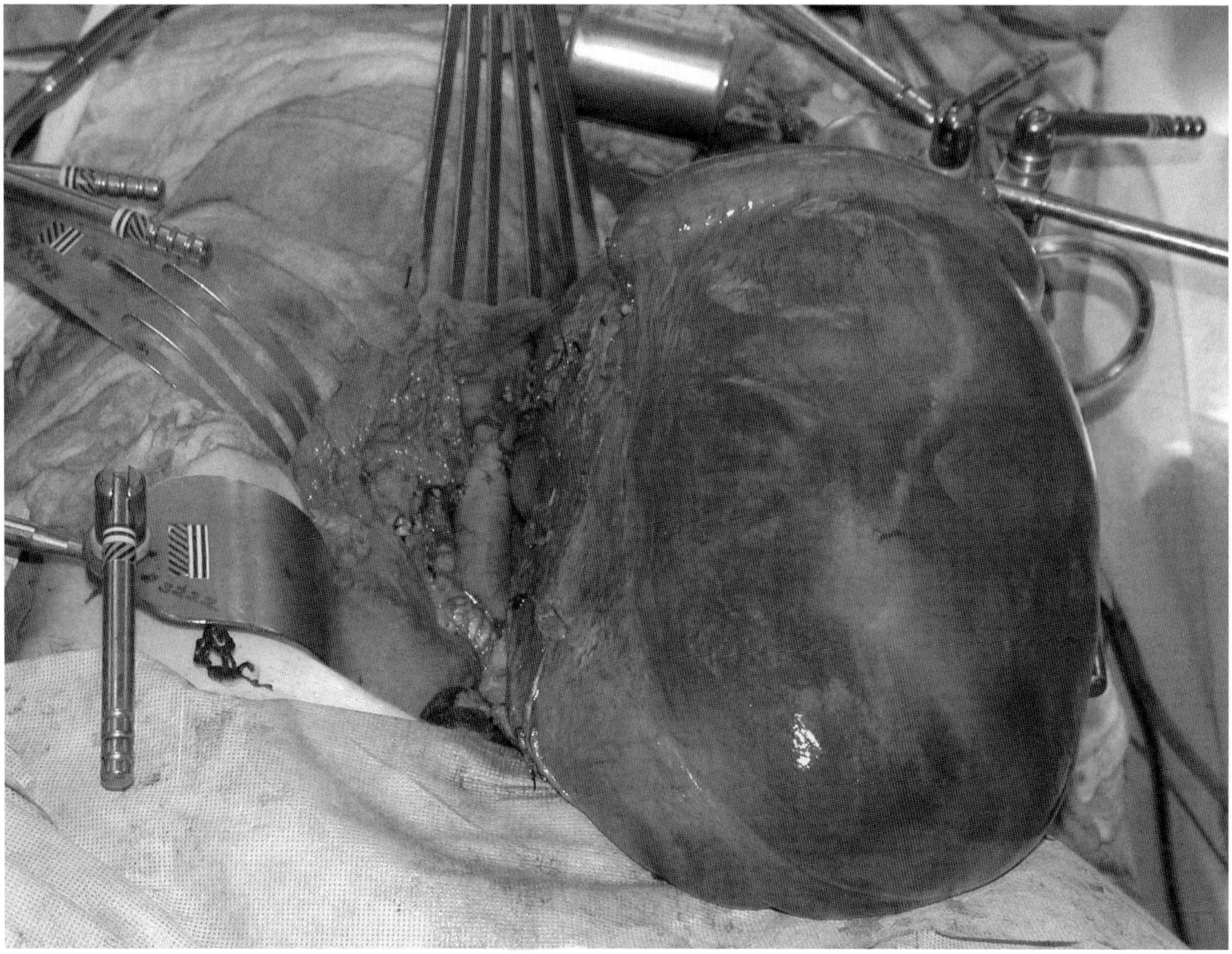

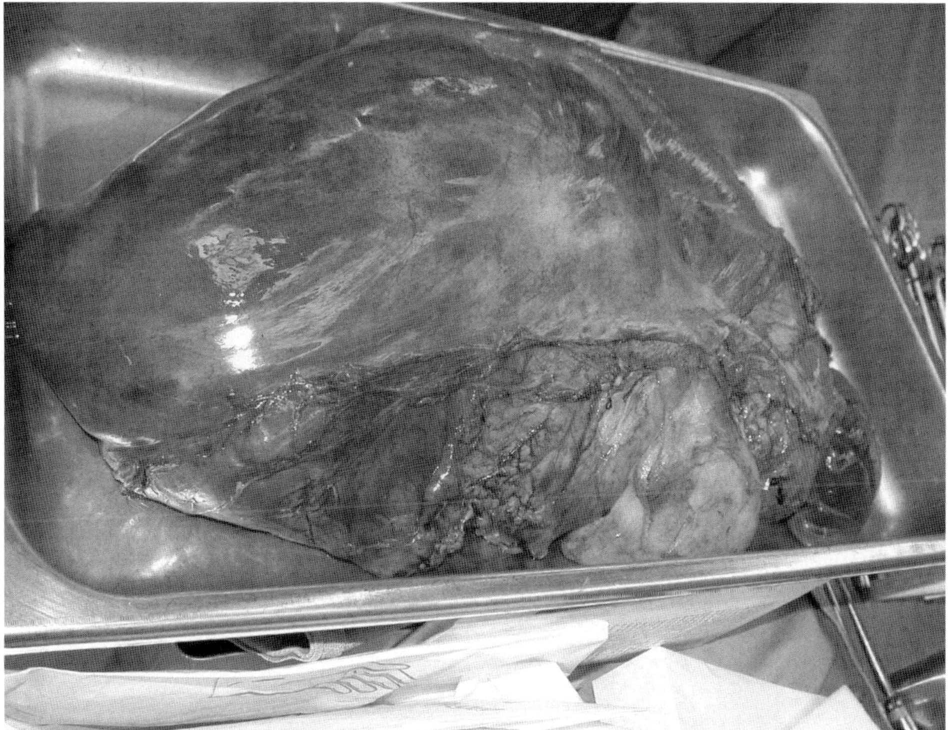

Figure 62.3B

Figure 62.3C

◼ Surgical Approach (Continued)

A midline abdominal incision is performed. The tumor is noted to push tightly against the anterior abdominal wall, hindering wide exposure, particularly of the left upper quadrant. Hence, a left oblique thoracoabdominal T-incision is added **(A).** The entire descending colon is densely adhered to the anterior surface of the mass, which is noted to extend from the left diaphragm to the pelvic brim, and medially it extends well past the level of the aorta. After careful mobilization **(B),** the patient undergoes resection of the retroperitoneal sarcoma **(C)** with en bloc left extended hemicolectomy, splenectomy, distal pancreatectomy, and left nephroureterectomy.

Discussion

The reported overall survival rates at 5 years range from 40% to 50%. Prognosis for patients with retroperitoneal sarcomas is dependent on the grade of the tumor and whether complete resection with negative margins can be achieved. In a Canadian series, the 5-year disease-free survival rate was 50% for patients who had margin-negative resections, as compared with 28% for patients who had undergone incomplete resections. Review of 500 cases of retroperitoneal sarcoma at Memorial Sloan-Kettering reported a median survival of 103 months in those who underwent complete resections, and only 18 months in those who underwent either incomplete resections or observation without resection. However, the same group recently emphasized that in select patients with unresectable retroperitoneal liposarcoma, partial resection was an independent predictive factor for survival as compared with biopsy alone (median survival 26 vs 4 months) and led to successful palliation of symptoms in 75% of patients. Median survival for patients with low-grade sarcomas was 80 months, compared to 20 months for high-grade sarcomas.

Suggested Readings

Heslin MJ, Lewis JJ, Nadler E, et al. Prognostic factors associated with long-term survival for retroperitoneal sarcoma: implications for management. *J Clin Oncol* 1997;15:2832–2839.

Jaques DP, Coit DG, Hajdu SI, et al. Management of primary and recurrent soft-tissue sarcoma of the retroperitoneum. *Ann Surg* 1990;212:51–59.

Kinsella TJ, Sindelar WF, Lack E, et al. Preliminary results of a randomized study of adjuvant radiation therapy in resectable adult retroperitoneal soft tissue sarcomas. *J Clin Oncol* 1988;6:18–25.

Pisters PWT, O'Sullivan B. Retroperitoneal sarcomas: combined modality treatment approaches. *Curr Opin Oncol* 2002;14: 400–405.

Singer S, Eberlein TJ. Surgical management of soft-tissue sarcoma. *Adv Surg* 1997;31:395–420.

Singer S, Corson JM, Demetri GD, et al. Prognostic factors predictive of survival for truncal and retroperitoneal soft-tissue sarcoma. *Ann Surg* 1995;221:185–195.

Storm FK, Mahvi DM. Diagnosis and management of retroperitoneal soft-tissue sarcoma. *Ann Surg* 1991;214:2–10.

Presentation

The patient is a 42-year-old woman complaining of vague lower abdominal pain for approximately 4 to 6 months with a recent increase in pain and left thigh sciatica. There is no history of trauma to the anatomical region. There are no systemic symptoms such as weight loss, anorexia, or fever. Physical examination reveals a large mass in the lower portion of the abdomen. The patient's abdomen appears obviously distended and a 10 × 20-cm mass is palpated. This nontender mass is quite firm and appears fixed to the underlying left pelvis. A pelvic examination shows a large extravaginal mass to both the right and left sides of the uterus. The ovaries are not palpable. Neurological examination reveals no evidence of neuropathy, although there is a positive straight leg raising sign on the left side. There is no sensory or reflex loss appreciated in this extremity. Her history is negative for other gastrointestinal or genitourinary complaints, and she is not pregnant.

Recommendation

Plain radiograph of the pelvis, computed tomography (CT) scan and magnetic resonance imaging (MRI) of the pelvis are recommended.

Pelvic X-Ray

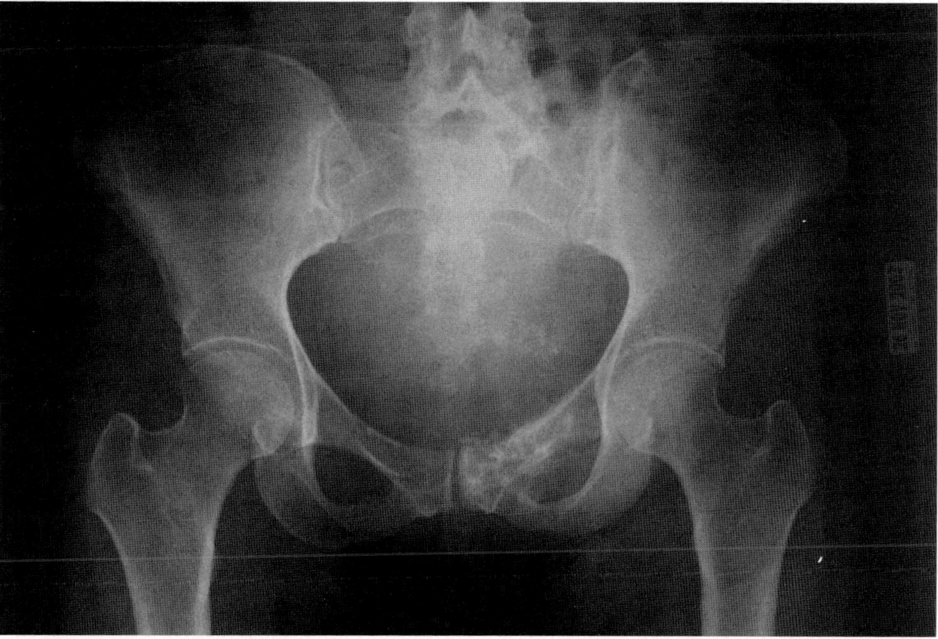

Figure 63.1A

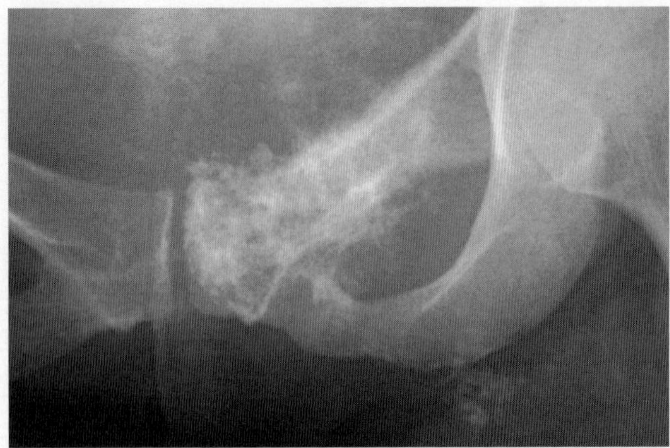

Figure 63.1B

◼ CT Scan

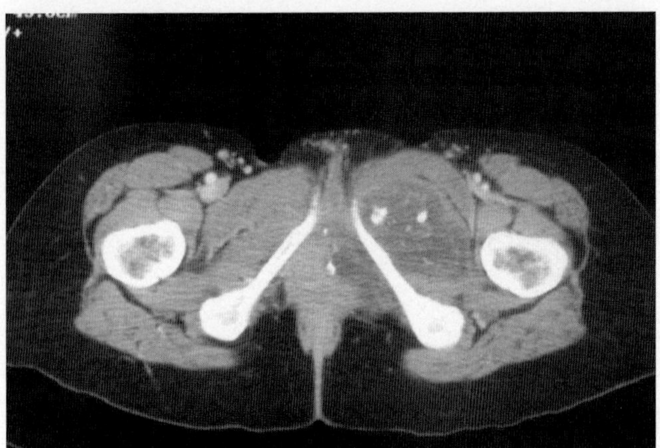

Figure 63.2A

Pelvic X-Ray Report

Plain radiograph of the pelvis with a coned-down view of the left superior ramus shows a stippled calcification in the soft tissues adjacent to the left superior pubic ramus **(A).** There is some calcification with extension into the adductor region of the thigh. Close-up radiograph of the pelvic floor shows stippled calcification and destruction of the left superior pubic ramus, suggesting that the pubic ramus is the primary origin of the tumor **(B).** This type of calcification is typical of cartilage-forming tumors. The pelvis is the most common site of primary chondrosarcomas. The hip and remaining ilium are unaffected.

CT Scan Report

CT scan of the pelvis shows an extremely large mass involving the true pelvis, extending from the left superior pubic ramus to the left pelvic wall and acetabulum. It then extends across to the right acetabulum, although there is no direct visualized destruction to either acetabuli. This mass shows a marked increase in stippling (calcification) in the inferior portion of the lesion, although the predominant component of the mass shows no matrix formation. The bladder is displaced medially and is compressed. The uterus is displaced anteriorly to the left. The rectum is markedly displaced anteriorly and to the left. Chondrosarcomas of the pelvis typically have an

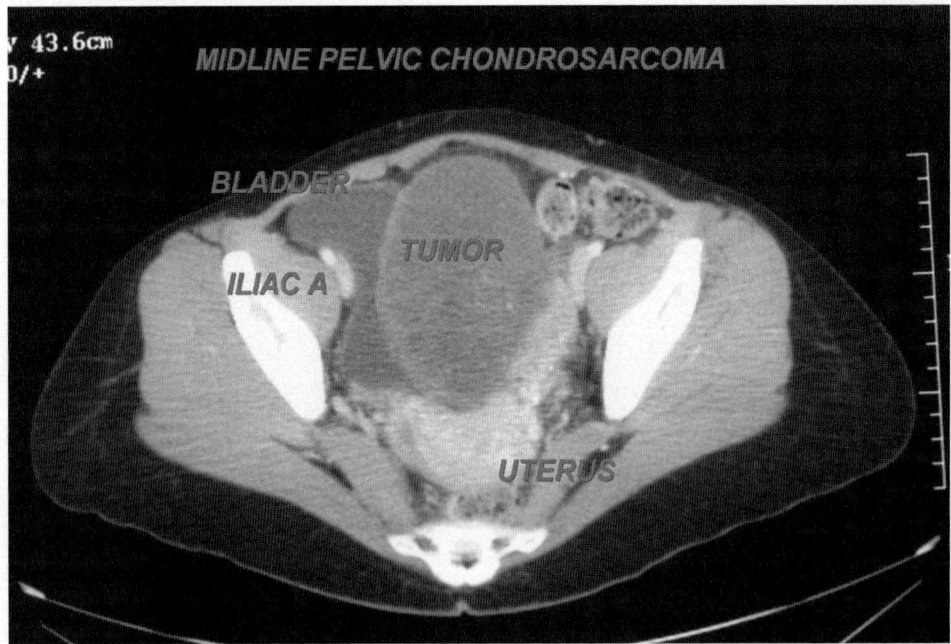

Figure 63.2B

extremely large soft tissue (extraosseous) component. The "water" density of the tumor suggests a myxoid type of chondrosarcoma. Note the tumor density is similar to that of the bladder. Axial CT below the true pelvis shows tumor and calcification extending into the left adductor region as well as the ischiorectal space. Pelvic chondrosarcomas that extend into the ischiorectal space often involve the urethra and bladder neck. The surgeon must be prepared to resect these structures.

MRI

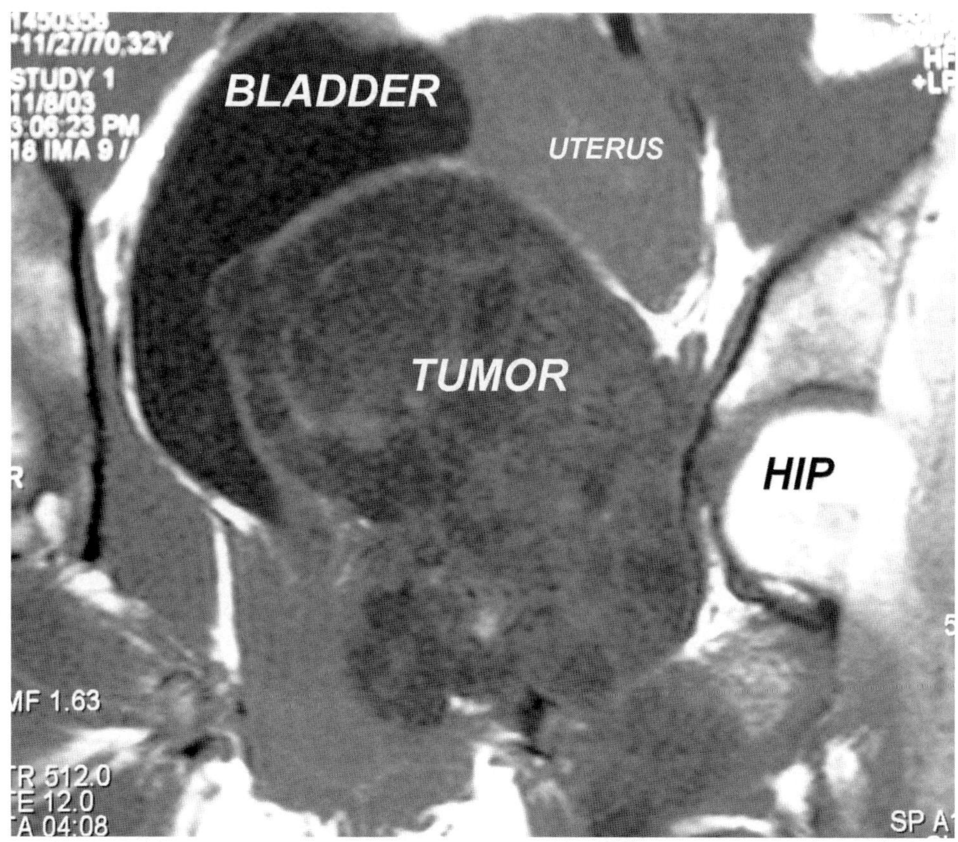

Figure 63.3

MRI Report

The T1 coronal view shows an extremely large mass arising from the left superior pubic ramus with large intrapelvic and extrapelvic components and extending well above the level of the iliac crests, involving both the left and right acetabular walls with extension into the left adductor muscle group and destruction of the left superior pubic ramus. The tumor extends across the midline, displacing the bladder and uterus, and lies against the left inner wall of the acetabulum with extension into the ischiorectal space. This mass demonstrates heterogeneosity with some areas of matrix formation. T2 coronal MRI *(not shown)* reveals obvious extension of the extraosseous component of the tumor arising from the superior pubic ramus. This mass fills the pelvis and extends above the iliac crests. There is obvious extension into the adductor compartment below the left superior pubic ramus.

Differential Diagnosis

The differential diagnosis of a primary tumor of the superior pubic ramus that fills the entire pelvis and has extension into the adductor group muscle is suspicious for a bone sarcoma in this middle-aged patient. This tumor is most likely a chondrosarcoma or one of its variants, although the differential includes metastatic carcinoma (unlikely, because most metastatic carcinomas are not accompanied by large extraosseous components) and osteosarcoma (usually found in adolescents). The other primary bone tumors do not demonstrate such an extensive extraosseous component. Lymphomas of bone may demonstrate extraosseous involvement; however, the CT scan and MRI show matrix (calcification) formation, which is characteristic of a cartilage tumor. Most chondrosarcomas of the pelvis are extremely large and present with very few symptoms related to the compression of the pelvic contents. The patient's presenting complaint of pain is nonspecific, and left-sided sciatica is most likely related to compression of portions of the lumbosacral plexus on the left side due to the large tumor mass. Despite the large size of the tumor, this patient had no complaints of urinary or rectal incontinence.

Multiple core needle biopsies were performed through a single puncture site. This was performed using CT guidance above the left superior pubic ramus, taking care to avoid the external iliac vessels and the femoral triangle.

Diagnosis

Chondrosarcoma, low-grade, with an extremely large extraosseous component, arising from the left superior pubic ramus.

Case Continued

Chest CT scan is performed, and is negative for pulmonary nodules. A three-phase bone scan shows only minimal radioisotopic uptake in the left superior pubic ramus with no uptake in the extraosseous component (this is explained because this tumor is producing cartilage and not osteoid).

■ Approach

Once diagnosis of chondrosarcoma is established, the patient requires complete local staging to evaluate the regional anatomy in preparation for either surgical resection or amputation, and systemically to exclude metastatic disease. Chondrosarcomas typically spread hematogenously and locally by invasion. The treatment of chondrosarcoma of bone is surgical resection or amputation. Radiation therapy has no role in the primary treatment of this tumor type and is only rarely used for palliation of metastatic disease. Chemotherapy is not utilized unless the tumor is a high-grade variant (mesenchymal or dedifferentiated chondrosarcoma). Most large chondrosarcomas are extremely low grade with a large component of myxoid tissue. This patient had a large myxoid low-grade chondrosarcoma and the method of treatment would be surgical resection. Because of the extremely large size of this tumor and the proximity to multiple visceral structures and iliac vessels, it is almost unresectable. A multidisciplinary surgical oncology team evaluated this patient. The team consisted of an orthopaedic oncologist, urologic oncologist, and gynecologic oncologist for surgical planning purposes.

■ Preoperative Photograph

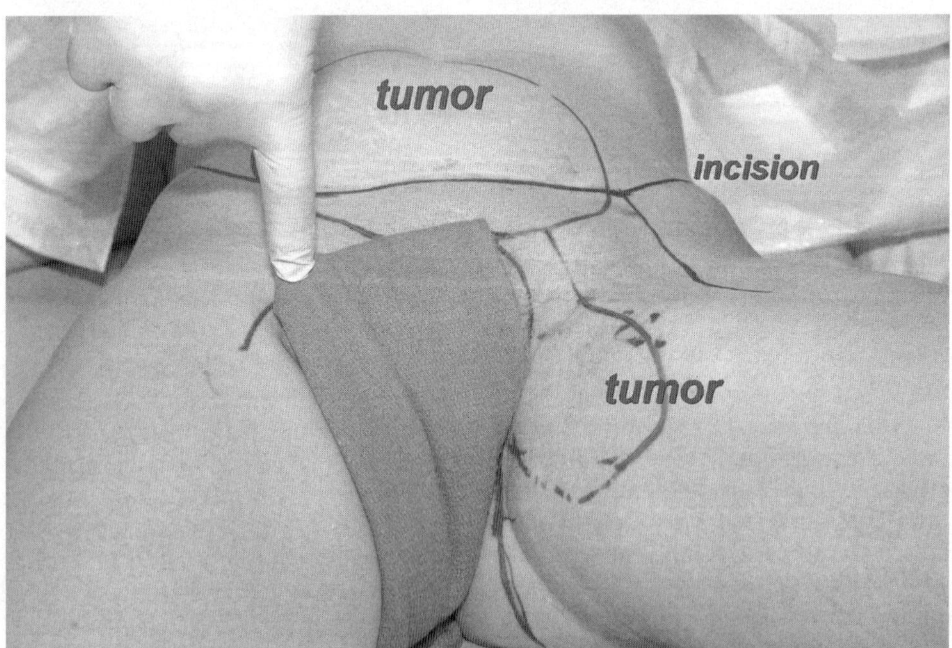

Figure 63.4

Preoperative Report

There is large cephalad tumor extension above the iliac crests with palpable tumor in the left adductor region that corresponds to the preoperative CT and MRI. The extended ilioinguinal incision is used to detach the entire abdominal wall from the anterior pelvis bilaterally as well as the rectus abdominis muscles from the body of the symphysis pubis. This approach provides a safe exposure to the tumor as well as the iliac vessels bilaterally, and permits removal of both lower pelvic floors en bloc with the tumor. In general, pelvic chondrosarcomas are resected through the retroperitoneal space without entering the abdomen.

Surgical Approach

Tumors that involve the pelvis are usually approached in a retroperitoneal manner. Due to the large size of this tumor, it was exposed through an extended ilioinguinal incision, which allowed complete exposure of the right and left pelvis retroperitoneally. The rectus abdominus muscles were released from the pubic rami bilaterally, and the entire abdominal wall was retracted proximally to expose the large tumor mass. Intraoperatively, the iliac vessels were exposed both proximally and distally to obtain vascular control and were easily mobilized away from the tumor mass. Similarly, the uterus was easily mobilized through one tissue plane away from the tumor. The bladder was juxtaposed to the tumor, and a portion of the bladder wall was resected and left attached to the tumor mass. In addition, this tumor extended into the left adductor muscles and involved the left superior pubic ramus. Therefore, the left pelvic floor and portions of the right pelvic floor were removed en bloc with the tumor and with a portion of the adductor musculature. Complete resection included bilateral pubic superior and inferior pubic ramus, as well as the adductor muscles and the retroperitoneal component of the tumor with a portion of the bladder attached. Reconstruction consisted of closing the main pelvic floor muscles by suturing them to the abdominal wall musculature to aid in closure of a large pelvic "dead" space. Both ureters were easily identified and were preserved, as was the rectum. In addition, the peritoneal cavity was opened prior to the reconstruction and the omentum was used to occupy the vacant space within the pelvis. Large chest tubes were utilized for drainage because the most common complications following large pelvic resections are seromas and hematomas.

Specimen Photograph

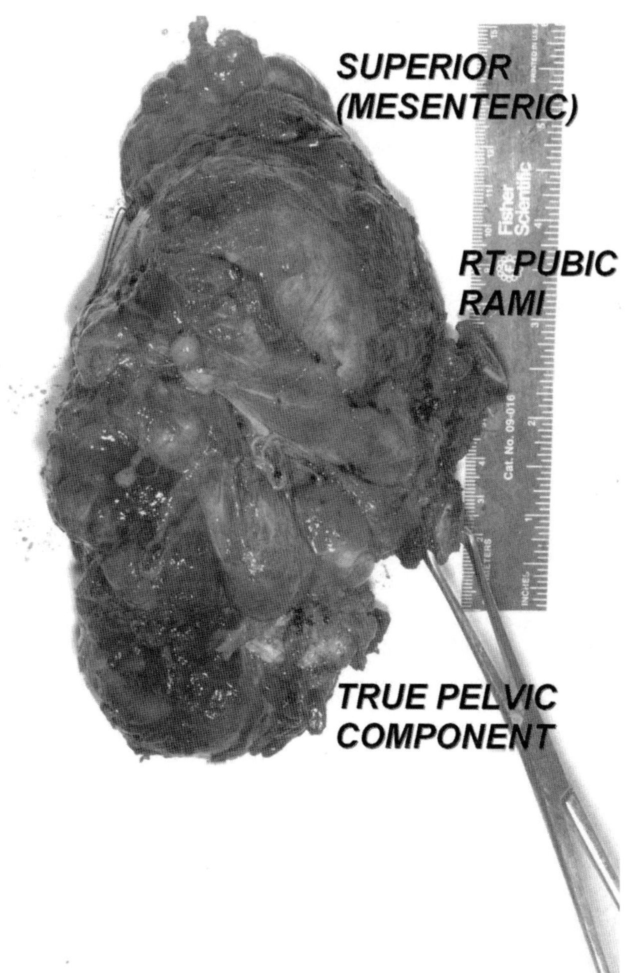

Figure 63.5

Specimen Report

The tumor is removed en–bloc, and measured 8 × 6 inches. The right (contralateral) pubic ramus is visible. This tumor corresponded well to the coronal MRI.

▩ Pelvic X-Ray

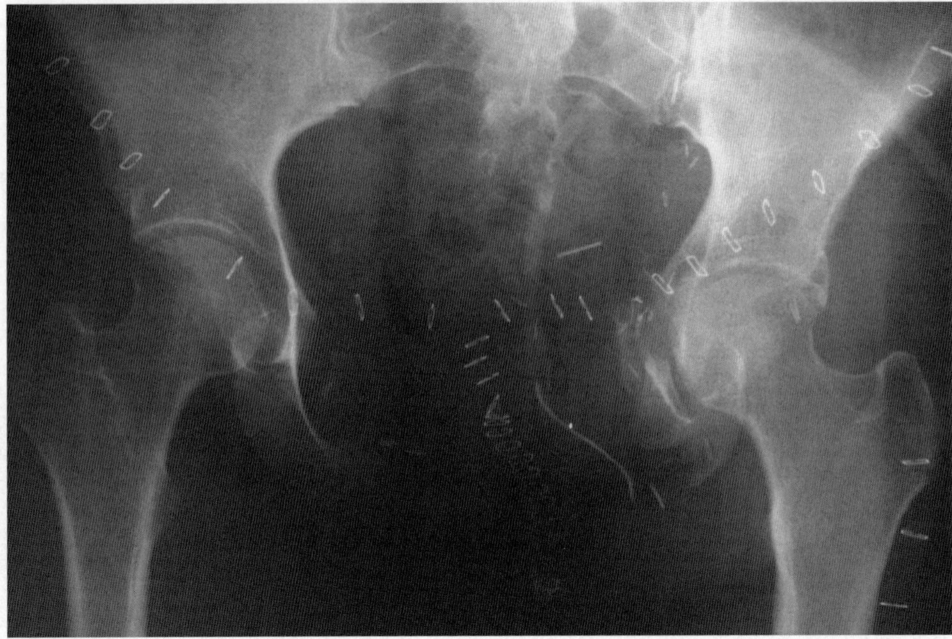

Figure 63.6

Pelvic X-Ray Report

Postoperative pelvic radiograph demonstrates the extent of the resection. Both the right and left pubic rami were resected en bloc with the tumor. The uterus, rectum, and urethra were preserved. A portion of the left medial acetabular wall was removed.

Case Continued

Postoperatively, the patient requires approximately 6 units of blood in addition to the 6 units of blood that were given intraoperatively. She is hemodynamically stabilized within 24 hours. No coagulation problems are encountered. The wound heals well. Bowel and bladder function are normal. Pain management postoperatively is achieved by utilizing perineural catheters in the left lumbosacral plexus and a patient-controlled analgesia pump. This patient begins ambulation with the assistance of two canes at 2 weeks. She uses an abdominal binder for a period of 2 to 3 months postoperatively for additional support. She now ambulates without the assistance of external supports.

Case Continued

This patient is followed every 3 months with MRI, serial CT scans of the chest and pelvis, and three-phase bone scans. There is no evidence of local recurrence or metastatic disease. At 5 years postoperatively, the patient remains free of disease. She continues to be followed yearly with imaging studies including CT scan, plain radiographs, and three-phase bone scans.

Discussion

Chondrosarcoma is the second most common primary malignant spindle-cell tumor of bone. Chondrosarcomas form a heterogeneous group of tumors. The basic neoplastic tissue is cartilaginous without evidence of direct osteoid formation. The case presented here showed a large pelvic chondrosarcoma with no osteoid formation but with marked displacement of the pelvic viscera. This is a typical presentation for pelvic chondrosarcomas. Many pelvic chondrosarcomas have a large component of myxoid tissue, accounting for their large sizes.

Chemotherapy and radiation therapy were not used for this patient, because her tumor was classified as a low-grade myxoid chondrosarcoma. Chemotherapy is only effective for high-grade or spindle-cell variant chondrosarcomas, or those of mesenchymal origin. Radiation therapy is utilized only for palliation or unresectable disease.

The classic chondrosarcomas are central (arising within a bone) or peripheral (arising from the surface of a bone). The other three chondrosarcoma variants have distinct histologic and clinical characteristics.

Central and peripheral chondrosarcomas can arise as primary tumors or secondary to other underlying neoplasms. Approximately 75% of chondrosarcomas arise centrally, that is, involving the shoulder girdle or pelvic girdle. Secondary chondrosarcomas most often arise from benign osteochondromas.

Approximately 50% of central chondrosarcomas occur in patients older than 40. Only 3.8% of chondrosarcomas arise in patients under 20 years of age. Chondrosarcomas are the most common malignant tumors of the sternum, scapula, and pelvic bone. Their clinical presentation varies, but in general they are minimally painful and cause local symptoms due to mechanical compression or irritation of adjacent structures. Chondrosarcomas only rarely directly invade adjacent nerves; typically, these nerves can be spared, as in the case presented here. Occasionally, urinary symptoms due to bladder neck involvement and distal edema due to iliac vein obstruction occur, but were not present in this patient.

Central chondrosarcomas have two distinct radiological patterns. One is a small, well-defined lytic lesion within the bone and may appear to be a benign lesion. The second type has a sclerotic border with a large extraosseous component, and it is difficult to localize.

The metastatic potential of chondrosarcomas tends to correlate with the histological grade of the tumor. Chondrosarcomas are graded I to III, with the survival rates being 47%, 38%, and 15% at 5 years. There is a small drop-off in survival between 5 and 10 years; therefore, patients should be followed carefully for at least a 10-year period.

Chondrosarcomas of the pelvis were typically treated with hemipelvectomy until the 1970s, when the technique of limb-sparing surgery and internal pelvic resections was developed. There are three types of pelvic resection. Type I involves resection of the ilium only. Type II involves resection of the acetabular area and the hip joint, and type III removes the pelvic floor. These may be combined for type I/II, type II/III, or type I/II/III pelvic resections. Type I and II have minimal functional loss for the patient. Functional loss for patients is contingent on the extent of resection required. The most important aspect in the treatment of pelvic chondrosarcomas is to determine the local anatomical extent prior to surgical resection. The indications for amputation, that is, an external hemipelvectomy, essentially include involvement of the iliac vessels and the iliac lumbosacral plexus in conjunction with a high-grade malignancy.

This presented case was extremely difficult and required bilateral type III resection in conjunction with adductor muscle group resection due to extraosseous tumor extension. The large retroperitoneal component was extremely difficult to approach, but the technique of an extended ilioinguinal incision and initial exposure of the femoral vessels enabled a safe resection. Despite the magnitude of this surgery, this patient only had some adductor weakness, and was able to ambulate free of all external aids within 2 to 3 months.

Suggested Readings

Enneking WF. *Musculoskeletal tumor surgery.* Vol. 1. New York, NY: Churchill Livingstone; 1983.

Jelinek JS, Mike V, Hutter RV, et al. Diagnosis of primary bone tumors with image-guided percutaneous biopsy: experience with 110 tumors. *Radiology* 2002;223:731–737.

Kawai A, et al. Prognostic factors for patients with sarcomas of the pelvic bones. *Cancer* 1998;82:851–859.

Malawer M, Bickels J. Pelvic resections and internal hemipelvectomies. In: Malawer M, Sugarbaker PH, eds. *Musculoskeletal cancer surgery: treatment of sarcomas and allied diseases.* Dordrecht: Kluwer Academic Publishers; 2000:405–414.

Marcove RC. Chodrosarcoma: diagnosis and treatment. *Orthop Clin North Am* 1977;8:811–820.

Marcove RC, et al. Chondrosarcoma of the pelvis and upper end of the femur. An analysis of factors influencing survival time in one hundred and thirteen cases. *J Bone Joint Surg Am* 1972;54:561–572.

case 64

Presentation

This patient is a 16-year-old girl with a 3-month history of right shoulder pain. The pain is described as occurring intermittently throughout the day. It is not related to any specific activities and tends to be worse at night. There is no history of a traumatic injury to this extremity. Physical examination demonstrates a significant asymmetry when compared with the contralateral shoulder. The right shoulder has a soft-tissue mass adhered to the underlying humerus. It is easily palpable and minimally tender. There are some dilated veins in the skin overlying the right proximal humeral mass. There is no fever or other notable systemic symptoms such as anorexia or weight loss.

Recommendation

Routine blood tests should be performed, including alkaline phosphatase. Perform chest radiograph, anteroposterior (AP) and lateral radiographs of the right proximal humerus and shoulder girdle, bone scan, and computed tomography (CT) or magnetic resonance imaging (MRI) scan of the shoulder girdle. Biopsy should be done to establish tissue diagnosis.

Case Continued

Laboratory examinations including a complete blood cell count (CBC), blood urea nitrogen (BUN), and electrolytes (e.g., alkaline phosphatase, calcium, and phosphorous) are performed, and the alkaline phosphatase is the only result not within normal limit ranges. The reported value of the alkaline phosphatase was markedly high at 600 units. The patient's white blood count was normal and the sedimentation rate was 18.

A posteroanterior (PA) chest radiograph is normal, but a lytic destructive lesion of the right proximal humerus is easily visualized. AP and lateral radiographs of the right proximal humerus and shoulder girdle show a large, destructive osteolytic and osteoblastic lesion of the proximal third of the humerus. Cortical destruction is observed in these studies. There is a significant soft-tissue component underlying the deltoid muscle, with evidence of extraosseous bone formation arising from the proximal humerus. There is marked periosteal elevation, though the joint space appears to be normal.

CT scans of the right humerus and shoulder girdle show a destructive lesion arising from the right proximal humerus, with a significant soft-tissue component under the deltoid muscle with extraosseous bone formation. The subchondral bone of the humerus is intact without any evidence of destruction or joint involvement by the soft-tissue mass.

MRI examination of the right shoulder girdle demonstrates extensive involvement of the intramedullary space, involving half of the proximal humerus. There is marked cortical destruction corresponding to the finding noted on the CT scan, but a large extraosseous component appears laterally, arising underneath the deltoid. The tumor also extends along the joint capsule. A right shoulder axillary angiogram is performed and demonstrates a hypervascular lesion arising from the right proximal humerus corresponding to the soft-tissue component and bony lesion. There is no obvious evidence of arterial involvement.

◼ Bone Scan

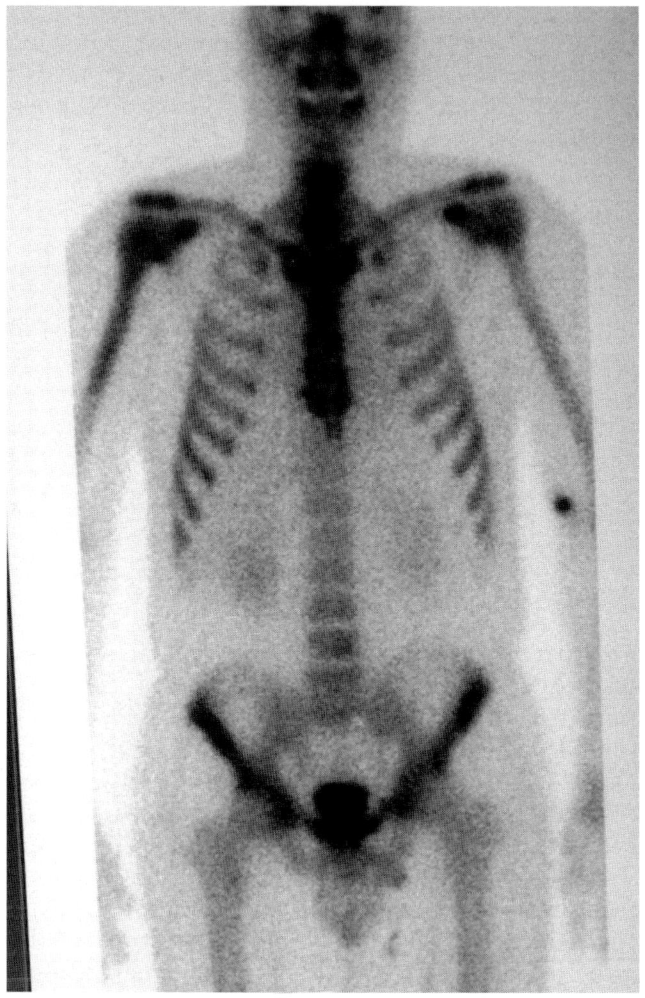

Figure 64.1

Bone Scan Report

The late phase of a three-phase bone scan shows increased radioisotopic uptake within the proximal right third to half of the proximal humerus, with normal uptake in the ipsilateral glenoid. There is no abnormal uptake in the remaining skeletal system. The most common differential in adolescence is a primary malignant tumor of bone (osteosarcoma vs Ewing sarcoma) or infection. The bone scan is a good study to determine the intraosseous extent of tumor within the medullary canal.

Case Continued

A biopsy is performed under CT guidance with a large needle trocar through a single stab wound through the anterior deltoid. Multiple cores are ob-

tained through this puncture site. A frozen pathology section is obtained at the same time, which demonstrates viable spindle-cell tumor with evidence of osteoid formation. There is no evidence of round cells, giant cells, inflammatory cells, or infection.

Differential Diagnosis

The differential diagnosis of a destructive lesion of the long bones in an adolescent is very suspicious for a primary malignancy. The most common primary malignant bone tumors are osteosarcomas, Ewing sarcomas, and less often, chondrosarcomas or giant cell tumors. In the adolescent population, the most common malignant bone tumors include osteosarcomas and Ewing sarcomas. A finding of a large soft-tissue mass is characteristic of osteosarcomas. Approximately 95% of osteosarcomas are accompanied by an extraosseous mass. This patient's history of pain is consistent with that of a primary bone tumor. Tumors arising from the skeletal system are often intermittently to excessively painful during the day, but are characteristically most painful at night. Night pain should be a strong warning for malignant bone pathology. It is rare for tumors arising from the bone to actually involve the neurovascular structures, as seen on the angiogram, but often the major vessels are displaced by the tumor mass itself. The alkaline phosphatase values were markedly elevated. This is a hallmark of, and a tumor marker for, osteosarcoma.

A large core needle biopsy harvested several cores (with CT guidance) through the anterior one third of the deltoid muscle. The soft-tissue component was biopsied, not the bone itself. A frozen section of one core showed high-grade spindle-cell sarcoma. The final pathology showed a highly malignant spindle-cell tumor with the tumor stroma making malignant osteoid.

Diagnosis

Osteosarcoma, stage IIB, arising in the right proximal humerus.

◼ Approach

Treatment of osteosarcoma requires a multimodality approach. This includes induction (preoperative) chemotherapy, surgical removal of the tumor by either a limb-sparing procedure or an amputation, and postoperative chemotherapy. Occasionally, the chemotherapy regimen is modified postoperatively (tailoring), depending on the response of the tumor to the induction chemotherapy. The pathological response is determined by evaluating the amount of tumor necrosis by careful examination and study of the resected tumor mass by a standard pathological technique (i.e., Huvos). Approximately 90% to 95% of all osteosarcomas can today be removed via limb-sparing surgery instead of an amputation. The indications for amputation include massive tumors with neurovascular involvement, pathological fracture, infection, or the occurrence of a tumor in an extremely young (skeletally immature) child.

The specific recommendation for this patient is induction chemotherapy followed by a limb-sparing surgical resection of the right proximal shoulder girdle. There are several different chemotherapy protocols. Typically, the induction phase lasts 12 to 16 weeks. The most common drugs used include doxorubicin (Adriamycin), cisplatin, ifosfamide, and high-dose methotrexate. The tumor is clearly resectable following induction chemotherapy as demonstrated by restaging studies, including repeat CT, MRI, and angiogram of the shoulder. The major nerves and vessels to the arm can be preserved, and the bony resection site can be reconstructed with a metallic endoprosthesis. A modular segmental prosthesis is presently being used for most patients with osteosarcomas. Following surgery and wound healing, patients with osteosarcomas are treated with postoperative chemotherapy for 6 to 12 months, depending upon various protocols.

◼ Axillary Angiogram

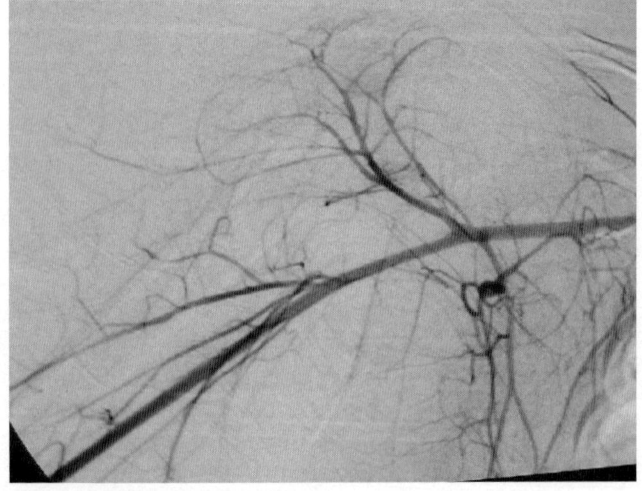

Figure 64.2

Axillary Angiography Report

Angiogram (midarterial phase) is performed with the arm placed in the abduction position following induction chemotherapy. Note there is no uptake of contrast within the proximal humerus or the extraosseous component.

Discussion

Angiography following induction chemotherapy is one of the most reliable imaging techniques to determine the impact (i.e., percent tumor necrosis) of preoperative chemotherapy. The absence of any uptake correlates with a good tumor response (i.e., >90% tumor necrosis). In addition, preoperative angiography is helpful to the surgeon in planning the definitive resection.

◼ Surgical Approach

This patient undergoes an extra-articular resection of the shoulder girdle including the proximal humerus, the lateral portion of the scapula including the glenoid, and the lateral one third of the clavicle. The proximal humeral prosthesis is then cemented in place, and the head is placed anterior to the remaining scapula. It is suspended from the scapula and remaining clavicle by Dacron tape. The reconstruction also consists of multiple muscle transfers, especially the pectoralis major and the trapezius. The deltoid muscle is the main muscle that is resected at the time of surgery because it typically provides an adjacent covering for the tumor mass. Shoulder girdle function is stable immediately following reconstruction. There is no need for arterial grafts or nerve reconstruction. Elbow and hand function are normal.

Discussion

Approximately 90% to 95% of all osteosarcomas of the proximal humerus can be treated by a limb-sparing resection instead of an amputation. The tumor is resected and the defect is reconstructed with a segmental modular prosthesis. The resection can either be intra-articular (through the joint) or extra-articular (en bloc removal of the proximal humerus including the glenoid). All muscles attaching to or arising from the proximal humerus are considered at risk for tumor spread. In general, tumors of the proximal humerus are best treated by extra-articular resections when undertaking a limb-sparing procedure, because there is a high incidence of local recurrence when joint preservation is attempted.

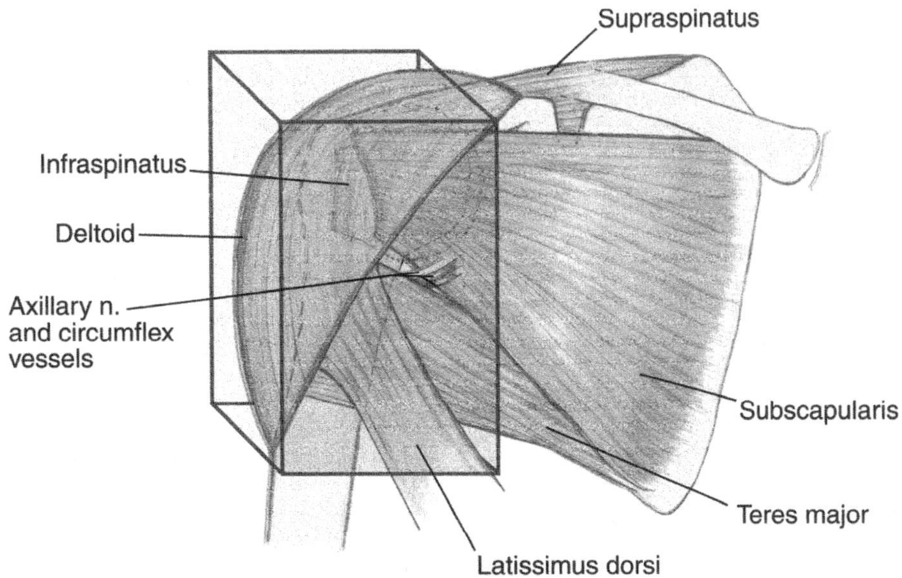

Figure 64.3 Surgical anatomy of the shoulder girdle.

Case Continued

The wound heals well except for a small area of flap necrosis, which requires debridement and secondary skin closure. Wound necrosis following limb-sparing surgery is one of the most common complications and should be treated aggressively to avoid a second-ary infection, especially with adjuvant chemother-apy. Following complete wound healing, the patient begins a postoperative chemotherapy regimen that includes doxorubicin (Adriamycin), cisplatin, and ifosfamide. She is examined every 3 months and un-dergoes CT scans, three-phase bone scans, and plain bone radiographs prior to each clinical evaluation.

Postoperative X-Ray

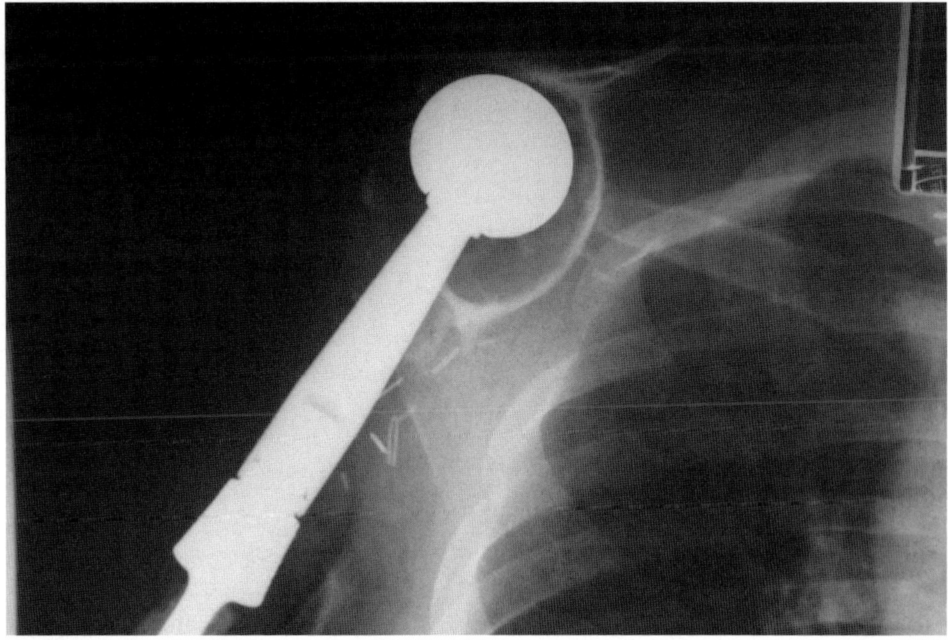

Figure 64.4

Postoperative X-Ray Report

A large segmental prosthesis is used to reconstruct the segmental defect. Note the absence of the glenoid. The area of semicircular ossification around the head of the prosthesis is a common finding after several years; it represents metaplastic new bone and is an attempt to create a "new" glenoid.

■ Specimen Photograph and X-Ray

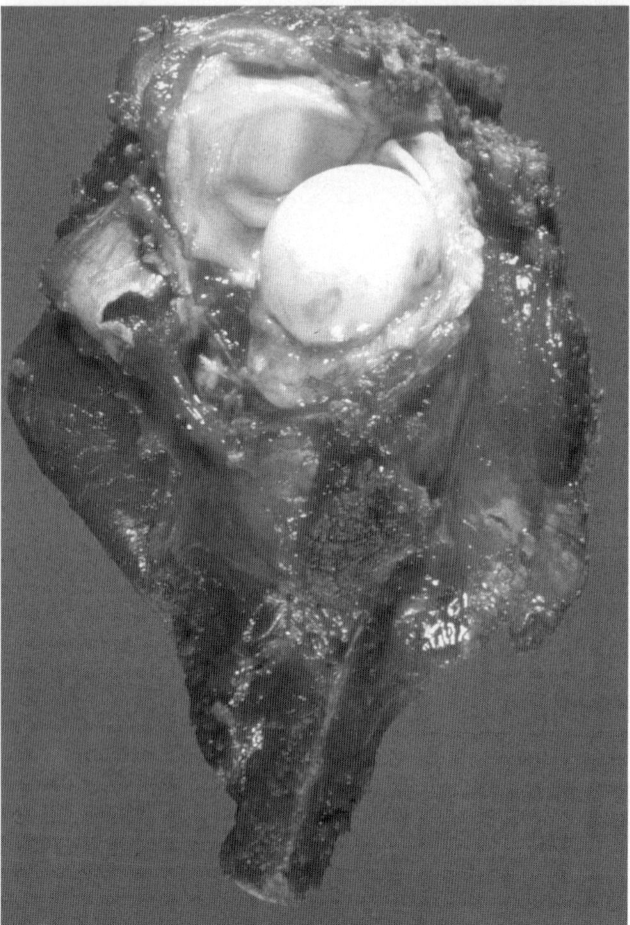

Figure 64.5A

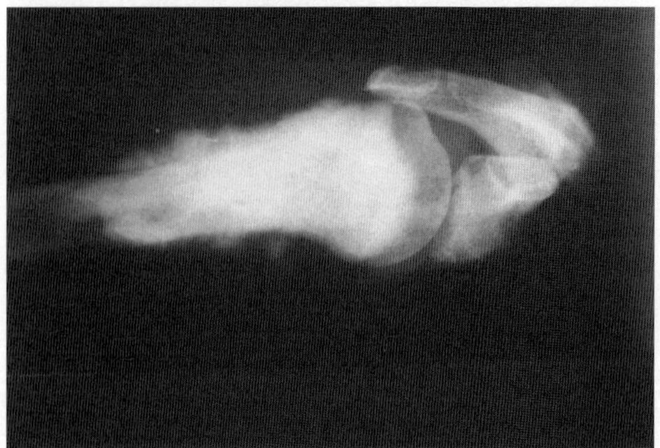

Figure 64.5B

Specimen Report

The gross resected specimen consists of one third of the proximal humerus along with the glenohumeral joint, deltoid, and other attaching muscles. This is classified as a type VB resection. Local recurrence following this type of resection for high-grade bone sarcomas is less than 5%. Plain radiograph of the specimen shows the proximal humerus, which is sclerotic (area of osteosarcoma), and the attached glenoid and acromion, demonstrating a complete extra-articular resection.

■ Histopathology Slides

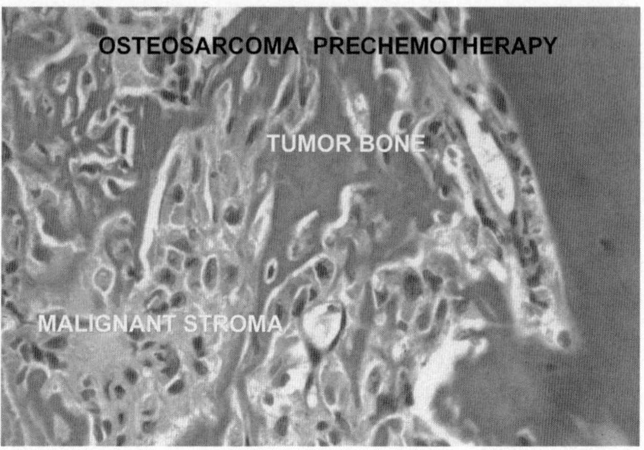

Figure 64.6A

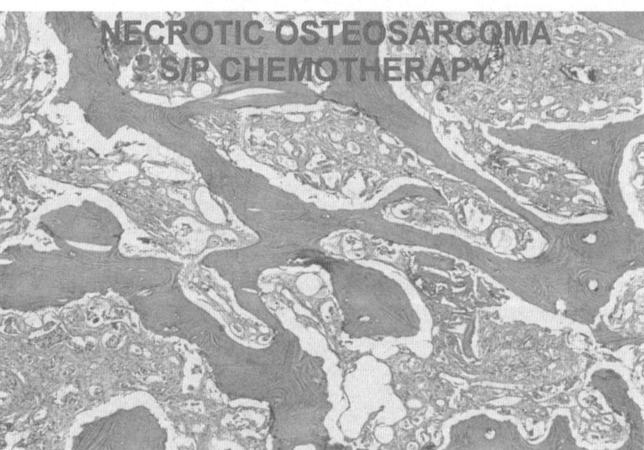

Figure 64.6B

Histopathology Report

Prechemotherapy histology **(A)** shows a typical high-grade osteosarcoma. The pink material represents malignant osteoid made by the malignant stroma cells. Following induction (preoperative) chemotherapy, examination of the removed specimen **(B)** shows complete stroma (cellular) necrosis with reparative granulation tissue. No viable tumor cells are seen. The remaining tumor osteoid *(pink)* remains with no viable cells seen between them. Tumor osteoid does not disappear following tumor necrosis. This patient had 98% tumor necrosis. Tumor necrosis greater than 90% is the most important predictor of survival.

Discussion

Patients with osteosarcomas are followed extremely carefully to rule out local recurrence or metastatic disease. If a bone sarcoma metastasizes, it almost always results in pulmonary nodules initially, with occasional metastatic nodules to the skeletal system. Metastases from osteosarcomas are almost always hematogenously spread. CT scans are the most accurate method of evaluating the lungs for pulmonary disease. Bone scans are also performed with special attention paid to increased abnormal uptake. Approximately 5% to 10% of patients with metastatic osteosarcomas relapse in bony sites initially prior to detection of pulmonary disease. Occasionally, an increase in alkaline phosphatase (tumor marker for malignant osteosarcoma cells) activity signifies local recurrence or metastatic disease; therefore, laboratory testing should be performed at regular intervals. In general, 50% of patients with osteosarcomas have an initial elevated alkaline phosphatase level.

Case Continued

Ten months postoperatively, chest CT scans show bilateral pulmonary nodules interpreted as metastatic osteosarcoma. At this point, this patient is treated with thoracotomy with resection of all four nodules. She is restarted on a chemotherapy regimen, and at 24 months postthoracotomy she remains disease free. This patient is followed for 24 months with no evidence of additional pulmonary disease or metastatic bony disease. Her shoulder girdle is functioning extremely well with normal elbow and hand function.

Discussion

There are approximately 1,000 new cases of primary malignant bone tumors diagnosed in adolescents in the United States each year. The most common malignant bone tumor is osteosarcoma. Ewing sarcoma is a round cell tumor of bone, which typically occurs in a slightly younger age group, but may occur up to the age of 30. These patients also often present with large soft-tissue masses. Ewing sarcomas occur at about half the incidence of osteosarcomas. Generally, osteosarcomas occur at the ends of long bones, whereas Ewing sarcomas occur in the axial skeleton, pelvis, scapula, and proximal femur. It is often difficult to distinguish between the two malignancies utilizing radiographs alone. The diagnostic clue on the initial radiograph for this patient was the evidence of new bone formation (extraosseous bone formation) in the soft tissues. This is pathognomonic for an osteosarcoma. The additional clue is an elevated alkaline phosphatase value, which occurs in 40% to 50% of all osteosarcoma patients but not in Ewing sarcoma patients. Alkaline phosphatase is a good tumor marker for malignant osteoid (i.e., osteosarcoma). This patient did not have any systemic symptoms, such as anorexia, fever, or weight loss. Sarcomas in general do not produce systemic complaints except for Ewing sarcoma, with reports of approximately 20% to 30%.

A needle biopsy with multiple core samples is utilized to confirm the diagnosis and is the preferred method of definitive diagnosis. A pathologist is present to perform a frozen section to determine if viable tissue (not necrotic tissue) is obtained and interpretable. An incisional biopsy is not indicated due to the high likelihood of local wound contamination by tumor cells. Open biopsies are performed only when inadequate tissue is obtained with the core needle biopsy.

The biopsy for patients with suspected musculoskeletal tumors is the first invasive procedure, but it is extremely important. Inappropriate biopsy can contaminate tissue planes, which may jeopardize the ability to perform a limb-sparing procedure. Today, most biopsies are performed under CT guidance utilizing a large core needle. Multiple cores are obtained in the presence of an experienced pathologist to ensure that adequate tissue is harvested. Often, necrotic cores are obtained, requiring additional samples. An incisional biopsy is rarely indicated, but when performed, should be in the line of dissection of any planned future incision for a resection or amputation. Therefore, the person performing the biopsy should consult with the orthopaedic oncologist. Tumors of the shoulder girdle should not be biopsied through the deltopectoral groove, because this would contaminate the pectoralis major muscle as well as the axillary space and vessels. It is strongly recommended that instead, biopsies be performed through the anterior one third of the deltoid with a core needle. The anterior one third of the deltoid can be resected at the time of definitive resection. The axillary nerve of the deltoid originates in a posterior position and will not be disturbed if the anterior portion of the muscle is resected.

Enneking established staging of musculoskeletal tumors, and these tumors are classified according to the Musculoskeletal Tumor Society Classification System. Stage I is a low-grade malignant tumor of bone; stage II is a high-grade malignant tumor of bone. An "A" designation refers to a tumor that is confined to the compartment (intracompartmental or intraosseous), whereas the "B" designation refers to a tumor that arises extraosseously or extracompartmentally. The patient described in this case report had a stage IIB lesion, that is, a high-grade bone sarcoma with an extraosseous component. Approximately 90% to 95% of all osteosarcomas present as stage IIB lesions.

Prior to the advent of adjuvant chemotherapy in the mid-1970s and early 1980s, 85% of patients with osteosarcomas died of their disease within 2 years due to pulmonary metastases. The lungs are the primary sites of metastatic spread, and 50% of patients had metastatic disease within 12 to 18 months. Chemotherapy has dramatically changed this dismal prognosis for patients with pediatric primary sarcomas of bone, especially osteosarcoma and Ewing sarcoma.

The chemotherapy utilized for osteosarcoma patients includes doxorubicin (Adriamycin), cisplatin, and ifosfamide, and sometimes high-dose methotrexate. There are several protocols available. Routinely, these drugs are utilized preoperatively (induction). Most tumors respond to induction chemotherapy with tumor shrinkage and a marked decrease in pain.

Induction chemotherapy was initially developed to shrink the tumor prior to surgery while giving manufacturers time to create custom endoprostheses for skeletal reconstruction. Today, modular segmental prostheses are readily available and can be custom fit in the operating room. Surgeons and oncologists have learned that the main advantage of induction chemotherapy is that it reduces the size of the tumor, making limb-sparing surgery possible and avoiding the need for amputation. In addition, evaluation of the tumor following resection provides the treating medical oncologists prognostic information regarding tumor response to the chemotherapy.

In general, tumor necrosis >90% is considered a good response. Approximately 10% of all patients have 100% tumor necrosis. The overall survival rate of patients with >90% tumor necrosis is between 70% and 80%. Patients with <90% tumor necrosis have only a 40% to 60% survival rate. Those with no tumor necrosis have a dismal prognosis.

Endoprosthetic replacements for large bony defects have been developed since the early 1980s. The changes in the development of the prostheses and improved surgical techniques have led to true evolution in the treatment of primary bony sarcomas, both in adolescents and adults. The primary bone tumors that occur in adults most commonly include chondrosarcoma and malignant fibrous histiocytoma of bone. Metastatic neoplasms of bone are the most common bone tumors in adults. The primary bone sarcomas in adults are treated using principles similar to those established for adolescents (i.e., induction chemotherapy followed by surgery and postoperative chemotherapy). Radiation therapy is not utilized for spindle-cell sarcomas in children or adults, except for palliation.

The treatment regimens of metastatic osteosarcoma to the lungs are variable. The patient described in this case report developed several pulmonary nodules at 10 months. The mainstay of treatment in her case was thoracotomy with the removal of all palpable disease. If there are four or fewer nodules, approximately 20% to 25% of the lung can be salvaged. The reinstitution of chemotherapy or a change to second-line drugs has not been standardized at the present time.

Suggested Readings

Enneking WF, Spanier SS, Goodman MA. A system for the surgical staging of musculoskeletal sarcoma. *Clin Orthop* 1980;153:106–120.

Jelinek JS, Murphy MD, Welker JA, et al. Diagnosis of primary bone tumors with image-guided percutaneous biopsy: experience with 110 tumors. *Radiology* 2002;223:731–737.

Malawer M, Wittig J. Overview of resections around the shoulder girdle: anatomy, surgical considerations, and classification. In: Malawer M, Sugarbaker PH, eds. *Musculoskeletal cancer surgery: treatment of sarcomas and allied diseases.* Dordrecht: Kluwer Academic Publishers; 2000:179–202.

Malawer M, Wittig J. Proximal humerus resection: the Tikhoff-Linberg procedure. In: Malawer M, Sugarbaker PH, eds. *Musculoskeletal cancer surgery: treatment of sarcomas and allied diseases.* Dordrecht: Kluwer Academic Publishers; 2000:519–552.

Malawer MM, Sugarbaker PH, Lampert M, et al. The Tikhoff-Linberg procedure: report of ten patients and presentation of a modified technique for tumors of the proximal humerus. *Surgery* 1985;97:518–528.

Wittig JC, Bickels J, Kellar-Graney KL, et al. Osteosarcoma of the proximal humerus: long-term results with limb-sparing surgery. *Clin Orthop* 2002;397: 156–176.

Wittig JC, Bickels J, Priebat D, et al. Osteosarcoma: a multidisciplinary approach to diagnosis and treatment. *Am Fam Physician* 2002;65:1123–1132.

Wodajo FM, Bickels J, Wittig J, et al. Complex reconstruction in the management of extremity sarcomas. *Curr Opin Oncol* 2003;15:304–312.

Presentation

An 18-year-old boy with pain in the right thigh presents to your office after his general practitioner treated him for a "pulled muscle" 6 weeks ago. On examination, the right thigh is swollen and slightly red. Palpation is painful and shows increased temperature compared to the left thigh.

X-Rays

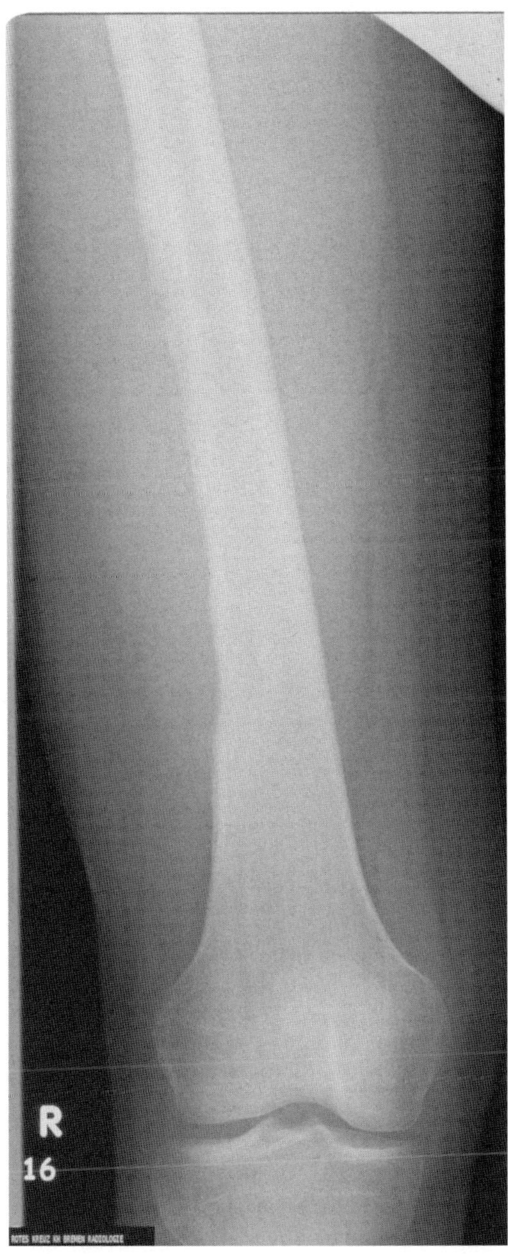

Figure 65.1A

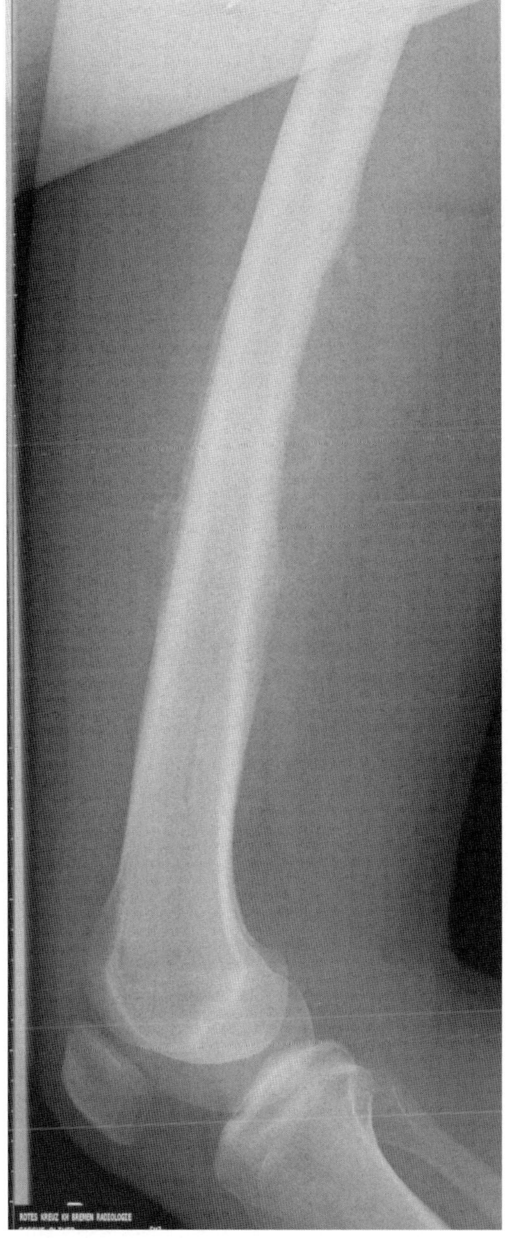

Figure 65.1B

X-Ray Report

On x-ray, an indistinct lesion of the medullary canal with mottled destruction pattern is seen. There is some reactive bone in the midportion of the lesion, some endosteal reaction, and a soft-tissue mass.

Differential Diagnosis

The differential diagnosis for an intramedullary lesion of the femur in adolescents includes osteo-myelitis, lymphoma, and Ewing sarcoma. Clinical and radiological symptoms of Ewing sarcoma show a large variability. It is a "chameleon," imitating almost all kinds of lesions of the bone. Therefore, it is most important to keep Ewing sarcoma in mind. Further imaging of the lesion should include the whole affected bone, because sometimes this tumor may grow as "skip lesions" in the compartment.

MRI

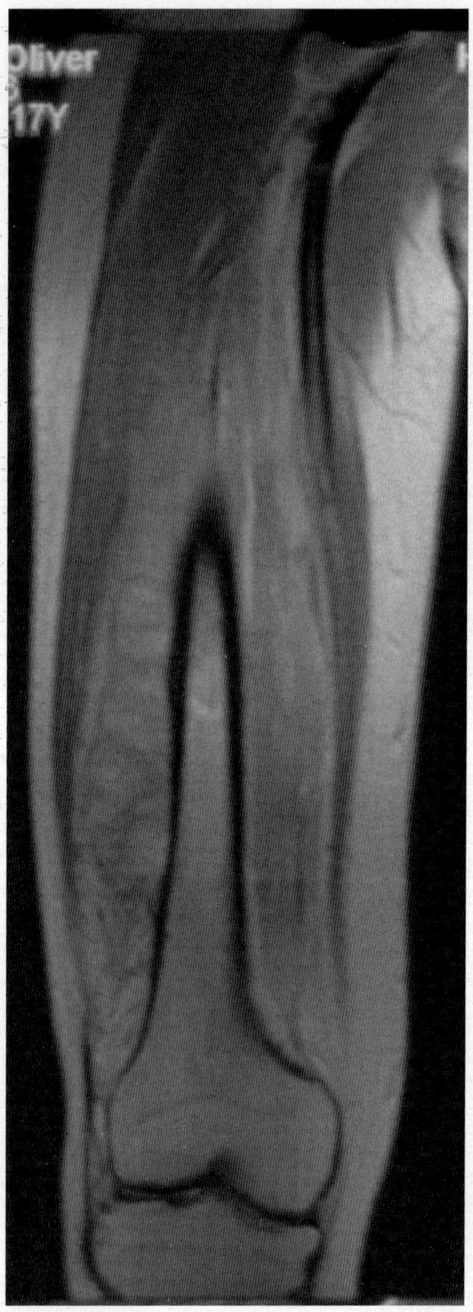

Figure 65.2A

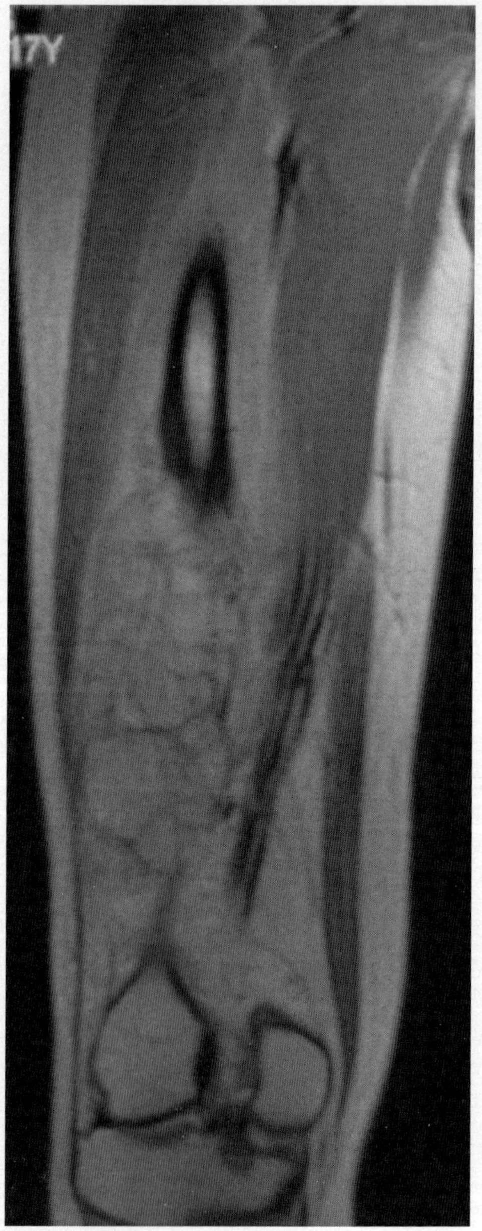

Figure 65.2B

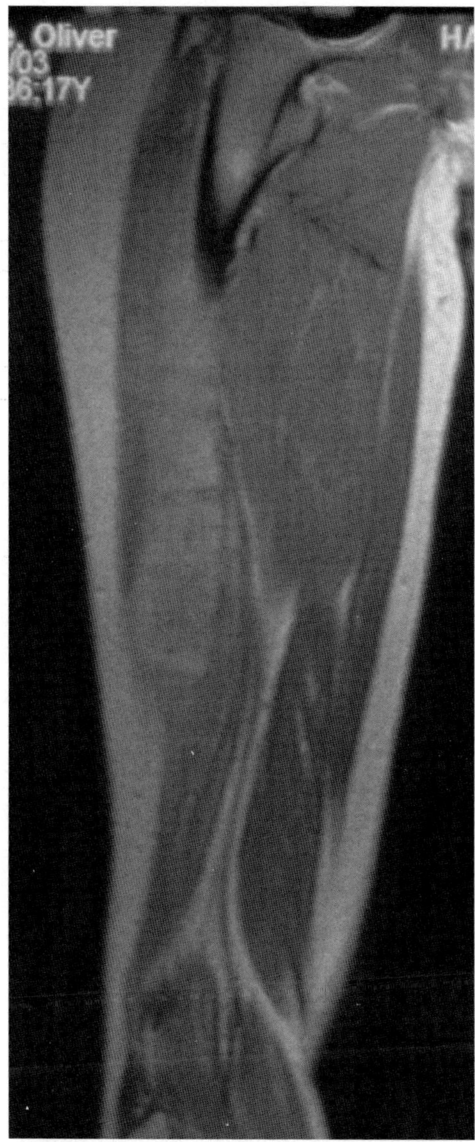

Figure 65.2C

MRI Report

On magnetic resonance imaging (MRI), a 19×6.5-cm heterogenous mass is seen lateral and dorsal to the diaphyses of the femur. Enhancement is present inside the intramedullary canal. Just below the lesser trochanter, a 1-cm suspicious lesion is detected.

Recommendation

Open biopsy or needle biopsy is recommended.

Discussion

Needle biopsy is almost always sufficient to establish the diagnosis. In difficult cases, an open biopsy is strongly recommended because additional studies may be necessary, especially evaluation for chromosomal translocations. A frozen section during surgery can determine if the biopsy material is adequate in quantity and quality. Furthermore, a bone marrow biopsy can be performed under general anesthesia.

Case Continued

The frozen section shows a tumor with small blue round cells. Further histological examination is periodic acid-Schiff (PAS) positive, CD 99 (MI-2) positive, vimentin positive, and the neuronal markers neuron-specific enolase (NSE) positive and S100 negative. The (11;22) translocation is positive. Further tumor staging includes bone marrow examination, computed tomography (CT) scan of the chest, and bone scan, and reveals no systemic tumor.

Diagnosis and Recommendation

Localized Ewing sarcoma of the right femur. Surgical staging reveals an extracompartmental aggressive bone tumor without systemic metastasis (stage IIb, according to Enneking). The patient is enrolled into the **Euro**pean **E**wing tumor **W**orking **I**nitiative of **N**ational **G**roups Study (Euro EWING) protocol. After six cycles of VIDE (vincristine, ifosfamide, doxorubicin, and etoposide), a repeat MRI scan is performed and local therapy is discussed with the patient.

▍ MRI

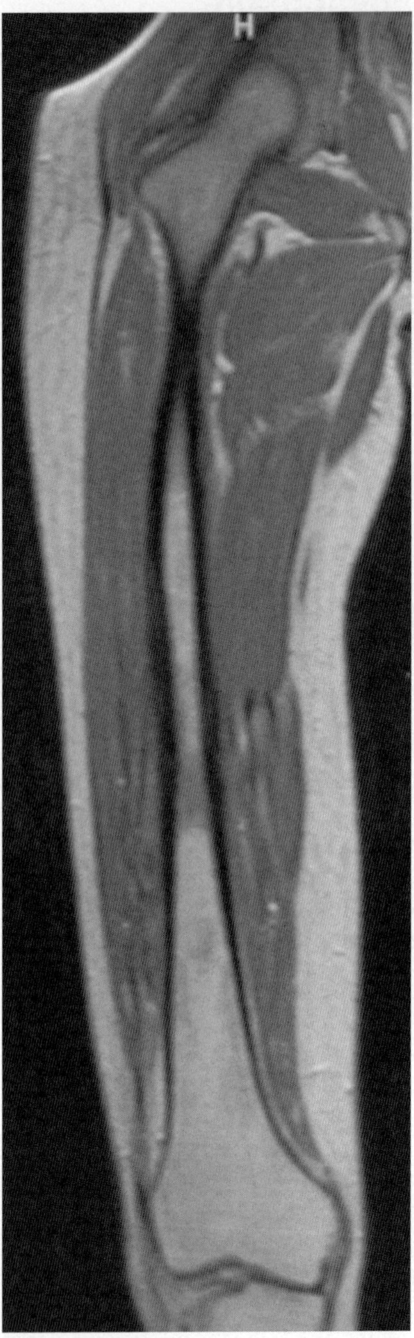

Figure 65.3A

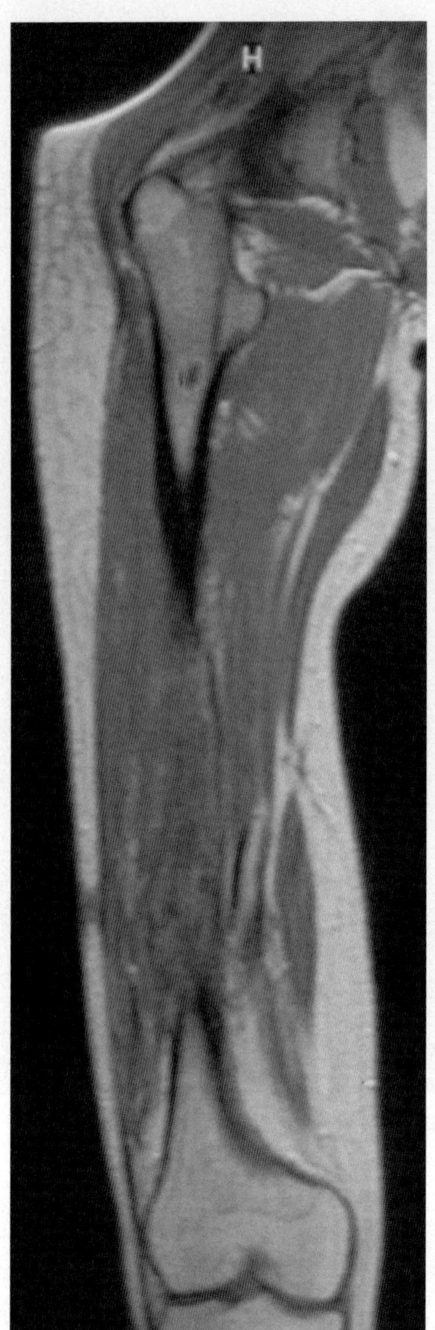

Figure 65.3B

MRI Report

After chemotherapy, the soft-tissue component of the tumor has disappeared almost completely. The intramedullary component of the tumor and lesion just below the lesser trochanter remain unchanged. The lesions still show enhancement in the dynamic contrast examination.

▍ Approach

The patient is offered a wide tumor resection to achieve adequate local tumor control. Because of the disseminated intramedullary growth of the tumor, the whole femur compartment should be resected. Endoprosthetic reconstruction would be performed by implantation of a total femur prosthesis with knee and hip arthroplasty. The complications mentioned to the patient are bleeding, femoral and sciatic nerve palsy, infection, local recurrence, limp, hip disarticulation, and death.

Discussion

It was discussed with the patient that local therapy of Ewing sarcoma is an important factor for local tumor control and overall survival. Radiotherapy increases the survival rate of Ewing sarcoma up to 24%. But even after combined chemotherapy and radiotherapy, two thirds of cases show persistent viable cancer. In general, surgery achieves better local control and survival figures than radiotherapy. Regarding overall survival, the efficacy of radiotherapy as compared to surgery varies among studies and seems to be dependent on patient selection and sequencing with chemotherapy. Although not proven by randomized studies, an impact on survival is likely, and in the long run overall survival cannot be improved without adequate local tumor control.

Surgical Approach

From a lateral approach, the incision starts 10 cm proximal to the greater trochanter along the lateral aspect of the femur and curves anteriorly to end 2 cm distal to the tibial tuberosity. The peroneal nerve is identified near the biceps femoris tendon. The biceps femoris is detached from the proximal fibula. The lateral head of the gastrocnemius muscle is divided at its femoral origin and the popliteal vessels are located. Branches to the distal femur are identified and ligated. The vascular bundle is traced to the adductor hiatus, which is incised. The peroneal nerve is followed to its junction with the sciatic nerve. The gluteus maximus tendon and the external rotators are detached from their femoral insertions, and the proximal portion of the sciatic nerve is located. The gluteus medius and minimus are divided near the greater trochanter. The branches of the medial femoral circumflex artery and vein are ligated, and the adductor muscles are detached from the femur.

The knee joint is opened laterally and the cruciate ligaments are detached. The vastus intermedius is left attached to the femur. The other portions of the quadriceps are resected due to tumor extension. The patella is dislocated medially and the joint is opened by incising the dorsal capsule, popliteus and plantaris tendons, and the medial iliotibial band and capsule. The medial head of the gastrocnemius is released. After disarticulation, the distal femur is elevated and the remaining muscles are detached. The hip joint capsule is opened, and the specimen is removed.

A modular total femur prosthesis is implanted, and the hip joint and capsule are reconstructed with a double cup and a trevira tube to prevent dislocations.

Postoperative X-Ray

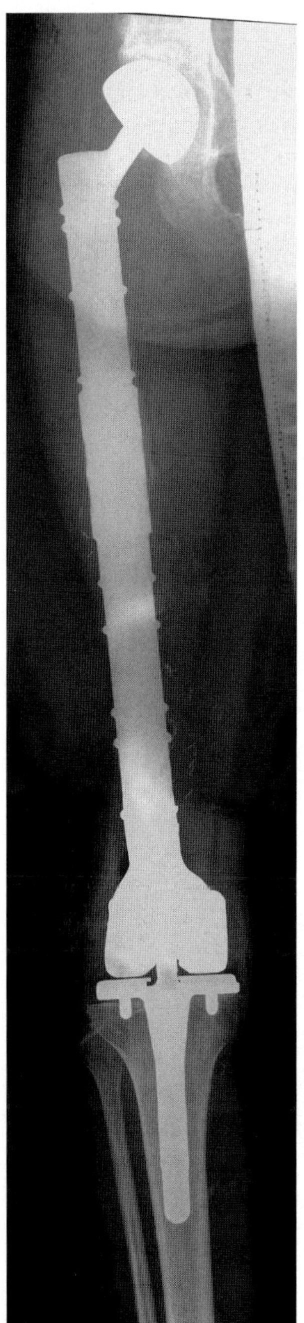

Figure 65.4

Postoperative X-Ray Report

The modular total femur prosthesis is seen and the hip and knee joint are intact.

Case Continued

Histology of the resected specimen shows <1% viable tumor, which is classified as a good response. All margins are "wide."

Discussion

Combined local therapy (surgery plus postoperative radiotherapy) has shown excellent local control rates, and it is offered to patients with high-risk lesions (e.g., pelvic tumors and poor responders). Because of the good response of the tumor and the primary tumor site, no postoperative radiotherapy is advised.

Case Continued

Further chemotherapy according to the Euro EWING protocol is administered. The patient is allowed to mobilize immediately. No hip exercises are allowed for 6 weeks, and walking on crutches is permitted until muscular stability of the leg is regained.

Suggested Readings

Dunst J, Schuck A. Role of radiotherapy in Ewing tumors. *Pediatr Blood Cancer* 2004;42:465–470.

Gosheger G, Hillmann A, Lindner N, et al. Soft tissue reconstruction of megaprostheses using a trevira tube. *Clin Orthop* 2001;393:264–271.

Mittermayer F, Krepler P, Dominkus M, et al. Long-term follow-up of uncemented tumor endoprostheses for the lower extremity. *Clin Orthop* 2001;388:167–177.

Nakamura S, Kusuzaki K, Murata H, et al. More than 10 years of follow-up of two patients after total femur replacement for malignant bone tumor. *Int Orthop* 2000;24:176–178.

Presentation

A 59-year-old man with no previous medical history complains of persistent dull abdominal pain that extends to the perineum. He reports that his bowel function has worsened slightly over the last couple of years. On rectal examination, a firm mass is palpable on the posterior aspect of the rectal ampulla; the superior margin of the mass is not appreciable. On neurologic examination, S2-S3 dysesthesia is detected. The patient has already undergone an abdominal ultrasound showing a presacral solid mass.

Differential Diagnosis

Metastatic tumor is the most frequent sacral lesion, particularly in adults older than 30 years, and should be excluded primarily. Among primitive sacrococcygeal masses, chordoma is the most frequent malignant disease, and the most common benign lesion is giant cell tumor.

Discussion

Among sacral primary tumors, 40% are chordomas, 12% are giant cell tumors, 8% are myelomas, 8% are lymphomas, 8% are Ewing sarcomas, 5% are chondrosarcomas, 4% are osteosarcomas, 4% are fibrosarcomas, and 3% are aneurysmatic bone cysts.

Chordoma is a rare neoplasm arising from aberrant primitive notochord remnants, localized to the midline spine, in the sacrococcygeal region and at the skull base. Tumor burden ranges from 2 to 30 cm maximum diameter at diagnosis. Symptoms are nonspecific, median age of presentation is 50 to 60 years, and there is a male predominance.

Recommendation

Biopsy to establish tissue diagnosis is recommended.

Discussion

Transrectal needle biopsy should be avoided (unless a rectal resection has already been planned) due to possible neoplastic seeding of the pelvis and viscera. Transperitoneal surgical biopsy must be avoided as well. Computed tomography (CT)-guided fine-needle biopsy or core needle biopsy by a posterior approach should be discussed with the operating surgeon, and the biopsy site should be tattooed. If needle biopsy is not feasible or the material obtained is not sufficient, surgical biopsy is indicated, with posterior small midline access to permit subsequent excision of scar.

Histopathology Slides

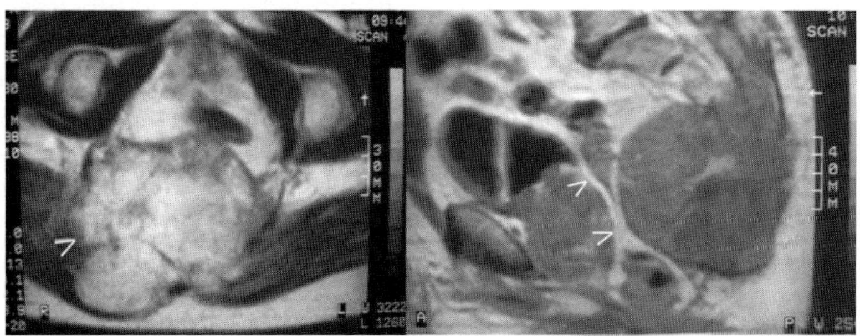

Figure 66.1

Histopathology Report

Neoplastic proliferation of large-sized cells organized in cord-like strands, with abundant myxoid substance consistent with a chordoma.

MRI

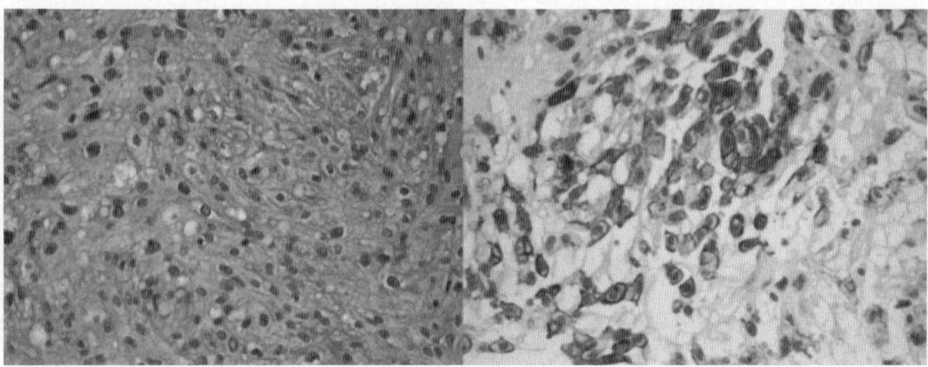

Figure 66.2 A   B

MRI Report

Axial T2 MRI **(A)** reveals an expansive pelvic mass measuring 12×12 cm involving the higher sacral vertebrae and coccyx. The rectum is displaced anteriorly without any evidence of invasion. There is posterior and caudal extension of the lesion toward the buttocks with muscle infiltration bilaterally. **(B)** On sagittal T1, bone structure is disrupted, and the rectum is displaced by tumor mass.

Case Continued

The patient has a normal CT scan of the chest, and hence has chordoma with extension to higher sacrum.

Approach

Chordoma is a low-grade and slow-growing malignant tumor. Responsiveness to chemotherapy and radiotherapy is poor; resection with a wide margin is the mainstay of treatment.

The patient should be informed of the major surgical concerns, including bone and possible muscle resections, sacral nerve roots sacrifice, and the need for reconstruction. Immediate surgical complications include bleeding and infections. Perioperative mortality should be mentioned. Mid- and long-term possible surgical sequelae are prolonged seroma, wound

Diagnosis and Recommendations

Chordoma. Complete staging with abdominopelvic magnetic resonance imaging (MRI) and CT scan of the chest to evaluate local extent of disease and presence of metastases.

infection, fecal incontinence, urinary retention, erectile impotence, and relative ischiatic deficiency.

The goal of surgical therapy is to perform an en bloc resection with wide bone and soft-tissue margins, to provide optimum local control. Preoperative surgical planning should be meticulous, with special regard to bone level resection, sacral roots sacrifice, and reconstructive time.

If bone resection is not higher than the inferior plate of the first sacral vertebra, an exclusive posterior approach is feasible, satisfactory, and safe. After skin flap preparation, the sacrum is exposed, and the sacroiliac and sacrotuberous ligaments as well as gluteus maximus are divided. At a deeper level, the piriformis muscles and sacrospinous and anococcygeal ligaments are identified and divided. The rectum is gently detached from the presacral lamina and the tumor, with great care to avoid the hemorrhoidal plexus, which may bleed profusely. At the chosen level for sacrum resection, a careful digital dissection of the anterior soft tissue is performed on both sides through the greater ischiatic notch. The body of the sacrum is cut through with an osteotome. The higher nerve roots are visualized and preserved; the lower roots, including S3, are removed en bloc with the tumor.

A combined abdominosacral approach is advocated for total sacrectomy: the anterior approach permits safe control of internal iliac vessel branches and the sacral roots that need to be preserved, and the rectum is mobilized or removed as necessary.

Bone resection is performed by a subsequent posterior approach with vertical osteotomy of sacroiliac joints. Laparoscopically assisted sacrectomy has been reported.

The pelvic girdle maintains stability if the first sacral vertebra is preserved; otherwise, continuity between the spine and iliac bones should be restored. Synthetic mesh may be necessary to avoid posterior herniation of the viscera. In the case of skin infiltration by tumor mass, musculocutaneous flap reconstruction may be necessary.

Neurological outcome correlates with root resection level: if bilateral S3 roots are preserved, usually normal urinary and bowel function are maintained; if bilateral S2 roots are preserved, temporary urinary retention, fecal incontinence, or both may be experienced. In case of preservation of only S1 roots, definitive bowel and urinary dysfunction are always present and diversion might be needed.

The patient should be referred to a tertiary care center, because the initial surgical procedure provides the best chance of cure. A multispecialist surgical team is sometime needed. Surgical planning should consider that the more sophisticated the reconstruction, the higher the risk of infection, with the resulting possibility of delay in treatment.

Intraoperative Photographs

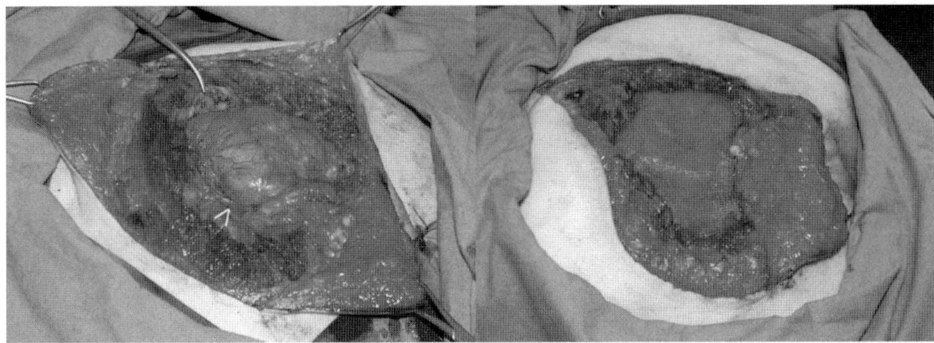

Figure 66.3A   **B**

Surgical Approach

A posterior approach is performed with a "reverse Y" skin incision. High sacrectomy with bone section at the S1 level is performed. Gluteus maximus and piriform muscles are resected en bloc with the tumor mass. Note the divided gluteus maximus muscles, sacral stump *(clamp tip)*, and left S2 nerve **(A)**, which is the highest nerve root preserved. Reconstruction with nonabsorbable polypropylene mesh is necessary **(B)**. The surgical specimen is microscopically marginal at the level of S1 bone resection. Surgical resection lasts 6 hours; 3 units of packed red blood cells are transfused perioperatively. Postsurgical cutaneous flaps healed after 4 months, requiring hyperbaric oxygen therapy. The patient experienced long-term and definitive urinary retention. No fecal incontinence is observed; only a slightly hypotonic sphincter was appreciated on rectal examination. Relative hyposthenia of the lower limbs was present.

Discussion

Mortality for chordoma is primarily due to locally recurrent disease. Disease-free survival and overall survival rates at 10 years are 20% to 25% and 50%, respectively. In our series, local relapse rates were related to microscopic margin status, with 54.5% in negative-margin operations, 50% in the positive margin resection with adjuvant radiation therapy, and 100% for patients operated upon with positive margins.

Local recurrence more frequently involves soft tissue surrounding the sacrum, the rectum, and the perianal and gluteal areas, than the sacral stump. Complete resection of recurrent disease is difficult, and sometimes palliative treatment is the only feasible procedure.

Distant metastases occur in 10% of patients, with the lungs being the most common site, followed by other vertebral bodies, liver, and soft tissues.

Follow-up should include clinical examination, supplemented with pelvic and thoracic imaging.

Case Continued

The patient receives adjuvant radiation therapy with a total dose of 60 Gy. He develops lung metastasis 60 months after primary surgery. He therefore undergoes complete resection of an isolated 4-cm lung nodule by thoracotomy. He is alive and disease free 74 months after initial surgery.

Suggested Readings

Baratti D, Gronchi A, Pennacchioli E, et al. Chordoma: natural history and results in 28 patients treated at a single institution. *Ann Surg Oncol* 2003;10:291–296.

Catton C, O'Sullivan B, Bell R, et al. Chordoma: long-term follow-up after radical photon irradiation. *Radiother Oncol* 1996;41:67–72.

Dorfmann HD, Czerniak B. Chordoma and related lesions. In: *Bone tumors*. St. Louis, MO: Mosby; 1998:974–1007.

Gennari L, Azzarelli A, Quagliolo V. A posterior approach for the excision of sacral chordoma. *J Bone Joint Surg Br* 1987;69: 565–568.

Localio SA, Eng K, Ranson JHC. Abdominosacral approach for retrorectal tumors. *Ann Surg* 1980;191:555–560.

Malawer MM, Link MP, Donaldson SS. Sarcomas of bone. In: DeVita VT Jr, Hellman S, Rosenberg SA, eds. *Cancer: principles and practice of oncology.* 6th ed. Philadelphia, PA: Lippincott Williams & Wilkins; 2001:1928–1929.

Sundaresan N, Huvos AG, Krol G, et al. Surgical treatment of spinal chordomas. *Arch Surg* 1987;122:1479–1482.

Presentation

A 41-year-old man is referred for management of a newly diagnosed melanoma on his left chest. The pathology report describes a 0.9-mm melanoma, Clark's level III. He has light red hair, pale skin, and numerous freckles, and reports that his skin burns easily. He notes that his brother was treated for melanoma about 5 years ago and is now free of disease. On examination, he has a healing punch biopsy site on the left chest approximately 4 cm below the nipple, and no evidence of satellite lesions or in-transit disease. Regional node basins are clinically negative.

Clinical Photograph

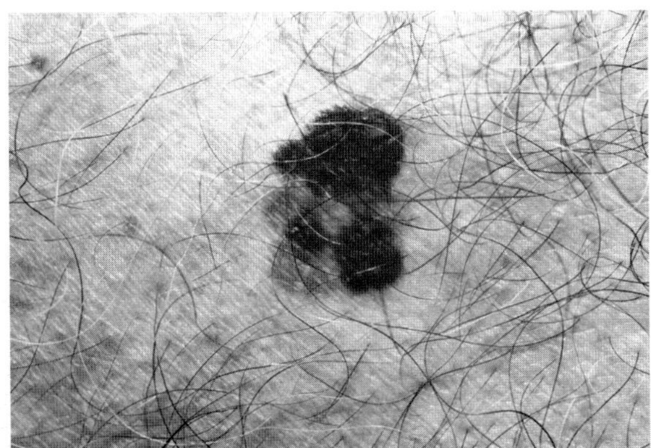

Figure 67.1

Physical Examination Report

On skin examination, a flat, irregularly shaped, pigmented lesion with color variegation is noted on the right side of his back.

Discussion

Most newly diagnosed melanoma patients present with thin (<1 mm) to intermediate (1 to 4 mm) Breslow thickness lesions. Treatment decisions are based on the pathology of the primary lesion, and review of the pathology slides by an experienced dermatopathologist is useful. Clinical evaluation includes an examination of node basins for evidence of lymphadenopathy, and skin examination for evidence of other suspicious skin lesions. For patients whose clinical examination reveals no evidence of distant disease, preoperative testing can be limited to standard chest x-ray and liver enzyme levels including lactate dehydrogenase (LDH).

Case Continued

Review of the outside pathology slides of the left chest lesion confirms the diagnosis of melanoma, 0.9 mm, Clark's level III, and additionally notes the presence of histologic ulceration. A punch biopsy of the dark lesion on his right back shows melanoma in situ.

Diagnosis and Recommendation

This patient has two primary melanomas without clinical evidence of regional disease. He needs to undergo complete blood cell (CBC) count, evaluation of liver enzyme levels, and a chest x-ray as a basic staging work-up to exclude distant disease.

Case Continued

Chest x-ray and liver enzymes are normal.

Approach

The melanoma in situ on his back should be excised with a measured margin of 5 mm. The melanoma on his chest is 1 mm or less in thickness, so a 1-cm measured margin is recommended. However, this thin, or T1, melanoma also has the feature of histologic ulceration, a poor prognostic feature. This is, therefore, a T1b melanoma, and lymphatic mapping and sentinel node excision is also recommended to stage the regional nodes.

Discussion

Every primary melanoma requires wide local excision for local control. Margin width is determined by the thickness of the primary lesion. Melanoma in situ is conventionally excised with a 5-mm margin, although there are no prospective studies evaluating margin width for melanoma in situ, and it is unknown if narrower margins might be sufficient. A thin (1 mm or less) invasive melanoma is excised with a measured 1-cm margin, largely based on the results of the World Health Organization study. Intermediate thickness (1 to 4 mm) melanoma is preferably excised with a 2-cm measured margin, based on the Intergroup trial of 2-cm vs 4-cm margins for this group of patients. Thick (>4 mm) melanoma should be excised with a minimum 2-cm margin; it is unknown whether wider margins would be advantageous, and no prospective randomized trial is available to guide the choice of margin width.

The status of the regional nodes is the most important prognostic factor for patients with newly diagnosed melanoma. Sentinel node biopsy is a minimally invasive method of evaluating the regional nodes and should be offered to patients with melanomas >1 mm in thickness, and to patients with thinner melanomas (T1b) if they display adverse features of ulceration or deeper Clark's level (IV or V). Sentinel node biopsy provides excellent prognostic information and aids in making appropriate treatment decisions. Knowledge of the pathologic nodal status is particularly important in patients who enter clinical trials of systemic adjuvant therapy to assure homogeneity of treatment groups.

Preoperative lymphatic mapping is essential for accurate sentinel node biopsy. An intradermal injection of technetium sulfur colloid is made in the nuclear medicine suite in normal-appearing skin directly adjacent to the biopsy site. Planar images are accrued to observe the accumulation of tracer in the sentinel nodes. For truncal primaries it is important to image all four node basins, because drainage to more than one basin is common. It is also important to look for unusual sites for the sentinel nodes: they have occasionally been described at sites outside of conventionally defined node basins, such as the triangular intramuscular space, the popliteal or epitrochlear fossa, and sites in the subcutaneous tissues between the primary site and the nearest node basin. The site of the sentinel node(s) detected on lymphoscintigraphy is marked on the overlying skin. In the operating room, a hand-held gamma probe is used to detect gamma emission from the technetium trapped in the node; this allows retrieval of the node through a small incision. Isosulfan blue 1% is injected intradermally around the original primary biopsy site to function as a visual aid in identifying the sentinel node.

Case Continued

The patient has a lymphoscintigraphy, which results in rapid identification of a sentinel node in the left axilla. No other hot spots are seen.

▌ Surgical Approach

The patient is brought to the operating room for wide local excision of the two primary melanomas and for the sentinel node biopsy. The gamma probe is sterilely draped and is used to scan the trunk for other hot spots and to confirm the presence of the hot signal in the left axilla. A single hot spot is found in the left axilla. About 1 mL of isosulfan blue 1% is injected intradermally around the biopsy site on the left chest. Approximately 5 minutes after injection, a small incision is made in the left axilla at the site of the hot spot. The gamma probe is used to help guide the dissection. Deep in the mid axilla a hot, blue node is encountered; this node is resected by clamping, dividing, and ligating small lymphatic tributaries. The node is intensely blue and is counted with the gamma probe ex vivo to confirm its identity as the sentinel node. It is placed in formalin and sent to pathology for permanent section. The operative procedure now continues with the wide local excisions. The 0.9-mm invasive melanoma on the chest is excised with a measured 1-cm margin. The excision is carried down to, but not through, the underlying muscle fascia. The excision is fashioned as an ellipse with a length:width ratio of 3:1. To achieve closure without undue tension, advancement flaps are created by lifting a flap just superficial to the superficial fascia. The wound is closed with a series of interrupted inverted absorbable sutures in the dermis and a running subcuticular absorbable suture. The in situ melanoma on the right back is excised in the subcutaneous plane with a 5-mm measured margin.

Case Continued

The patient recovers uneventfully from his surgery. The pathology of the wide excisions shows no further melanoma at either primary site.

Histopathology Slides

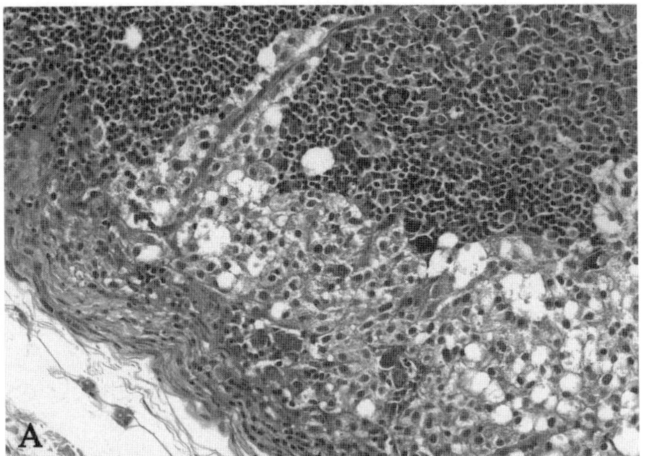

Figure 67.2A

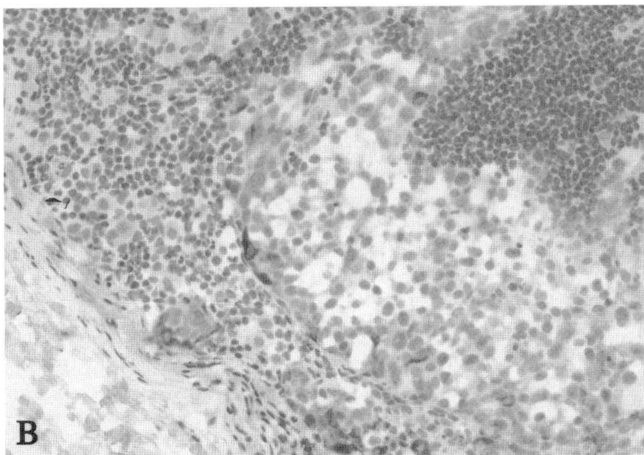

Figure 67.2B

Histopathology Report

The sentinel node is found to have a microscopic deposit of metastatic melanoma, which is recognized on hematoxylin and eosin stains and confirmed by immunohistochemistry with Melan-A and HMB-45.

Diagnosis and Recommendation

Based on the result of the pathologic examination of the sentinel node, this patient has stage III disease. He has a T1b primary and a single node with microscopic disease, so he is classified as having stage IIIB and can be expected to have a 5-year chance of survival of approximately 53% and a 10-year chance of survival of approximately 38%. A complete left axillary dissection is recommended to decrease his risk of regional recurrence, to complete his staging by determining if other nodes in that basin are positive, and to give him an opportunity for overall control.

Surgical Approach

A complete axillary dissection is performed. The dissection is carried out through a broad curved incision in the lower axilla, fashioning the incision to include the sentinel node biopsy scar in an incorporated ellipse. All three levels of axillary nodes are included in the dissection in their entirety. The arm is rotated forward and the pectoralis minor muscle is retracted sharply to facilitate access to the level 3 nodes, which are dissected down in continuity with the lower nodes. A closed suction drain is placed. Postoperatively, he is given passive range-of-motion exercises to perform, beginning on the first postoperative day.

Discussion

For patients with regionally metastatic melanoma, factors strongly associated with outcome are the number of metastatic nodes, whether the tumor burden in the nodes is microscopic or macroscopic, and whether the primary is ulcerated. Therapeutic node dissection is done for known positive regional lymph nodes. Because current systemic therapies are of little documented survival benefit, complete surgical resection of the regional node basin is sometimes the only active treatment for stage III melanoma. In general, node dissection for melanoma should be anatomic and complete. In the axilla, this includes complete dissection of levels I, II, and III. It is worth noting that the extent of the dissection for melanoma is substantially more than the dissection that has been commonly performed as a staging dissection for breast cancer. The postoperative course is usually uneventful. A closed suction drain is left in place until it puts out 40 mL or less per day. Range-of-motion exercises can be started the day after surgery. The risk of infection is low, and antibiotics are not continued beyond the perioperative period. The risk of lymphedema following complete axillary dissection is 10% to 15%.

Case Continued

The patient recovers uneventfully from the axillary dissection. Twenty-five lymph nodes in the axillary specimen are negative. His staging is therefore T1b N1a M0, or stage IIIB. No further staging studies are needed outside of a clinical trial. He consults with the medical oncologist, and his case is presented at the multidisciplinary tumor conference. He is eligible for treatment with interferon-alpha or may enroll in a vaccine trial. He decides to enroll in a vaccine trial.

Recommendation

The estimated prognosis of this patient was changed dramatically by his staging with sentinel node biopsy. In the absence of the sentinel node information, he would have been misclassified as having clinical stage I melanoma, and would not have had the opportunity to have his nodal disease resected, nor would he have been offered systemic therapy. This patient has now had complete resection of all identifiable disease and is considered to be at high risk of systemic recurrence. He has chosen to participate in a clinical trial of vaccine therapy.

Discussion

Until the results of an ongoing randomized trial are reported, it is unknown whether knowledge of the nodal status influences subsequent chance of survival. Sentinel node staging for patients who may be considered for clinical trials is essential for ensuring homogeneous experimental groups. Enrollment in clinical trials should be especially encouraged in patients with high-risk, resected disease, because current therapies are minimally effective.

Case Continued

After completing treatment, he returns for routine follow-up. He has had two primary melanomas and is at substantial risk of recurrence; he needs two types of follow-up. He plans to return for routine examination for his risk of recurrence every 3 to 4 months in the first 2 years, and then every 6 months up to year 5, and then annually. He is counseled that he needs to remain in routine skin screening indefinitely for his risk of another primary skin cancer. He also has a family history of melanoma. His family is counseled about prevention measures, including sunburn avoidance as well as routine screening for skin cancers at 6- to 12-month intervals. Routine skin screening for his children should begin no later than the age of puberty, or earlier if concerning pigmented lesions are present.

Discussion

Patients who have been treated for melanoma need follow-up both for their risk of melanoma recurrence and for their risk of a second primary skin cancer. Skin examination is preferably performed no less than once a year by a dermatologist with specific interest in skin cancers; skin examination may be warranted more often if there are many atypical pigmented lesions or if the patient is unable to assess their own skin. First-degree relatives should also seek routine skin screening. The most important element of the follow-up plan regarding the risk of melanoma recurrence is the history and physical examination, with a focus on the wide excision site, potential sites of in-transit disease, and the node basins. For asymptomatic patients, some oncologists choose to obtain yearly chest x-rays and liver enzyme measurements, including LDH. In general, computed tomography scans or positron-emission tomography scans are not performed unless there are specific concerning symptoms or signs of recurrence.

Suggested Readings

Balch CM, Buzaid AC, Soong SJ, et al. Final version of the American Joint Committee on Cancer staging system for cutaneous melanoma. *J Clin Oncol* 2001;19:3635–3648.

Balch CM, Houghton A, Sober AJ, et al. *Cutaneous melanoma.* 4th ed. St Louis, MO: Quality Medical Press; 2003.

Balch CM, Soong S, Ross MI, et al. Long-term results of a multi-institutional randomized trial comparing prognostic factors and surgical results for intermediate thickness melanomas (1.0 to 4.0 mm): Intergroup Melanoma Surgical Trial. *Ann Surg Oncol* 2000;7:87–97.

Balch CM, Soong SJ, Gershenwald JE, et al. Prognostic factors analysis of 17,600 melanoma patients: validation of the American Joint Committee on Cancer melanoma staging system. *J Clin Oncol* 2001;19:3622–3634.

Gershenwald JE, Thompson W, Mansfield PF, et al. Multi-institutional melanoma lymphatic mapping experience: the prognostic value of sentinel lymph node status in 612 stage I or II melanoma patients. *J Clin Oncol* 1999;17:976–983.

Kirkwood JM, Strawderman MH, Ernstoff MS, et al. Interferon alfa-2b adjuvant therapy of high-risk resected cutaneous melanoma: The Eastern Cooperative Oncology Group Trial EST 1684. *J Clin Oncol* 1996;14:7–17.

Morton DL, Wen DR, Wong JH, et al. Technical details of intraoperative lymphatic mapping for early stage melanoma. *Arch Surg* 1992;127:392–399.

Poo-Hwu JJ, Ariyan S, Lamb L, et al. Follow-up recommendations for patients with American Joint Committee on Cancer Stages I-III malignant melanoma. *Cancer* 1999;86:2252–2258.

Veronesi U, Cascinelli N. Narrow excision (1-cm margin): a safe procedure for thin cutaneous melanoma. *Arch Surg* 1991;126:438–441.

Presentation

A 47-year-old man with a history of a melanoma excised from his distal right calf 18 months earlier returns for routine follow-up. The pathology for that lesion was a 1.33-mm thick, Clark's level IV, nonulcerated melanoma that was vertical growth phase positive. He underwent a wide local excision with sentinel lymph node mapping and biopsy that showed no residual melanoma and no tumor in two sentinel lymph nodes. He now presents with a 6-week history of a 2-cm area of reddish-tinted nodules proximal to his melanoma scar that was nontender. He does not feel that the nodules have changed in the 6 weeks since he noticed them.

Clinical Photograph

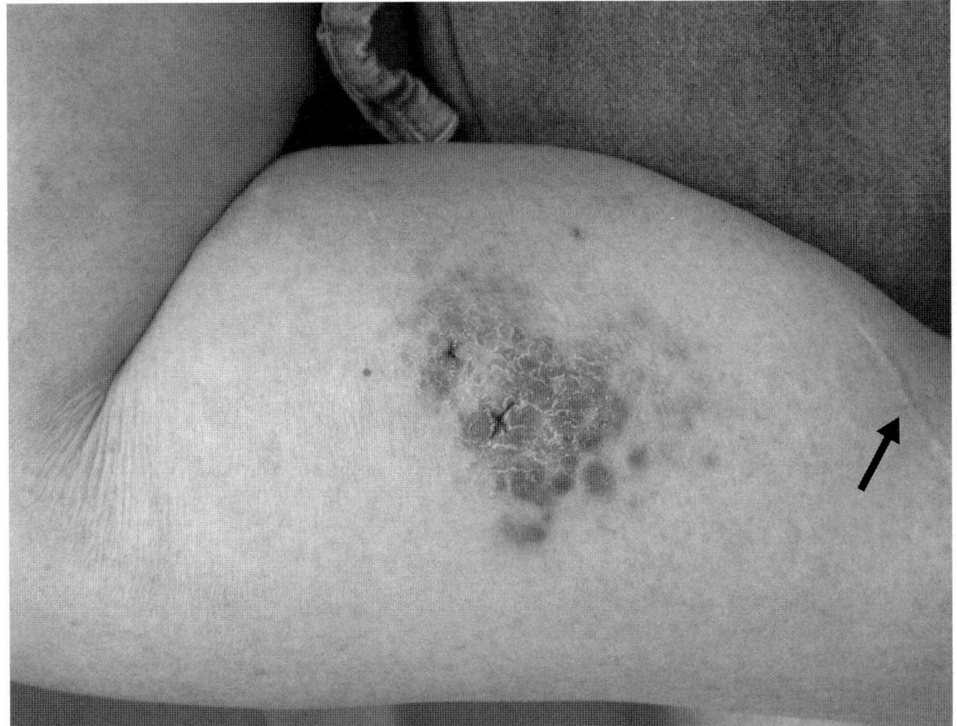

Figure 68.1

Physical Examination Report

The raised erythematous lesions are visible proximal to the scar *(arrow)*.

Differential Diagnosis

There are a variety of nonneoplastic and benign cutaneous conditions that can explain a subcutaneous nodule, including dermatofibroma, angiolipoma,

307

and folliculitis. However, any nodule presenting within the lymphatic drainage field of a previously resected melanoma should be considered a potential in-transit metastasis. In-transit metastases develop within the lymphatic vessels of the skin and can be either intradermal or subcutaneous. Although typically pigmented (pink or red in color), in-transit nodules may be nonpigmented. Also, although in-transit disease typically occurs between the site of the primary melanoma and the draining nodal basin, lesions can appear distal to the primary scar, often in the lower extremities.

Approach

Nodules that are suspected to be in-transit melanoma can be confirmed pathologically by either excisional biopsy or fine-needle aspiration. For the initial lesion, in which the level of suspicion and the certainty of the diagnosis is less secure, a simple excision of the nodule under local anesthesia is appropriate. For recurrent disease, the diagnosis is more obvious because multiple similar-appearing nodules may be present. Fine-needle aspiration can establish the diagnosis of in-transit melanoma if the nodule has enough bulk to allow insertion of the needle into the mass. Although the margin of excision is well defined for primary melanomas, there are no clear guidelines for the margin of excision of in-transit nodules. A simple excision with 3 to 5 mm of normal tissue around the melanoma is adequate because local recurrence of the resected in-transit nodule is not an important clinical issue. The entire region of the body is at significant risk for new lesions. Wide excisions, particularly with skin grafts or attempts to obtain margins of 2 to 4 cm, should not be performed. Patients suffer significant morbidity for no benefit, because the disease can recur anywhere within the skin drained by that lymphatic basin. Similarly, there is no role for adjuvant radiation therapy because radiation cannot be given circumferentially to an extremity, and there is no defined margin for the radiation field.

Another point of surgical management of an initial isolated in-transit melanoma nodule is whether a sentinel lymph node mapping and biopsy should be done at the area of the in-transit nodule. This technique will map a lymph node or nodes at that site, and there is a possibility of defining microscopic spread to the draining nodal basin. However, it is not standard of care to perform sentinel node mapping with resection of in-transit melanoma. Arguments against adding a node biopsy are that patients already have stage III by having an in-transit lesion, and patients in this situation are more likely to recur with other in-transit nodules or systemically. It is appropriate after identifying in-transit disease to stage a patient with computed tomography (CT) scans of the chest, abdomen, and pelvis, or with a positron-emission tomography (PET) scan.

After resection of the initial in-transit nodule, and assuming that the staging studies are negative, the patient is eligible for adjuvant treatment appropriate for resected stage III melanoma. This would include adjuvant interferon-alpha or a variety of experimental vaccines. There is no role for an adjuvant isolated limb perfusion in this setting because the toxicity of that procedure outweighs any potential benefits. Patients should be instructed to perform self-examinations of the area involved and to notify their physicians if any new nodules appear. They should be followed closely in clinic, such as at 3-month intervals.

Case Continued

The patient does well for 4 months after he undergoes excision of the nodules, and then he notices diffuse edema of the extremity. The primary care physician orders a venous Doppler, which does not demonstrate any venous thrombosis. Two weeks later, the patient notices several areas of new reddish nodules distributed throughout the lower extremity. He comes for an examination, and lesions similar to the initial in-transit nodule are present.

His leg from the knee down shows moderate swelling, and he has numerous tender masses of the lower extremity. A fine-needle aspiration of one of the masses documents melanoma.

The patient now presents with both superficial and subcutaneous melanoma that is too extensive to completely resect short of an amputation.

Clinical Photograph

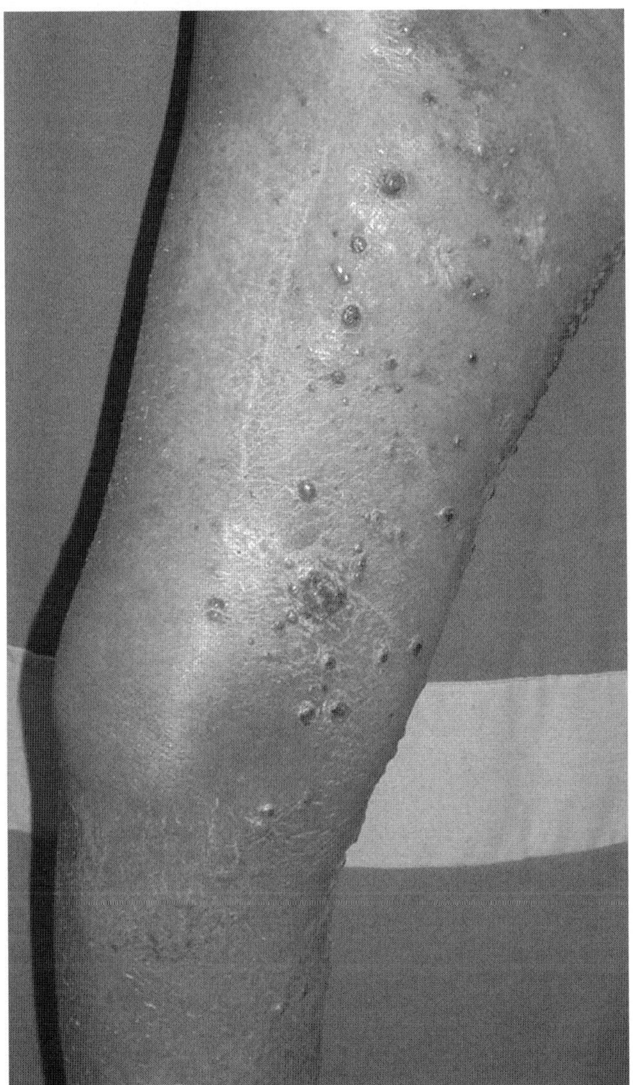

Figure 68.2

Physical Examination Report

There are multiple cutaneous and subcutaneous nodules of varying sizes involving the lower extremity.

Diagnostic Testing

The important distinction in this setting is to determine if there is disease outside the extremity, so the patient needs to be restaged. CT scans of the chest, abdomen, and pelvis and magnetic resonance imaging (MRI) of the head are done and show no evidence of distant metastases. He has a PET scan that shows no disease outside the extremity but very extensive disease in the right calf. This patient has developed unusual in-transit metastases that are deep within the subcutaneous tissue resting on the fascia. About 2% to 4% of in-transit nodules follow this pattern, as opposed to lesions that can be seen or easily palpated on the skin. In this setting, it is appropriate to obtain either an MRI or an ultrasound of the extremity to measure the size of the deep in-transit lesions to be able to accurately measure response to therapy.

Recommendation

This patient is an ideal candidate for regional therapy with isolated limb perfusion (ILP) because he has disease isolated to the extremity with no local resection options.

Surgical Approach

The optimal regimen is a 60-minute perfusion with melphalan and mild hyperthermia. The melphalan dose is based on limb volume, giving 10 mg/L limb volume for lower extremities and 13 mg/L for upper extremities. Hyperthermia is achieved by heating the perfusate and the leg by a warming blanket to achieve tissue temperatures between 38.5°C and 40.0°C. The operation involves dissecting either the common femoral vessels or the external iliac vessels, cannulating the artery and vein, and then utilizing a cardiopulmonary bypass circuit to recirculate heated, oxygenated perfusate with high-dose melphalan. The limb is isolated by placing a tourniquet at the base of the limb. The drug level of the melphalan in the extremity is very high because of the large dose given and because the organs of drug metabolism (liver and kidneys) do not eliminate this agent recirculating in the extremity. After a 60-minute treatment period, the circuit is interrupted and the melphalan is flushed from the extremity.

Discussion

Alternative treatments are systemic therapy or a new, less invasive, therapy of isolated limb infusion. However, ILP has been used to treat in-transit melanoma for over 40 years.

The response rates for this regimen are between 80% and 100%, with complete response rates reported as between 50% and 65%. This complete response rate is 10-fold higher than what can be achieved with the best systemic treatment. Combination biochemotherapy has complete response rates of 3% to 5% and high-dose IL-2 has complete response rates of 5% to 8%. The duration of response has been reported to be between 9 and 13 months. Approximately 25% of patients have sustained complete responses with this local therapy. No other chemotherapeutic has shown this level of response given during ILP. Recent efforts to enhance this response by adding high-dose tumor necrosis factor have not shown significant improvement over melphalan alone in randomized trials. There is no adjuvant therapy given after melphalan ILP that is of any proven benefit.

In follow-up, if patients achieve a significant partial response and have only a small volume of residual disease, it is appropriate to resect that disease, because patients may have no other viable tumor. If patients develop recurrent disease in the extremity after a significant prolonged response, it is appropriate to offer a repeat ILP. Regional failure in this setting is not equivalent to failure of systemic therapy in which there is specific drug resistance, and response rates for reperfusion are similar to response rates for initial perfusion. An alternative in the retreatment setting is the new technique of isolated limb infusion. This is a percutaneous catheter technique in which cannula are passed from the contralateral groin into the midthigh. A pneumatic tourniquet provides isolation, and drug is slowly recirculated by syringe under hypoxic conditions as opposed to an oxygenated perfusion. Initial response rates have been reported as high as 60% to 80%, but the proportion of complete responses is less than that of ILP. In the reoperative setting, where surgical approach is more difficult with added potential complications, isolated limb infusion may provide an alternative regional treatment.

Suggested Readings

Fraker DL. Management of in-transit melanoma of the extremity with isolated limb perfusion. *Curr Treat Options Oncol* 2004; 5:173–184.

Lens MB, Dawes M. Isolated limb perfusion with melphalan in the treatment of malignant melanoma of the extremities: a systematic review of randomized controlled trials. *Lancet Oncol* 2003;4:359–364.

Noorda EM, Vrouenraets BC, Nieweg OE, et al. Isolated limb perfusion: what is the evidence for its use? *Ann Surg Oncol* 2004; 11:837–845.

Noorda EM, Vrouenraets BC, Nieweg OE, et al. Isolated limb perfusion for unresectable melanoma of the extremities. *Arch Surg* 2004;139:1237–1242.

Zogakis TG, Bartlett DL, Libutti SK, et al. Factors affecting survival after complete response to isolated limb perfusion in patients with in-transit melanoma. *Ann Surg Oncol* 2001;8: 771–778.

Presentation

A 45-year-old woman presented to her dermatologist after noticing a suspicious lesion on her left thigh. An excisional biopsy performed in the office demonstrated a 1.8-mm superficial spreading melanoma with ulceration. The patient now presents to your office for definitive surgical management. On physical examination, there is a well-healed longitudinal scar on the right thigh and a palpable 1.5-cm, mobile, firm lymph node in the left groin.

Differential Diagnosis

Any patients diagnosed with invasive melanoma should undergo a thorough physical examination, paying particular attention to the regional draining lymph node basins. Approximately 5% of patients will present with clinically apparent regional lymph node involvement at the time of diagnosis. Still others develop palpable lymphadenopathy months or years after excision of a primary melanoma, while occasional patients present with nodal metastasis in the absence of a detectable primary tumor. Regional lymph nodes may become enlarged due to infection, inflammation, or reactive hyperplasia, particularly after a biopsy of the primary tumor has been performed. However, any palpable nodes that are larger than 1 to 1.5 cm in size, hard, or fixed to adjacent structures must be considered suspicious for metastatic involvement. Metastatic nodal involvement can be reliably verified in most cases with a fine-needle aspiration biopsy. Excisional biopsy should be reserved for situations in which the node is clinically suspicious but the aspiration biopsy is negative or indeterminate, because the complications of an open biopsy (including seroma, infection, and scarring) can interfere with the performance of a subsequent lymph node dissection. If an excisional biopsy is performed, it is important to orient the incision so that it can be readily re-excised during the complete lymph node dissection if the node proves to be involved with tumor.

Diagnosis

Fine-needle aspiration biopsy confirms the presence of metastatic melanoma.

Approach

Unfortunately, once melanoma has spread to the lymph nodes, there is a steep drop-off in survival. The 5-year survival rate for patients with node-positive melanoma (American Joint Committee on Cancer [AJCC] stage III) is 49%, and declines to 37% at 10 years. Not all stage III melanoma patients, however, have the same outlook: 5-year survival rates range from 13% for patients with a combination of poor risk factors (ulceration, high regional lymph node burden) to 69% for patients with a more favorable profile. It is imperative to keep in mind that node-positive melanoma is a potentially curable disease, and an aggressive surgical approach is warranted. A patient such as this one, with biopsy-proven palpable nodal involvement, should undergo wide local excision of the primary tumor and complete lymph node dissection if there is no radiologic evidence of distant metastasis.

In the presence of metastatic disease, however, the value of regional node dissection is limited, and should be restricted to selected patients with present or impending symptoms from their nodal disease. Metastatic workup should be performed to evaluate any patient presenting with clinical stage III disease. The most important part of this workup is a detailed history and physical examination. The history should include a thorough review of symptoms, focusing on symptoms consistent with metastatic disease, including any neurologic symptoms from possible brain metastases. The presence of any unusual symptoms should prompt the appropriate imaging and, where appropriate, histologic confirmation. The physical examination should include a careful search for in-transit metastases, distant skin or subcutaneous metastases, or lymphadenopathy outside of the regional basin(s).

In addition to the history and physical examination, all patients with stage III disease should have a chest radiograph and a serum lactate dehydrogenase (LDH) level measurement. Patients with abnormalities on chest x-ray or an elevated LDH level should undergo a further search for metastatic disease. This should consist of a computed tomography (CT) scan of the chest, abdomen, and pelvis and magnetic resonance imaging (MRI) or CT of the brain. The use of positron-emission tomography (PET) scanning has also been advocated; the value of this technique is discussed in more detail subsequently.

More controversial is the extent of further imaging studies required in the asymptomatic patient with a normal chest x-ray and LDH level. When the chest x-ray is normal, a chest CT scan adds little value. CT scan or MRI of the brain is not routinely necessary in asymptomatic patients. For patients such as the present case with palpable inguinal adenopathy, a CT of the abdomen and pelvis will not only evaluate for the presence of intra-abdominal metastasis, but can also identify enlarged pelvic lymph nodes that might convert a superficial inguinal node dissection to a superficial and deep dissection. For patients with palpable axillary or cervical lymph nodes, the added value of further imaging is less clear.

Whole-body PET scanning has emerged as a potentially valuable tool for preoperative evaluation of melanoma patients. In patients with stage III disease, PET scanning has been reported to be superior to CT scans, upstaging patients to stage IV (and hence altering therapy) in 16% to 28% of cases. Combination PET/CT scans are now becoming available and may ultimately prove to be superior to either modality alone, although prospective studies are currently ongoing. Unfortunately, others have not found PET scanning to be reliable, with high false-positive rates. It is important to remember that both CT scans and PET scans can have false-positive findings; histologic confirmation of an abnormal lesion should be obtained whenever feasible before concluding a patient has stage IV melanoma and abandoning a surgical approach.

Recommendation

Chest x-ray, LDH measurement, and CT scan of the abdomen and pelvis are recommended. Further imaging should be done only if positive findings are encountered.

Case Continued

The patient is asymptomatic and physical examination shows no evidence of metastatic disease. The chest x-ray and LDH level are also normal. A CT scan of the abdomen and pelvis shows no areas suspicious for metastatic disease and no enlarged pelvic lymph nodes. However, the metastatic inguinal lymph node was visualized.

Abdomen/Pelvis CT Scan

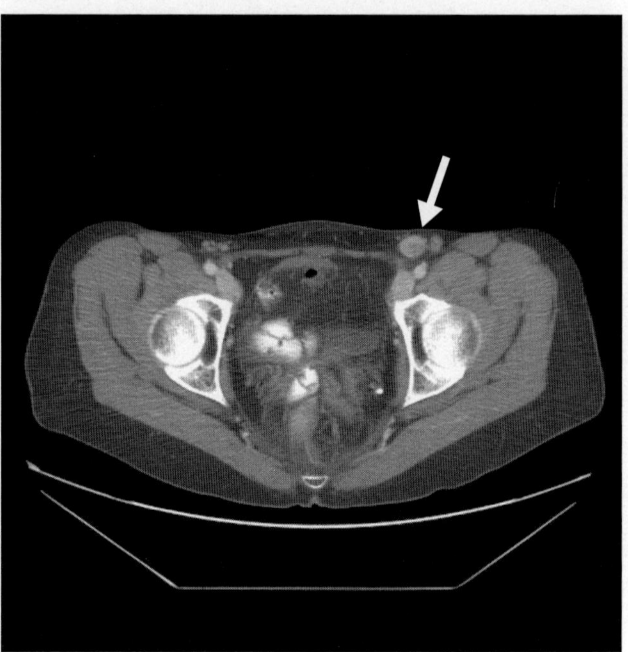

Figure 69.1

Abdomen/Pelvis CT Scan Report

There is an enlarged lymph node seen in the left groin *(arrow)*.

Surgical Approach

For patients with palpable inguinal disease, the extent of lymphadenectomy ("superficial" only versus "superficial and deep") is controversial, given the higher rate of complications involved with deep inguinal lymph node dissections. Some surgeons advocate complete superficial and deep inguinal lymph node dissections in all patients with palpable adenopathy. Others reserve deep inguinal node dissection to those patients with a positive Cloquet's node or three or more involved nodes. Still others do not perform deep dissections in the absence of clinical or radiographic evidence of pelvic adenopathy. If a deep groin dissection is to be performed together with a superficial dissection, this can be accomplished through one skin incision by obliquely dividing the external and internal oblique muscles to expose the pelvic retroperitoneum, or alternatively by dividing the inguinal ligament. Dividing the ligament is particularly useful in cases of extensive disease low in the pelvis along the distal external iliac vessels. Although it is simpler to divide the ligament over the femoral vessels, wound healing may be improved if the inguinal ligament is detached from the anterior superior iliac spine.

Discussion

For patients with palpable disease in the axilla, a complete axillary lymph node dissection should include levels I, II, and III to provide the best regional control. In a relatively thin person, with anterior retraction of the pectoralis major and minor muscles, it is often possible to adequately dissect the level III nodes without dividing the pectoralis minor muscle. In many patients, however, especially if the level III nodes are involved by tumor, it is necessary to divide the pectoralis minor. To do so, the pectoralis major is retracted anteriorly and the fascia on either side of the tendon of the pectoralis minor is incised. With a finger behind the muscle to protect the axillary nerve, artery, and vein posteriorly, the insertion of the pectoralis minor is divided with electrocautery. To improve access to the upper levels of the axilla, the lateral pectoral neurovascular bundle can be ligated at the posterolateral aspect of the pectoralis major muscle. Whenever possible, the medial pectoral nerve should be preserved to maintain innervation of the pectoralis major muscle.

Case Continued

The patient undergoes a wide radical excision of the melanoma with 2-cm margins and a superficial inguinal lymph node dissection. Three of 11 inguinal nodes are positive for lymph node metastases. There is no evidence of extracapsular extension.

Intraoperative Photographs

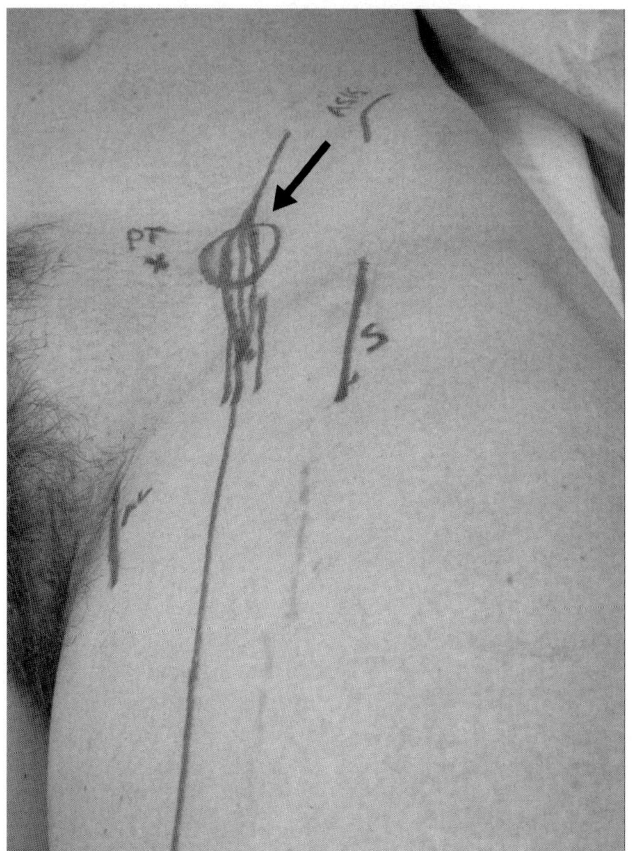

Figure 69.2A

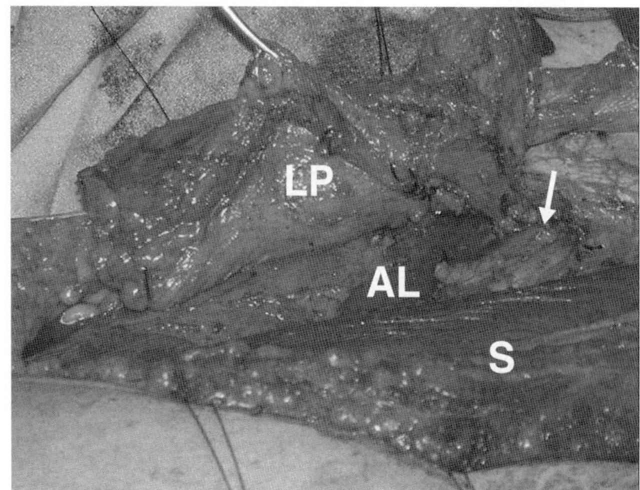

Figure 69.2B

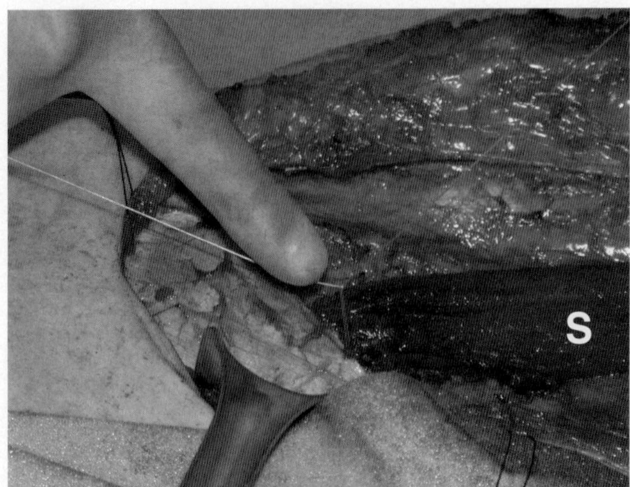

Figure 69.2C

Intraoperative Report

The enlarged lymph node is outlined along with the proposed incision **(A)**. The inguinofemoral lymph node package has been dissected, revealing the femoral vessels, adductor longus medially, and sartorius laterally **(B)**. The sartorius flap to cover the exposed femoral vessels is seen **(C)**.

Discussion

Even after a complete node dissection, there is a risk of recurrence in and around the dissected bed. This risk of regional recurrence is increased with large-sized nodes, multiple involved nodes, or extracapsular extension. Many series indicate that the risk of regional recurrence is particularly high in the neck.

Some have advocated adjuvant radiation therapy to the dissected nodal basin, although its indications have not been clearly defined. Several nonrandomized studies have suggested that postoperative radiation after radical lymph node dissection decreases regional recurrence rates in node-positive patients. To date there is no convincing randomized data on which to make a recommendation, although randomized trials are presently under way. Until more data are available, the risks and potential benefits of adjuvant radiation therapy must be carefully weighed. It is reasonable to consider postoperative radiation therapy in patients with gross extracapsular extension or multiple involved lymph nodes, which some define as four or more while others consider 10 or more pathologically involved nodes. Given the higher risk of recurrence and the lesser morbidity of radiation therapy after a neck dissection, the threshold for adjuvant radiation for cervical metastases is lower. On the other hand, adjuvant radiation after an inguinal node dissection is associated with significant morbidity, and should be reserved for patients with a very high risk of regional relapse.

Case Continued

The patient recovers well from her operation and the decision is made not to pursue radiation therapy. She returns to the office to discuss adjuvant therapies.

Discussion

Even more worrisome than the risk of regional relapse in this patient is the potential for the development of distant metastases. In this patient, with three macroscopically evident nodal metastases and an ulcerated primary tumor (stage IIIC), the estimated risk of distant metastasis exceeds 60%. Most patients with distant metastases ultimately die of their disease. Over the years there have been multiple trials involving a variety of drugs tested in the adjuvant setting, but none had demonstrated a benefit in reducing the risk of relapse or death for high-risk melanoma patients. Examples include single-agent chemotherapy (primarily DTIC, or dacarbazine), combination chemotherapy, retinoids, and non-specific immunostimulants (bacille Calmette-Guérin vaccine [BCG], Cryptosporidium parvum, levamisole, and others). This changed with the publication of the Eastern Cooperative Oncology Group (ECOG) trial E1684, a randomized trial of high-dose interferon alfa-2b (IFNα-2b) for patients with high-risk melanoma (defined as any node-positive patients or node-negative patients with melanomas 4.0 mm or greater). This was the first trial to demonstrate a statistically significant benefit to an adjuvant therapy, and led to approval by the Food and Drug Administration (FDA) of high-dose IFNα-2b as adjuvant therapy for high-risk melanoma. Unfortunately, significant toxicities combined with less unequivocal results of subsequent trials have made its use more controversial.

The E1684 trial compared high-dose interferon with observation after complete node dissection in a randomized trial, and while this regimen was toxic, the results were positive. The treatment group showed a significant improvement in disease-free and overall survival compared with the control group. High-dose interferon significantly increased median survival by 1 year and produced a 24% relative improvement in the 5-year survival rate (46% for IFN-α2b patients versus 37% for observation patients).

A follow-up Intergroup trial, E1690, compared adjuvant high-dose interferon, as well as a 2-year low-dose IFNα-2b regimen, with observation. Although the results of this trial confirmed the disease-free survival advantage for high-dose IFNα-2b seen in

E1684, there was no overall survival advantage. It is possible that the reason why E1690 failed to demonstrate a survival advantage is the result of differences in eligibility criteria and, more importantly, the subsequent availability of postrelapse IFN-α2b crossover therapy in the E1690 trial compared to E1684, but there is no way to prove this. A third trial, Intergroup E1694, compared 1 year of high-dose IFNα2b with 2 years of a ganglioside vaccine called GMK. In designing this trial, high-dose interferon was considered the standard of care, and there was no observation arm. This trial was stopped early when it was apparent that the high-dose interferon arm was associated with significantly greater relapse-free and overall survival compared with the vaccine arm. Although it is conceivable that the GMK vaccine had a deleterious effect, the likelihood of this seems extremely low. Thus, of the three trials examining high-dose interferon in the adjuvant setting, all demonstrated improvement in relapse-free survival, while two of the three demonstrated an improvement in overall survival. In contrast, multiple trials utilizing low-dose interferon have shown an inconsistent or transient effect on relapse-free survival and no overall survival benefit.

Although high-dose interferon clearly improves disease-free survival, the question of overall survival remains subject to debate. The potential benefits must be weighed against the toxicity of high-dose interferon, which is substantial. Serious side effects include fatigue, flu-like symptoms (malaise, fevers, chills, arthralgias), liver function abnormalities, neutropenia and infectious complications, nausea and vomiting, and psychiatric symptoms including depression and suicide. Treatment lasts a full year, although most patients relate that the toxicity is worst during the 1-month intravenous induction phase. Successful administration of high-dose IFNα-2b adjuvant therapy requires a committed team, including oncologists, nurses, pharmacists, social workers, and psychiatrists/psychologists.

Based on the available data, all patients with high-risk melanoma should have a balanced discussion concerning the potential risks and benefits of adjuvant high-dose interferon. Participation in clinical trials is always encouraged, and patients who opt not to be treated with IFNα-2b should be informed about participating in randomized trials of alternative adjuvant therapies, including studies of melanoma vaccines.

Recommendation

Adjuvant high-dose interferon alfa-2b (Intron A). This regimen involves an "induction" phase of IFNα-2b 20 mu/m^2 intravenously 5 days a week for 4 weeks followed by a "maintenance" phase of 10 mU/m^2 subcutaneously 3 days a week for the remainder of a full year after starting treatment. Upon completion of therapy, maintain close clinical follow-up, including periodic complete skin examinations.

Discussion

Any patient with a history of melanoma has a substantial risk of developing a second melanoma in addition to the risk of recurrence of their original melanoma, and will need appropriate education and lifelong surveillance. They must be instructed in avoiding sun exposure and sunburn and minimizing solar or ultraviolet light exposure, and they should be taught to perform lifelong self-examination of the skin and lymph nodes. Patients with stage III melanoma should have a history and physical examination (including regional lymph nodes, skin inspection, and palpation of the primary tumor location) performed every 3 to 4 months for the first 2 years, every 6 months for the next 3 years, and every 12 months thereafter. There is no evidence to date to support the role of blood tests or radiologic examinations as part of the routine surveillance of asymptomatic patients, although some clinicians advocate periodic chest x-ray and evaluation of LDH level. Any atypical signs or symptoms on history and/or physical examination should prompt a metastatic workup, because there may be a potential benefit to the surgical resection of stage IV disease.

Suggested Readings

Ballo MT, Ang KK. Radiation therapy for malignant melanoma. *Surg Clin North Am* 2003;83:323–342.

Johnson TM, Bradford CR, Gruger SB, et al. Staging work-up, sentinel node biopsy, and follow-up tests for melanoma: update of current concepts. *Arch Dermatol* 2004;140:107–113.

Morton DL, Wanek L, Nizze JA, et al. Improved long-term survival after lymphadenectomy of melanoma metastatic to regional nodes. Analysis of prognostic factors in 1134 patients from the John Wayne Cancer Clinic. *Ann Surg* 1999;214:491–501.

Pawlik TM, Sondak VK. Malignant melanoma: current state of primary and adjuvant treatment. *Crit Rev Oncol Hematol* 2003;45:245–264.

Sabel MS, Sondak VK. Pros and cons of adjuvant interferon in the treatment of melanoma. *Oncologist* 2003;8:451–458.

Tyler DS, Onaitis M, Kherani A, et al. Positron emission tomography scanning in malignant melanoma. Clinical utility in patients with stage III disease. *Cancer* 2000;89:1019–1025.

Presentation

A 69-year-old woman presents to her primary care physician after she notices a firm, nontender, red mass on her left forearm. She first noticed it several weeks ago, and in the interval since it has grown rapidly. An excisional biopsy performed under local anesthesia demonstrates a Merkel cell carcinoma. She is referred to your office for further treatment. A thorough history and physical examination reveals the patient is asymptomatic and has no evidence of clinically involved lymph nodes.

Clinical Photograph

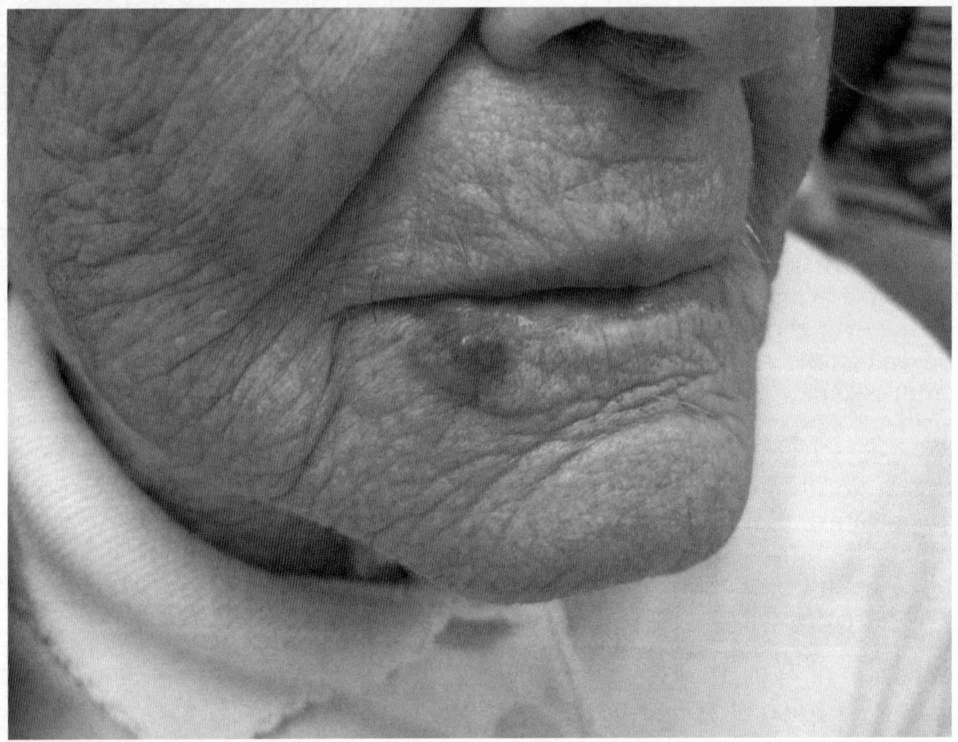

Figure 70.1

Physical Examination Report

Typical appearance of Merkel cell carcinoma (although not of the patient in this discussion).

Discussion

Merkel cell carcinoma is a rare but aggressive skin cancer. Merkel cells are primary neural cells, found either alone within the basal layer of the epidermis or in groups as a component of the tactile hair disc of Pinkus. Merkel cell carcinoma was originally called *trabecular cell carcinoma* and was thought to be derived from sweat glands. However, electron microscopy demonstrated dense-core granules typical of Merkel cells and other neuroendocrine cells within these tumors, suggesting (although not proving) their origin was from Merkel cells. Merkel cell carcinoma is also called *neuroendocrine carcinoma of the skin* or *small cell carcinoma of the skin.*

Merkel cell carcinoma is rare, with only approximately 500 new cases each year and an annual incidence based on Surveillance, Epidemiology, and End-Results data of 0.23 per 100,000 for whites. This tumor is typically considered a disease of the elderly, with an average age at diagnosis of 69 years and only 5% of patients below the age of 50 years. The incidence is higher in males than in females. Merkel cell carcinomas most commonly present as an intracutaneous nodule or plaque that has grown rapidly over a few weeks to months. It can be flesh colored, red, or purple, and it sometimes ulcerates. Merkel cell carcinoma appears to be related to sun exposure, and as such is more common on sun-exposed areas, with approximately 50% on the face and neck, 40% on the extremities, and 10% on the trunk.

Merkel cell tumors arise in the dermis and frequently extend into the subcutaneous fat with an intact epidermis. The tumor is composed of small blue cells with hyperchromatic nuclei and minimal cytoplasm. Lymph-vascular invasion is commonly present. There are three variants: intermediate (the most common), small cell, and trabecular. The small cell variant is identical to other small cell carcinomas and must be distinguished from metastatic small cell carcinoma. This can be accomplished through immunohistochemistry. Merkel cell tumors express CAM 5.2 and cytokeratin (CK) 20. CK7 and thyroid transcription factor, which are typically found on bronchial small cell carcinomas, are absent on Merkel cell carcinomas.

Histopathology Slides

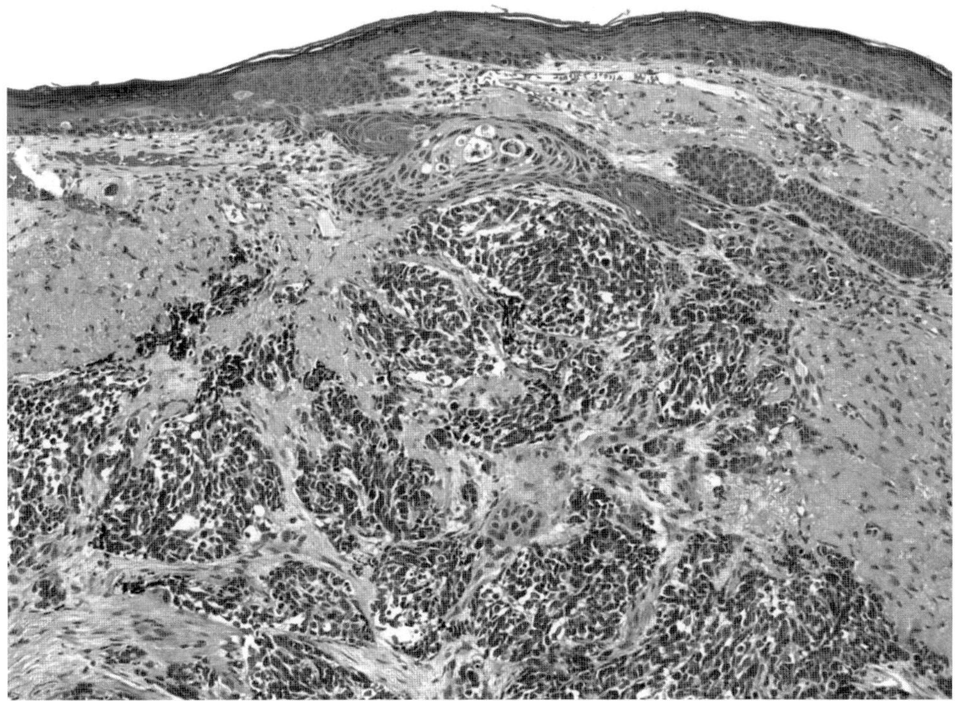

Figure 70.2A

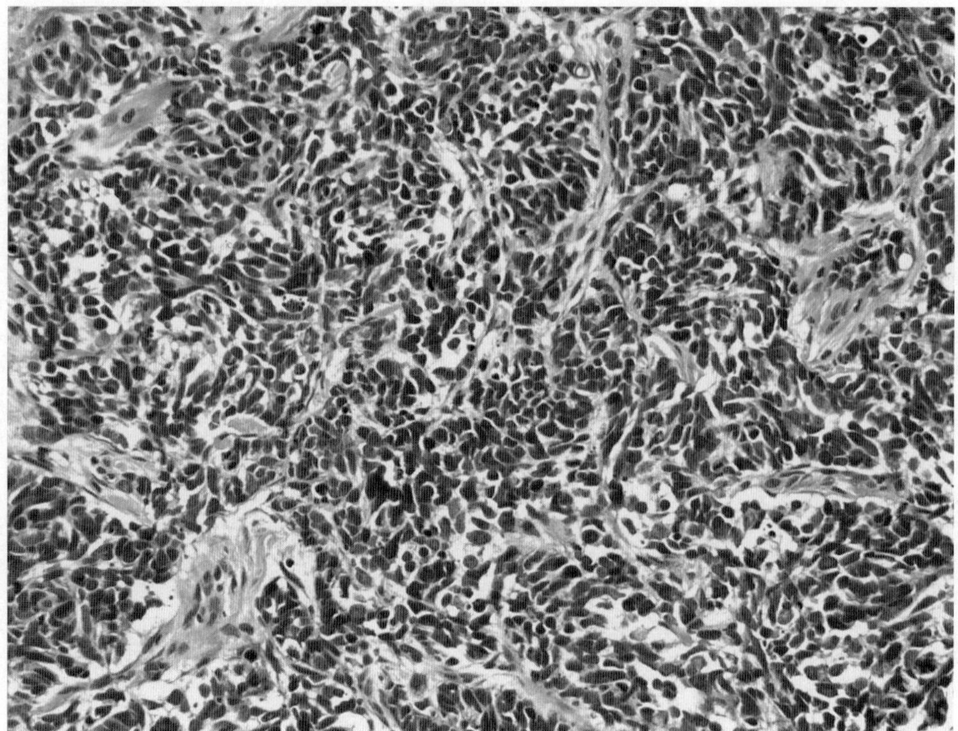

Figure 70.2B

Histopathology Report

Histology of Merkel cell carcinoma.

Discussion

Approximately 70% to 80% of patients present with localized disease. Ten percent to 30% have regional lymph node involvement, and 1% to 4% have distant disease at presentation. In addition to the regional lymph nodes, Merkel cell carcinoma also frequently metastasizes to skin; all patients should have a thorough skin and lymph node examination. Other sites of metastasis include the liver, lung, bones, and brain. Patients with clinically involved lymph nodes or symptoms suggestive of distant metastases should have a computed tomography (CT) scan of the chest, abdomen, and pelvis. CT scan of the chest should also be considered in patients with the small cell variant to exclude the presence of a lung mass suspicious for small cell lung cancer. Both positron emission tomography (PET) and octreotide scans have also been described as useful in select situations. Bone scans and magnetic resonance imaging (MRI) of the brain are not indicated in the absence of specific symptoms.

Recommendation

Wide excision of the primary tumor with intraoperative lymph node mapping and sentinel lymph node biopsy is recommended.

Approach

Because of the high rate of local recurrence, the standard recommendation for the excision of Merkel cell carcinoma has been to obtain 2- to 3-cm margins around the apparent edge of the primary tumor and extend the resection down to and including the underlying fascia. Although some studies have reported lower local recurrence rates with wider margins, other studies have shown no difference in outcome based on margin status. Because Merkel cell carcinoma is so rare, optimal treatment remains unclear. When feasible, wide excision with 2-cm margins should be obtained unless this will result in a suboptimal functional or cosmetic result. In these cases, a narrower margin may be acceptable, particularly if it is combined with postoperative radiation, as discussed subsequently. For patients with Merkel cell carcinomas in cosmetically sensitive areas, where even 1-cm margins would be difficult, Mohs micrographic surgery has been proposed. Early reports demonstrate good local control, but definitive trials have not been conducted.

The regional lymph nodes are pathologically involved in 10% to 30% of patients with clinically localized Merkel cell carcinomas. Regional node involvement is an important prognostic factor. Sentinel lymph node biopsy (SLNB) allows for accurate staging of clinically node-negative patients with Merkel cell carcinoma without the morbidity of a full lymph node dissection. Several studies have confirmed the ability of sentinel node biopsy to successfully identify extremely minute foci of metastatic Merkel cell carcinoma within clinically and even histologically negative sentinel nodes. Because Merkel cell carcinomas have a histologic appearance of a small blue cell malignancy approximately the size of a lymphocyte, detection of small deposits of metastatic Merkel cell carcinoma within lymph nodes is extremely difficult using standard hematoxylin and eosin (H&E) examination. Merkel cell carcinoma cells, however, can be readily distinguished from lymphocytes by their characteristic immunohistochemical-staining pattern, particularly by the use of anticytokeratin antibodies. The sentinel node biopsy technique allows the identification of a small number of lymph nodes that can be extensively evaluated by serial sectioning and immunohistochemistry, permitting the detection of a very small volume of nodal metastatic disease. The natural history and optimal therapy of such small-volume metastatic disease remains completely uncertain. The relatively short median disease-free interval in patients with initially localized tumors that relapse in regional nodes suggests that even small-volume nodal disease is clinically important and likely to be associated with a significant risk of ultimate metastasis.

Surgical Approach

The patient is taken to the operating room for wide excision and sentinel lymph node biopsy after injection of perilesional technetium sulfur colloid. First, 1 mL of 1% isosulfan blue (Lymphazurin) is injected in the intradermal location. A small incision is made in the axilla and the blue lymphatic channel is followed to a blue/hot lymph node(s). Following completion of the sentinel lymph node biopsy, the lesion should be excised with 2.0-cm margins and skin flaps elevated to allow primary wound closure. If considerable tension is present, then reconstruction with either a split-thickness skin graft or a rotational flap should be considered.

Case Continued

The patient undergoes wide resection without the need for a skin graft. Two axillary sentinel nodes are identified. The final pathology examination reveals no residual Merkel cell carcinoma in the primary specimen, and two of two lymph nodes are positive for metastatic disease, evident on both the H&E and immunohistochemistry analyses.

Histopathology Slide

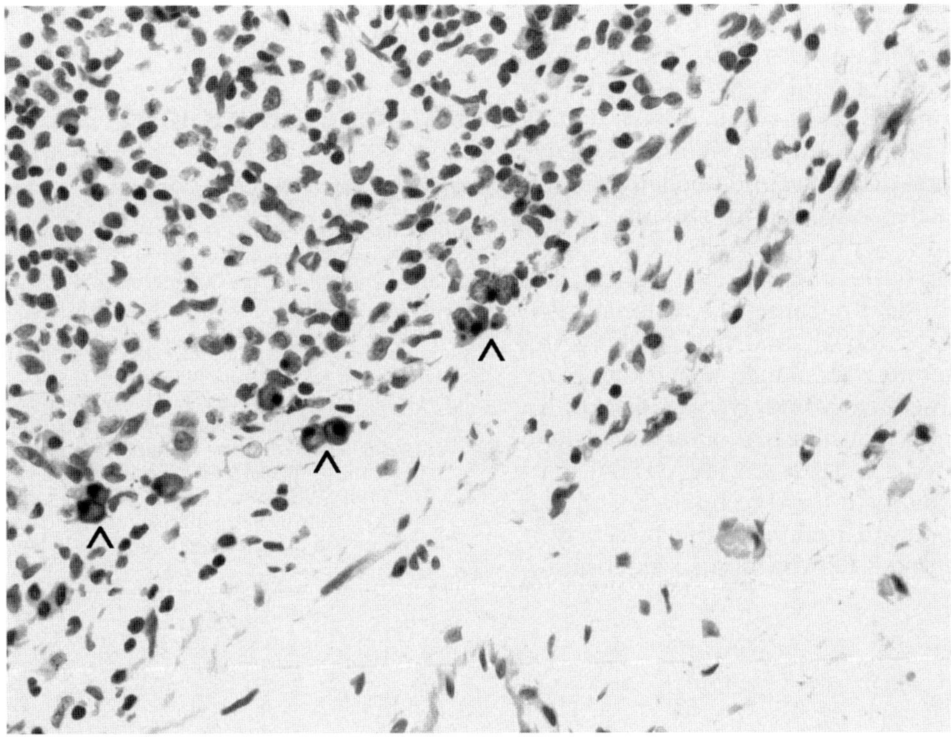

Figure 70.3

Histopathology Report

Anticytokeratin immunohistochemistry detection of Merkel cell cancer micrometastases *(arrowheads)* in a sentinel lymph node.

Discussion

When the sentinel lymph node is found to contain metastatic Merkel cell carcinoma, a complete lymph node dissection is recommended. Regional recurrence for patients with microscopically positive sentinel nodes after complete node dissection is rare, but after sentinel node biopsy alone is expected to occur frequently. On the other hand, Merkel cell carcinoma is a radiosensitive tumor. Although there are limited data as to whether surgery or radiation is more efficacious, some have suggested that for patients with minimal tumor burden in the sentinel node (particularly for scattered foci of disease detected only by immunohistochemistry), radiation to the nodal basin, instead of a complete node dissection, may be adequate.

Adjuvant radiation may be used for both local and regional control. Recommendations for postoperative radiation vary; however, radiation therapy carries additional morbidity, and the management of patients with local or regional recurrences in radiated fields can be difficult. Therefore, adjuvant radiation should be applied selectively. In this patient, who had wide margins obtained around the Merkel cell, adjuvant radiation therapy to the primary site is not necessary. Adjuvant radiation to the primary site should be strongly considered in patients in whom wide surgical margins are not feasible or in whom the margins are close or positive after optimal excision. For a patient with small-volume nodal disease found at sentinel node biopsy, for whom the choice between completion dissection and nodal irradiation is being contemplated, the need for radiation of the primary site should factor into the decision. If postoperative radiation to the primary site is indicated, it makes sense to consider radiating the regional basin at the same time, as an alternative to undergoing completion dissection with radiation to the primary administered subsequently. Adjuvant radiation to the regional basin is not necessary after a complete node dissection for a microscopically positive sentinel node. It should be utilized to improve regional control after a node dissection in the presence of multiple positive nodes or extracapsular extension.

Chemotherapy is typically used in patients with advanced disease or distant metastases. Response rates are high, but the duration of response is typically short and cures are exceedingly rare. Thus, given the high rate of recurrence for node-positive patients, there is interest in adjuvant chemotherapy. To date, no prospective randomized trials of adjuvant chemotherapy have been performed. Despite this, it is reasonable to consider adjuvant systemic chemotherapy after resection of node-positive Merkel cell cancers, particularly if the nodal metastases were clinically evident or there are multiple metastatic lymph nodes. The chemotherapy regimens employed are similar to those used for patients with small cell lung cancer. Generally, these regimens include combination therapy with cisplatin and etoposide or carboplatin and paclitaxel. A prospective study of adjuvant chemotherapy and radiation in patients with high-risk Merkel cell carcinoma by the Trans-Tasman Radiation Oncology Group (TROG) demonstrated excellent locoregional control and survival after 3 years in patients treated with synchronous carboplatin/etopside and radiation.

Case Continued

The patient returns to the operating room for a completion node dissection. None of the 24 axillary nodes had metastatic Merkel cell carcinoma. She is then referred to a medical oncologist for consideration of adjuvant chemotherapy.

Suggested Readings

Agelli M, Clegg LX. Epidemiology of primary Merkel cell carcinoma in the United States. *J Am Acad Dermotol* 2003;49: 832–841.

Brady MS. Current management of patients with Merkel cell carcinoma. *Dermatol Surg* 2004;30:321–325.

Goessling W, McKee PH, Mayer RJ. Merkel cell carcinoma. *J Clin Oncol* 2002;20:588–598.

Mendenhall WM, Mendenhall CM, Mendenhall NP. Merkel cell carcinoma. *Laryngoscope* 2004;114:906–910.

Poulsen M, Rischin D, Walpole E, et al. High-risk Merkel cell carcinoma of the skin treated with synchronous carboplatin/ etoposide and radiation: a Trans-Tasman Radiation Oncology Group study—TROG 96:07. *J Clin Oncol* 2003;21: 4371–4376.

Tai PT, Yu E, Winquist E, et al. Chemotherapy in neuroendocrine/Merkel cell carcinoma of the skin: case series and review of 204 cases. *J Clin Oncol* 2000;18:2493–2499.

Presentation

A 58-year-old white man, human immunodeficiency virus (HIV)-positive since 1989, is referred for evaluation of squamous cell carcinomas of the right forehead, scalp vertex, and left lower eyelid. In the previous 4 years, the patient has been treated for seven cutaneous squamous cell cancers and three recurrences on the scalp, face, and trunk. Past treatment modalities include electrodesiccation and curettage, cryosurgery, surgical excision, Mohs micrographic surgery, and local radiation therapy. He has also started treatment with oral isotretinoin (80 mg/day).

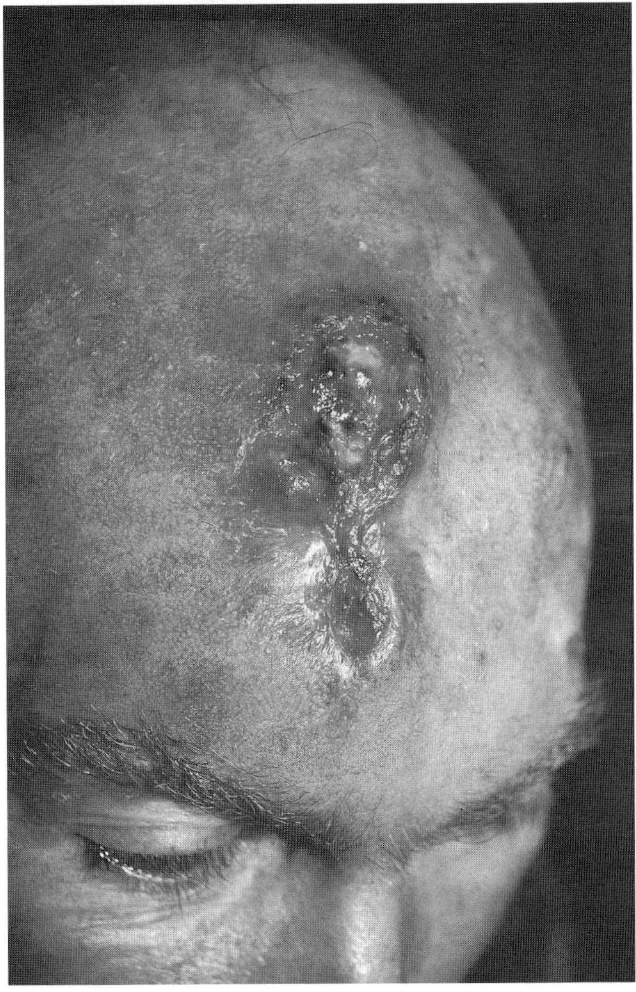

Figure 71.1

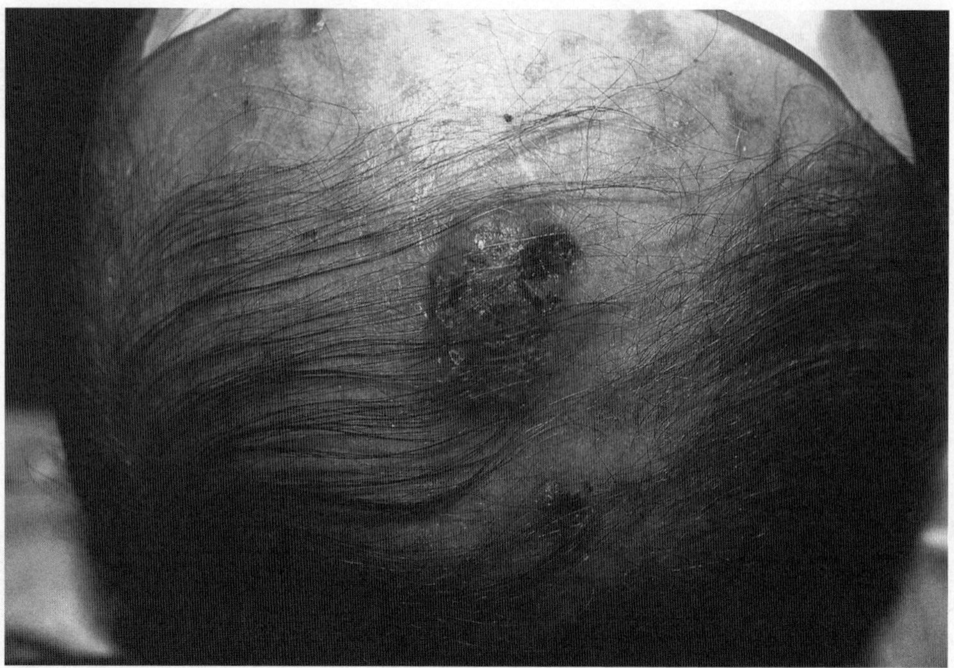

Figure 71.2

Physical Examination Report

Skin examination on the day of presentation reveals two contiguous erythematous nodules with central keratotic plugs, measuring 6.4 × 3.2 cm in total size, located on the right forehead. The tumors were ulcerated prior to surgery. There is a 1.7 × 1.7-cm erythematous nodule on the left lower lateral canthus and a 3.2 × 2.5-cm nodule on the scalp vertex. Innumerable erythematous patches and plaques on the scalp and forehead are also noted. There were healed scars on the left lower forehead, right upper lip, left shoulder, and central chest. The right forehead tumor was treated 1 year previously with local radiation, but recurred a few months prior to presentation. The left lower eyelid lesion had been treated previously with cryosurgery.

Case Continued

As part of the evaluation, a contrast magnetic resonance imaging (MRI) study of the head shows an ill-defined enhancing process of the anterior scalp extending from the midline to the right and reaching the soft tissue of the face. No bone or intracranial involvement is appreciated.

Differential Diagnosis

Clinically, the differential diagnosis of squamous cell carcinoma (SCC) is broad. Lesions can present with any of various morphologies, most commonly as verrucous, scaly, or ulcerated papules, plaques, or nodules. The clinician may need to differentiate SCC from verruca vulgaris, seborrheic keratosis, actinic keratosis, melanocytic nevus, subcutaneous fungal infection, basal cell carcinoma, melanoma, keratoacanthoma, trauma, herpes virus infection, and primary syphilis, among others. The need for a diagnostic biopsy should be guided by the clinical suspicion for malignancy.

The histology of SCC usually consists of downwardly proliferating masses of epithelial cells that contain atypical squamous cells and horn pearls. These features may vary depending on the tumor subtype and the degree of tumor differentiation. Other commonly recognized histologic subtypes of SCC include spindle-cell, acantholytic (adenoid), mucin-producing, and verrucous carcinomas.

Discussion

Skin cancer is the most common malignancy in humans. More than 1 million new cases of nonmelanoma skin cancer are diagnosed each year. SCCs account for about 20% of all nonmelanoma skin cancers in whites. In the United States, SCC is estimated to cause between 1,500 and 2,500 deaths per year. The most important etiologic factor for SCC is exposure to ultraviolet radiation, especially during childhood. Exposure to ionizing radiation and chemical carcinogens like arsenic and tar, certain genodermatoses such as xeroderma pigmentosum, human papillomavirus infection, immunosuppression, and chronic skin injury also increase the risk of developing SCC. Fair skin, light hair, and blue eyes are other risk factors for SCC development.

Actinic keratoses (AK) are considered precursor lesions of cutaneous SCC, and some authors even describe them as a type of carcinoma in situ. Persons with multiple AKs have a 6% to 10% lifetime risk of developing an invasive SCC. Bowenoid papulosis and epidermodysplasia verruciformis are two other conditions that may evolve into invasive SCC and should be followed closely. Squamous cell carcinoma in situ, such as Bowen's disease (sun-exposed areas) and erythroplasia of Queyrat (glans penis), may also progress to invasive disease if not treated completely.

Although SCC can exhibit a variety of clinical behaviors, including local tissue destruction and metastatic spread, the overall rate of local recurrence and metastasis is <10%. However, a subset of these tumors behaves even more aggressively. This high-risk subset can have rates of recurrence and metastasis up to 47%. Features that correlate with higher risk include diameter >2 cm, rapid tumor growth, location such as the ear or lip, local recurrence, host immunosuppression, poor histologic differentiation, depth of 4 mm or greater, and evidence of perineural invasion.

It is well established that organ transplant recipients, especially those who are fair skinned, have a much higher risk of developing skin cancer than the general population. Basal cell carcinoma (BCC) and SCC account for >90% of all posttransplant skin cancers. The SCC:BCC ratio (1:4 in non-transplant patients) is reversed in organ transplant recipients. SCCs in transplant recipients occur at a younger age and are more likely to be multiple tumors and behave more aggressively. The risk of developing posttransplant SCC is directly proportional to the degree and duration of immunosuppression.

In contrast to posttransplant immunosuppression, the relationship of SCC to HIV is not clear. The major risk factors for developing SCC in HIV patients are similar to those of non-HIV patients and include fair skin type and sun exposure. An increase in the SCC:BCC ratio of the HIV population has not

been demonstrated. The number of tumors, local recurrences, metastasis, and survival do not correlate with more advanced disease or lower CD4+ cell counts. However, SCCs in patients with HIV have occurred at a younger age and have been associated with significant morbidity and mortality. Management of high-risk tumors in HIV patients should be analogous to that of organ transplant recipients.

Diagnosis

High-risk invasive squamous cell carcinoma.

Recommendation

Consider options of Mohs micrographic surgery versus excision with wide margins.

Surgical Approach

In 1992, Brodland and Zitelli proposed the currently accepted guidelines for the margins of resection of primary cutaneous SCC. For low-risk tumors, they recommended excision to the level of the subcutaneous fat with margins of no less than 4 mm beyond the clinically definable tumor border. For high risk tumors, a 6-mm margin was recommended. Their study did not include recurrent SCC, for which Mohs micrographic surgery is considered the treatment of choice.

Mohs surgery is performed in stages. The first stage begins with curettage of the visible tumor to define its gross limits. The area to be excised is then mapped and recorded. The tumor is excised with a narrow margin around the initial curetted site. The resulting specimen is color coded to record the orientation of the tumor. Frozen sections of the entire specimen margin are analyzed for the presence of tumor. If any tumor is present, subsequent stages are performed until the margins are clear. Once clear margins are achieved, the wound may be repaired or, less commonly, allowed to heal by secondary intention, depending on the size and the site of the defect.

Case Continued

The patient first undergoes Mohs micrographic surgery for the tumor on the right forehead.

Perioperative Images

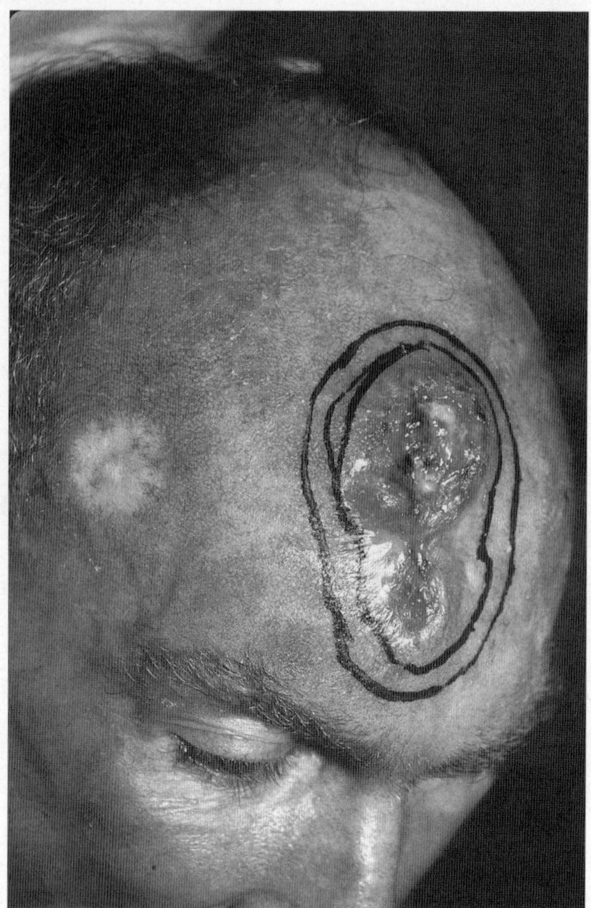

Figure 71.3

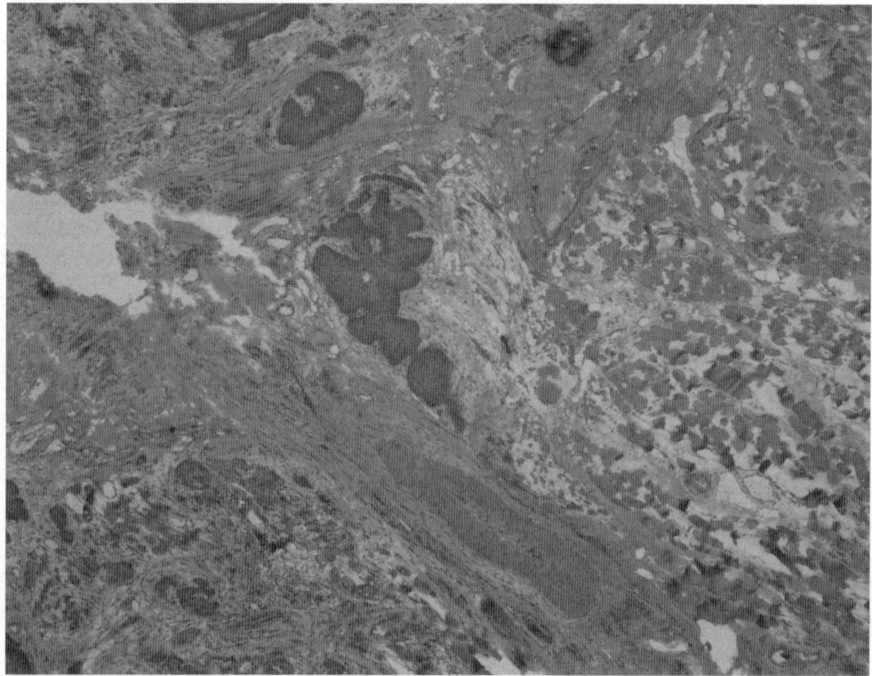

Figure 71.4A

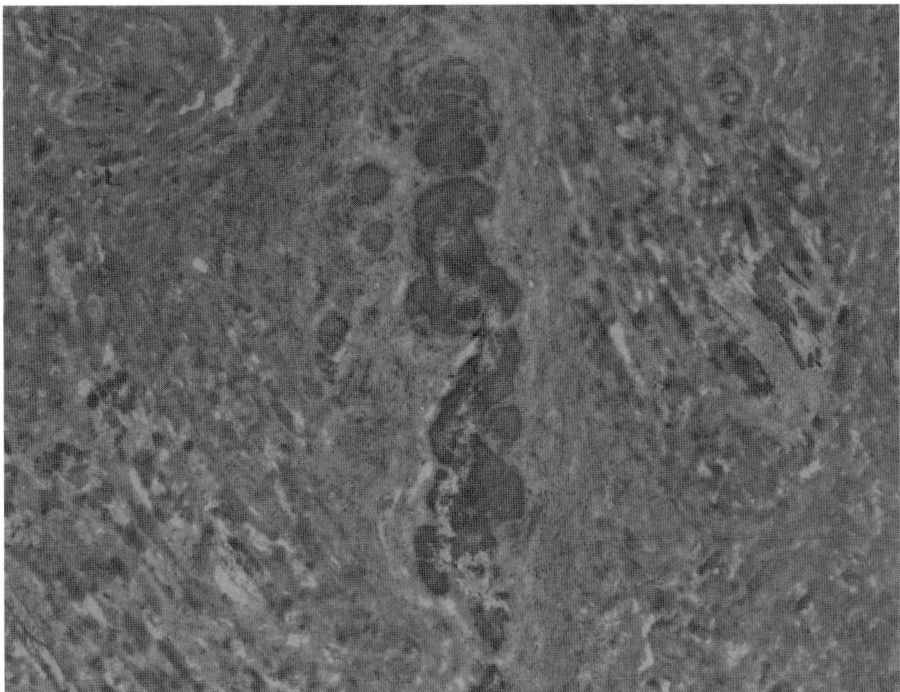

Figure 71.4B

Perioperative Report

A 1-cm margin was outlined around the tumor. Peripheral margins were still positive after two surgical stages. Hematoxylin and eosin staining revealed clusters of squamous cells proliferating and invading deep subcutaneous tissue and clusters of atypical squamous cells invading muscle.

Perioperative Image

Case Continued

The patient returns 1 week later and undergoes one more stage to achieve clear peripheral and deep margins.

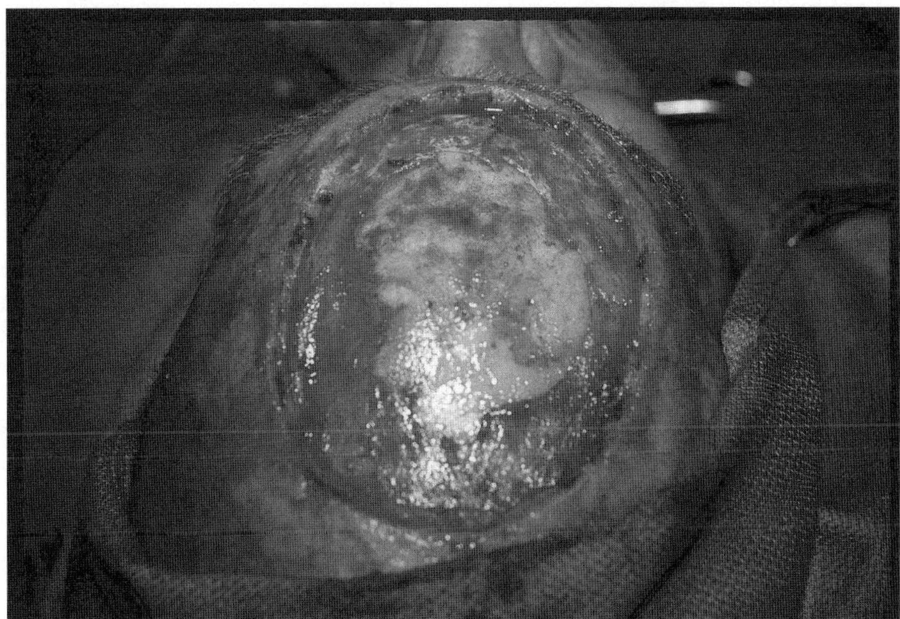

Figure 71.5

Perioperative Report

The resulting defect measured 8.4 × 10.5 cm and extended to the level of the bone.

Case Continued

On that same day, the patient underwent Mohs surgery for the lesions on the left lateral canthus and scalp vertex. One stage of Mohs surgery led to clearance of the left canthal tumor, whereas the scalp vertex tumor required two stages for clearance. The final lateral canthal defect extended from the left lower eyelid onto the cheek and down to the level of the muscularis, and measured 3.0 × 2.1 cm. The final defect size on the scalp vertex was 4.2 × 5.0 cm. The defect extended to the bone at its right anterior portion, and to the level of the periosteum in all other areas. The patient was referred to facial plastic surgery for repair of all three defects. The scalp vertex defect was closed with a combination of local rhomboid rotational flaps and a split-thickness skin graft. The forehead and the left upper cheek defects were repaired with split-thickness skin grafts. The postoperative course was complicated by a wound infection with *Pseudomonas* organisms, which was treated with ceftazidime, tobramycin, and ciprofloxacin.

Approach

The management of high-risk SCC is controversial, especially in the absence of clinical or radiologic evidence of metastasis. Mohs micrographic surgery is the preferred treatment for high-risk SCC, but the concomitant use of sentinel lymphadenectomy has been advocated in patients with a clinical N0 status. Sentinel lymph node (SLN) biopsy, a technique used to identify the first lymph node that receives lymph flow from a primary tumor, has been used in the management of oral, oropharyngeal, and genital SCC. Proponents of the use of SLN biopsy for high-risk cutaneous SCC believe that it may contribute to better staging and assessment of prognosis in these tumors. This technique may help identify patients who could benefit from therapeutic lymph node dissection, radiation, or chemotherapy, while sparing lower risk patients from the morbidity of these additional procedures.

Adjuvant modalities should be considered in the treatment of high-risk SCC. Surgery followed by adjuvant radiotherapy (wide-field irradiation with or without lymph node irradiation) has been shown to be more effective and have fewer adverse effects than radiotherapy alone and is reasonable to use in the treatment of difficult tumors. Intralesional or systemic interferon alfa-2b and alfa-2c can also be considered in combination with surgical modalities. Other adjuvant therapies that have been reported include photodynamic therapy, hyperthermia, cisplatin cytotoxic chemotherapy, and retinoids.

Topical and systemic retinoids have been used in the treatment of precancerous and cancerous lesions in nonimmunosuppressed individuals. These vitamin A analogs are of limited efficacy against existing skin cancers, but they appear to have chemopreventive effects. Studies suggest a beneficial effect of systemic retinoids in the prevention of skin cancer in patients at risk for developing large numbers of tumors, such as organ transplant recipients. Initial studies in the transplant population used etretinate, a systemic retinoid that is no longer marketed. Acitretin is now the most commonly utilized retinoid for cancer chemoprevention in immunosuppressed transplant patients, followed by isotretinoin. Most studies with isotretinoin have been performed in immunocompetent individuals, but similar results are inferred for immunosuppressed patients. The benefit of these medications is only present during treatment; as a result, long-term therapy is usually required. Unfortunately, the therapy may be limited by side effects, including dry skin and mucous membranes, hair loss, hyperlipidemia, skeletal toxicity, and osteoporosis.

Stasko et al. published the most recent guidelines for the management of SCC in organ transplant recipients. These guidelines are based on a retrospective review of the available literature and the collective clinical experience of the International Transplant-Skin Cancer Collaborative and the European Skin Care in Organ Transplant Patients Network. They emphasize the importance of patient education regarding sun exposure and protection, screening for high-risk cases, close follow-up, early treatment of precancerous lesions, and low threshold for skin biopsy. Suspected or proven SCC with clinically less aggressive qualities, such as smaller size, slow growth, and low-risk location, can be treated promptly with electrodesiccation and curettage, cryosurgery, or surgical excision, with Mohs micrographic surgery for moderate-risk lesions. Aggressive, nonmetastatic SCC should be completely excised, ideally with the Mohs micrographic technique, although wide excision with careful margin control is also acceptable. Inoperable tumors may require primary radiation therapy. Adjuvant radiation therapy should be considered if clear margins are not achieved or if there is significant perineural invasion. Metastatic SCC in transplant recipients is treated in the same manner as nonimmunosuppressed patients, with additional attention to reducing immunosuppression. Lesions with satellite metastases should be excised, and adjuvant radiation, chemotherapy, and/or chemoprophylaxis should be considered. Tumors with lymph node metastases require excision and therapeutic lymphadenectomy with or without adjuvant radiation to the tumor site and lymph node basin. Standard chemotherapy based on fluorouracil, methotrexate, paclitaxel, or cisplatin has limited efficacy, but can be used for relapsed nodal metastatic or systemic metastatic SCC. Substantial reduction of immunosuppressive therapy in these patients may lead to a reduction in the formation of new cutaneous SCCs.

Rapamycin and its derivatives, the mTOR protein inhibitors, are a promising class of immunosuppressive agents that exhibit antineoplastic properties. Clinical data suggest that transplant patients treated with rapamycin have a lower incidence of skin malignancy. When to introduce these agents to allow for both the best graft function and the prevention of skin cancer is still a topic of controversy. Some investigators suggest switching to rapamycin after the occurrence of the first skin tumors. Future clinical studies are needed for the accurate assessment of skin cancer prevention with the use of mTOR inhibitors.

Clinical Photograph

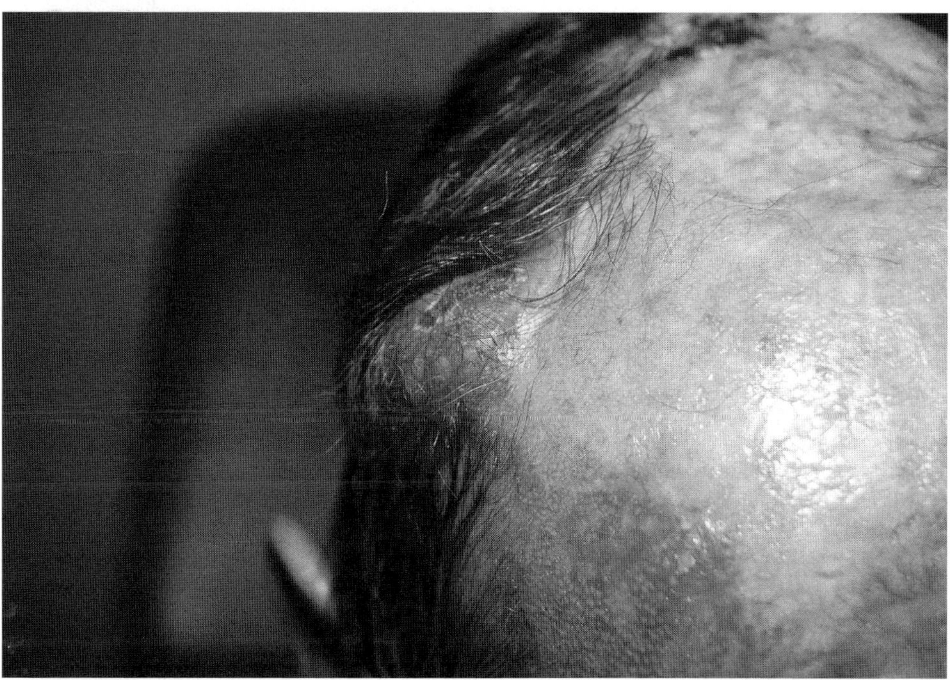

Figure 71.6

Physical Examination Report

One month after Mohs surgery, the patient is noted to have two new 1-cm nodules on the right anterior frontal scalp. Biopsy of one nodule was consistent with metastatic SCC.

Case Continued

The patient underwent Mohs excisional surgery for the metastatic nodules, and he was referred to medical and radiation oncology for opinions on adjuvant therapeutic options. Radiotherapy was not recommended because of the patient's previous radiation history; given the patient's immunosuppressed status and lack of other clinical evidence of regional or distant disease, systemic chemotherapy was not recommended. Oral isotretinoin (60 mg/day) was restarted.

Clinical Photograph

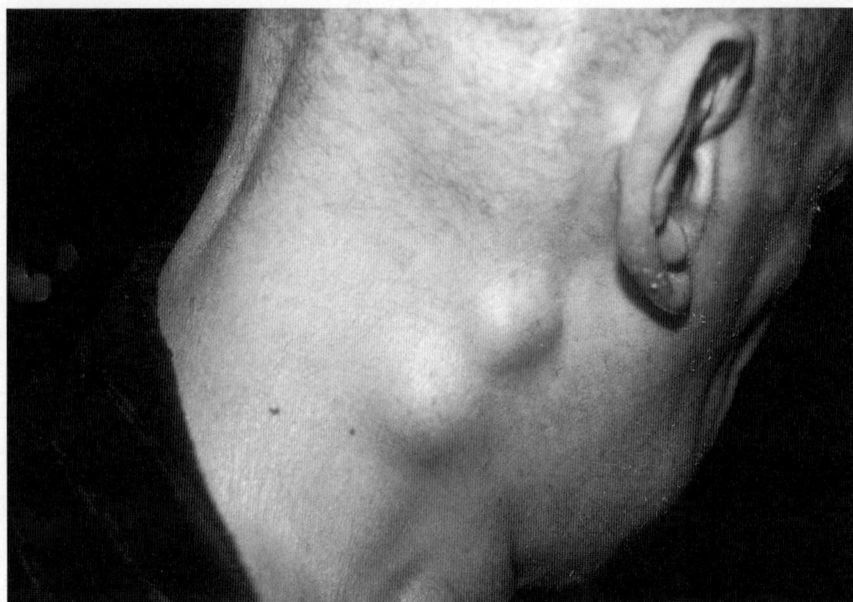

Figure 71.7

Physical Examination Report

The patient's disease progressed, and prominent cervical lymphadenopathy developed despite 5 months of isotretinoin chemoprophylaxis.

Case Continued

He was then started on 5-fluorouracil (5-FU) and cisplatin, and there was evidence of improvement after three cycles. His treatment was changed to outpatient leucovorin and 5-FU, but his cancer progressed while on this therapy. Two cycles of docetaxel and carboplatin followed, but he developed severe stomatitis and neutropenia without any response to treatment. At this point, he again received two cycles of 5-FU and cisplatin and one cycle of 5-FU and gemcitabine, but his tumors and lymphadenopathy continued to worsen. He received aggressive palliative radiation to the scalp and the cervical and preauricular lymph node regions.

Clinical Photograph

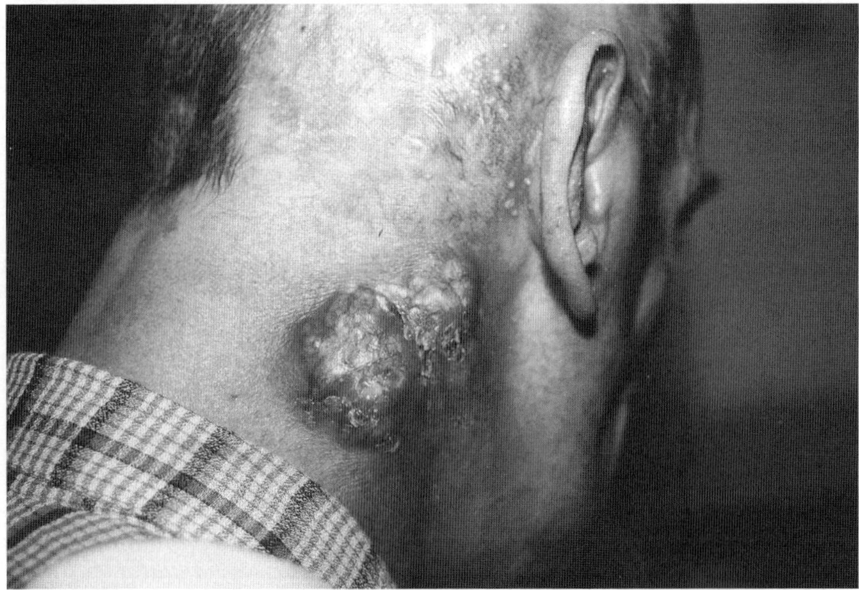

Figure 71.8

Physical Examination Report

Severe cervical lymphadenopathy persisted after palliative radiation therapy.

Case Continued

He suffered severe radiotherapy mucositis and weight loss that required gastric tube placement for nutritional support. Despite a reasonable palliative response to the radiation, he eventually died of his disease.

Discussion

In-transit metastasis, a concept widely accepted in melanoma, has been recently described in SCC, especially in the setting of organ transplantation. These metastases lack epidermal connection to the nearby primary tumor and are thought to represent metastasis in the surrounding skin via lymphatic spread. They are associated with high-risk SCC and imply increased risk for distant metastasis and a poor prognosis in transplant patients. The management of in-transit metastasis should include surgical excision and broad-field radiation with or without retinoid chemoprophylaxis and follow-up examinations every 1 to 3 months.

Suggested Readings

Alam M, Ratner D. Cutaneous squamous-cell carcinoma. *N Engl J Med* 2001;344:975–983.

Berg D, Otley C. Skin cancer in organ transplant recipients: epidemiology, pathogenesis, and management. *J Am Acad Dermatol* 2002;47:1–13.

Brodland D, Zitelli J. Surgical margins for excision of primary cutaneous squamous cell carcinoma. *J Am Acad Dermatol* 1992;27:241–248.

De Graaf Y, Euvrard S, Bouwes Bavinck J. Systemic and topical retinoids in the management of skin cancer in organ transplant recipients. *Dermatol Surg* 2004;30:656–661.

Euvrard S, Kanitakis J, Claudy A. Skin cancers after organ transplantation. *N Engl J Med* 2003;348:1681–1691.

Geohas J, Roholt N, Robinson J. Adjuvant radiotherapy after excision of cutaneous squamous cell carcinoma. *J Am Acad Dermatol* 1994;30:633–636.

Jensen P, Hansen S, Moller B, et al. Skin cancer in kidney and heart transplant recipients and different long-term immunosuppressive therapy regimens. *J Am Acad Dermatol* 1999;40:177–186.

McKenna D, Murphy G. Skin cancer chemoprophylaxis in renal transplant recipients: 5 years of experience using low-dose acitretin. *Br J Dermatol* 1999;140:656–660.

Nguyen P, Vin-Christian K, Ming M, et al. Aggressive squamous cell carcinomas in persons with the human immunodeficiency virus. *Arch Dermatol* 2002;138:758–763.

Reschly M, Messina J, Zaulyanov L, et al. Utility of sentinel lymphadenectomy in the management of patients with high-risk cutaneous squamous cell carcinoma. *Dermatol Surg* 2003;29:135–140.

Rowe D, Carroll R, Day C. Prognostic factors for local recurrence, metastasis, and survival rates in squamous cell carcinoma of the skin, ear, and lip. *J Am Acad Dermatol* 1992;26:976–990.

Stasko T, Brown M, Carucci J, et al. Guidelines for the management of squamous cell carcinoma in organ transplant recipients. *Dermatol Surg* 2004;30:642–650.

Weisberg N, Bertagnolli M, Becker D. Combined sentinel lymphadenectomy and Mohs micrographic surgery for high-risk cutaneous squamous cell carcinoma. *J Am Acad Dermatol* 2000;43:483–488.

case 72

Presentation

The patient is an 80-year-old woman from the Dominican Republic who had a biopsy-proven basal cell carcinoma (BCC) on the left lateral nose 1 year prior to presentation. She underwent excision of the tumor in the Dominican Republic 1 month after biopsy, and was repaired with a full-thickness skin graft that covered the entire dorsum of the nose. The pathology specimen from the excision was noted to have tumor present at the margins. Repeat biopsy of the nose in the United States 1 month prior to presentation confirmed the presence of BCC.

Clinical Photograph

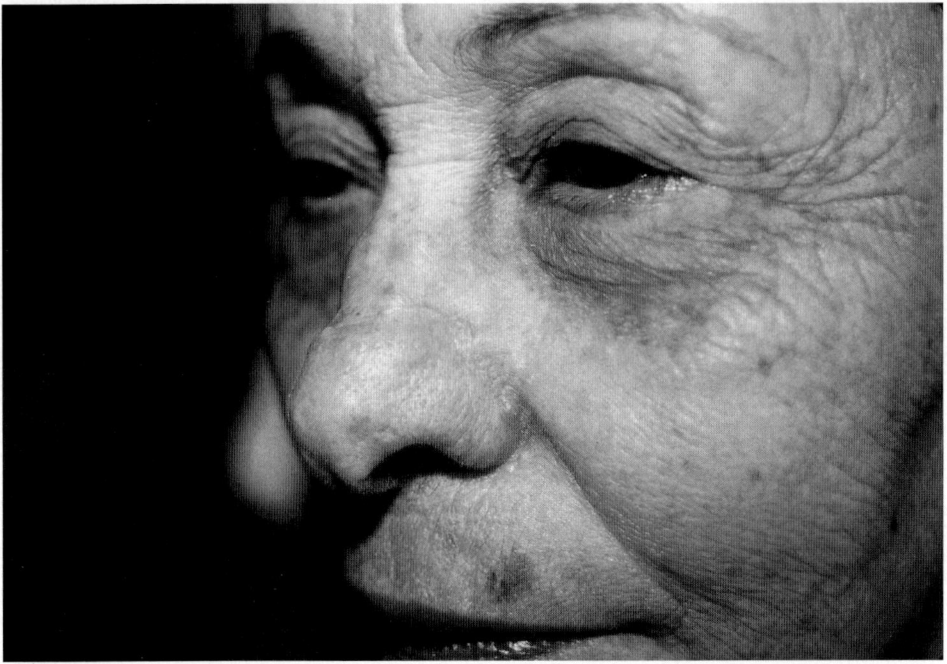

Figure 72.1

Physical Examination Report

On the day of presentation, she has a 0.7 × 0.5-cm ill-defined erythematous plaque on the left lower nasal sidewall adjacent to the skin graft. A newly developed papule of 0.3 × 0.3 cm in the left lower nasolabial fold is biopsied and found to be BCC.

Differential Diagnosis

The histologic characteristics of BCC are distinctive, with uniform aggregates of basaloid epithelial cells exhibiting peripheral palisading of their nuclei. The basaloid aggregates often lie within a mucinous stroma, and may show retraction from the surrounding dermal connective tissue. Once a biopsy specimen

"

showing BCC is obtained, there is usually no differential diagnosis between BCC and another tumor because the pathology is unambiguous. The histologic presentation of this tumor is variable, however, and multiple BCC subtypes have been described. The most commonly recognized subtypes of BCC include nodular, superficial, pigmented, micronodular, morpheaform, infiltrative, and basosquamous types. Often a particular biopsy specimen will not show only a single specific subtype of BCC, but rather a combination of subtypes.

Discussion

BCC is the most common malignancy of the skin. Worldwide, Australia is the country with the highest incidence of this tumor. It is thought that the principal risk factor for the development of BCC is exposure to ultraviolet radiation. Although BCC can be found on any part of the body, the most common locations are in photodistributed areas. Patients who have been treated for psoriasis with psoralens and ultraviolet A light (PUVA) are at a higher risk for developing BCC. Physical risk factors for the development of this tumor include light skin (with a tendency for sunburns instead of tanning), presence of red or blond hair, and blue or green eyes. It is uncommon to diagnose BCC in patients with dark skin. Treatment for prior BCC or for other malignancies with ionizing radiation increases the risk for new tumor formation in the exposed treatment areas. Patients with inherited skin diseases such as xeroderma pigmentosum, Gorlin syndrome (basal cell nevus syndrome), Bazex syndrome, and Rombo syndrome are also at risk for developing BCC. Exposure to environmental arsenic, such as from well water, increases the risk of developing BCC. Prior development of a BCC is also a risk factor for developing additional tumors. Recent studies have shown this risk to be between 33% and 77%.

Studies have shown that the subtype of BCC can be important in prognosis. In general, the nodular and superficial types of BCC are the least biologically aggressive, while the morpheaform, infiltrative, and micronodular subtypes are considered to be aggressive growth pattern tumors, with a greater risk for subclinical extension and recurrence. For this reason, the aggressive growth pattern subtypes of BCC are considered to be high-risk lesions.

Molecular analyses of BCCs have shown mutations in the Patched 1 (PTCH1) gene, which is a component of the Hedgehog signaling pathway. This is the same germline mutation found in patients with Gorlin syndrome. Other genes in this pathway, including Smoothened and Sonic Hedgehog, have also been found to be mutated in BCC. Mutations in the p53 gene have been found in up to 50% of BCCs.

Diagnosis

BCC, aggressive histologic growth pattern.

Recommendation

Mohs micrographic surgery.

Approach

Although BCC rarely metastasizes, it can be locally aggressive as well as destructive, with the potential to invade both soft tissues and bone. In general, a variety of treatment options exist for basal cell carcinoma, including electrodesiccation and curettage, cryotherapy, traditional surgical excision, radiotherapy, and surgical excision utilizing the Mohs micrographic surgery technique.

For most BCCs on the face, Mohs micrographic surgery is the treatment of choice because of its precise control of surgical margins and concurrent maximum viable tissue preservation. Indications for Mohs surgery for BCC include large tumor size (>2 cm), anatomic areas associated with high risk of recurrence (mainly head and neck, especially around the eyes, lips, and ears, i.e., the H-zone of the face), incompletely excised tumors, tumors with aggressive growth pattern histology, such as morpheaform or infiltrative features, tumors with ill-defined borders, recurrent tumors, neurotropic tumors, tumors arising in areas previously treated with ionizing radiation, and the need for maximum tissue preservation. In the case presented here, Mohs micrographic surgery was the treatment of choice for many of the reasons listed above.

Surgical Approach

Mohs micrographic surgery is performed by first curetting any visible tumor, to define the gross margins of the lesion. These curettings may be processed by the on-site laboratory staff and examined in frozen section as a reference for tumor growth pattern. After the gross extent of the tumor is defined, a map of the surgical area to be excised is recorded. A 2- to 3-mm margin around the initial curetted site is removed, and the specimen is marked to record the orientation of the tumor to correspond with the map marked on the patient. The entire margin of the surgical specimen is examined for the presence of tumor. If tumor is present at the surgical margin, additional surgical sections are removed until the margins are clear. Finally, the resulting wound is repaired. Options for repair depend on the size and location of the surgical defect and include primary closure and the use of skin grafts and flaps, as well as allowing wounds to heal by secondary intention. The overall estimated 5-year cure rate reported in the literature for primary BCC treated by Mohs micrographic surgery is 99%. For recurrent tumors, the estimated cure rate is 95%.

Perioperative Images

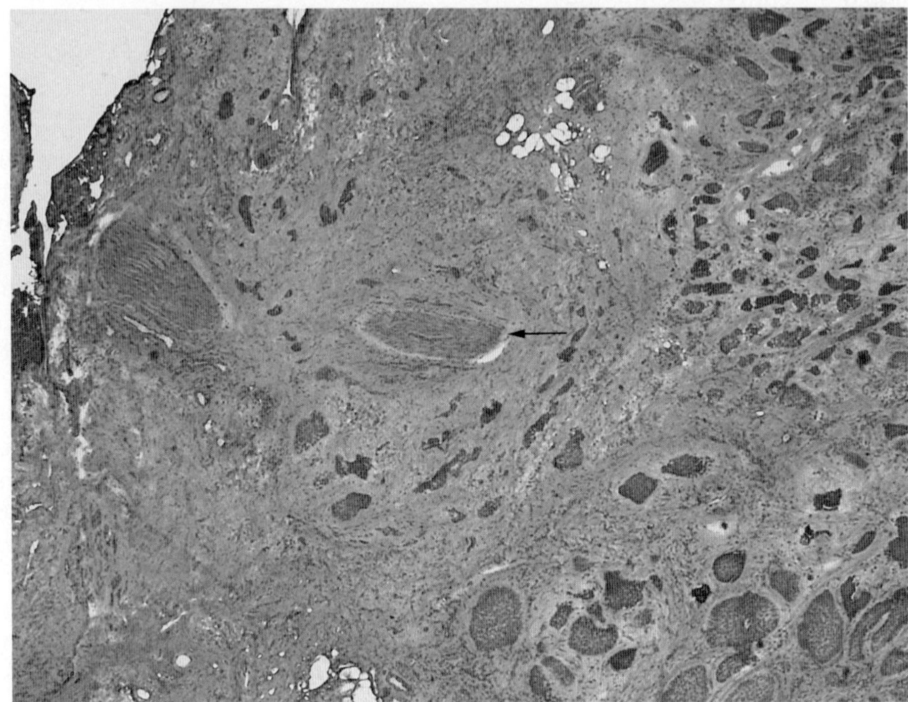

Figure 72.2

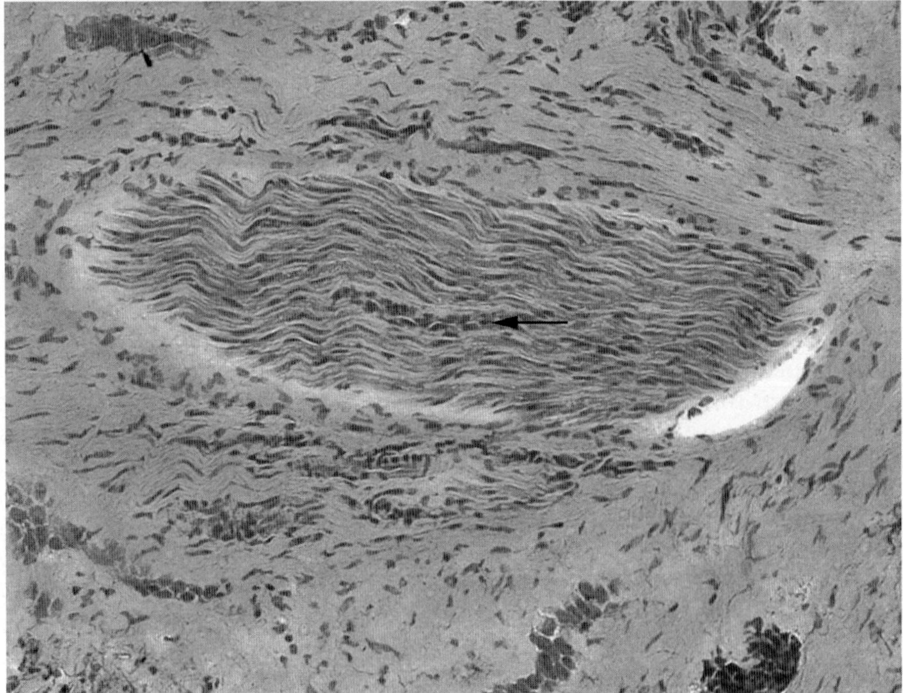

Figure 72.3

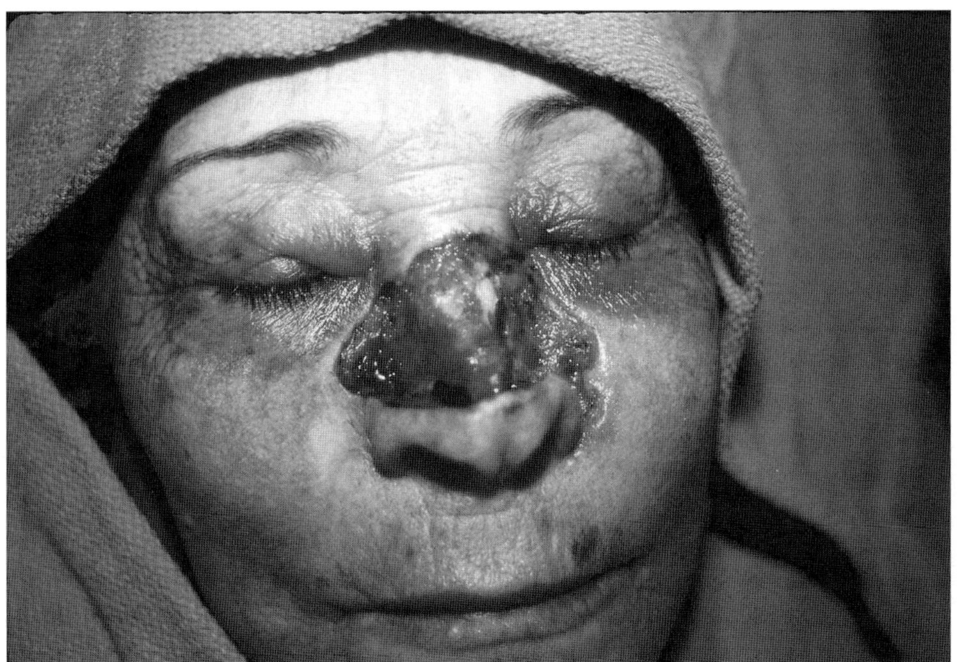

Figure 72.4

Perioperative Report

Using the Mohs micrographic surgical technique, a total of nine stages are performed. This is accomplished over a 2-day period, with the patient resting at home overnight after the first day. As is suspected in this case, the patient's initial lesion on the nose is contiguous with the tumor confirmed by biopsy on the day of surgery. The tumor extends along and between the medial and lateral crural cartilages and beneath the left side of the nasal bone. The tumor also extends to the upper aspect of the left nasal sidewall, onto the medial aspect of the left cheek, and onto the left nasal ala sparing the alar rim. Histologically, the tumor is noted to have perineural invasion, and a diffuse micronodular and morpheaform growth pattern on hematoxylin and eosin stain. The nerve indicated by an *arrow* in Figure 72.2 is shown on a high-power view in Figure 72.3, revealing its invasion by tumor *(arrow)*. At the end of the ninth stage, persistent tumor is seen tracking between the medial crura of the nasal tip toward the columella. The total defect measures 6.3 × 4.1 cm.

Discussion

This case is an exceptional example of the destructive potential of BCC. Most cases of BCC treated by Mohs micrographic surgery have tumor-free margins after one to three surgical stages. Curettage has been shown to be an effective method of defining the gross margins of BCC before Mohs micrographic surgery. Although most BCCs can be easily treated with standard techniques that include surgical resection with a 1-cm margin, Mohs micrographic surgery is the treatment of choice for aggressive, large tumors, such as this patient's, with ill-defined borders.

Perineural invasion of BCC has a higher rate of recurrence and complications as compared to tumors without perineural spread. The cleavage plane between the nerve and nerve sheath provides an area of low resistance for the tumor to spread. Involvement of the facial nerves can give direct access to the central nervous system. Among patients with tumors of the face with perineural spread, 60% to 70% are asymptomatic. Complications of BCC with perineural spread include blindness, stroke, and sinus involvement. Rates of perineural invasion of BCC are low, with a study by Mohs reporting an incidence of 0.92%. A more recent prospective study of 434 patients with BCC by Ratner et al. showed that 6.7% had perineural inflammation, perineural tumor invasion, or both. The mean postoperative defect area of tumors with perineural invasion was 17.85 cm^2, which was 605% greater than that of tumors without any perineural involvement. Mohs surgery alone is effective for early-stage BCC with perineural involvement. Postoperative radiation therapy should be considered for those patients with late-stage disease or those showing frank cranial nerve involvement.

Case Continued

Because of the anticipated large facial defect, the patient is referred preoperatively to plastic surgery for consultation about repair.

▮ Perioperative Image

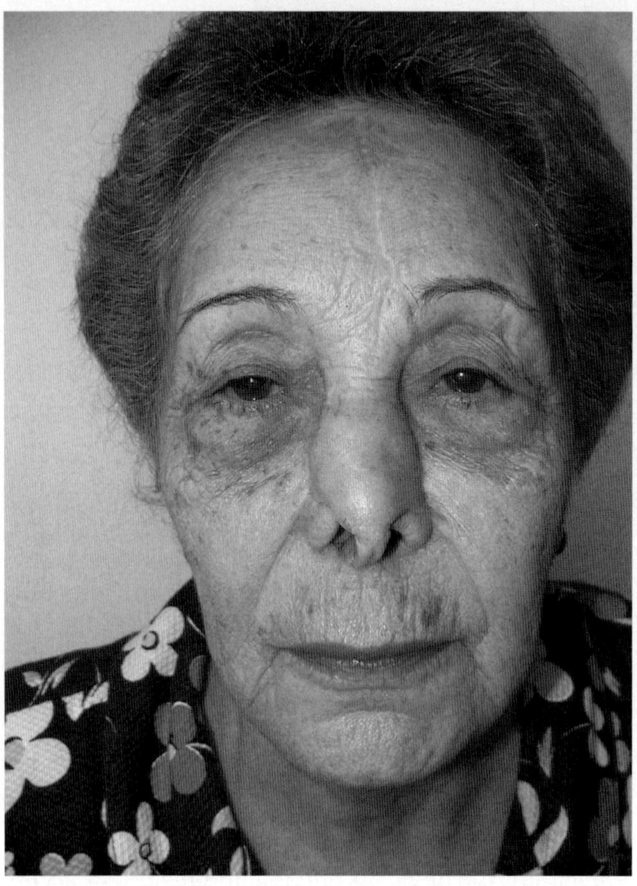

Figure 72.5 Photograph courtesy of Dr. Arnold Breitbart.

Perioperative Report

Tissue from the columella and nasal tip is removed, and these tissues are tumor free by histologic examination. The reconstruction is accomplished under general anesthesia by a combination of bilateral cheek advancement flaps, intranasal lining flaps, auricular cartilage grafts, and a forehead flap.

Case Continued

The flaps and grafts heal well, and the patient remains disease free 3 years after her surgery.

Suggested Readings

Barrett TL, Greenway HT, Massullo V, et al. Treatment of basal cell carcinoma and squamous cell carcinoma with perineural invasion. *Adv Dermatol* 1993;8:277–305.

Dicker T, Siller G, Saunders N. Molecular and cellular biology of basal cell carcinoma. *Austral J Dermatol* 2002;43:241–246.

Lawrence CM. Mohs' micrographic surgery for basal cell carcinoma. *Clin Exp Dermatol* 1999;24:130–133.

Maloney ME. Histology of basal cell carcinoma. *Clin Dermatol* 1995;13:545–549.

Ratner D, Bagiella E. The efficacy of curettage in delineating margins of basal cell carcinoma before Mohs micrographic surgery. *Dermatol Surg* 2003;29:899–903.

Ratner D, Lowe L, Johnson T, et al. Perineural spread of basal cell carcinomas treated with Mohs micrographic surgery. *Cancer* 2000;88:1605–1613.

Saldanha G, Fletcher A, Slater DN. Basal cell carcinoma: a dermatopathological and molecular biological update. *Br J Dermatol* 2003;148:195–202.

Thissen M, Neumann M, Schouten L. A systematic review of treatment modalities for primary basal cell carcinomas. *Arch Dermatol* 1999;135:1177–1183.

Wong CSM, Strange RC, Lear JT. Basal cell carcinoma. *BMJ* 2003;327:794–798.

Presentation

A 38-year-old man presents with multiple firm, purple-reddish-brown nodules and plaques on the lower extremities. The patient had been diagnosed with human immunodeficiency virus (HIV) 5 months before and had a history of hepatitis B infection. The patient has been treated for 4 months with highly active antiretroviral therapy (HAART), which has not improved his current disease.

Clinical Photograph

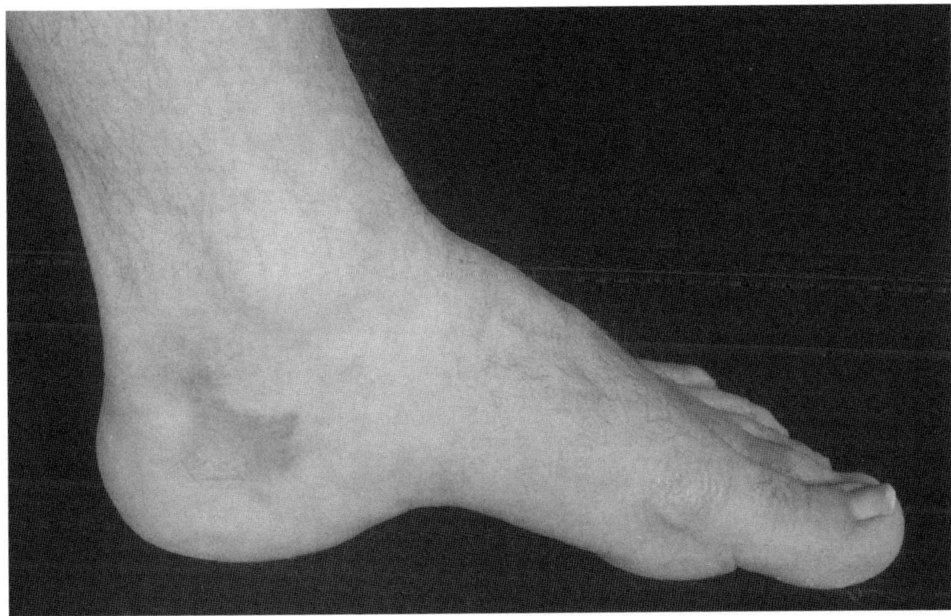

Figure 73.1

Physical Examination Report

Kaposi sarcoma (KS) on the medial aspect of the foot before chemotherapy: purple-reddish-brown nodules and plaques.

Differential Diagnosis

The differential diagnosis of reddish nodules on the extremities in adults includes lymphoma, KS, bacillary angiomatosis, cat-scratch disease, hemangioma, and angiosarcoma, as well as basal cell cancer and amelanotic melanoma.

Discussion

KS is a multifocal, polyclonal, hyperplastic neoplasm arising from lymphatic endothelial cells. KS is the most common tumor occurring in HIV-positive patients. Human herpes virus 8 (HHV-8) or KS-associated herpes virus (KSHV) together with cytokine-induced endothelial cell growth and some state of immunocompromise represent important conditions for its development. HHV8 DNA sequences have been shown to be associated with all different forms of KS, including the HIV-positive and HIV-negative forms.

In the United States, the risk for KS in patients with acquired immunodeficiency syndrome (AIDS) was estimated to be more than 20,000 times that of the general population and 300 times that of other immunosuppressed patients. KS has been reported among all risk groups for HIV infection and in both sexes.

AIDS-KS commonly presents multifocally and symmetrically. Lesions may begin as macules, frequently evolving to papules and tumors. Before the HAART era, oral KS lesions represented the first clinical manifestation in about one quarter of AIDS patients. In the HAART era, the incidence of KS in HIV-infected patients has decreased in the western world. In the United States, the AIDS-KS incidence has declined from 4.8 cases/100 persons/year in 1990 to 1.5 cases/100 persons/year in 1997. Once the diagnosis of KS is clinically suspected, it is confirmed by biopsy and histological examination.

Recommendation

Biopsy of thigh and laboratory tests.

Case Continued

The results of routine laboratory studies were within normal limits, including CD4+ and CD8+ lymphocyte counts and the CD4/CD8 ratio. HIV-RNA quantification revealed <50 copies/mL. HHV-8 was positive in the KS biopsy as assessed by polymerase chain reaction (PCR). The patient had IgG antibodies against HHV8, cytomegalovirus, and Epstein-Barr virus. He also had antibodies against the hepatitis B surface and core proteins (HBc-Ag and HBs-Ag).

Histopathology Slide

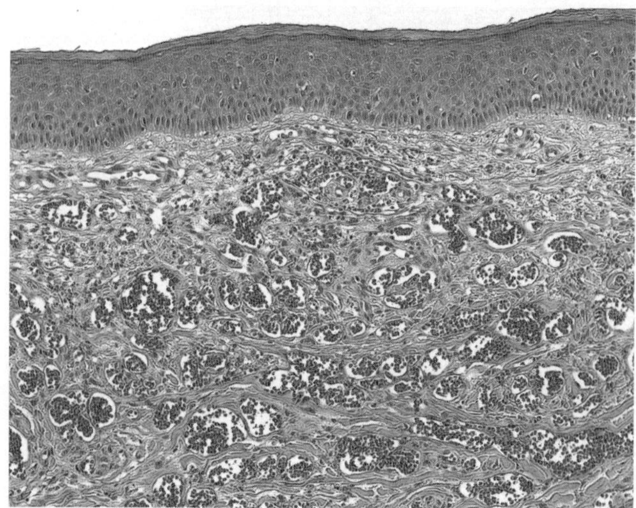

Figure 73.2

Histopathology Report

A specimen of the excised nodule reveals spindle-like tumor cells and numerous vascular spaces with extravasated erythrocytes. Spindle cells are dispersed throughout dermal collagen bundles forming irregular proliferations.

Diagnosis

Kaposi sarcoma.

Discussion

The histological results support the clinical diagnosis of KS. Histologically, KS is characterized by a proliferation of spindle cells and cleft-like vascular structures with vascular channel formation. In this patient, AIDS-KS occurred at normal CD4 cell counts, suggesting that HIV does contribute more than just immunodeficiency to the pathogenesis of KS. In this regard, the HIV transactivating protein (tat) has been proposed. HAART typically causes profound and sustained suppression of viral replication, reducing morbidity and prolonging life in patients with HIV infection. It is noteworthy that upon the initiation of HAART, the KS lesions in our patient did not disappear.

Recommendation

Endoscopy, rectoscopy, chest x-ray, assessment of lymph node status.

Pathology Report

KS of the duodenal tract. Histological examination of the excised mucosa revealed numerous spindle-shaped tumor cells, a lymphocytic and granulocytic infiltrate, and endothelial expression of CD34.

Discussion

CD34 is an endothelial marker, expressed at relatively high levels in many KS tumor cells. Recently, the antibody D2-40 has been introduced; it stains lymphatic endothelia and has proven the lymphatic origin of KS lesions. Visceral involvement, as in our patient, is common but is often asymptomatic. The most commonly affected sites of systemic KS involve the oral cavity, gastrointestinal tract, lungs, and lymph nodes. AIDS-KS causes significant mortality and morbidity, with organ dysfunction such as lymphatic obstruction or rapidly progressive pulmonary failure. Sometimes hyperkeratotic KS develops following lymphatic edema.

Approach

Treatment options depend on the type of KS, the extent of the tumor, the organs involved, the HIV-1 viral load, and the $CD4^+$ T-lymphocyte count. This patient was offered therapy with liposomal doxorubicin (Doxil). It was explained to the patient that no curative therapy exists for AIDS-KS. Neither local nor systemic treatments have been shown to prolong survival. The goal of KS treatment is to provide safe and effective palliation of symptoms and further spread.

Case Continued

Chemotherapy was initiated with six cycles of doxorubicin at 20 mg/m^2 every 3 weeks.

Discussion

For patients with more widely disseminated, progressive, or symptomatic disease, systemic therapy with cytotoxic chemotherapy or interferon-α is generally warranted. The current first-line therapy for advanced KS consists of liposomal Adriamycin, especially when CD4 counts are low. A retrospective analysis has addressed the outcome, survival, adverse events, and clinical complications of long-term (up to 4 years) chemotherapy for AIDS-KS with pegylated liposomal doxorubicin. Although 66% of patients responded to treatment, the most common adverse events included pancytopenia and abnormal liver function tests.

Case Continued

Laboratory abnormalities did not occur in the patient. Six months later, the patient's response to therapy was assessed. The gastrointestinal and cutaneous lesions showed an excellent clinical response. On the skin, postinflammatory hyperpigmentation was observed. In addition, the patient's blood was tested for the presence of HHV8 DNA in peripheral blood mononuclear cells (PBMCs) by nested PCR. The PBMCs and the plasma were found to be negative for the presence of HHV8 DNA upon completion of six cycles of chemotherapy. One year after the chemotherapy, no clinical recurrence had occurred.

Clinical Photograph

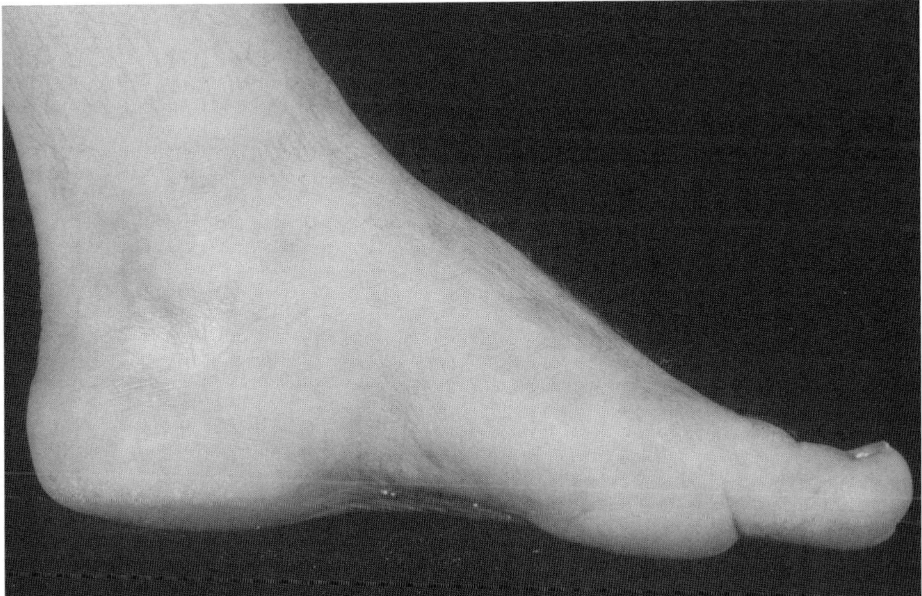

Figure 73.3

Physical Examination Report

KS after the chemotherapy showing scar tissue.

Acknowledgment

We are grateful to Dr. Vivian Kouri, Institute Pedro Kouri, Havana, Cuba, for establishing the nested KSHV-PCR and real-time KSHV-PCR.

Suggested Readings

Ascoli V, Scalzo CC, Andreoni M, et al. Kaposi's sarcoma following malignant mesothelioma. *Virchows Arch* 1999;435:612–615.

Beral V, Peterman TA, Berkelman RL, et al. Kaposi's sarcoma among persons with AIDS: a sexually transmitted infection? *Lancet* 1990;335:123–128.

Dezube BJ. AIDS-related Kaposi sarcoma. *Arch Dermatol* 2000; 136:1554–1556.

Hengge UR, Brockmeyer NH, Rasshofer R, et al. Fatal hepatic failure with liposomal doxorubicin. *Lancet* 1993;341:383–384.

Hengge UR, Esser S, Rudel HP, et al. Long-term chemotherapy of HIV-associated Kaposi' s sarcoma with liposomal doxorubicin. *Eur J Cancer* 2000;37:878–883.

Hengge UR, Franz B, Goos M. Decline of infectious skin manifestations in the era of highly active antiretroviral therapy. *AIDS* 2000;14:1069–1070.

Hengge UR, Ruzicka T, Tyring SK, et al. Update on Kaposi's sarcoma and other HHV8 associated diseases. Part 1: epidemiology, environmental predispositions, clinical manifestations, and therapy. *Lancet Infect Dis* 2002;5:281–292.

Hengge UR, Ruzicka T, Tyring SK, et al. Update on Kaposi's sarcoma and other HHV8 associated diseases. Part 2: pathogenesis, Castleman's disease, and pleural effusion lymphoma. *Lancet Infect Dis* 2002;6:344–352.

Hengge UR, Stocks K, Goos M. Acquired immune deficiency syndrome-related hyperkeratotic Kaposi's sarcoma with severe lymphoedema: report of five cases. *Br J Dermatol* 2000; 142:501–505.

Jones JL, Hanson DL, Dworkin MS, et al. Effect of antiretroviral therapy on recent trends in selected cancers among HIV-infected persons. Adult/Adolescent Spectrum of HIV Disease Project Group. *J Acquir Immune Defic Syndr* 1999;21:11–17.

Kahn HJ, Bailey D, Marks A. Monoclonal antibody D2-40, a new marker of lymphatic endothelium, reacts with Kaposi's sarcoma and a subset of angiosarcomas. *Mod Pathol* 2002; 15:434–440.

Sepkowitz KA. Effect of HAART on natural history of AIDS-related opportunistic disorders. *Lancet* 1998;351:228–230.

Silverman S Jr, Migliorati CA, Lozada-Nur F, et al. Oral findings in people with or at high risk for AIDS: a study of 375 homosexual males. *J Am Dent Assoc* 1986;112:187–192.

Zong JC, Ciufo DM, Alcendor DJ, et al. High-level variability in the ORF-K1 membrane protein gene at the left end of the Kaposi's sarcoma-associated herpesvirus genome defines four major virus subtypes and multiple variants or clades in different human populations. *J Virol* 1999;73:4156–4170.

Presentation

A 41-year-old woman is admitted to your hospital with hypertension and severe headache. Workup shows an increased level of noradrenaline in urine, 15 times greater than the reference level. Computed tomography (CT) scan reveals a large tumor close to the right adrenal expanding into the hilus of the liver.

CT Scan

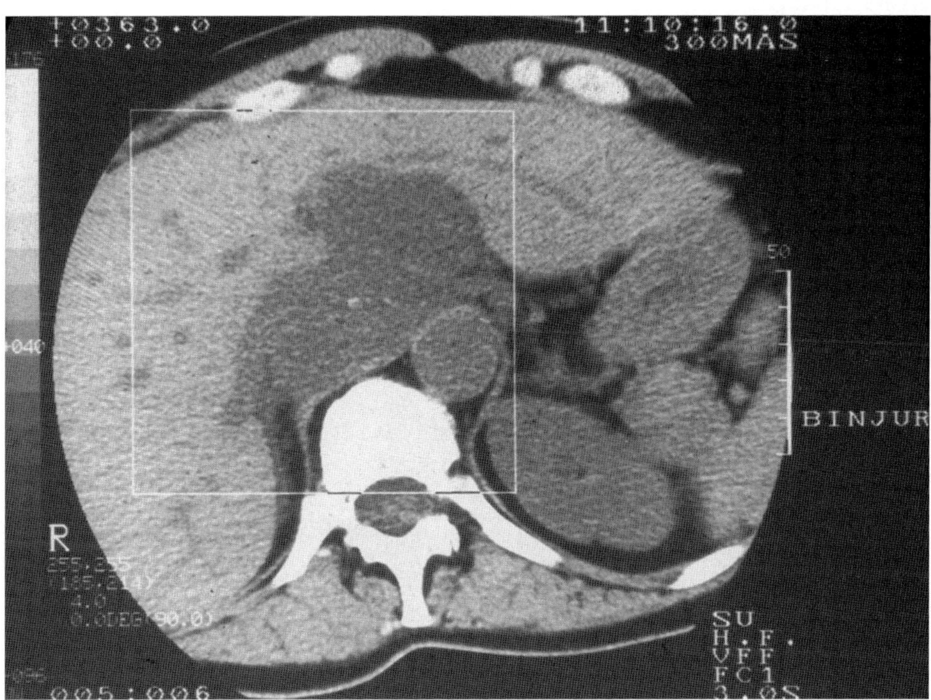

Figure 74.1

CT Scan Report

A large tumor is seen close to the right adrenal, bulging into the liver.

Differential Diagnosis

This patient has a large tumor in close proximity to the liver and the right adrenal. The tumor produces noradrenaline and dopamine. It is evidently a paraganglioma; whether it is adrenal or extra-adrenal may be difficult to discern, but magnetic resonance imaging (MRI) is often helpful. It is hard to know preoperatively if this tumor is malignant, but the location and size strongly suggest a malignant tumor.

Recommendations

Patients with catecholamine-producing tumors are usually advised to have preoperative treatment with alpha-receptor blocking agents to reduce the vascular sensitivity to circulating catecholamines. Phenoxybenzamine 30 to 200 mg daily has been widely used. Doxazosin 4 to 12 mg can also be recommended. Other agents also have been used. So far, there are no studies done to compare the efficiency of various types of drugs used for preoperative treatment.

Case Continued

For alpha-receptor blockade, you chose to use phenoxybenzamine. This patient is treated with phenoxybenzamine 160 mg daily, which results in an orthostatic reaction and a stuffy nose. This is a high dose expected to cause hypotension when the tumor has been removed.

Surgical Approach

The patient is explored through a thoracoabdominal incision. During the operation, periods of hypertension are treated with adenosine infusion, and similarly, periods of hypotension are treated with noradrenaline infusion. The venous drainage is carefully isolated and ligated in continuity and divided. Next, the arterial blood supply is controlled. Following this, the tumor is resected en bloc.

Case Continued

The tumor is 10 cm in diameter, highly vascularized, and difficult to resect. The perioperative blood loss was 6 liters. Postoperatively, the patient spends 48 hours in intensive care and is discharged from the hospital on postoperative day 15. The resected specimen is sent to pathology.

Perioperative Image

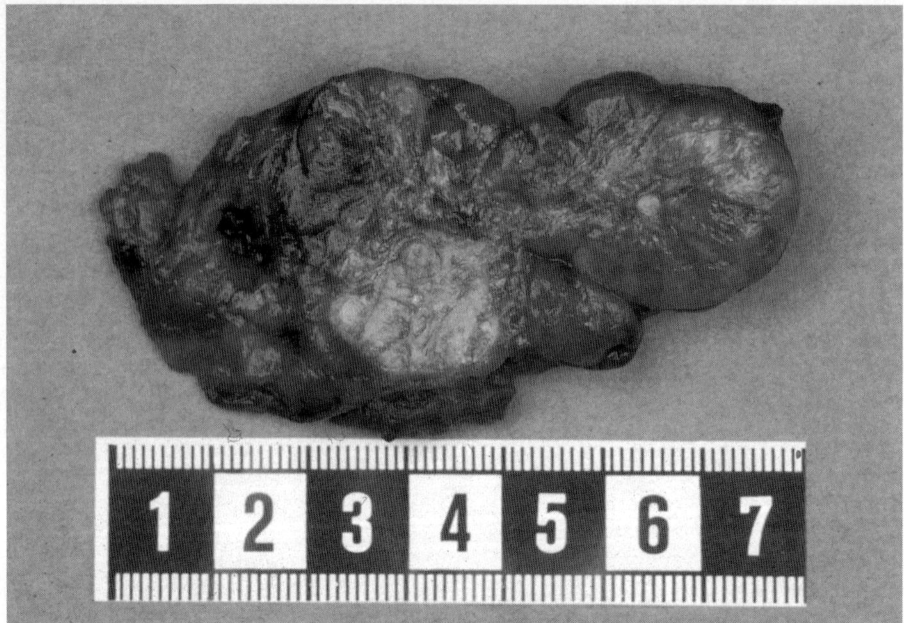

Figure 74.2

Perioperative Report

A gross view of the resected specimen reveals a large irregular tumor with macroscopic as well as microscopic suspicion of malignancy.

Pathology Report

Microscopic examination reveals a paraganglioma with high suspicion of being malignant, although this diagnosis is often difficult without evidence of metastatic growth.

Case Continued

The patient is followed in the outpatient clinic. She has a normal urinary level of catecholamines and overall is in good general condition. Surveillance metaiodobenzylguanidine (MIBG) scintigraphy is negative.

Recommendation

Follow-up of patients operated for pheochromocytoma with suspicion of malignancy should include regular control of urinary catecholamines, abdominal CT scan, and lung x-ray.

Case Continued

Two years after the operation, the patient again returns for follow up. Urinary catecholamines have increased and are 50% above the normal level. In searching for metastatic disease, MIBG scintigraphy is not valuable. CT scan reveals at least three liver metastases and chest x-ray shows two pulmonary metastases.

Diagnosis and Recommendation

The patient evidently has metastatic disease. When distant metastases appear, it is important to evaluate whether these are resectable for cure. In the case of a catecholamine-producing tumor, it is always valuable to attempt cytoreduction to avoid development of hypertension.

Case Continued

You decide to resect the liver metastases and the patient is again preoperatively prepared with the alpha-receptor blocking agent phenoxybenzamine. This time the dose used is much lower, only 30 mg. This was due to the hypotensive periods that had occurred postoperatively after the first operation. At operation, the prior incision is used. After a time-consuming dissection, three metastatic nodules are removed from the liver. Postoperatively, the patient recovers well, and 2 months later she is admitted to the thoracic service, where the two pulmonary metastases are removed. Postoperatively now, 2.5

years after the primary operation, the patient has no evidence of disease. She is working full time, with normal levels of urinary catecholamines.

The patient again presents 1 year later with slightly increased levels of noradrenaline in urine. Abdominal CT scan reveals liver metastases in the right lobe, which are treated with angiographic embolization. She tolerates this well except for some right upper quadrant pain, which eventually resolves.

The patient again is shown to have a rising noradrenaline level in urine 18 months later. The hypertension is more difficult to control and workup with MIBG scintigraphy is negative. The CT scan now reveals numerous liver metastases.

Discussion

The patient now has recurrent metastatic malignant paraganglioma where surgery is no longer possible. At this stage, other treatment modalities must be used. The first line of treatment of metastatic paraganglioma after surgery is treatment with MIBG-^{131}I if the tumor demonstrates uptake of this drug. The next step will be chemotherapy, although the experience is limited.

Case Continued

The patient is started on a combination chemotherapy regimen of cyclophosphamide, vincristine, and dacarbazine. This results in a complete response lasting for 32 months, and the noradrenaline levels are normal during this time. Ten years after the initial operation and 5 years after the start of chemotherapy treatment, the patient had normal noradrenaline levels and no sign of metastatic disease.

The patient presents again with signs of metastatic disease, including increased blood pressure, and workup reveals metastatic disease to the liver, pelvis, and hip.

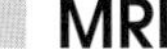 **MRI**

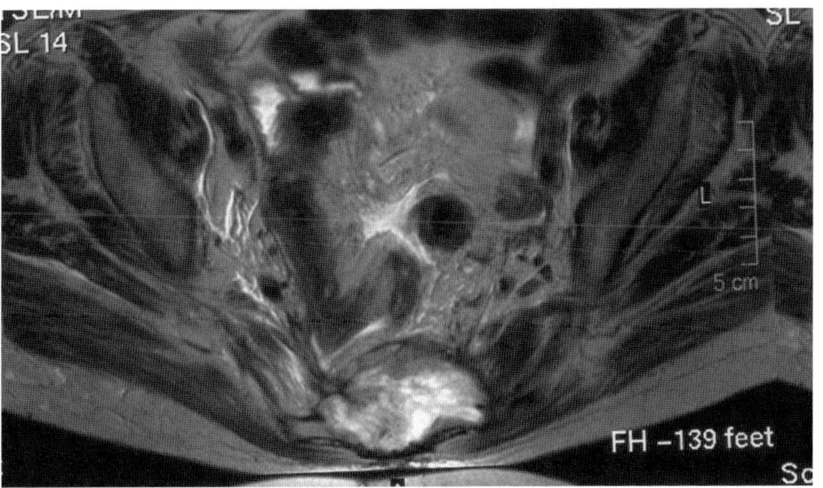

Figure 74.3

MRI Scan Report

Presence of a large metastasis in sacrum.

Case Continued

The patient receives external-beam radiation therapy for pain relief and chemotherapy is reinstituted. The patient dies 12.5 years after the initial operation.

Discussion

Malignancy in paraganglioma, including pheochromocytoma, is difficult to diagnose. In the absence of metastatic disease, it is possible to predict metastatic behavior if local invasion is also accepted as a criteria for malignancy. The treatment should always be primary surgery, but if surgical removal of all metastatic tissue is not possible, the tumor will recur and eventually cause the death of the patient. In metastatic disease, it is worthwhile to attempt MIBG-^{131}I treatment, if scintigraphy is positive, and chemotherapy, as some patients have favorable responses. Radiation is mainly indicated when the patient has local pain, for instance from skeletal metastases. Treatment of malignant paraganglioma is best handled in a multidisciplinary fashion.

Suggested Readings

Averbuch SD, Steakley CS, Young RC, et al. Malignant pheochromocytoma: effective treatment with a combination of cyclophosphamide, vincristine, and dacarbazine. *Ann Intern Med* 1988;109:267–273.

Edström Elder E, Hjelm Skog A-L, Höög A, et al. The management of benign and malignant pheochromocytoma and abdominal paraganglioma. *Eur J Surg Oncol* 2003;29:278–283.

Gröndal S, Bindslev L, Sollevi A, et al. Adenosine: a new antihypertensive agent during pheochromocytoma removal. *World J Surg* 1988;12:581–585.

Lack EE. *Tumors of the adrenal gland and extra-adrenal paraganglia.* Washington, DC: Armed Forces Institute of Pathology; 1997.

Schlumberger M, Gicquel C, Lumbroso J, et al. Malignant pheochromocytoma: clinical, biological, histologic and therapeutic data in a series of 20 patients with distant metastases. *J Endocrinol Invest* 1992;15:631–642.

Sisson JC, Shapiro B, Shulkin BL, et al. Treatment of malignant pheochromocytomas with 131-1 metaiodobenzylguanidine and chemotherapy. *Am J Clin Oncol* 1999;22:364–370.

Presentation

A 45-year-old woman with a history of node-negative breast cancer undergoes a computed tomography (CT) scan as part of her routine follow-up. The CT scan was supposed to be of the chest, but the upper abdomen was imaged and a 6-cm tumor was seen in the right adrenal gland. Her physician ordered a magnetic resonance imaging (MRI) scan, which further delineated a 7-cm tumor in the right adrenal gland. She is referred to you for management of this incidentaloma. She is not cushingoid, nor does she have any evidence of virilization. Her pulse equals 100 beats per minute and blood pressure is 145/95 mm Hg. She is not taking any blood pressure medications. She does not have headaches or spells of nervousness.

MRI

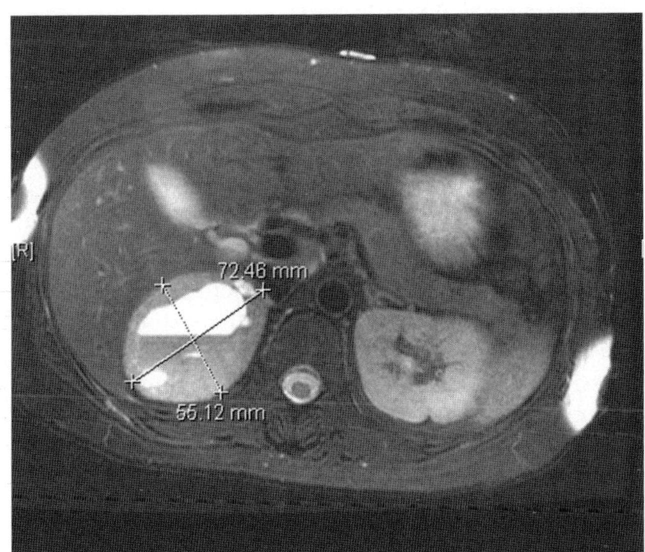

Figure 75.1A

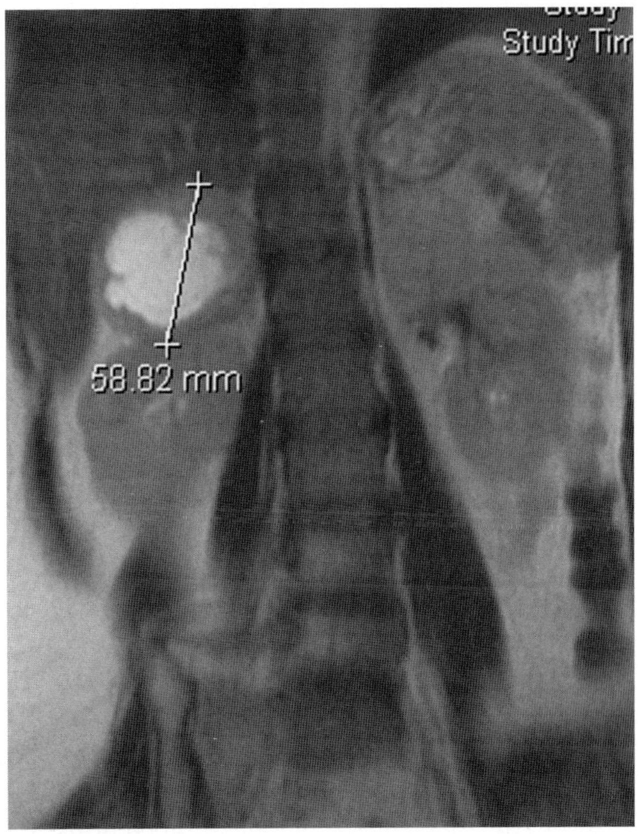

Figure 75.1B

MRI Report

The MRI scan reveals a right adrenal tumor *(cross markings)*. The tumor measures 7.2 cm by 5.5 cm. It is heterogeneous. On sagittal images of the same tumor *(line markings)*, it is seen to be suprarenal and pushing on the inferior vena cava and liver.

Differential Diagnosis

The differential diagnosis includes benign and malignant adrenal medullary and cortical tumors as well as metastatic breast cancer to the adrenal gland.

The workup of an incidentaloma is designed to address two issues that may require surgical intervention. First is the presence of a hormonally functional adrenal tumor. Second is whether or not the adrenal tumor is malignant. Hormonally functional tumors include those with excessive secretion of aldosterone, cortisol, male or female hormones, and catecholamines. Aldosteronoma is excluded by measuring serum levels of potassium (K^+), as long as the patient is not taking any blood pressure medications. If the serum K^+ is >3.5 mEq/L, aldosteronoma is excluded. This patient had a serum K^+ of 4 mEq/L. Hypercortisolism can be identified by its signs and symptoms. Moreover, 24-hour urine levels of hydrocortisone or free cortisol should be measured before and following low-dose dexamethasone. Patients with Cushing syndrome will not suppress levels following low-dose dexamethasone, while normal individuals will. This patient did not have elevated urinary levels of free cortisol and reduced levels after dexamethasone. Finally, pheochromocytoma should be excluded by measuring a 24-hour urine concentration of vanillylmandelic acid (VMA), metanephrine, normetanephrine, and total catecholamines. A newer study designed to rule out pheochromocytoma is measurement of blood levels of plasma-free metanephrine and normetanephrine which have an accuracy of over 95%. This patient had elevated levels of plasma-free normetanephrine and elevated urinary levels of VMA and total catecholamines consistent with the diagnosis of pheochromocytoma.

The issue of malignancy is determined primarily by the size of the adrenal tumor. A critical criterion for the diagnosis of adrenal cortical cancer is tumor weight >100 g, which equals a diameter of 6 cm. Tumors that are >4 cm in diameter should be removed based on the possibility that they may be malignant. Smaller tumors that are nonfunctional should be re-imaged by CT or MRI in 6 months; if they have increased in size, they should be removed. For this patient with a history of breast cancer, if the biochemical studies exclude pheochromocytoma and there is no other site of disease, the tumor could be aspirated to diagnose breast cancer metastases to the adrenal. Resection of metastatic cancer to the adrenal may be indicated if there is a long disease-free interval and it is the sole site of tu-

mor. Beware of needle aspiration of unexpected pheochromocytoma because sudden death has been reported in this context.

Case Continued

This patient has elevated urinary and plasma-free levels of catecholamines.

Diagnosis and Recommendation

The diagnosis is pheochromocytoma. The patient should be prepared with alpha-blockade followed by beta-blockade and scheduled for right adrenalectomy.

Approach

The patient is started on phenoxybenzamine at 10 mg orally twice daily, and is instructed to drink at least 2 liters of liquid per day. After 3 to 5 days, the dose of phenoxybenzamine is increased to 10 mg three times daily. At that point, approximately 1 week later, her pulse rate increases to 120 beats per minute and propranolol is started and increased to get the pulse to approximately 80 beats per minute. Propranolol should not be used unless the patient has had alpha-blockade. The blood pressure should be titrated with phenoxybenzamine to normal range. After approximately 2 to 3 weeks, the patient is ready for surgery.

Surgical Approach

This is a large potentially malignant pheochromocytoma, so an open right adrenalectomy is chosen. The anesthesiologist has placed an arterial catheter and a central venous catheter. The operation is done through a bilateral subcostal incision, and the right lobe of the liver is completely mobilized to expose the right adrenal gland. The adrenal vein is ligated early in the operation to avoid episodes of severe hypertension. Hypertension is treated with nitroprusside and hypotension is treated with vasopressin. Alternatively, a laparoscopic right adrenalectomy may be used because it results in less pain postoperatively and is associated with a more rapid recovery. However, it may not be indicated for large tumors that are potentially malignant. Pheochromocytomatosis has been reported as a complication of laparoscopic resection of pheochromocytomas. This means that tumor was spilled and seeded throughout the abdominal cavity.

Discussion

Pheochromocytomas are rare tumors that secrete excessive catecholamines. Pheochromocytomas may be intra-adrenal or extra-adrenal and benign or malignant. Early diagnosis and therapy improve the prognosis. The incidence of malignancy is as low as 5% and as high as 46% in different series. Extra-adrenal tumors are more likely to be cancerous. Pheochromocytomas may be associated with endocrine and nonendocrine inherited disorders. Bilateral adrenal medullary pheochromocytomas are components of multiple endocrine neoplasia (MEN) type 2a and MEN-2b. Some families have bilateral adrenal pheochromocytomas and no other manifestation of MEN. In other families, only extra-adrenal pheochromocytomas have been reported. Pheochromocytomas occur in approximately 25% of patients with von Hippel-Lindau (VHL) disease and in 1% of patients with neurofibromatosis and von Recklinghausen disease.

Pheochromocytomas cause intermittent, episodic, or sustained hypertension. Pheochromocytomas also cause insulin resistance and diabetes. Following resection of the tumor, the insulin sensitivity improves. Extra-adrenal pheochromocytomas may arise anywhere, including the carotid body, intra-cardiac, along the aorta (both thoracic and abdominal), and within the urinary bladder. The most common extra-adrenal location is the organ of Zuckerkandl, which is near the origin of the inferior mesenteric artery to the left of the aortic bifurcation. Data from series of patients with sporadic pheochromocytomas indicate that the right adrenal gland harbors a tumor more often than the left gland. Pheochromocytomas usually measure between 3 and 5 cm in diameter and weigh <100 g. Tumors are tan to gray in color and have a soft consistency. Larger tumors are cystic and have necrosis or calcification. Microscopically, pheochromocytomas are usually arranged in cords or alveolar patterns. Tumors are generally clearly separated from the adrenal cortex by a thin band of fibrous tissue. Extension into the cortex or vascular invasion may occur.

The pathologic distinction between benign and malignant pheochromocytomas is not clear. The only absolute criterion for malignancy is the presence of secondary tumors in sites where chromaffin cells are not usually present and visceral metastases. Malignant tumors tend to be larger and weigh more.

Patients with pheochromocytomas can present with a range of symptoms, from mild labile hypertension to sudden death secondary to severe hypertension, myocardial infarction, or cerebral vascular accident. The classic patient describes "spells" of paroxysmal headaches, pallor, palpitations, hypertension, and diaphoresis. In 50% of patients, the hypertension is intermittent, but it may be sustained. In children, hypertension is sustained. Patients may have lactic acidosis. Patients may have weight loss and hyperglycemia.

The diagnosis of pheochromocytoma is based on measuring catecholamines and metabolites in the urine. This requires a 24-hour urine for VMA, metanephrine, and catecholamines. However, plasma-free metanephrines and normetanephrine have been used recently to reliably diagnose pheochromocytoma. Certainly the blood measurement greatly facilitates the workup and is accurate.

CT and MRI are the two nonnuclear-medicine imaging studies to localize pheochromocytomas. Both are noninvasive and sensitive, being able to reliably detect tumors 1 cm in diameter. MRI may be more specific because of findings with different sequences. CT detects more than 95% of pheochromocytomas including nine of 10 bilateral tumors. CT also detects most extra-adrenal retroperitoneal tumors. However, MRI has similar sensitivity. Moreover, MRI also imaged all pheochromocytomas demonstrated on CT, plus metastases to the chest, retroperitoneum, and liver that were not seen. Because it has no radiation exposure, MRI can be performed during pregnancy.

Another excellent test for localization of pheochromocytomas is nuclear scanning after the administration of labeled metaiodobenzylguanidine (MIBG). The compound is similar to norepinephrine and is taken up by vesicular monoamine transporters. The sensitivity of MIBG scanning with I-131 for pheochromocytoma is 100% and the specificity is 95%.

Once the diagnosis is established and the tumor localized, preoperative preparation includes alpha-adrenergic blockade. Patients are started on phenoxybenzamine, 10 mg orally two or three times daily. If tachycardia develops, beta-adrenergic blocking agents (propranolol) are added. Propranolol should never be started before alpha blockade because unopposed vasoconstriction may worsen hypertension. Phenoxybenzamine increases the total blood and plasma volume and reduces lactic acidosis. Appropriately used calcium channel antagonists and selective alpha$_1$-receptor blockers are also effective and safe.

Small (<6 cm) intra-adrenal pheochromocytomas are removed using laparoscopic techniques. However, larger tumors should be removed by open surgery. Laparoscopic procedures appear to decrease pain and shorten the time to recovery. However, iatrogenic pheochromocytomatosis has been described as a possible complication of laparoscopic removal. Whichever method is used to remove the tumor, the patient should be followed up with repeat imaging and biochemical studies because tumors may be malignant or incompletely resected.

Suggested Readings

Grumbach M, Biller M, Baunstein G, et al. Management of the clinically inapparent adrenal mass. *Ann Intern Med* 2003;138:424–429.

Honigschnabl S, Gallo S, Niederle B, et al. How accurate is MR imaging in characterization of adrenal masses: update of a long-term study. *Eur J Rad* 2002;41:113–122.

Li M, Fitzgerald P, Price D, et al. Iatrogenic pheochromocytomatosis: a previously unreported result of laparoscopic adrenalectomy. *Surgery* 2001;130:1072–1077.

Sawka A, Jaeschke R, Singh R, et al. A comparison of biochemical tests for pheochromocytoma: measurement of fractionated plasma metanephrines compared with the combination of 24-hour urinary metanephrines and catecholamines. *J Clin Endocrinol Metab* 2003;88:553–558.

Weise M, Merke D, Pacak K, et al. Utility of plasma free metanephrines for detecting childhood pheochromocytoma. *J Clin Endocrinol Metab* 2002;87:1955–1960.

Presentation

The patient is a 52-year-old man who has severe epigastric pain and diarrhea. He is treated with 20 mg omeprazole daily without resolution of the pain. He has lost 10 pounds. Upper gastrointestinal endoscopy shows a duodenal ulcer and a question of a tumor in the duodenum. He is *Helicobacter pylori* negative.

Endoscopic Image

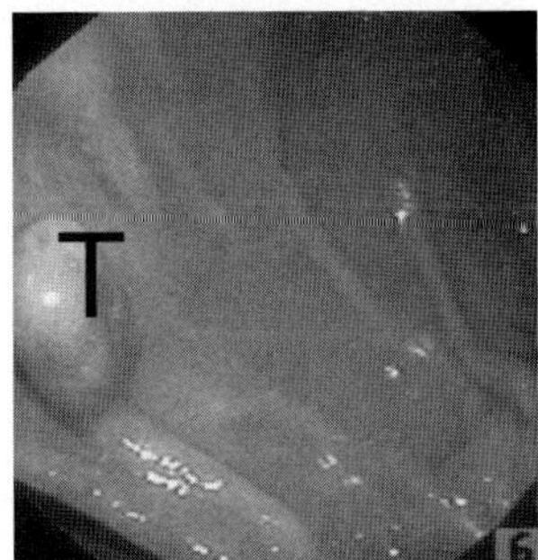

Figure 76.1

Endoscopy Report

An upper gastrointestinal endoscopy shows a duodenal gastrinoma *(T)* in the second portion of the duodenum.

Differential Diagnosis

The differential diagnosis includes peptic ulcer, food poisoning, Zollinger-Ellison syndrome (ZES), antral G-cell hyperplasia, and gastric outlet obstruction. Multiple endocrine neoplasia type 1 (MEN-1) should be considered.

Medications that inhibit gastric acid secretion, like omeprazole, should be discontinued for at least 7 days prior to testing. These medications cause achlorhydria and can cause a false elevation in the serum level of gastrin. Similarly, if the patient has evidence of gastric outlet obstruction from ulcer disease or scarring, a nasogastric tube should be inserted to reduce gastric antral distension that can also result in hypergastrinemia. A fasting serum level of gastrin and gastric acid output are measured. Patients with ZES have an elevated fasting serum concentration of gastrin (>100 pg/mL) and an elevated basal acid output (>15 mEq/h). This combination is diagnostic for ZES. A secretin test may also be done, in which 2 U/kg of secretin is administered intravenously and serum levels of gastrin are obtained prior to secretin and at 1, 5, 10, and 15 minutes later. An increase >200 pg/mL in the serum level of gastrin following secretin is consistent with ZES. However, this is not an absolute criterion for the diagnosis, as only 85% of patients with ZES will have a positive secretin stimulation test. Antral G-cell hyperplasia should be excluded by measuring serum levels of gastrin before and after a protein meal. Patients with ZES do not have the gastrin level changed by dietary manipulation. Once the diagnosis of ZES is obtained, the presence of MEN-1 should be excluded. Approximately 20% of patients with ZES have MEN-1. MEN-1 is diagnosed by obtaining a careful family history for the clinical manifestations of MEN-1, examining for lipomas (which are common in MEN-1), and measuring serum levels of prolactin, pancreatic polypeptide, chromogranin A, ionized calcium, and intact parathyroid hormone. Most (95%) patients with MEN-1/ZES have primary hyperparathyroidism at the time of the diagnosis of ZES.

Case Continued

The patient has an elevated serum level of gastrin (950 pg/mL), an elevated basal acid output (100 mEq/h), and an abnormal secretin test (>600 pg/mL incremental increase in gastrin following secretin). There is no family history of endocrine tumors and there are normal serum levels of calcium, parathyroid hormone, prolactin, and pancreatic polypeptide such that MEN-1 is excluded. Serum levels of chromogranin A are elevated, and this is consistent with ZES.

Diagnosis and Recommendation

The diagnosis of sporadic Zollinger-Ellison syndrome means that there is a gastrin-secreting neuroendocrine tumor that is causing the severe peptic ulcer disease, diarrhea, and weight loss. The next step in management is to control the acid hypersecretion with medication and to perform localizing studies to try to image the tumor. The key to controlling the symptoms of ZES is to measure the acid output and administer a proton-pump inhibitor at doses that normalize the acid secretion. This typically requires omeprazole at 60 to 80 mg every 12 hours. The acid output should be <10 mEq/h prior to the dose of omeprazole. If the patient has gastroesophageal reflux disease (GERD), the acid output should be kept lower than 5 mEq/h. If the acid output is controlled in this manner, the peptic ulcer disease will heal, the diarrhea will stop, and the patient will gain weight. The next step is to try to image the tumor. High-resolution pancreatic protocol computed tomography (CT) should be performed to try to image the primary tumor and possible liver metastases. Tumors larger than 1 cm are imaged. However, primary gastrinomas may be small and not identified. Somatostatin receptor scintigraphy (SRS), also known as octreotide scan, should also be done. It is a whole-body scan that images the tumor based on the density of type 2 somatostatin receptors. Approximately 90% of gastrinomas will be imaged, and SRS is more sensitive than CT and MRI combined. However, in this particular patient, both CT and SRS failed to identify any gastrinoma.

Approach

In patients with sporadic ZES, even with negative imaging studies, surgical exploration for removal of the gastrinoma is indicated because approximately 40% to 50% of patients will be cured of ZES.

Surgical Approach

A bilateral subcostal incision is made in the upper abdomen. The entire abdomen is carefully explored, including the liver, small bowel, and ovaries (in women). Primary gastrinomas have been reported within the liver and the ovary. If a gastrinoma is in the ovary, a total abdominal hysterectomy is indicated. The gastrocolic ligament is divided to expose the lesser sac. A Kocher maneuver is performed. The inferior border of the pancreas is mobilized by dividing the inferior attachments so that the pancreas can be palpated with the index finger underneath and the thumb on top. Lymph nodes around the porta hepatis, celiac axis, and head of the pancreas are systematically sampled to document the presence of lymph node metastases or lymph node primary gastrinomas. Intraoperative ultrasound of the pancreas and liver is performed to image tumor within either organ. Tumors appear sonolucent compared to the more echo-dense pancreas and liver. The duodenum is opened to identify gastrinomas within the duodenum, the most common site of missed tumors. In this patient, a gastrinoma is identified within the duodenum and it is excised with a small rim of normal intestine around the tumor.

Intraoperative Image

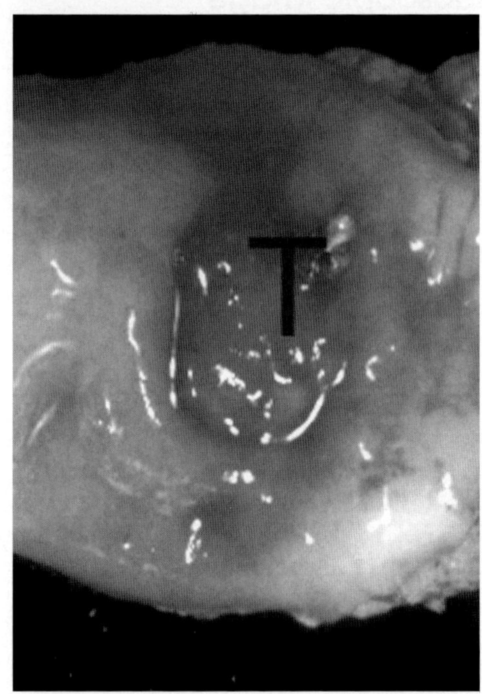

Figure 76.2

Intraoperative Report

The gross appearance of the excised gastrinoma *(T)* at the time of surgery is shown. The tumor measures 6 mm in diameter and is excised with a normal full-thickness bowel rim around it.

Discussion

Gastrinomas occur in the gastrinoma triangle (triangle including the head of the pancreas and the duodenum) approximately 80% of the time. The duodenum is the most common site of a primary tumor (incidence of approximately 50% to 60%), with the pancreas the second most common site. Duodenal tumors are more common in the first portion of the duodenum, and occur with decreasing frequency throughout the entire duodenum. Pancreatic tumors more commonly metastasize to the liver, whereas duodenal primaries commonly spread to adjacent lymph nodes. Tumors in the tail of the pancreas should be resected by a distal pancreatectomy splenectomy. Tumors within the head of the pancreas should be enucleated. Tumors within the duodenum should be removed with a small rim of normal duodenum around the tumor. Bulky large tumors in the head of the pancreas region with significant nodal metastases should be removed with a proximal pancreaticoduodenectomy (Whipple procedure).

Gastrinomas are most commonly within the duodenum. Duodenotomy (opening the duodenum) identifies more tumors and results in a greater cure rate, indicating that it should be done routinely in all operations for gastrinoma. These tumors are frequently small, most commonly found in the proximal duodenum, and associated with lymph node metastases in 60% of patients. Resection of primary gastrinoma has been shown to decrease the probability of liver metastases. The long-term cure rate with gastrinoma resection is 40% in patients with sporadic ZES. Even localized liver metastases can be removed for apparent amelioration of symptoms and prolongation of survival. Serum levels of chromogranin A and gastrin can be used to assess curative resection, but minor changes in levels are not sensitive enough to assess tumor regression or progression. A secretin stimulation test is generally positive prior to other signs of tumor recurrence. Repetitive imaging with CT and SRS can be used to image recurrent tumor. Aggressive surgery, including Whipple pancreaticoduodenectomy, has been performed for locally advanced neuroendocrine tumors of the pancreas. However, because the prognosis is good with pancreatic neuroendocrine tumors, the operative death rate and morbidity of surgery should be low. A recent report shows that the Whipple for neuroendocrine tumors had an operative mortality of 10% and a complication rate of 30%. However, the long-term survival was also excellent in that 81% and 70% of patients were alive at 5 and 10 years, respectively.

Suggested Readings

Abou-Saif A, Gibril F, Ojeaburu JV, et al. Prospective study of the ability of serial measurements of serum chromogranin A and gastrin to detect changes in tumor burden in patients with gastrinomas. *Cancer* 2003;98:249–261.

McIntyre TP, Stahfels KR, Sell HW Jr. Gastrinoma. *Am J Surg* 2002;183:666–667.

Norton JA, Alexander HR, Fraker D, et al. Does the use of routine duodenotomy (DUODX) affect rate of cure, development of liver metastases or survival in patients with Zollinger-Ellison syndrome (ZES)? *Ann Surg* 2004;239:617–625; discussion 626.

Norton JA, Fraker DL, Alexander HR, et al. Surgery to cure the Zollinger-Ellison syndrome. *N Engl J Med* 1999;341:635–644.

Norton JA, Warren RS, Kelly MG, et al. Aggressive surgery for metastatic liver neuroendocrine tumors. *Surgery* 2003; 134:1057–1065.

Sarmiento JM, Farnell MB, Que FG, et al. Pancreaticoduodenectomy for islet cell tumors of the head of the pancreas: long-term survival analysis. *World J Surg* 2002;26:1267–1271.

Zogakis TG, Gibril F, Libutti SK, et al. Management and outcome of patients with sporadic gastrinoma arising in the duodenum. *Ann Surg* 2003;238:42–48.

Presentation

The patient is a 45-year-old woman who has been found to be occasionally unarousable by her husband in the early morning hours. She will become coherent if he gives her orange juice to drink. She had a seizure spell that lasted for several minutes when she missed lunch while shopping at the mall one Saturday afternoon. She has gained 20 pounds recently and would like to lose weight. She works as a nurse at a home health agency.

Differential Diagnosis

The differential diagnosis includes insulinoma, fasting hypoglycemia, surreptitious hypoglycemia, and seizure disorder.

The initial diagnostic test is measurement of fasting morning levels of glucose and insulin. The glucose level is 50 mg/dL and the insulin level is 10 microIU/mL. These levels are suggestive of an insulinoma, and the patient is admitted to the hospital to undergo a supervised 72-hour fast. She is placed in the intensive care unit (ICU), where she can be carefully observed. The observation is important to be certain that during the fast she does not develop severe symptoms of neuroglycopenia and that she does not administer any medications or insulin that may induce hypoglycemia. A 24-hour urine for sulfonylurea levels is obtained to rule out the use of oral hypoglycemic drugs. At the start of the fast, a venous catheter is placed to allow administration of dextrose-50 if hypoglycemic symptoms occur. Further, an arterial line is placed to obtain blood samples for insulin and glucose determination. As the test continues, serum levels of glucose and insulin are measured every 6 hours. If the patient develops confusion, slurred speech, altered mental status, or inability to answer simple questions, then serum levels of glucose, insulin, C-peptide, and proinsulin are measured and an ampoule of D-50 is administered to see if the neuroglycopenic symptoms resolve. Patients with

insulinoma will develop neuroglycopenic symptoms at approximately 12 to 24 hours during the fast. At that time of symptoms, glucose levels should be <45 mg/dL and insulin levels will be inappropriately elevated to >5 IU/mL in patients with insulinoma. Patients with insulinoma will also have elevated levels of proinsulin and C-peptide. The nurse administers the dextrose intravenously and the neuroglycopenic symptoms should rapidly resolve. Patients with surreptitious hypoglycemia will have normal levels of C-peptide and proinsulin. Whipple's triad includes neuroglycopenic symptoms, hypoglycemia, and relief of symptoms with glucose administration. These findings are consistent with the diagnosis of insulinoma. Patients with surreptitious hypoglycemia are typically female health care workers who have access to insulin or oral hypoglycemic drugs. They are excluded by careful supervision during the fast, and by measuring C-peptide, proinsulin, and urinary sulfonylurea levels.

Case Continued

At 12 hours into the fast, the patient developed confusion and tremulousness. Serum glucose levels were 35 mg/dL and serum insulin levels were 7 microIU/mL. C-peptide and proinsulin levels were also elevated.

Diagnosis and Recommendation

The findings are diagnostic of insulinoma. Management of the hypoglycemia and localization of the tumor are the next two priorities.

■ Approach

The next step is to maintain normal blood glucose levels by asking the patient to set the alarm clock at night to awaken from sleep and eat a snack. It is best to mix cornstarch with some of the food so that slower absorption of carbohydrates will allow less frequent feeding. These two maneuvers will usually keep the blood glucose level in the normal range and avoid neuroglycopenic symptoms. Insulinomas are generally small (<2 cm), benign, and located within the pancreas. The final step is to try to localize the insulinoma. The initial study is a high-resolution computed tomography (CT) scan of the pancreas with intravenous contrast.

CT Scan

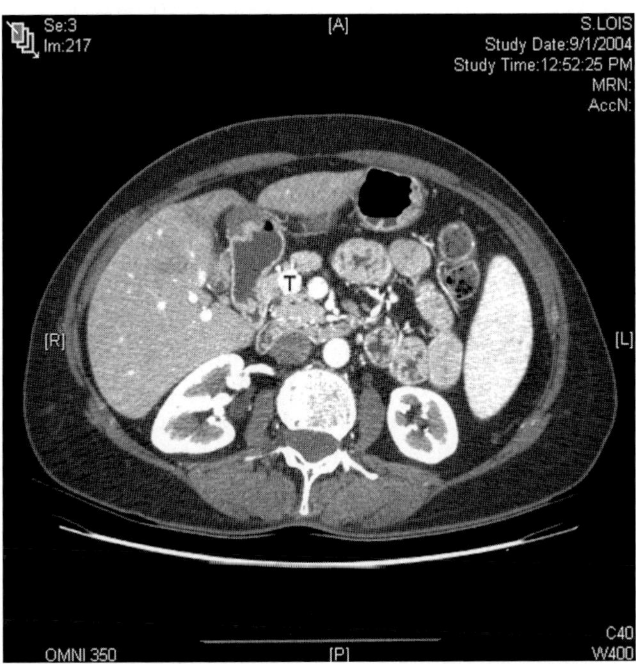

Figure 77.1A

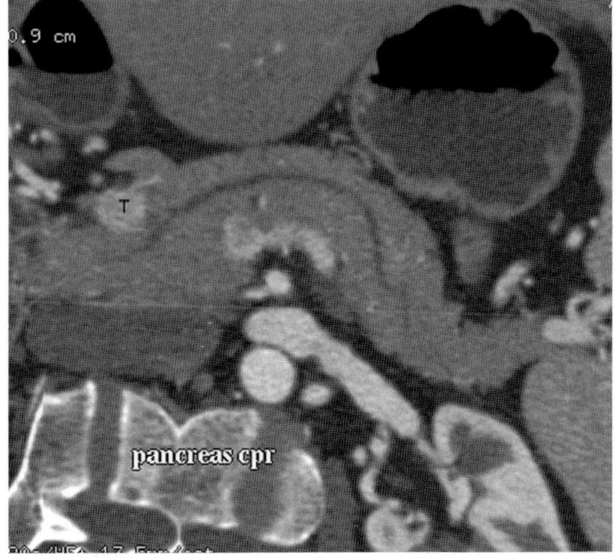

Figure 77.1B

CT Scan Report

High-resolution CT scan identified a small hypervascular insulinoma within the head of the pancreas *(T)*. It is bright on CT with intravenous contrast because of increased vascularity. Special computer formatting was done to localize the tumor to the uncinate process of the head and show the relationship of the insulinoma *(T)* to the pancreatic duct.

Case Continued

No additional localization procedures were necessary in this case.

Discussion

In some patients, the CT scan is negative and the tumor can still be localized by endoscopic ultrasound and/or calcium angiogram. Endoscopic ultrasound is performed by gastroenterology, and the tumor is imaged by a high-resolution transducer that is placed in the stomach for the body and tail and in the duodenum for the head of the pancreas. Insulinomas appear sonolucent compared with the more echo-dense pancreas. This study is supposed to have a high sensitivity and specificity, but it is very observer dependent, and false-positive and false-negative results may occur. Another study that is designed to regionally localize tumor in patients with insulinomas that cannot be imaged is the calcium angiogram. A standard angiogram is performed to determine the arteries that perfuse the various sections of the pancreas (head, body, and tail). During the angiogram, 60% of the time the insulinoma will be imaged as a blush in the pancreas. Calcium is injected sequentially into the different pancreatic arteries and insulin levels are measured in the hepatic vein. When the area of the pancreas with the insulinoma is injected with calcium, the insulin levels in the hepatic vein increase within seconds following the injection. This study then localizes the tumor to the head, body, or tail of the pancreas. It is positive in 90% of patients with insulinoma. If no tumor is clearly identified at surgery, the region with the step-up can be removed.

Intraoperative Ultrasonogram

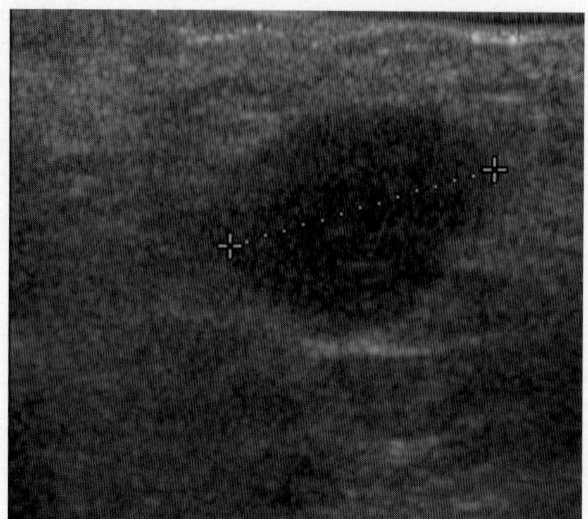

Figure 77.2

Intraoperative Ultrasonography Report

On intraoperative ultrasound of the insulinoma, two crosses identify the tumor. It is sonolucent on ultrasound compared with the more echo-dense pancreas.

Surgical Approach

The surgical approach and mobilization of the pancreas are identical to that described for gastrinoma, except insulinomas are always within the pancreas itself. The major breakthrough during surgery is the use of intraoperative ultrasound that identifies the tumor and guides the enucleation. Because these tumors are generally small and benign, the tumor should be enucleated, preserving as much pancreas and adjacent organs as possible. Sometimes the tail of the pancreas and spleen must be removed if the tumor is near the pancreatic duct. Blind subtotal pancreatectomy should be avoided. Proper operative identification with ultrasound will facilitate excision and allow the safest route to avoid injury to the bile duct or pancreatic duct. Well-localized tumors like the one imaged here may be able to be removed by laparoscopic techniques using laparoscopic ultrasound to guide the procedure.

Discussion

Insulinomas occur in the pancreas and are evenly distributed among the head, body, and tail. Insulinomas are most often benign, but 5% to 10% of the time they are malignant. Insulinoma is diagnosed by a 72-hour fast with the development of neuroglycopenic symptoms. Insulinoma is proven by hypoglycemia (glucose level >45 mg/dL) and hyperinsulinism (insulin level >5 microIU/mL). Close supervision is necessary to exclude factitious hypoglycemia, which is the use of medications to falsely decrease blood glucose levels. After the diagnosis of insulinoma is made based on the results of the fast, localization studies are used to try to image and identify the tumor. CT correctly images approximately 50% of these tumors. In a recent study with multiphasic helical CT, 19 of 30 insulinomas were correctly identified. There were no false positives. Most experts agree that multiphasic CT is the imaging study of choice for pancreatic neuroendocrine tumors. It can image all large tumors (>2 cm) and it images approximately 50% of tumors as small as 1 cm. Tumors appear as a blush on CT because of increased vascularity. Somatostatin receptor scintigraphy is the imaging study of choice for all pancreatic neuroendocrine tumors except insulinomas. Endoscopic ultrasound is able to identify most insulinomas, and identifies more of them preoperatively than all other studies. However, occasionally it may have false-positive results that lead to misguidance of the surgery. Pancreatic nodules and accessory spleens have been confused with insulinoma. Specificity of endoscopic ultrasound can be improved by needle biopsy that is used for pancreatic tumors and lymph nodes. The best results are seen when one combines thin-section helical CT with endoscopic ultrasound. In a study of 18 consecutive patients, this combination identified an insulinoma in each patient. Preoperative calcium angiogram has been shown to localize most (>90%) insulinomas. Similar studies have been done with secretin injection for gastrinomas. However, recently calcium angiogram has been shown to effectively localize most gastrinomas as well.

Because insulinomas are generally benign and located within the pancreas, the goal of surgery is to precisely identify the tumor and remove it while preserving as much pancreas as possible. Intraoperative ultrasound has been useful for precise operative localization. It can identify the tumor and its relationship to vital structures like the common bile duct and the pancreatic duct. It allows the surgeon to decide the best way to remove the tumor and avoid complications. Further, modern methods have allowed laparoscopic enucleation of insulinomas based on laparoscopic ultrasound done during the surgery. If it can be done, this procedure results in less pain and a more rapid recovery. However, similar complications, like pancreatic fistula and abscess, may occur with laparoscopic pancreatic operations and must be considered. Because of this fact, the length of stay with laparoscopic surgery for insulinoma has not been dramatically different than open operations.

Suggested Readings

Fernandez–Cruz L, Saenz A, Astudillo E, et al. Outcome of laparoscopic pancreatic surgery: endocrine and nonendocrine tumors. *World J Surg* 2002;26:1057–1065.

Gouya H, Vignaux O, Augui J, et al. CT, endoscopic sonography and a combined protocol for preoperative evaluation of pancreatic insulinomas. *AJR Am J Roentgenol* 2003;181:987–992.

Hiramoto JS, Feldstein VA, LaBerge JM, et al. Intraoperative ultrasound and preoperative localization detects all occult insulinomas. *Arch Surg* 2001;136:1020–1026.

Jaroszewski DE, Schlinkert RT, Thompson GB, et al. Laparoscopic localization and resection of insulinomas. *Arch Surg* 2004;139: 270–274.

Tagaya N, Kasama K, Suzuki N, et al. Laparoscopic resection of the pancreas and review of the literature. *Surg Endosc* 2003;17: 201–206.

Turner JJ, Wren AM, Jackson JE, et al. Localization of gastrinomas by selective intra-arterial calcium injection. *Clin Endocrinol* 2002; 57:821–825.

case 78

A 25-year-old woman who is a medical student presents with a history of routine physical examination performed at the time of entry to medical school. The patient is totally asymptomatic. The routine physical examination reveals a well-defined mass involving the right lobe of the thyroid. It measures 2.5 × 2.5 cm, moves very well with swallowing, and does not appear to be fixed to the trachea or surrounding structures. The trachea is central. Careful examination of the neck does not reveal any suspicious lymphadenopathy. Examination of the oral cavity, larynx, and pharynx is within normal limits. Both vocal cords are normal and mobile. There is no past history of thyroid disease or history of radiation as a child. The family history does not define any thyroid-related problem or thyroid cancer in the family. The patient does not give any history of radiation to the neck as a child.

Differential Diagnosis

This young female patient presents with a mass in the thyroid, which measures approximately 2.5 cm and does not appear to be fixed to the surrounding structures. This is a classical presentation of a solitary thyroid nodule. The differential diagnosis includes multinodular goiter with a prominent right thyroid nodule, Hashimoto thyroiditis, carcinoma of the thyroid, medullary carcinoma of the thyroid, and benign follicular adenoma of the thyroid.

The most common thyroid swelling in a young woman is a classic presentation of solitary thyroid nodule. Even though the patient is totally asymptomatic, this requires further investigations. The differential diagnosis includes a benign follicular lesion, such as follicular adenoma, or it may be follicular carcinoma based in capsular invasion, which is documented only in the permanent histology after surgery (Table 78.1). The patient has no history of radiation, which is generally a major carcinogenic etiology for development of thyroid cancer.

A solitary thyroid nodule is quite a rare presentation for Hashimoto thyroiditis. The diagnosis of medullary carcinoma of the thyroid should be rare, but needs to be considered, and obtaining a careful family history is crucial. If any of the family members had medullary carcinoma of the thyroid, this would be the most important history. Metastatic tumors to the thyroid at this age are extremely rare and need not be considered in the differential diagnosis. History of residence of the patient in an endemic area is important to distinguish other conditions such as nodular goiter. However, in a young woman with a solitary thyroid nodule that is firm, the most important diagnosis is to exclude papillary carcinoma of the thyroid.

A variety of diagnostic tests are available in this patient including blood studies, imaging studies, and needle biopsy. The question is not what is available, but what is necessary. The most important diagnostic study in this patient is fine-needle aspiration biopsy. In a patient who presents with a well-defined solitary thyroid nodule, a fine-needle aspiration biopsy would be the first diagnostic study. The accuracy of fine-needle aspiration biopsy is over 95% and it can be reliably used in the evaluation and management of this patient.

Table 78.1: Various Stages of Follicular Lesions

Follicular adenoma
Atypical follicular adenoma
Encapsulated well-differentiated follicular neoplasm of
  low malignant potential
Follicular neoplasm without capsular invasion
Follicular neoplasm with minimal capsular invasion
Follicular neoplasm with major capsular invasion
Follicular neoplasm with vascular invasion minor/major
Follicular carcinoma
Poorly differentiated follicular carcinoma
Anaplastic carcinoma

Case Continued

The fine-needle aspiration biopsy in this patient was reported to show papillary carcinoma of the thyroid.

Diagnosis and Recommendation

Other diagnostic tests include thyroid function tests. Most of the patients with solitary thyroid nodules are euthyroid, and thyroid function tests are rarely helpful. However, the thyroid-stimulating hormone (TSH) value may be helpful to rule out a "hot" or hyperfunctioning thyroid nodule. If the TSH value is very low, thyroid scan is indicated to see if the patient has a "hot" thyroid nodule. However, the workup probably will remain the same in a well-defined, firm, solitary thyroid nodule. The incidence of multinodular goiter in a patient who presents with a solitary thyroid nodule is quite small and the patient can be evaluated with an ultrasound. The ultrasound is a very useful diagnostic tool to define the size of the thyroid nodule and to see if any other nodules are present in the opposite lobe. It also defines any enlarged or suspicious lymph nodes. Ultrasound is also very helpful to define whether there are any punctate calcifications suggestive of papillary carcinoma of the thyroid or pericapsular hypervascularity. These investigations are quite helpful. An ultrasound-guided fine-needle aspiration biopsy can also be performed to direct the needle in the most suspicious area of the nodule. Thyroid scan is rarely of any help. It will define this nodule to be cold, which is hypofunctioning thyroid nodule, and does not help make a decision whether it is benign or malignant. The incidence of malignancy in cold thyroid nodules is approximately 16% to 20%. Similarly, the incidence of malignancy in solid thyroid nodules is between 16% and 20%. These investigations do not define whether the patient has a benign or malignant process. However, the fine-needle aspiration biopsy will be very suspicious. The other imaging studies, such as computed tomography (CT) scan and magnetic resonance imaging (MRI), are rarely of help in a well-defined solitary thyroid nodule. These investigations are of great help in patients who present with large thyroid nodules or large substernal pathologies.

Routine use of calcitonin assay is not helpful unless the family history is strongly suggestive of medullary carcinoma of the thyroid, or the patient has any other suspicious findings such as unexplained hypertension or any other characteristics suspicious for multiple endocrine neoplasia (MEN).

Once the diagnosis of papillary carcinoma is made with fine-needle aspiration biopsy, the patient should be considered for surgery. In a young woman, it is always important to rule out pregnancy prior to any surgical intervention. Careful preoperative evaluation of the vocal cords is essential. Indirect laryngoscopy with a mirror will generally define the condition and mobility of the vocal cords. However, if the mirror examination is difficult, fiberoptic laryngoscopy should be performed. Evaluation of the vocal cords for their mobility should be routine in the evaluation and management of thyroid nodules both preoperatively and postoperatively. An informed consent should be obtained after discussing the complications of surgery, such as scar formation, hematoma, hoarseness of voice, inability to raise the voice, and need for calcium supplementation, depending upon the extent of surgery. The overall incidence of these complications is <3% to 4%; however, some of these complications can be quite distressing to the patient, especially hoarseness of voice, or the inability to raise the voice may jeopardize the patient's singing abilities. If the patient undergoes total thyroidectomy, there is approximately a 10% to 15% chance of developing temporary hypoparathyroidism and a 2% to 3% chance of developing permanent hypoparathyroidism. These issues need to be discussed with the patient in detail.

Approach

This patient with a papillary carcinoma of the thyroid that is 2.5 cm at the age of 25 falls into classic low-risk thyroid cancer where the overall chance of a good outcome exceeds 98% to 99%. It is important to discuss the surgical approach to this problem along with complications. The surgical approach includes thyroid lobectomy or total thyroidectomy. There is no role for a subtotal thyroidectomy in patients suspected to have papillary carcinoma of the thyroid. The patient needs a detailed explanation of the controversy in relation to the management of thyroid nodule and the extent of thyroidectomy. The issues related to lobectomy versus total thyroidectomy need to be discussed with the patient and with the referring endocrinologist. Most of these patients will do extremely well with lobectomy alone. The major advantage of lobectomy includes a lower incidence of complications related to parathyroid and recurrent laryngeal nerve injury. The advantages of total thyroidectomy include ease of follow-up of the patient with thyroglobulin levels and ability to perform radioactive iodine dosimetry and iodine ablation. However, in young patients with low risk, there is hardly any need for submitting these patients to radioactive iodine ablation. The overall outcome in these patients is so good that any additional treatment is essentially overtreatment. It is important to discuss all these issues with the patient, and even though a physician will give definite recommendations, it is important that the patient is made aware of the pros and cons of the treatment approaches.

Surgical Approach

The patient is placed in the supine position with the neck in extension. A skin crease neck incision is made and subplatysmal flaps are created. The midline is identified and the strap muscles are elevated off the thyroid gland and retracted laterally. The middle thyroid vein is divided and ligated, which allows the thyroid lobe to be retracted medially. The branches of the superior thyroid are individually ligated and divided to avoid injury to the superior laryngeal nerve. The branches from the inferior thyroid artery are also divided while preserving the parathyroid glands. The recurrent laryngeal nerve is identified and preserved. The inferior thyroid vein is ligated. The thyroid lobe is dissected off the trachea along with the isthmus. The opposite thyroid lobe is carefully palpated, and if no nodules are felt, then the thyroid lobectomy and isthmusectomy is completed. If a total thyroidectomy is to be performed, then the same dissection is completed on the opposite side.

Discussion

Well-differentiated thyroid carcinoma is probably the most rapidly increasing thyroid cancer in the United States. This may be related more to the early diagnosis of these lesions with incidentalomas than a true increase in the incidence of thyroid cancer. Approximately 24,000 new patients with thyroid cancer are seen every year in the United States. There clearly is an increasing incidence of thyroid cancer in women; however, what is interesting is the mortality from thyroid cancer has essentially remained unchanged over the past 25 years. Approximately 1,000 patients die of thyroid cancer every year in the United States. However, a majority of the deaths are related to either anaplastic or medullary thyroid cancer. Death from well-differentiated thyroid cancer is quite rare, especially in young individuals. There appears to be an increasing incidence of incidentalomas diagnosed with routine evaluation of the neck with ultrasound, CT scan, or MRI. CT or MRI for other head and neck pathologies, such a motor vehicle accident, carotid problems, or chest problems,

may reveal an incidental thyroid nodule. A majority of these nodules are generally benign; however, they do require further evaluation. Generally, nodules smaller than 1 cm can be observed and followed closely. However, if there is a clinical concern, an ultrasound-guided fine-needle aspiration biopsy, which is quite helpful, should be considered. Recently, there appears to be an increasing incidence of positron-emission tomography (PET) incidentalomas; PET scan being performed routinely for other malignant tumors may reveal an increased uptake in the thyroid lobe suggestive of incidental thyroid nodularity. These patients need to be evaluated further with the use of ultrasound and ultrasound-guided needle biopsy. If the ultrasound-guided needle biopsy is negative, the patient can be observed and followed on a routine basis. Obviously, if the fine-needle biopsy is suspicious or reported to be malignant, the patient needs surgical intervention.

It is very important for the treating physician to appreciate the pitfalls of fine-needle aspiration biopsy. Even though the accuracy of fine-needle aspiration biopsy exceeds 90% to 95%, certain pitfalls, such as the presence of Hürthle cells or a follicular lesion, are very important. A solitary thyroid nodule may be reported as a follicular lesion on fine-needle aspiration biopsy. The only way one can distinguish a benign follicular lesion from one that is malignant is to look at the entire capsule, which will require surgical resection of the thyroid lobe. The presence of Hürthle cells in the fine-needle aspiration biopsy can also be quite confusing in relation to suspicion of Hürthle cell lesion. However, a large number of these patients may have Hashimoto thyroiditis, confusing the presence of Hürthle cells.

It is vitally important to understand the biology of thyroid cancer, prognostic factors, and risk groups prior to considering any definitive treatment of suspected thyroid cancer. Thyroid cancer is a unique human neoplasm. It is the only cancer where age is the most important prognostic factor. Patients below the age of 45 behave remarkably well compared to patients above the age of 45. There is no stage III and IV thyroid cancer in patients below the age of 45 simply because, even with pulmonary metastasis, the outcome is very good and these patients have stage II thyroid cancers. This is the only human cancer where age is included in the staging system of thyroid cancer by the American Joint Committee on Cancer (AJCC) and Union Internationale Contre le Cancer (UICC). The presence of nodal metastasis has no implication in the overall outcome of patients with thyroid cancer. This is probably the most unique feature of thyroid cancer compared to any other human tumors. The multicentricity of thyroid cancer is well known and extends between 30% and 60%. However, the presence of multicentric microscopic papillary carcinoma of the thyroid (laboratory cancer) has no clinical implications. The presence of extrathyroidal extension and involvement of the surrounding structures, such as strap muscles, recurrent laryngeal nerve, tracheal wall, or esophageal musculature, are the most important clinical prognostic factors to be evaluated during the surgery. If these structures are involved, the patient requires appropriate surgical intervention with gross resection of all extrathyroidal extension of the disease. If gross tumor is left behind, disease will recur in the central compartment, at which time the surgical salvage may be quite difficult.

The management of solitary thyroid nodule generates considerable debate and controversy, with extremely strong feelings about either total thyroidectomy or less than total thyroidectomy. Obviously the decision regarding the extent of thyroidectomy should be based on the extent of the disease, condition of the opposite lobe, age of the patient, size of the tumor, and presence or absence of extrathyroidal extension. Routine total thyroidectomy is rarely indicated in all patients with papillary carcinoma of the thyroid. However, if gross extrathyroidal extension has occurred or disease is present in the opposite lobe, obviously one would consider total thyroidectomy. In high-risk group patients, total thyroidectomy should be considered so that radioactive iodine can be used as an adjuvant treatment modality. However, a majority of the young patients who belong to low-risk groups have excellent survival, up to 99%, and will do very well with lobectomy alone, with an obviously lower incidence of complications. Every patient with thyroid cancer, especially a young patient, does not require radioactive iodine ablation. The role of thyroid-suppressive therapy remains controversial in a young patient. However, most of the patients are placed on thyroid-suppressive therapy to maintain TSH levels below 0.5.

Presentation: Case 78B

A 65-year-old man who is a professor of English presents with a history of a right thyroid mass, which the patient has noted for almost 2 years. He did not seek any medical attention until his voice recently became hoarse. The patient now has trouble teaching in the classroom due to severe hoarseness of voice. He presented to his family practitioner for hoarseness of voice, and was initially treated under the presumed diagnosis of laryngitis. When his symptoms did not improve after 3 weeks, he was referred to a head and neck surgeon.

Differential Diagnosis

The presence of an enlarging mass in the thyroid with a change in voice is essentially diagnostic for carcinoma of the thyroid. The presence of vocal cord paralysis in thyroid mass is suggestive of tumor extending out of the thyroid gland and invading the surrounding structures, such as the recurrent laryngeal nerve. A patient like this will benefit most from a thorough evaluation by a head and neck surgeon to evaluate the size of the thyroid nodule, fixity of the thyroid nodule to the central compartment, and presence of any nodal metastasis, and indirect or fiberoptic laryngoscopy to evaluate vocal cord function.

Clinical Photograph

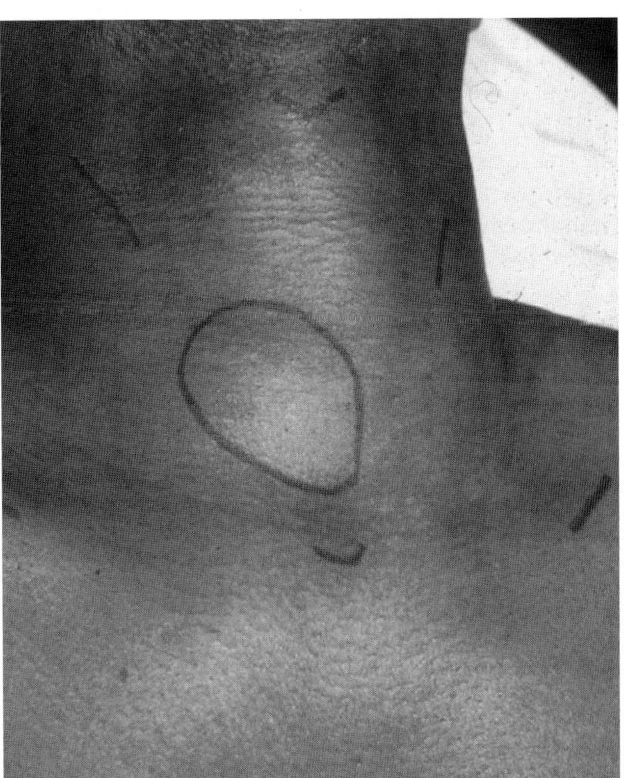

Figure 78.1

Physical Examination Report

Clinical examination in this patient reveals a firm mass measuring 4 cm, which appears to be semi-fixed to the central compartment. However, there is no cervical lymphadenopathy and the fiberoptic examination reveals a paralyzed right vocal cord in the midabduction position.

Recommendation

Fine-needle aspiration biopsy of the thyroid nodule and CT scan of the neck.

Discussion

A fine-needle aspiration biopsy should be evaluated by an experienced pathologist to see whether this is papillary carcinoma or poorly differentiated carcinoma. Fine-needle aspiration biopsy may not be helpful in distinguishing papillary carcinoma from other forms. However, it is helpful to distinguish anaplastic thyroid carcinoma. Clearly, the history of the presence of a growing thyroid mass over 2 years is generally not suggestive of anaplastic thyroid carcinoma. However, this diagnosis must be ruled out.

A further imaging study, such as an ultrasound, is quite helpful; however, a CT scan should be considered in this patient because the vocal cord is paralyzed, and the anatomic extent of the disease must be defined and whether there is any involvement of the trachea must be determined. It is important to perform a CT scan without contrast in this individual because it is likely that he will require radioactive iodine postoperatively, and if iodinated contrast dye is used for evaluation, the radioactive iodine treatment will have to be postponed for 6 months. An MRI scan may be considered with gadolinium; however, the CT scan without contrast will give a better anatomical definition of the extent of the disease.

CT Scan

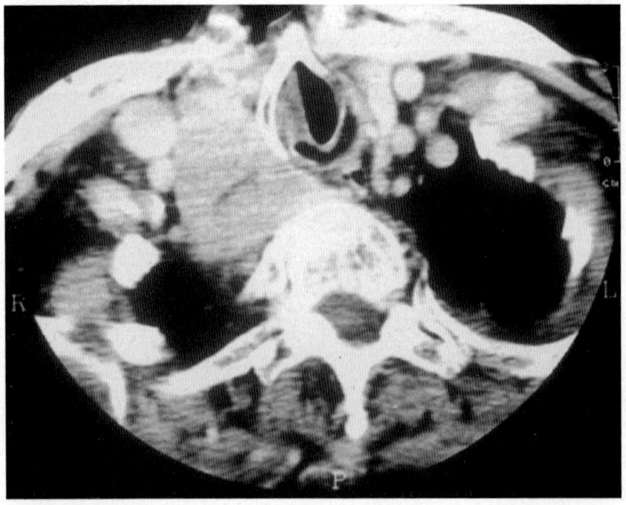

Figure 78.2

CT Scan Report

A CT scan of the neck in this patient revealed a tumor adherent to the trachea and a paralyzed vocal cord; however, the tracheal lumen and the tracheal wall appeared to be within normal limits. There was no intratracheal extension of the disease.

Histopathology Slide

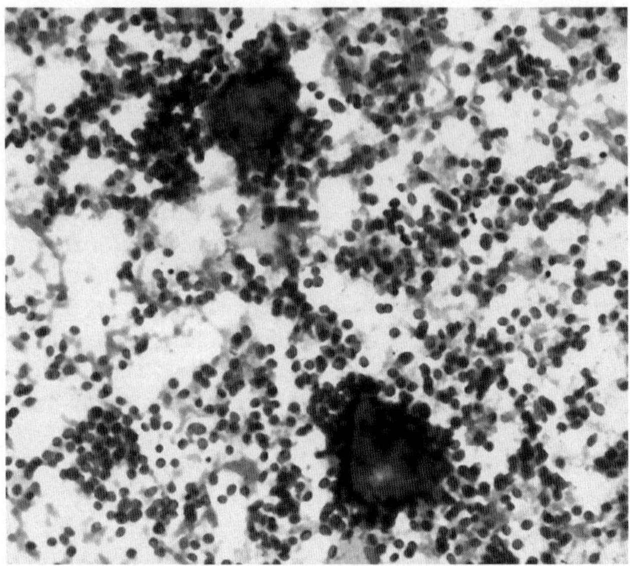

Figure 78.3

Histopathology Report

Fine-needle aspiration biopsy was suggestive of papillary carcinoma of the thyroid; however, the cytologist could not rule out the tall cell variety of papillary carcinoma of the thyroid. Classic psammoma bodies were seen.

Surgical Approach

The patient who has a proven diagnosis of papillary carcinoma with a tumor measuring 4 cm with extrathyroidal extension will definitely require total thyroidectomy. This patient requires a satisfactory surgical approach for his extrathyroidal extension of the disease, including sacrifice of the recurrent laryngeal nerve and careful preservation of the left recurrent laryngeal nerve. Because the patient's one vocal cord is paralyzed, it is vitally important at the time of surgery to identify the opposite recurrent laryngeal nerve and carefully preserve it. Any injury to the opposite recurrent laryngeal nerve will result in paralysis of the opposite vocal cord, leading to airway problem and tracheostomy. At the time of surgery, the strap muscles should be sacrificed because the tumor is bulky with extrathyroidal extension. However, the tumor can be shaved off the trachea and the esophagus. The central compartment should be evaluated for the presence of lymph nodes, and if any enlarged nodes are noted, paratracheal clearance should be considered. Superior mediastinal clearance should also be undertaken to remove grossly enlarged lymph nodes. It is vitally important to identify the parathyroid glands and preserve them carefully. Should any of the parathyroid glands appear to be devascularized, a frozen section of a portion of the parathyroid should be obtained to confirm whether the tissue in question is parathyroid and the remaining parathyroid gland should be autotransplanted, preferably in the sternomastoid muscle.

Discussion

This patient clearly falls into the group of high-risk thyroid cancer, where the patient is elderly with a large tumor with extrathyroidal extension. One of the most important prognostic factors in this patient is the presence of extrathyroidal extension. It is vitally important at the time of initial surgery to resect all gross tumor. If macroscopic tumor is left behind, the disease will recur in the central compartment, upon which the surgical salvage is very difficult, and overall there is an almost 50% mortality in patients with recurrence in the central compartment, especially in the high-risk category. At the time of surgery, it is important to evaluate the extent of the disease and resect all the surrounding structures. The strap muscles can be easily resected. The extrathyroidal extension is most detrimental in the posterior extension into the recurrent laryngeal nerve, tracheoesophageal groove, and esophageal musculature. If the tumor is adherent to the trachea, most often it can be shaved off the trachea. It is very important to evaluate the extent of the disease preoperatively to assess if there is any intraluminal disease in the trachea. The esophageal musculature can be easily resected; however, if the tumor is extending into the lumen of the trachea, it will require appropriate preoperative evaluation including tracheoscopy and bronchoscopy. If the tumor extends into the lumen of the trachea, the patient will require tracheal resection. Approximately five to six rings of the trachea can be easily resected and a primary anastomosis can be performed.

The majority of these tumors are also generally poorly differentiated thyroid cancers. Thyroid cancer is a spectrum of diseases: at one end of the spectrum are papillary and follicular cancers, with an extremely good prognosis; however, at the other end of the spectrum, there is undifferentiated or anaplastic thyroid cancer. The majority of these tumors in the elderly are poorly differentiated thyroid cancers, which include tall cell, insular, trabecular, and angioinvasive cancers. It is very important for the pathologist to differentiate among the well-differentiated and poorly differentiated thyroid cancers. It is also important to rule out anaplastic thyroid carcinoma, where the surgical resection is almost always incomplete and surgery is generally not indicated. Once the high-risk nature of the thyroid cancer is detected, it is appropriate to consider total thyroidectomy so that radioactive iodine can be utilized in the postoperative period. Even with poorly differentiated thyroid cancer, there may be an element of well-differentiated thyroid cancer, which can be treated with radioactive iodine ablation. Generally a large dose of radioactive iodine is used in the postoperative period. In this patient, because one vocal cord is paralyzed, it would be easy to sacrifice the recurrent laryngeal nerve on the side of the larger disease. However, it is vitally important to protect the opposite recurrent laryngeal nerve to avoid any injury to the opposite vocal cord.

Most of the patients with poorly differentiated thyroid cancer generally do not respond to radioactive iodine; however, radioactive iodine scanning is performed, and approximately 150 to 200 mCi of radioactive iodine is given as a single dose to determine if there is any uptake in the neck, cervical lymph nodes, or mediastinum, or pulmonary metastasis. If there is no uptake after a large dose of radioactive iodine, a second radioactive iodine treatment is generally not indicated. These patients are best followed with thyroglobulin and PET scan. PET scan is generally positive in patients with poorly differentiated thyroid cancer, especially if distant metastases are present. Most of these tumors are nonradioavid; however, there is a high glucose metabolism, and fluorodeoxyglucose (FDG) will detect such instances of metastatic disease. The PET positivity increases as the tumor de-differentiates. The patient in whom the PET scan is positive for distant disease behaves much more poorly than those who are PET negative. Thyroglobulin is a sensitive tumor marker in patients who have undergone total thyroidectomy and radioactive iodine ablation of the residual thyroid tissue, and these patients are best monitored with PET scan and thyroglobulin assay. The central compartment is best evaluated with clinical examination, CT scan, and ultrasound. Ultrasound is a relatively easy and very effective way to follow these patients to see if there is any obvious recurrent disease in the central compartment. Ultrasound is also helpful in performing a fine-needle aspiration biopsy of a suspicious lesion in the thyroid bed. If any recurrent disease is noted, surgical salvage may be considered. The principles of surgery in locally advanced thyroid cancer include removal of all gross disease, preservation of the vital structures, preservation of the functioning recurrent laryngeal nerve, and resection of the tumor, shaving the tumor off the trachea and esophagus. Primary laryngectomy or tracheal resection is rarely required unless the tumor is invading the lumen of the trachea or destroying the larynx. However, it is rare to perform primary total laryngectomy in patients with locally aggressive thyroid cancer. Most often, the tumor can be shaved off the tracheal and laryngeal cartilage.

Presentation: Case 78C

A 33-year-old woman presents with a right thyroid nodule. She is essentially asymptomatic. The patient had noted a thyroid nodule approximately 2 years previously. Initially, it measured approximately 2.5 cm; however, over time it increased in size. The fine-needle aspiration biopsy that was performed 2 years ago was suggestive of a follicular lesion. However, the patient elected to remain under observation only. Because the thyroid nodule increased in size recently, she opted for surgical intervention. At the time of surgery, the left lobe appears to be within normal limits and a right thyroid lobectomy and isthmusectomy is performed. The frozen section is reported to be a follicular lesion and because the opposite lobe is normal, the patient only undergoes right thyroid lobectomy.

■ Histopathology Slide

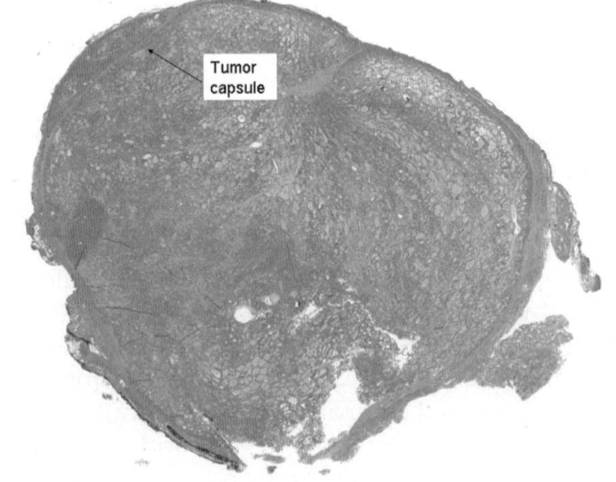

Figure 78.4

Histopathology Report

The final pathology report reveals a follicular carcinoma with minimal capsular invasion and no vascular invasion.

Discussion

It is a common clinical scenario where the patient undergoes a thyroid lobectomy for a follicular lesion, the frozen section is reported to be either benign or suspicious of follicular lesion, and the final pathology report, upon review of the entire capsule, reveals minimal capsular invasion. The typical reaction is to bring the patient back to the operating room for completion thyroidectomy. However, it is very important to discuss the case with the pathologist to see whether there is minimal capsular invasion or major vascular invasion. Obviously, if the patient has a major vascular invasion or major capsular invasion, or gross extrathyroidal extension of the disease, a completion thyroidectomy should be considered so that the patient can be treated with radioactive ablation. However, if there is minimal capsular invasion, it is a minimally invasive follicular carcinoma of the thyroid, popularly known as nonthreatening malignancy, and the survival in this group is excellent. A case like this generates considerable debate and controversy; however, understanding the biology of the tumor and discussion with the pathologist assist with further management decisions. Every patient with a follicular carcinoma who has minimal capsular invasion does not require completion thyroidectomy. However, those with a large tumor, major angioinvasion, or gross extrathyroidal extension require a completion thyroidectomy. The purpose of completion thyroidectomy in these individuals is to allow the use of radioactive iodine for ablation. However, in minimal capsular invasion, generally the outcome is so good that these patients do not require additional treatment. In this patient, the decision was made to observe the patient carefully. The role of suppressive therapy using thyroxine in such patients also generates considerable debate and controversy. Even though there are no good data to suggest that suppressive therapy is helpful, most physicians will place the patient on suppressive therapy to maintain low TSH values. The TSH values are maintained between 0.1 and 0.5 mg/mL. Excess suppressive therapy has deleterious effects, such as osteoporosis and occasionally cardiac arrhythmias.

Summary

These cases are common clinical scenarios seen in patients with papillary and follicular thyroid cancers. Even though there is considerable debate and controversy in the management of thyroid cancer, especially related to the extent of thyroidectomy, the decision should be made based on the understanding of the biology of the tumor, prognostic factors, and risk group analysis. In the low-risk group, the outcome is excellent and the long-term survival is 98% to 99%, and the decision regarding the extent of thyroidectomy should be based on the gross extent of the disease rather than a philosophy of routinely performing total thyroidectomy. However, in high-risk patients, a total thyroidectomy generally is indicated to promote the role of radioactive iodine. It is vitally important to minimize the complications related to nerve injuries and permanent hypoparathyroidism. If a parathyroid gland is identified at the time of surgery, and appears as devascularized, a small portion of the parathyroid should be submitted for frozen section; after confirming the frozen section of the tissue to be parathyroid, the remaining parathyroid gland should be auto-transplanted, preferably in the sternomastoid muscle. Paratracheal clearance should be routinely considered if there are suspicious or enlarged paratracheal lymph nodes. However, lateral neck dissection is generally reserved for clinically palpable or obvious metastatic nodes in the jugular chain or in the lateral neck. It is very important for the treating physician to discuss the biology, risk groups, and prognostic factors with the patient before making any definitive decisions.

Suggested Readings

Fuchshuber P, Loree TR, DeLacure MD, et al. Differentiated thyroid carcinoma: risk group assignment and management controversies. *Oncology (Huntingt)* 1998;12:99–106; discussion 106, 112, 115.

Kuriakose MA, Hicks WL Jr, Loree TR, et al. Risk group-based management of differentiated thyroid carcinoma. *J R Coll Surg Edinb* 2001;46:216–223.

Loree TR. Therapeutic implications of prognostic factors in differentiated carcinoma of the thyroid gland. *Semin Surg Oncol* 1995;11:246–255.

Shah JP, Loree TR, Dharker D, et al. Prognostic factors in differentiated carcinoma of the thyroid gland. *Am J Surg* 1992; 164:658–661.

Shah JP, Loree TR, Dharker D, et al. Lobectomy versus total thyroidectomy for differentiated carcinoma of the thyroid: a matched-pair analysis. *Am J Surg* 1993;166:331–335.

Shaha AR, Loree TR, Shah JP. Intermediate-risk group for differentiated carcinoma of thyroid. *Surgery* 1994;116:1036–1040; discussion 1040–1041.

Shaha AR, Loree TR, Shah JP. Prognostic factors and risk group analysis in follicular carcinoma of the thyroid. *Surgery* 1995;118:1131–1136; discussion 1136–1138.

Shaha AR, Shah JP, Loree TR. Patterns of nodal and distant metastasis based on histologic varieties in differentiated carcinoma of the thyroid. *Am J Surg* 1996;172:692–694.

Shaha AR, Shah JP, Loree TR. Low-risk differentiated thyroid cancer: the need for selective treatment. *Ann Surg Oncol* 1997;4:328–333.

Shaha AR, Shah JP, Loree TR. Patterns of failure in differentiated carcinoma of the thyroid based on risk groups. *Head Neck* 1998;20:26–30.

case 79

Presentation

A 25-year-old woman presents to the emergency room complaining of headache, palpitations, and anxiety. She has had similar symptoms several times over the past 3 months. On physical examination her blood pressure is 210/120 mm Hg in both arms and she is noted to have an enlarged thyroid. Chest x-ray is within normal limits. Complete blood cell (CBC) count and chemistry profile are unremarkable.

Differential Diagnosis

The differential diagnosis of hypertensive crisis in a young woman includes essential hypertension, stimulant abuse, renal artery stenosis, hyperthyroidism, pre-eclampsia, and pheochromocytoma.

Discussion

The episodic nature of the "spells" described by the patient suggests the possibility of pheochromocytoma. This is best evaluated by biochemical studies

CT Scan

including plasma and/or urinary catecholamines and metanephrines. These tests take several days to return, and therefore computed tomography (CT) or magnetic resonance imaging (MRI) of the adrenal glands is the quickest test to evaluate for the presence of adrenal pheochromocytoma.

Recommendation

CBC, electrolytes, thyroid function tests, drug screen, pregnancy test, and CT scan of the abdomen.

Case Continued

The patient has a normal CBC and electrolytes, negative pregnancy test, normal thyroid functions (T_4 and TSH), and negative drug screen. CT of the abdomen shows a 7-cm cystic mass in the right adrenal. Plasma metanephrines are elevated. Twenty-four-hour urine normetanephrine is 30 nmol/L (normal is <1 nmol/L), 24-hour urine metanephrine is 5 nmol/L (normal is <0.5 nmol/L), and 24-hour urine epinephrine and norepinephrine are elevated as well.

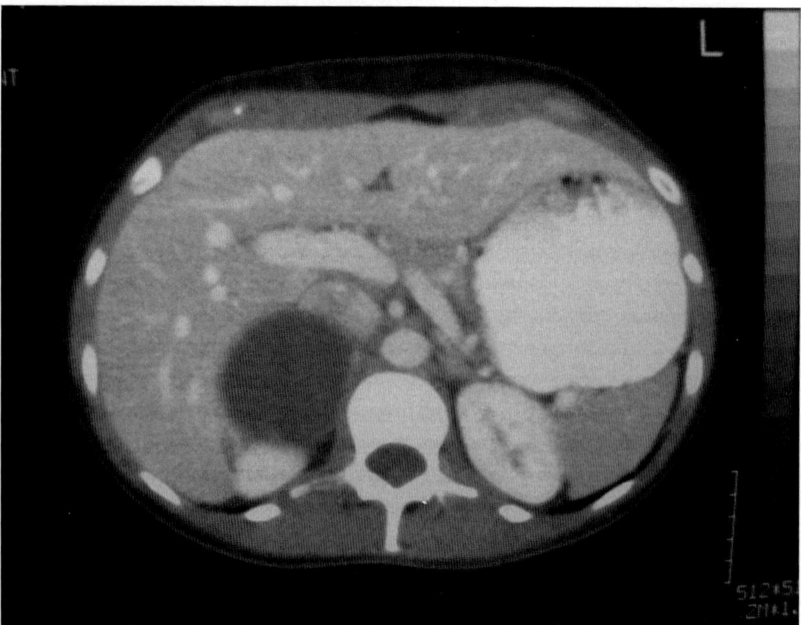

Figure 79.1

CT Scan Report

The CT scan shows a 7-cm cystic mass in the right adrenal with a thick enhancing rim. The left adrenal is normal.

Diagnosis and Recommendation

Right adrenal pheochromocytoma. Adrenalectomy is recommended, with preoperative preparation with alpha-blockade. The presence of a pheochromocytoma coexisting with a thyroid mass raises the possibility of multiple endocrine neoplasia (MEN) type 2a with medullary thyroid carcinoma (MTC). Measurement of serum calcitonin level and fine-needle aspiration (FNA) cytology of the thyroid mass are recommended after removal of the pheochromocytoma.

Surgical Approach

The patient is started on phenoxybenzamine 10 mg twice a day 1 week prior to surgery, and is admitted 4 days prior to surgery for increasing doses of phenoxybenzamine. The dosage is increased in 10-mg increments until postural hypotension is achieved. Preoperative hydration is given with intravenous fluids started the day prior to surgery. Laparoscopic adrenalectomy is performed using arterial and central venous monitoring lines. Pathology reveals pheochromocytoma.

Discussion

Preoperative alpha-blockade is critical to ensure the safe accomplishment of adrenalectomy. Laparoscopic adrenalectomy is safe in patients with small, asymptomatic lesions, and may be performed in symptomatic patients who have excellent control of hypertension and alpha-blockade. Open adrenalectomy is a reasonable option in this case as well. Following removal of the pheochromocytoma, the thyroid mass should be addressed, and thyroid surgery may be carried out after the patient has recovered from the adrenalectomy.

The rule of 10s is useful in describing the clinical presentation of pheochromocytoma. Approximately 10% are hereditary (von-Hippel-Lindau, neurofibromatosis type 1, MEN types 2a and 2b), 10% are bilateral, 10% are malignant, and 10% are extra-adrenal. In this case, the pheochromocytoma is cystic, which is not uncommon. In patients with bilateral hereditary pheochromocytomas, a cortical-sparing approach has been described, but success with this approach is not well documented.

Case Continued

Several weeks following adrenalectomy, thyroid FNA is performed and reveals a medullary thyroid carcinoma. The serum calcitonin level is 900 pg/mL. CT scan of the neck shows a large left thyroid tumor and smaller right-sided lesions. The patient then undergoes total thyroidectomy, central neck dissection, parathyroidectomy with autotransplantation, and left-sided functional neck dissection. Pathology reveals multifocal medullary thyroid carcinoma with 4 of 10 central nodes involved with metastatic MTC. Postoperatively, genetic counseling and genetic testing are done. Testing reveals the presence of a germline mutation in the RET proto-oncogene, confirming the diagnosis of MEN type 2a. Continued yearly surveillance for left-sided pheochromocytoma is carried out and first-degree family members are counseled and offered genetic testing as well.

Discussion

Familial forms of MTC are the MEN type 2a and 2b syndromes and the related disorder of familial non-MEN MTC (FMTC). In these autosomal dominant inherited disorders, multifocal bilateral MTC develops in all patients, usually at a young age. The mutations responsible for these disorders, in the RET gene, were identified in 1993, and current treatment of at-risk individuals relies upon the results of genetic testing.

In MEN 2a, patients may also develop pheochromocytomas, hyperparathyroidism, cutaneous lichen amyloidosis, and Hirschsprung disease. FMTC is characterized by the development of MTC without any other endocrinopathies. MTC in these patients has a later age of onset, and a more indolent clinical course than MTC in patients with MEN 2a and MEN 2b. In MEN 2b, MTC develops in all patients at a very young age (infancy). Patients may have pheochromocytomas, and all individuals have mucosal neuromas (lips, tongue, digestive tract, and conjunctiva) as well as megacolon, skeletal abnormalities, and markedly enlarged peripheral nerves. MEN 2b patients do not develop hyperparathyroidism. MTC in MEN 2b is rarely cured, possibly because it is rarely identified prior to metastasis.

Patients and at-risk family members who are found to have inherited the RET gene mutation are candidates for thyroidectomy regardless of their calcitonin levels. Individuals with MEN 2a and FMTC are virtually certain to acquire MTC at some point in their lives (usually before the age af 30 years). Genetic counseling should be provided to individuals and parents of children who are to undergo genetic testing. In order to test a patient for the presence of a mutation in the RET gene, peripheral blood is drawn and DNA is extracted and analyzed. It has been shown in several series that RET mutation carriers often harbor foci of MTC in the thyroid gland even when stimulated calcitonin levels are normal. Patients with MEN 2a and FMTC should have a thyroidectomy at age 5 to 6. Patients with MEN 2b should undergo thyroidectomy during infancy, because of the aggressiveness and earlier age of onset of MTC in these patients. It is advisable to follow the calcitonin level every 1 to 2 years. These patients must also continue to be followed for the development of pheochromocytomas and hyperparathyroidism.

Suggested Readings

Brandi ML, Gagel RF, Angeli A, et al. Guidelines for diagnosis and therapy of MEN type 1 and type 2. *J Clin Endocrinol Metab* 2001;86:5658–5671.

Brunt LM, Doherty GM, Norton JA, et al. Laparoscopic adrenalectomy compared to open adrenalectomy for benign adrenal neoplasms [see comment]. *J Am Coll Surg* 1996;183:1–10.

Dralle H. Lymph node dissection and medullary thyroid carcinoma. *Br J Surg* 2002;89:1073–1075.

Moley JF, DeBenedetti MK. Patterns of nodal metastases in palpable medullary thyroid carcinoma: recommendations for extent of node dissection. *Ann Surg* 1999;229:880–887; discussion 887–888.

Presentation

A 72-year-old woman with a history of diffuse osteopenia presents to your office after she was seen by her primary medical doctor and found to have elevated serum calcium on routine blood screening. Bone densitometry reveals the bone mineral density of the L2-L4 spine to be 2.2 standard deviations below age-matched controls.

She denies a history of nephrolithiasis, pathologic fractures, pancreatitis, peptic ulcer disease, fatigue, or depression. She does admit to occasional back pain. There is no family history of endocrinopathies, and she denies irradiation to her neck. On examination, there are no palpable masses in the neck. The serum calcium is 10.6 (normal, 8.5 to 10.4) mg/dL, and her corresponding intact parathyroid hormone (iPTH) level is 145 (normal, 10 to 65) pg/mL.

Differential Diagnosis

Contemporary series of patients with primary hyperparathyroidism are dominated by elderly women with mild to moderate degrees of hypercalcemia and few, if any, overt symptoms and signs of the disorder. These patients often have nonspecific symptoms such as depression, decreased cognitive ability, myalgias, and arthralgias. The women often exhibit mild skeletal complications of hyperparathyroidism (osteopenia or osteoporosis) and have a very low incidence of renal stones. Prospective analyses have suggested that even apparently asymptomatic patients with hyperparathyroidism may have subtle psychiatric symptoms, which can be reversed by treatment.

Among the differential diagnoses for hypercalcemia in an elderly woman, primary hyperparathyroidism is the most likely explanation. However, it is important to establish the biochemical diagnosis with additional testing and to exclude other possible diagnoses, including secondary hyperparathyroidism, benign familial hypocalciuric hypercalcemia (BFHH), malignancy (i.e., squamous cell, breast, or colon cancers), granulomatous disease (i.e., sarcoidosis, tuberculosis), and dietary (i.e., large amounts of supplemental calcium or vitamin D, yogurt and antacids, or betel nuts) and pharmacologic (i.e., lithium, thiazide diuretics) causes.

The most common pathologic cause of primary hyperparathyroidism is a parathyroid adenoma (85%). Adenomas are benign and typically affect only one gland, but in 5% of cases, there are two. Primary hyperparathyroidism is more frequent in women than in men, at a ratio of 3:1. Macroscopically, the affected adenoma is enlarged, tan-brown, ovoid, encapsulated, and occasionally has areas of hemorrhage or cystic spaces. Histologically, they are composed of cohesive sheets of chief cells, oncocytic cells, transitional oncocytic cells, or a mixture of these cells.

Parathyroid hyperplasia affects all glands and is the underlying cause of primary hyperparathyroidism in 10% of cases. It can be associated with the multiple endocrine neoplasia (MEN) 1 and 2a syndromes. MEN 1 includes hyperparathyroidism, pituitary adenoma, and pancreatic tumors (most commonly gastrinomas or insulinomas). MEN 2a includes hyperparathyroidism, medullary carcinoma of the thyroid, and pheochromocytoma. Parathyroid carcinoma is a rare (<1% of cases) cause of primary hyperparathyroidism.

The biochemical diagnosis is established with elevated serum calcium, elevated iPTH, normal blood urea nitrogen (BUN) and creatinine (to exclude secondary hyperparathyroidism), and normal or elevated 24-hour urinary calcium (to exclude BFHH). After the diagnosis is established, noninvasive preoperative imaging should be performed to facilitate minimally invasive parathyroidectomy (MIP). Localization can include Sestamibi-technetium 99 (Tc 99m) scintigraphy, ultrasonography, computed tomography (CT), or magnetic resonance imaging (MRI). There is a general consensus that the single best study is Sestamibi, especially when combined with single-photon emission computed tomography (SPECT).

Sestamibi scan utilizes Tc 99m, which diffuses into cells and concentrates in the mitochondria. Parathyroid adenomas have a generous blood supply, high metabolic rate, and an absence of p-glycoprotein on the cell surface, which allows for a rich uptake of Tc 99m. When combined with SPECT, Sestamibi is an especially powerful tool, because it allows for three-dimensional localization. Ultrasound of the neck is often combined with Sestamibi to exclude underlying thyroid abnormalities, which can distort Sestamibi findings. The combined specificity of the two studies is 90%.

Recommendation

Establish the biochemical diagnosis, and then perform imaging to localize the pathology.

Case Continued

The patient underwent additional laboratory and imaging tests. The patient had normal renal function; the BUN and creatinine were 15 (normal, 7 to 30) mg/dL and 0.8 (normal, 0.5 to 1.2) mg/dL, respectively. Her 24-hour urinary calcium excretion was 140 (normal, 50 to 400) mg/24 hours, with an adequate urine volume collected of 2500 mL. She then underwent a Sestamibi scan with SPECT and neck ultrasound.

Sestamibi With SPECT

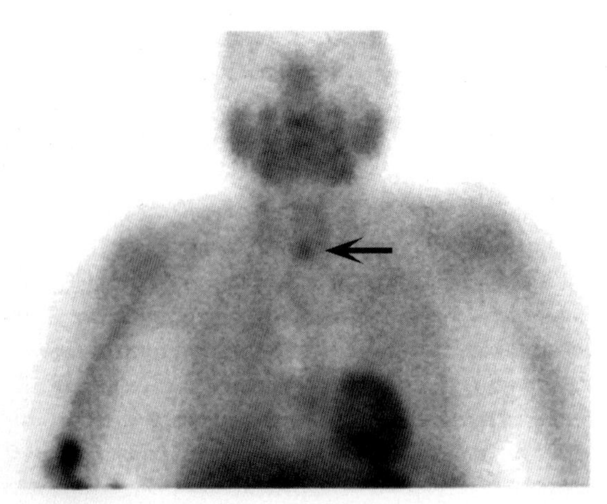

Figure 80.1

Sestamibi With SPECT Report

There is a mild focus of uptake *(arrow)* in the anterior portion of the right lower thyroid bed. These findings are consistent with a small parathyroid adenoma in the anterior, right lower thyroid bed.

Ultrasonogram

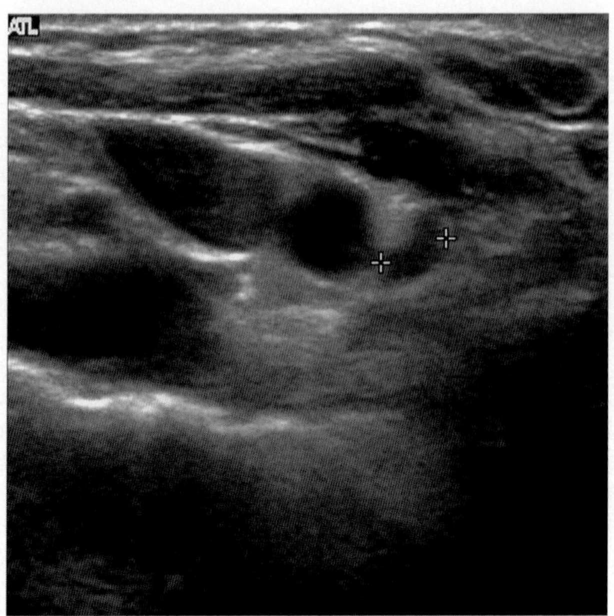

Figure 80.2

Ultrasonography Report

Inferior to the right lobe of the thyroid is a 0.9 × 0.3-cm hypoechoic, somewhat oval-shaped structure with vascular flow identified, raising the possibility of right lower parathyroid enlargement (marked).

Diagnosis and Recommendation

Primary hyperparathyroidism secondary to a right inferior parathyroid adenoma. The patient is offered a minimally invasive parathyroidectomy (MIP); that is, a unilateral neck exploration performed under cervical block with sedation through a small (1 to 4 cm) incision on an outpatient basis using the intraoperative parathyroid hormone assay.

Approach

Parathyroidectomy is curative and safe in the hands of experienced surgeons. The rate of complications is as low as 1.2%, and cure rates are as high as 98%. Parathyroidectomy also can be done safely in patients older than 80 years of age.

A National Institutes of Health (NIH) consensus panel in 2002 specified the indications for surgery in primary hyperparathyroidism. These include any of the following: (a) a serum calcium level 1 mg/dL or more above the normal range; (b) a 24-hour urinary calcium >400 mg; (c) a reduction of more than 30% in the creatinine clearance, compared with age-matched controls; (d) a bone density more than 2.5 standard deviations below the t-score; (e) age younger than 50 years; and (f) the presence of symptoms that can be ascribed to primary hyperparathyroidism, such as nephrolithiasis or fragility fractures.

Nonoperative treatment in asymptomatic primary hyperparathyroidism means conscientious, prolonged surveillance and medical control of the patient. The patient should be examined at least once a year, and serum calcium, renal function, bone density, and clinical manifestations should be documented. Hormone-replacement therapy should be considered in postmenopausal women to prevent osteoporosis and cardiovascular disease. Estrogens decrease the effect of parathyroid hormone on bone. Medications such as bisphosphonates, calcitonin, or mithramycin are not indicated in the treatment of asymptomatic patients.

Surgical Approach

The patient is brought to the ambulatory operating room, and her neck is placed in extension in the semi-Fowler position. Adequate intravenous access is obtained, and a baseline serum PTH level is 107 pg/mL. She is sedated with fentanyl and midazolam. A cervical block is performed by the surgeon with 20 mL of 1% lidocaine in three stages. First, a superficial block is placed posterior and deep to the sternocleidomastoid muscle on the ipsilateral side of the Sestamibi-localized adenoma. Next, the transverse cervical nerves are blocked along the anterior border of the sternocleidomastoid muscle. Finally, a local field block is infiltrated along the line of the incision.

A 1.9-cm transverse incision is made three fingerbreadths above the sternal notch. A focused exploration is made of the right inferior, anterior neck, and the culprit parathyroid adenoma is identified and removed with care not to violate the capsule of the gland or disturb the right recurrent laryngeal nerve. Intraoperative PTH levels are obtained at 0 and 5 minutes postexcision; these were 43 and 28 pg/mL, respectively.

The patient phonated normally in the operating room and is transferred to the recovery room, awake and alert. She is discharged home 1 hour later.

Discussion

The rapid intraoperative PTH assay can be used to confirm adequate removal of hypersecreting parathyroid glands and predict a curative procedure. Its use is associated with reduced operating time and reduced operative failure rates for parathyroidectomy.

The most commonly employed technique is a chemiluminescence immunometric assay available from Nichols Institute Diagnostics (San Juan Capistrano, CA). A certified clinical laboratory technician ideally performs the assay either inside the operating room or in direct proximity; results of the assay are available within 12 minutes. A peripheral blood specimen is obtained prior to surgery, immediately following resection of the enlarged gland, and then 5 and 10 minutes after the excision. A 50% reduction in the rapid PTH value from the baseline level into the normal range is used an as indication that the exploration has been successful, and this has been predictive of cure in 96% of cases. Intraoperative needle aspiration of suspected parathyroid tissue for a quick measurement of intraoperative PTH is a useful alternative to frozen section for parathyroid identification. Aspiration of parathyroid tissue yields substantially higher hormone values than the upper limit of the standard curve.

Case Continued

The patient returns to clinic 7 days postoperatively. Her phonation is normal, and she is off narcotic analgesics. She denies symptoms or signs of hypocalcemia, including perioral numbness or tingling; she has a negative Cvostek sign. Her calcium is 9.4 mg/dL, and her iPTH level is 12 pg/mL.

Her pathology demonstrates a 200-mg parathyroid adenoma without evidence of malignancy. Six months postoperatively, her serum calcium is 9.2 mg/dL. She is discharged from clinic.

Suggested Readings

Bergenfelz A, Lindblom P, Tibblin S, et al. Unilateral versus bilateral neck exploration for primary hyperparathyroidism: a prospective randomized controlled trial. *Ann Surg* 2002; 236:543–551.

Bilezikian JP, Potts JT Jr, Fuleihan Gel-H, et al. Summary statement from a workshop on asymptomatic primary hyperparathyroidism: a perspective for the 21st century. *J Clin Endocrin Metab* 2002;87:5353–5361.

Irvin GL 3rd, Sfakianakis G, Yeung L, et al. Ambulatory parathyroidectomy for primary hyperparathyroidism. *Arch Surg* 1996;131:1074–1078.

LoGerfo P, Kim LJ. Technique for regional anesthesia: thyroidectomy and parathyroidectomy. *Oper Tech Gen Surg* 1999; 1:95–102.

Sosa JA, Udelsman R. Minimally invasive parathyroid surgery. *Surg Oncol* 2003;12:125–134.

Udelsman R. Six hundred fifty-six consecutive explorations for primary hyperparathyroidism. *Ann Surg* 2002;235: 665–672.

Presentation

A 53-year-old woman with a past medical history of hypertension and depression undergoes a routine serum chemistry check and is found to have an elevated serum calcium level of 13.5 mg/dL (3.4 mmol/L), a mildly elevated serum alkaline phosphatase, and a low serum phosphorus level of 1.8 mg/dL (0.58 mmol/L). She complains of general fatigue and polyuria. On physical examination she has normal vital signs; head and neck examinations reveal no adenopathy, and a palpable 2-cm nodule is found in the right thyroid lobe. Heart and lung examinations are within normal limits.

Differential Diagnosis

The differential diagnosis of elevated serum calcium in a patient with normal renal function includes primary hyperparathyroidism, paraneoplastic syndrome, metastatic carcinoma with lytic bone metastases, granulomatous diseases, familial hypocalciuric hypercalcemia, and parathyroid carcinoma. In patients with renal failure, secondary or tertiary hyperparathyroidism must be considered. In this patient, given her age, mild symptoms, and the lack of history of renal failure, the most likely diagnosis is primary hyperparathyroidism. The relatively high presenting serum calcium level and the palpable neck mass raise the suspicion for parathyroid carcinoma.

Discussion

Primary hyperparathyroidism is the third most common endocrine disorder in postmenopausal women. Over 80% of the patients have solitary benign adenomas, while approximately 15% of cases harbor multigland hyperplasia. The usual presentation of this disease is mild to moderate hypercalcemia, with an elevated serum parathyroid hormone level and no significant physical findings on neck examination. The markedly elevated serum calcium and a palpable mass on neck examination raise the suspicion of parathyroid carcinoma. However, most patients who present with primary hyperparathyroidism and a palpable neck mass have both a routine parathyroid adenoma and a thyroid nodule.

The diagnosis of primary hyperparathyroidism necessitates the findings of elevated serum calcium, elevated or inappropriate intact serum parathyroid hormone (PTH) level, and normal serum creatinine level.

Preoperative localization studies can allow more directed surgical treatment. A technetium-99m-methoxy isobutyl isonitrile (Sestamibi) scan with single-photon emission computed tomography (SPECT) can identify the enlarged hyperfunctional gland in up to 80% of cases. Adding SPECT allows three-dimensional evaluation of the gland location in relation to other structures in the neck, such as the thyroid and esophagus. If a SPECT scan cannot be obtained, a dedicated parathyroid neck ultrasound can provide the anatomic detail to complement the Sestamibi scan.

Recommendation

Additional serum tests for intact PTH and creatinine levels as well as a Sestamibi scan with SPECT. Also, a high water intake and elimination of calcium from the diet is advised.

Case Continued

Serum intact PTH and creatinine levels are obtained. She has normal renal function, but the PTH level is elevated (370 pg/mL, normal range 10 to 60).

▉ Sestamibi Scan

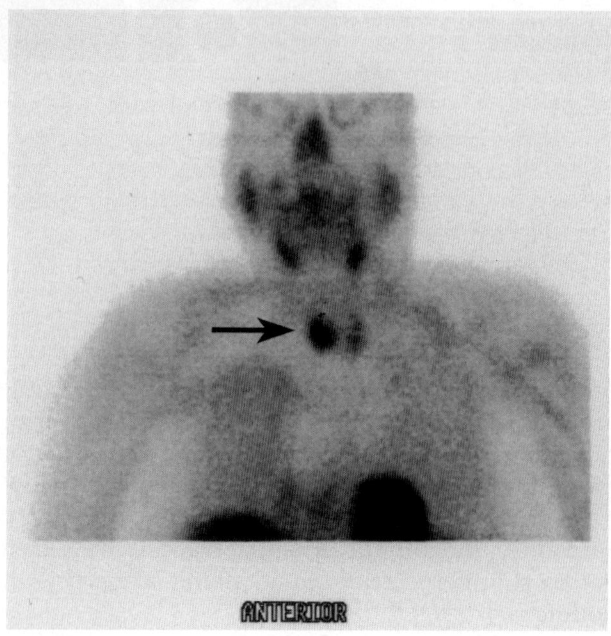

Figure 81.1

Sestamibi Scan Report

There is intense uptake of technetium-99m-labeled sestamibi in the right neck, inferior to the thyroid. suggestive of a right lower parathyroid adenoma.

Diagnosis and Recommendation

Primary hyperparathyroidism. Given the patient's high serum calcium, palpable neck mass, and hyperintense Sestamibi scan, parathyroid carcinoma may be suspected.

The patient is offered surgical resection with intraoperative PTH monitoring. The patient may be offered a minimally invasive parathyroidectomy under local anesthesia. However, if the surgeon encounters intraoperative findings suggestive of parathyroid carcinoma, the case may require conversion to general anesthesia to facilitate en bloc resection. She is told that a hemithyroidectomy and resection of local soft tissues may need to be performed if the diagnosis of carcinoma is suspected. The complications discussed are recurrent laryngeal nerve injury and bleeding.

▉ Surgical Approach

The patient is placed in the neck extension, semi-Fowler position and general endotracheal anesthesia is induced. A transverse anterior cervical incision is performed, subplatysmal flaps are created, and the strap muscles are divided in the midline and taken off the right thyroid capsule. The thyroid is medially rotated. In the thyrothymic tract, just inferior to the thyroid lobe in the paratracheal position, a 2.5-cm, firm, fibrotic mass is found, closely adherent to the thyroid lobe. There are no enlarged lymph nodes in the central neck. The superior parathyroid is normal appearing and is left in place. An en bloc resection of the mass and the right thyroid lobe is performed. All surgical margins are negative for parathyroid tissue. The recurrent laryngeal nerve is identified in the tracheoesophageal groove and appears uninvolved. It is preserved. A rapid intraoperative serum PTH measurement is obtained prior to surgical manipulation and at the time of resection as well as at 5-minute intervals postexcision. In this patient, the PTH level dropped at 5 minutes by more than 50% from baseline. No other masses are seen and the patient's incision is closed.

Discussion

Parathyroid carcinoma is rare, representing 0.1% to 3% of cases with primary hyperparathyroidism. The diagnosis of parathyroid carcinoma is usually made at the time of surgery based on clinical factors such as a hard, fibrosed gland adherent to neck structures. It is important that if such a gland is found, it should not be biopsied in vivo. Violating the parathyroid gland capsule spills cells and allows for implantation and spread of parathyroid cells, leading to parathyromatosis. This is particularly treacherous if parathyroid cancer is suspected. Pathologic frozen section is usually not helpful, because carcinoma is not easily distinguished from parathyroid adenomas with degenerative changes and fibrosis.

The diagnostic acumen therefore rests with the operating surgeon with a high index of suspicion. An en bloc resection of the ipsilateral thyroid lobe and any grossly involved structures, including the recurrent laryngeal nerve, if necessary, is performed.

The possibility of lymphatic spread has led to a controversy over whether prophylactic lymph node dissections should be undertaken. A central lymph node excision on the ipsilateral side should be done if clinically positive central lymph nodes are suspected. Lymph node metastases can be seen in up to 30% of patients.

Local recurrence is common, especially if the gland capsule is ruptured. The tumor metastasizes most commonly to lung, bone, and brain. If possible, palliative resections of local and distant metastases offer the best results.

The histologic diagnosis of carcinoma can be established by using Bondeson's criteria of invasive growth, extracapsular invasion, local recurrence, or the presence of distant metastases. Molecular indices, such as immunohistochemical staining for proliferating cell nuclear antigen and Ki-67, loss of the retinoblastoma tumor suppressor gene, and mutations in the HRPT2 gene seen in the familial hyperparathyroidism-jaw-tumor syndrome, appear promising in small studies in improving pathologic diagnosis and predicting tumor behavior.

Parathyroid carcinoma can vary in its aggressiveness. It may recur early or remain indolent for many years. Overall mortality rates in reported series range from 60% to 75% at 5 years. There seems to be no obvious relationship between age, gender, or preoperative calcium or PTH levels and prognosis.

In follow-up of patients, serum calcium and PTH levels are routinely measured. Imaging examinations are obtained according to clinical suspicion. Whole-body Sestamibi scans appear promising as first-line imaging studies, followed by CT or MRI scans.

Surgical resection is the most effective treatment. Palliative medical treatment of recurrent hypercalcemia due to residual parathyroid carcinoma is directed at reducing the serum calcium levels with hydration, furosemide, and bisphosphonate administration. Calcitriol inhibits cellular proliferation and may appear beneficial for short periods. Radiation therapy is usually ineffective. Calcimimetic agents may be employed in the future.

Ultrasonically guided injection of sclerosing agents may be tried in patients with inoperable recurrences.

Suggested Readings

Bondeson L, Sandelin K, Grimelius L. Histopathologic variables and DNA cytometry in parathyroid carcinoma. *Am J Surg Pathol* 1993;17:820–829.

Broadus A, Braaten K. Weekly clinicopathological exercises: a 47-year-old woman with late recurrent hyperparathyroidism. *N Engl J Med* 2002;346:694–700.

Cordeiro A, Montenegro F, Kulcsar M, et al. Parathyroid carcinoma. *Am J Surg* 1998;175:52–55.

Odoherty M, Kettle A. Symposium on parathyroid localization: parathyroid imaging and preoperative localization. *Nuclear Med Comm* 2003;24:125–131.

Shane E, Bilezikian J. Parathyroid carcinoma: a review of 62 patients. *Endocr Rev* 1982;3:218–226.

Presentation

The patient is a 79-year-old white male with a past medical history significant for repair of an abdominal aortic aneurysm, endovascular repair of a thoracic aneurysm, coronary artery disease, and carotid vascular disease. He was found 1 year ago to have an incidental 4.0-cm right adrenal mass on a computed tomography (CT) scan. The CT scan was performed for follow-up evaluation of his thoracic aneurysm. The patient was completely asymptomatic at the time, and underwent serum and urine cortisol tests as well as serum electrolyte and catecholamine tests, which were all negative.

The patient now presents to your office with a follow-up CT scan showing an increase in the size of the right adrenal mass and some right flank pain.

CT Scan

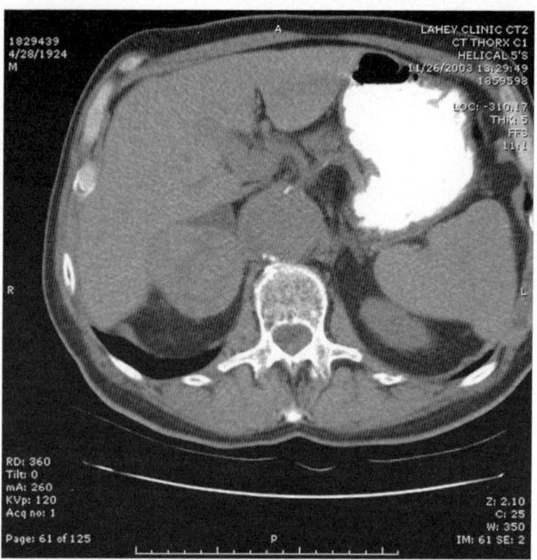

Figure 82.1A Copyright © 2004 Lahey Clinic.

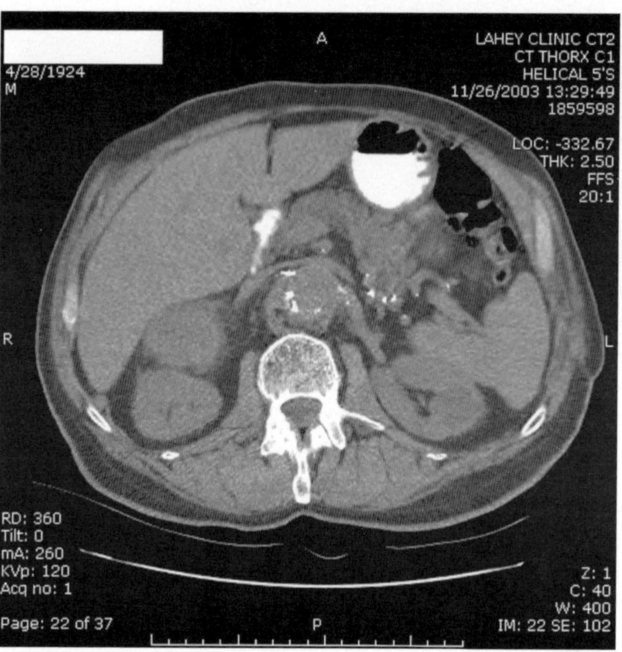

Figure 82.1B Copyright © 2004 Lahey Clinic.

CT Scan Report

A large 6 × 5.8-cm right adrenal mass is present, adjacent to a large aortic aneurysm. The mass does not appear to invade any surrounding structures, and a clear plane between the adrenal mass and the kidney exists. Multiple simple cysts are present in both kidneys. A large thoracic and abdominal aneurysm is evident

Differential Diagnosis

The differential diagnosis for adrenal masses includes adenomas, pheochromocytomas, myelolipomas, ganglioneuromas, adrenal cysts, hematomas, cortical carcinomas, and metastasis from other cancers.

Discussion

With the increase in the utilization of abdominal imaging techniques, such as ultrasonography and CT scanning, there has been a dramatic increase in incidentally discovered adrenal masses, also known as *incidentalomas*. Solid adrenal masses, regardless of symptoms, should undergo biochemical assessment and appropriate radiologic imaging.

In patients with a prior history of cancer, up to three fourths of asymptomatic adrenal masses will prove to be metastases. In cases of prior malignancy, a needle biopsy may be warranted. In patients with no history of cancer, two thirds of these tumors are benign lesions. The size of the adrenal mass is clinically important because the prevalence of adrenal cortical carcinoma is related to size. Although adrenal carcinoma accounts for <5% of all adrenal masses smaller than 4 cm, they can account for 25% of all adrenal lesions larger than 6 cm. Some series have demonstrated that over 90% of all adrenal carcinomas are 6 cm or larger.

Biochemical or hormonal evaluation includes 24-hour urine cortisol levels and determination of fractionated urinary and/or plasma metanephrines. Plasma-free metanephrines are also important because they are highly sensitive for detecting pheochromocytomas. In patients with hypertension, a potassium level and a plasma aldosterone concentration-plasma renin activity ratio should also be determined. Glucocorticoid evaluation should only be performed if Cushing syndrome or virilization are clinically evident.

Proper radiologic imaging with either CT scanning or magnetic resonance imaging (MRI) is necessary. As previously mentioned, adrenal malignancies are almost always larger than 6 cm, and CT scans provide a relatively accurate assessment of tumor size. CT scans are also useful for distinguishing benign lesions such as myelolipomas and cysts from malignant lesions.

MRI is also a valuable diagnostic tool, especially for tumors <5 cm. On T1-weighted images, most benign adenomas appear hypointense or isointense in relation to the spleen or liver, with little change in intensity on T2 images. Adrenal cortical carcinomas, however, are felt to be hypointense to the liver or spleen on T1 images but hyperintense on T2 images in relation to the liver or spleen. This finding, however, is not exclusive to adrenal cortical carcinomas because neural tumors, metastatic tumors, hemorrhage, and other lesions also have similar findings.

Newer applications of existing technologies, such as CT and MRI, as well as alternative studies, such as NP59 scanning, are enabling greater accuracy in differentiating between benign and malignant lesions.

There is little role for fine-needle aspiration (FNA) of adrenal masses unless a prior or concomitant history of cancer exists. The most common primaries that metastasize to the adrenal include melanoma, and lung, breast, and colon cancer.

In general, surgical extirpation is required for hormonally active adrenal lesions, for biochemically inactive adrenal lesions larger than 6 cm, and for adrenal lesions that grow in size or have radiographic evidence consistent with malignancy.

Recommendation

Anatomical imaging with MRI. Hormonal evaluation with 24-hour urine cortisol, serum catecholamines, and serum cortisol. Vascular surgery consultation is necessary to evaluate the stability of his aneurysms and determine a possible connection between the aneurysms and his recent right flank pain.

Case Continued

The patient has MRI of the chest and abdomen, which demonstrates a large right adrenal mass with an increase in signal in T2 images in relation to the liver. The vascular surgeon felt that the patient's aneurysms were stable and did not account for his recent flank pain. Repeat evaluations of urine and plasma cortisol levels as well as serum catecholamines were all negative.

Diagnosis and Recommendation

Large, growing, hormonally inactive adrenal mass, suspicious for malignancy. With the high suspicion for malignancy, chest x-ray should be obtained. If any abnormality is noted on chest x-ray, then CT scan of the chest is needed for further characterization.

Approach

Complete surgical resection is the best treatment option because other options, such as medical therapy and radiation therapy, have demonstrated little or no benefit in long-term survival. Adrenalectomy can be performed either as an open procedure (retroperitoneal approach, secondary to prior abdominal aneurysm repair) or with a laparoscopic approach.

Discussion

Adrenal carcinomas are extremely rare, with an incidence of only 1 per 1.7 million. There are only approximately 150 to 200 cases diagnosed in the United States each year. Like benign adenomas, cortical carcinomas may exhibit symptoms from the release of hormones. One quarter of all patients with adrenocortical carcinomas have clinically evident symptoms of Cushing syndrome as well as virilization. Patients with nonfunctioning or subclinically secreting tumors most commonly present with symptoms such as abdominal pain or a palpable mass.

Adrenal carcinomas commonly metastasize to lung, liver, and lymph nodes, and invade directly into surrounding structures such as the kidney, inferior vena cava, and spleen.

Complete surgical resection is the best treatment option because other options, such as medical therapy and radiation therapy, have demonstrated little or no benefit in long-term survival. The 5-year survival rate is only approximately 50% in cases with complete en bloc surgical resection. The overall 5-year survival rate ranges from 0% to 45% depending on stage (see below).

The mainstay of medical therapy for patients with unresectable disease or with recurrent/metastatic disease has been mitotane, a DDT derivative. The response rates for mitotane vary widely in the literature, and the toxicity is usually severe. In the majority of studies, there has not been any demonstrable improvement in survival. Alternate agents such as cisplatin, etoposide, doxorubin, and vincristine have been used with relatively little success.

Radiotherapy has generally been reserved for palliation in patients with bone metastases because these tumors are considered to be radio resistant.

Surgical Approach

As previously mentioned, complete surgical excision of the tumor is the only potentially curative treatment modality. Frequently, complete tumor resection involves removing not only the adrenal gland but also involved adjacent organs. In patients with an intracaval thrombus, cardiac bypass techniques may be employed to facilitate complete surgical extirpation.

There are several surgical approaches available to the surgeon. A laparoscopic approach can be utilized; however, these are usually reserved for small adrenal tumors with no evidence of invasion into adjacent organs and/or tumor thrombus. There are case reports that exist demonstrating the feasibility of performing laparoscopic adrenalectomy even with tumor thrombus in the adrenal vein.

Open adrenalectomy, however, remains the standard of care for the treatment of adrenal cortical carcinomas. The proper open approach depends on several factors including surgeon preference and experience, size and laterality of the tumor, and the body habitus of the patient. For larger tumors, a thoracoabdominal approach is frequently utilized. This incision is made above the 9th or 10th ribs and may involve detachment of the posterior segment of the rib if necessary.

Attention must be taken to avoid injuring the lung during the incision of the pleura. Incision of the diaphragm should stay posterior to avoid injuring branches of the phrenic nerve. This approach provides excellent exposure of the adrenal gland and its adjacent ipsilateral organs. Closure of the thoracoabdominal incisions requires careful repair of the diaphragm. Intercostal sutures and a chest tube should also be placed during closure.

For tumors with extra-adrenal or caval involvement, a transabdominal approach via a chevron or transverse incision is extremely useful. This approach allows for complete exposure of not only adjacent organs but also contralateral structures.

Other options include supracostal, subcostal, and posterior/modified posterior approaches. These approaches are best suited to smaller tumors. The posterior approach allows for rapid exposure of the adrenal gland and quick control of the vein, especially in cases of pheochromocytoma. In addition, this approach has a low degree of associated morbidity.

Regardless of the approach, certain principles are useful during adrenalectomy. Visualization is essential because the adrenal gland lies high and posterior in the retroperitoneum. Dissection of the adrenal gland is often started laterally and continued posteriorly. With gentle traction on the kidney, the cranial attachments and blood supply can be freed and the entire gland can be brought down inferiorly, allowing for identification of the adrenal vein, which is located posteriolaterally on the right side. This is in stark contrast to pheochromocytomas, which require immediate control of the adrenal vein.

The fragility of the adrenal gland and its propensity for bleeding are well documented. During dissection, tension should be maintained on the surrounding structures rather than the adrenal gland itself if possible. To emphasize this concept, many have often stated that "the patient should be dissected from the tumor," especially in patients with pheochromocytomas.

Case Continued

The surgical options were reviewed with the patient. Due to his prior surgical history, an open retroperitoneal approach via a supracostal 11th rib incision was performed. Because the mass was not unusually large, a supra-11th incision was made without injuring or entering the pleura. The mass was well demarcated and did not involve any of the surrounding structures. The pulse radiating from the underlying aortic aneurysm was easily apparent. Careful attention was paid to avoid disrupting the large aneurysm, and the adrenal mass was successfully completely resected.

Intraoperative and Specimen Photographs

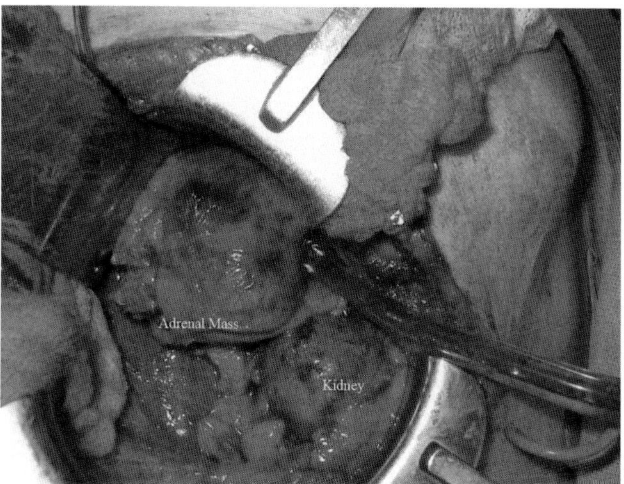

Figure 82.2A Copyright © 2004 Lahey Clinic.

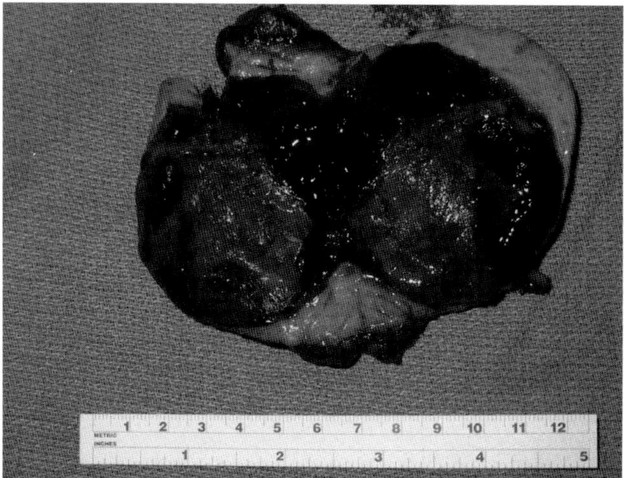

Figure 82.2B Copyright © 2004 Lahey Clinic.

Intraoperative Report

This intraoperative photo shows the adrenal mass in relationship to the kidney. There does not appear to be any local invasion from the mass. The large aneurysm lies directly posterior to the mass with radiating pulsations. The adrenal mass with central hemorrhage and necrosis is seen in the resected specimen.

Discussion

Staging of adrenal cortical carcinomas relies on tumor diameter, involvement of adjacent and distant organs, and nodal status.

In many larger series, stage was the most significant prognostic factor. The 5-year survival rate for stage I tumors was 30% to 45%, stage II tumors was 12.5% to 57%, stage III tumors was 5% to 18%, and stage IV tumors was 0%. Unresectable tumors progressed rapidly within a few months, with a median survival ranging from 3 to 9 months. For tumors with complete resection, the median survival time was 13 to 28 months.

Case Continued

The patient tolerated the procedure without any difficulty and was transferred to the postanesthesia care unit (PACU) in stable condition. In the PACU, the patient experienced persistent hypotension despite fluid resuscitation. A CT scan of the chest/abdomen was performed to exclude hemorrhage from his aneurysm. The CT scan was suggestive of a subacute thoracic aneurysm leak. A vascular surgery consultation was obtained, and conservative management was recommended. The patient was subsequently transfused 2 units of packed red blood cells and was transferred to a monitored floor in stable condition.

The rest of the patient's hospital course was uneventful, although he did develop *Clostridium difficile* colitis. This was successfully treated with oral metronidazole, and the patient was discharged home on postoperative day 8 in excellent condition.

Pathologic examination of this mass suggested T2 or stage II adrenal cortical carcinoma. The patient will be scheduled for follow-up in 3 months, and then every 6 months for reimaging.

Discussion

The postoperative management of adrenal cortical carcinoma is unclear. Although no definitive guidelines exist, this patient will need to undergo lifelong follow-up. Among patients with complete surgical resections, 80% will have recurrent disease, with documented cases occurring up to 10 years after presumed curative resection. Surgical re-exploration remains the only effective treatment for these patients.

Suggested Readings

Gill IS, Novick AC. Laparoscopic vs open adrenal surgery. *AUA Update* 1999;18:257–263.

Ng L, Libertino JA. Adrenocortical carcinoma: diagnosis, evaluation and treatment. *J Urol* 2003;169:5–11.

NIH state-of-the science statement on management of clinically inapparent adrenal mass ("incidentaloma"). *NIH Consens State Sci Statements* 2002;19:1–23.

Tritos NA, Cushing GW, Heatley G, et al. Clinical features and prognostic factors associated with adrenocortical carcinoma: Lahey Clinic Medical Center experience. *Am Surg* 2000 Jan;66:73–79.

Vaughn ED Jr, Blumenfeld JD, Del Pizzo J, et al. The adrenals. In: Walsh PC, Retik AB, Vaughan ED Jr, et al., eds. *Campbell's urology.* 8th ed. Philadelphia, PA: WB Saunders; 2002:3507–3569.

Vaughn ED Jr. Diagnosis of surgical adrenal disorders. *AUA Update* 1997;16:306–311.

Presentation

A 35-year-old man with no significant past medical history notices a right hemiscrotal mass on self-examination. The mass is painless, firm, and apparently intratesticular. The primary medical doctor orders a scrotal ultrasound and refers the patient to you.

Ultrasound Image

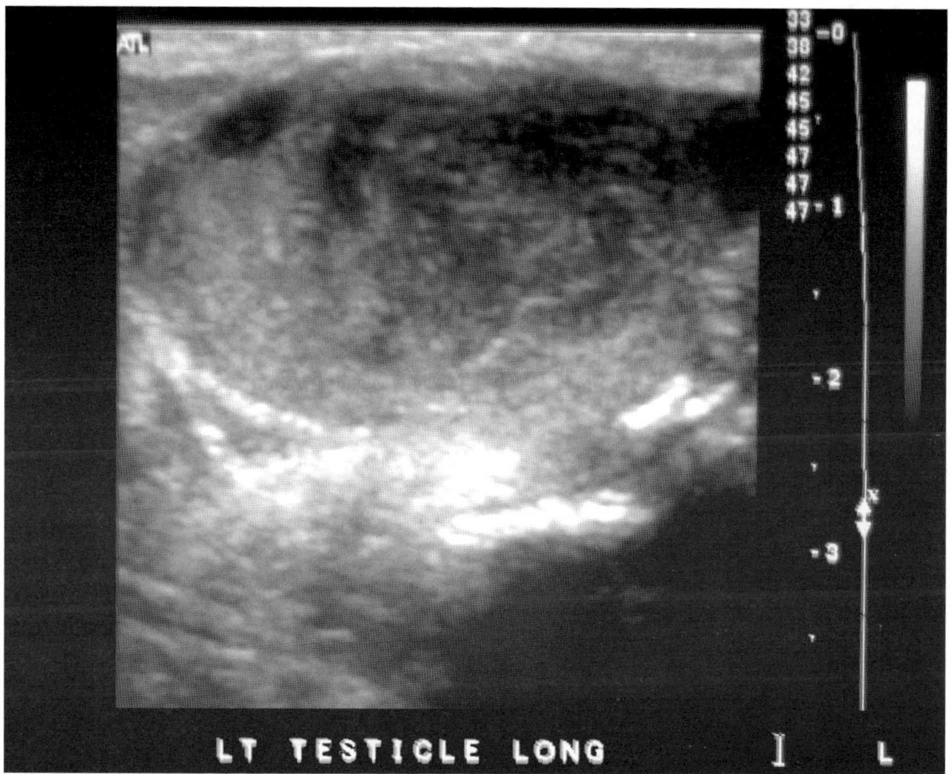

Figure 83.1

Ultrasonography Report

On ultrasound, the right testis and adnexal structures are normal. The left testis exhibits a solid hypoechoic intratesticular mass.

Differential Diagnosis

Most solid intratesticular masses represent germ cell testicular cancer. Two basic types exist: seminomas and nonseminomas. Seminoma is the most common single type, whereas nonseminomas typically consist of various components (embryonal carcinoma, yolk sac tumor, teratoma, and choriocarcinoma). Other possibilities include Leydig and Sertoli cell tumors, most of which behave in a benign fashion. Another possibility is an epidermoid cyst, which is a monolayer teratoma and is a benign lesion. In older men, lymphoma would be another consideration. Intratesticular inflammatory conditions are extremely rare, and a patient who presents with the ultrasound described in this case presentation usually has a tumor.

Recommendation

This patient should have a determination of serum alpha-fetoprotein, beta human chorionic gonadotropin (HCG), and lactate dehydrogenase (LDH). Approximately 10% of seminomas have a low-level elevation of beta HCG; an elevation of serum alpha-fetoprotein is synonymous with the diagnosis of nonseminoma. An elevation of serum LDH is not diagnostic but may aid in following the response to therapy.

Case Continued

In this particular patient, the alpha-fetoprotein, beta HCG, and LDH were normal.

Diagnosis

The probable diagnosis is a testicular tumor.

Recommendation

The patient is advised to undergo a right radical orchiectomy.

Surgical Approach

A right inguinal incision is made. The aponeurosis of the external oblique is opened and the spermatic cord is dissected to the internal ring. A soft clamp is placed on the cord at the level of the internal ring and the testis is delivered into the wound. A high ligation and division of the spermatic cord is performed and the cord and testis are removed as a single specimen. It is important to not cut into the tumor or spill tumor into the wound, as such spillage can contaminate a separate lymphatic drainage area. Another important point to emphasize is that any attempt to biopsy, either percutaneously or open, through the scrotum is contraindicated, as this can lead to scrotal recurrence and aberrant lymphatic metastases.

Case Continued

The pathologist reports that the tumor is a pure seminoma. The tumor is 2 cm in diameter and totally confined to the testis parenchyma. All surgical margins are clear. The patient is advised to undergo computed tomography (CT) scanning of the chest, abdomen, and pelvis in order to accurately stage the process.

The chest, abdomen, and pelvis are normal on CT scanning. There is no evidence of solid organ involvement, nor is there evidence of lymphadenopathy.

Approach

Testis tumors are staged clinically as stage I, II, and III. Stage I denotes no evidence of metastatic disease; stage II patients have metastatic disease to the abdomen; stage III patients have metastatic disease beyond the abdomen. This particular patient has a stage I seminoma. It is well recognized that patients with stage I seminomas have an approximately 15% chance of occult metastatic disease. Usually this disease is to the ipsilateral retroperitoneal nodes. Because seminoma is exquisitely sensitive to external-beam radiation, one management approach is to advise irradiation of the ipsilateral retroperitoneal lymphatics. After such treatment, a few patients will have a recurrence in the chest or mediastinum after therapy; these patients can be cured with three courses of cisplatin, etoposide, and bleomycin. The overall survival rate is 98%.

Because 85% of stage I seminoma patients are cured with radical orchiectomy alone, another approach is to observe the patient after radical inguinal orchiectomy. Frequent physical examinations, CT scans, and chest x-rays are performed; and if a patient shows evidence of metastatic disease, he is treated with either radiotherapy or cisplatin-based chemotherapy. With this approach, called surveillance, the overall survival rate is also 98%. Therefore, the choice of therapy is dependent upon local physician capabilities, patient choice, and potential side effects of the alternative treatments.

Suggested Readings

Aass N, Fossa SD, Host H. Acute and sub-acute side effects due to infradiaphragmatic radiotherapy for testicular cancer: a prospective study. *Int J Radiat Oncol Biol Phys* 1992;22:1057-1064.

Chung P, Parker MB, Panzarella T, et al. Surveillance in stage I testicular seminoma: risk of late relapse. *Can J Urol* 2002;9:1637-1640.

DeSantis M, Bokemeyer C, Becherer A, et al. Predictive impact of 2-fluoro-2-deoxy-D-glucose positron emission tomography for residual post chemotherapy masses in patients with bulky seminoma. *J Clin Oncol* 2001;19:4355.

Fossa SD, Horwich A, Russell JM, et al. Optimal planning target volume for stage I testicular seminoma: a Medical Research Council randomized trial. *J Clin Oncol* 1999;17:1146.

Hamilton C, Horwich A, Easton D, et al. Radiotherapy for stage I seminoma testis: results of treatment and complications. *Radiother Oncol* 1986;6:115-120.

<h1 style="text-align:right">case 84</h1>

Presentation

A 24-year-old man presents to his primary physician with severe back pain. Lumbosacral spine films are obtained, and are normal. The patient is treated with anti-inflammatories, but the pain worsens. Ultimately, the primary physician orders a computed tomography (CT) scan.

CT Scan

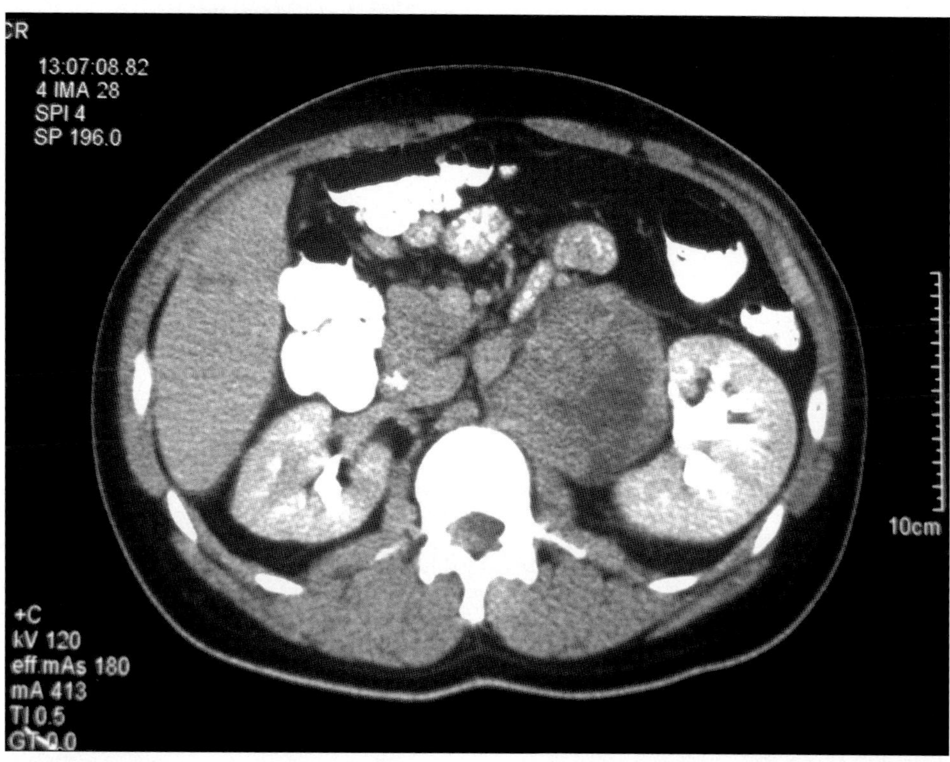

Figure 84.1

CT Scan Report

A large retroperitoneal mass is noted. The internal organs are normal.

Differential Diagnosis

Metastatic germ cell testicular cancer presents commonly with a retroperitoneal mass. Another possibility is lymphoma. Inflammatory or infectious retroperitoneal processes are extremely rare in young men who are otherwise healthy. Therefore, the most common diagnosis would be neoplasia. Please also refer to Case 62 on retroperitoneal sarcoma.

The patient should have determination of serum alpha-fetoprotein, beta human chorionic gonadotropin (HCG), and lactate dehydrogenase. Elevation of beta HCG or alpha-fetoprotein confirms the diagnosis as metastatic germ cell testicular cancer. If elevation of either of these markers is noted, a testicular ultrasound should be obtained because most germ cell tumors of the retroperitoneum are metastatic and not primary retroperitoneal tumors. In this particular patient, both alpha-fetoprotein and beta HCG were significantly elevated and the patient was noted to have a solid intratesticular mass.

Diagnosis

Metastatic nonseminomatous testicular cancer.

Recommendation

The patient is advised to undergo systemic chemotherapy with cisplatin, etoposide, and bleomycin.

Approach

Nonseminomatous germ cell testicular tumors are staged according to the presence of metastatic disease. Stage I denotes no evidence of metastasis. Stage II denotes retroperitoneal only tumor, and stage III designates metastasis beyond the retroperitoneum. Germ cell testicular tumors are usually sensitive to cisplatin-based chemotherapy. Additionally, they are frequently curable merely by surgical removal even after metastasis has occurred. Therefore, these patients are treated with surgery, chemotherapy, or a combination of surgery and chemotherapy. The current patient has a high-volume retroperitoneal-only tumor. His chance for cure with surgery alone is very low, and therefore the patient is advised to undergo systemic chemotherapy. Additionally, at some time he will need radical orchiectomy because there is a blood-testis barrier, and chemotherapy cannot reliably penetrate and eliminate the testicular primary.

Case Continued

The patient undergoes cisplatin-based chemotherapy. The serum alpha-fetoprotein and beta HCG normalize, and a CT scan is obtained after the completion of chemotherapy to restage the patient.

CT Scan

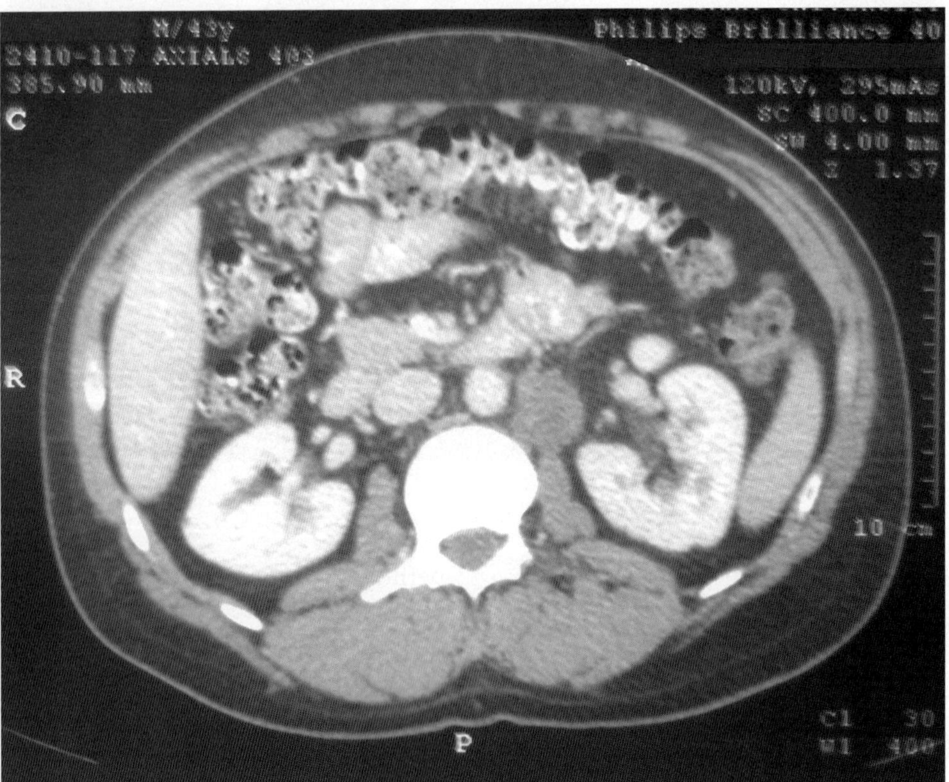

Figure 84.2

CT Scan Report

Shrinkage of the retroperitoneal mass has occurred; however, a definite mass remains after chemotherapy.

Diagnosis

Residual mass after chemotherapy.

Recommendation

Postchemotherapy retroperitoneal lymph node dissection.

Discussion

After chemotherapy, if alpha-fetoprotein and beta HCG normalize and a persistent radiographic mass is noted it should be surgically excised. Pathologically, these masses consist of teratoma, necrosis, active germ cell cancer, or any combination of these three entities. Surgical resection of necrosis confers no benefit to the patient; however, it is impossible preoperatively to determine who has only necrosis in the residual mass. Surgical removal of teratoma or active germ cell cancer is therapeutic, and therefore all residual masses after chemotherapy should be referred for postchemotherapy retroperitoneal lymph node dissection (RPLND).

Surgical Approach

Most postchemotherapy RPLNDs are done through a midline approach. The viscera are mobilized off the retroperitoneum, after which a complete surgical removal of residual tumor and retroperitoneal lymphatics is performed. Additionally, as noted above, in this patient a radical orchiectomy should be performed.

Case Continued

The patient underwent postchemotherapy RPLND. The resected tumor consisted of teratoma. As such, the patient has a good long-term prognosis but will have to be monitored for potential growth of unresected microscopic teratoma.

Suggested Readings

Baniel J, Foster RS, Rowland RG, et al. Complications of postchemotherapy retroperitoneal lymph node dissection. *J Urol* 1995;153:976-980.

Donohue JP, Foster RS. Management of retroperitoneal recurrences: seminoma and nonseminoma. *Urol Clin North Am* 1994;21:761-772.

Fossa SD, Qvist H, Stenwig AE, et al. Is postchemotherapy retroperitoneal surgery necessary in patients with nonseminomatous testicular cancer and minimal residual tumor masses? *J Clin Oncol* 1992;10:569-573.

Foster RS, Donohue JP. Retroperitoneal lymph node dissection. In: Vogelzang NJ, Scardino PT, Shipley WU, et al., eds. *Comprehensive textbook of genitourinary oncology*. Philadelphia, PA: Lippincott Williams & Wilkins; 1996; 955-961.

Sheinfeld J, Bajorin D. Management of the postchemotherapy residual mass. *Urol Clin North Am* 1993;20:133-143.

case 85

Presentation

A 53-year-old man with no significant past medical history is referred to your office with a 1-month history of intermittent gross hematuria and left flank pain. He is a nonsmoker and has had no prior surger-ies. Physical examination is notable only for a palpable left upper quadrant abdominal mass. His serum creatinine is 1.1 mg/dL, hematocrit is 35%, and liver function tests, coagulation panel, and prostate-specific antigen level are normal. Urinalysis and culture show no evidence of infection. An abdominal computed tomography (CT) scan is obtained.

CT Scan

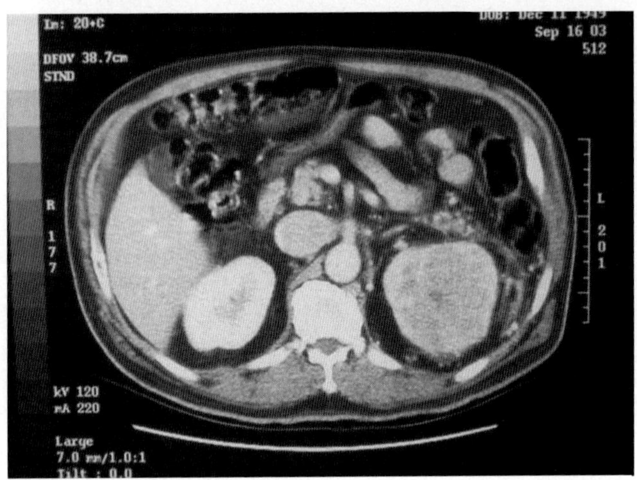

Figure 85.1A

Figure 85.1B

CT Scan Report

Large left renal mass with tumor thrombus extension into left renal vein and inferior vena cava.

Differential Diagnosis

The differential diagnosis for a renal mass in an adult can be broadly divided into benign (simple cyst, angiomyolipoma, oncocytoma) and malignant (renal cell carcinoma, sarcoma, metastasis) tumors. In light of a venous tumor thrombus, renal cell carcinoma should be the primary diagnosis.

Discussion

Renal cell carcinoma (RCC) is the most common malignant tumor of the kidney. Despite the increased incidence of small incidentally detected renal lesions, locally advanced tumors also continue to be diagnosed with increasing frequency. Of patients with RCCs, 4% to 10% demonstrate direct tumor extension into the vena cava. This form of tumor growth tends to be by expansion along the pathway of least resistance rather than by direct invasion, thus the vein wall itself is rarely involved. Most contemporary series have shown that tumor thrombus extension does not necessarily carry an ominous prognosis provided that complete surgical resection can be accomplished, and that there is no associated perinephric fat involvement, invasion of contiguous visceral structures or regional lymph nodes, or distant metastatic sites. Five-year survival rates for patients with vena caval extension without evidence of metastatic disease have been reported to be 30% to

70% following radical nephrectomy and tumor thrombectomy. Controversy exists regarding the prognostic significance of the level of vena caval tumor thrombus extension. The surgical management of RCC with tumor thrombus extension remains a technically challenging endeavor. Preoperative assessment of the cephalad extent of the thrombus is critical in planning the surgical approach. To that extent, magnetic resonance imaging (MRI) and transesophageal echocardiography are now commonly utilized in the preoperative planning.

MRI

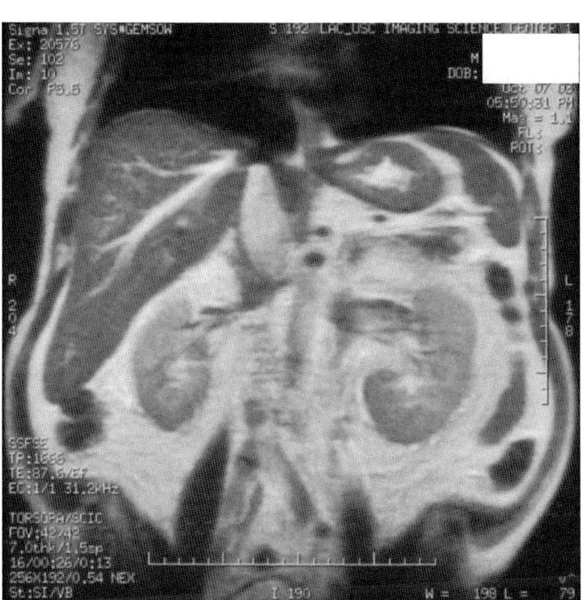

Figure 85.2A

MRI Report

Left renal mass with tumor thrombus extension into renal vein and vena cava up to the level of the diaphragm (level II).

Surgical Approach

A variety of surgical approaches has been described to deal with venous tumor thrombus extension, including a high right thoracoabdominal incision, chevron with median sternotomy, and midline transabdominal with median sternotomy. A thorough intra-abdominal exploration should be performed. A radical nephrectomy, including kidney and adrenal within Gerota's fascia, is performed, and retroperitoneal lymphadenectomy should be performed with early ligation of the renal artery. The kidney is completely mobilized until it is left

Recommendation

Staging evaluation and MRI of chest and abdomen. Transesophageal echocardiogram to assess level of tumor thrombus.

Case Continued

Chest x-ray and bone scan show no evidence of metastatic disease.

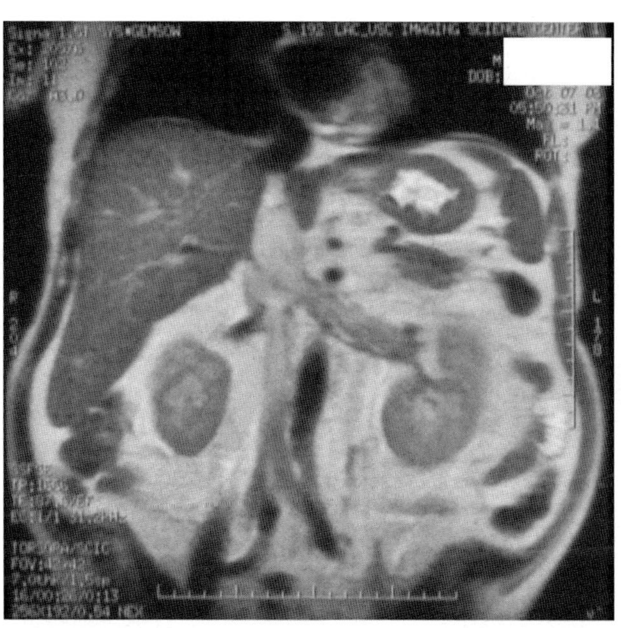

Figure 85.2B

attached only by the renal vein. All venous inflow into the cava above and below the thrombus must be controlled with vascular clamps or tourniquets. Cephalad caval control is accomplished by placing a tourniquet around the inferior vena cava (IVC) within the pericardium, and portal blood flow is temporarily controlled via a vascular clamp across the porta hepatis (Pringle maneuver). The right kidney should be on ice slush to prevent warm ischemia during clamping. A trial of caval occlusion is performed to ensure adequate intravascular fluid volume to maintain systemic blood pressure during the cavotomy. With the patient in the Trendelenburg position, the cavotomy should circumscribe the renal vein and extend longitudinally to allow gentle enucleation of the thrombus. The surgeon has approximately 20 minutes of warm hepatic ischemia time during which the tumor and thrombus can be extracted and the venotomy closed with vascular suture. The lumen of the cava is irrigated and inspected to ensure no residual thrombus before closing it with vascular suture. The clamps and tourniquets are released as the cavotomy is closed to flush out any thrombus or air. An external vena caval clip is applied to the infrarenal cava to prevent pulmonary emboli. A tube thoracostomy is placed in the hemithorax and the incision is closed.

Case Continued

An 8th rib thoracoabdominal incision is made with a T-extension to the left costochondral junction. Intraperitoneal exploration does not reveal any gross metastatic disease. A radical nephrectomy with en bloc caval thrombectomy and retroperitoneal lymphadenectomy is performed.

◾ Clinical Photograph

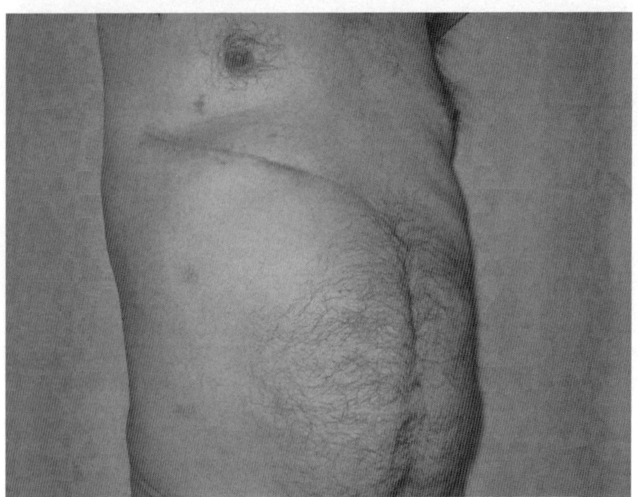

Figure 85.3A

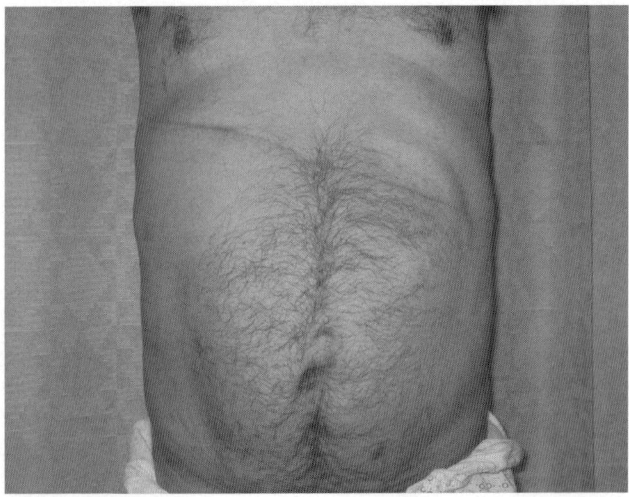

Figure 85.3B

Case Continued

Pathologic analysis reveals multifocal clear cell RCC, measuring 8 cm in greatest dimension, nuclear grade 4/4, extending through the renal capsule, but contained within Gerota's fascia. The tumor extends into the renal pelvis, though the ureteral margin is negative. The tumor thrombus is completely excised en bloc with the specimen. All surgical margins are negative, and there is no involvement of 66 retroperitoneal lymph nodes (pT3b N0 M0).

The patient has an uneventful hospital course. Two months later, the patient presents with worsening shortness of breath. A chest x-ray and subsequent chest CT scan are obtained.

◾ Chest X-Ray and CT Scan

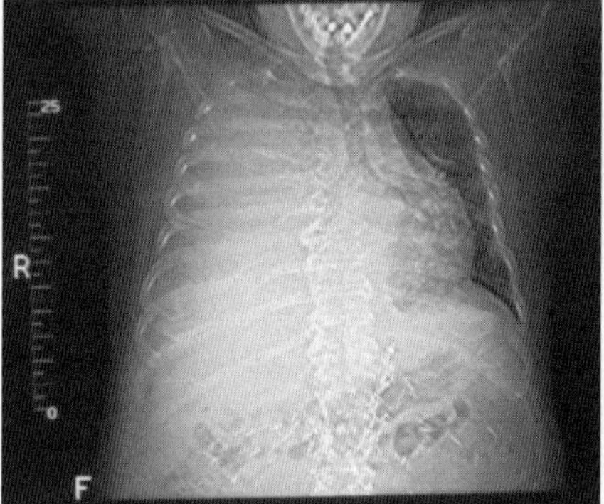

Figure 85.4A

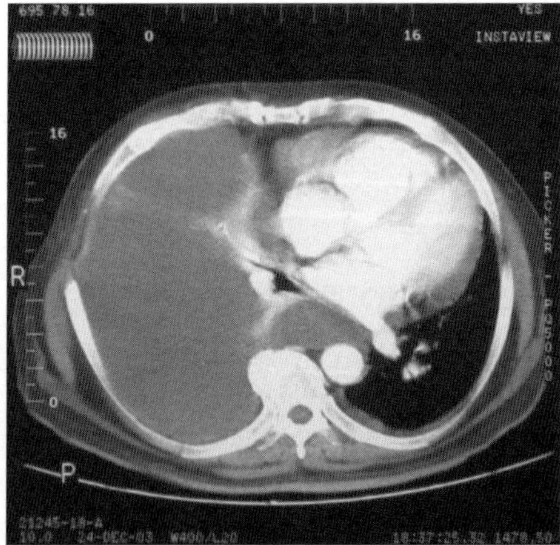

Figure 85.4B

Chest X-Ray and CT Scan Report

Large right pleural effusion.

Recommendation

CT-guided drainage of pleural fluid with cytologic analysis and follow-up postdrainage chest CT scan.

Case Continued

The patient undergoes CT-guided drainage of the pleural fluid. Cytology reveals only atypical cells, though the postdrainage CT scan reveals several small bilateral lung nodules, not previously seen, consistent with new metastatic lesions. Over the next few days, the drainage decreases and the pleural drain is removed. Biopsy of one of the lung nodules confirms metastatic RCC. He is scheduled to participate in a chemotherapy trial with the medical oncologist.

Discussion

Metastatic RCC has been considered to be resistant to both cytotoxic chemotherapy and radiation therapy, with responses observed in only limited numbers of patients. RCC has been shown to evoke an immune response, which investigators have attempted to augment by administering cytokines in doses above physiological levels. For this reason, therapeutic options have ranged from no treatment, to immunotherapy with cytokines such as interleukin-2 (IL-2) and interferon-alpha, to chemotherapy alone or in combination with cytokines. Objective tumor responses are seen only in a small fraction of patients (about 15% to 20%), with very few long-term survivors. Currently, the use of immunomodulating cytokines like interferon-alpha and IL-2, either alone or combined with chemother-apeutic agents, provides the best available results in routine clinical practice.

Recently, some new promising investigational approaches have been reported. Immunotherapy with novel cytokines, monoclonal antibodies, dendritic cell therapy, and allotransplantation offer some promise. Novel therapeutic strategies include combining cytokines, and antiangiogenic approaches such as thalidomide and antivascular endothelial growth factor therapy. Increasing understanding of cancer biology is beginning to allow for a more targeted approach to the therapy of metastatic RCC.

Similar to other malignancies, there are reports encouraging aggressive surgical resection of the clinically solitary metastasis, whether synchronous or metachronous. Prolonged survival has been observed following surgery and adjuvant immunotherapy in highly selected patients, though the morbidity associated with resection of known disease should be weighed against the potential benefit. Those patients with good performance statuses and solitary resectable metastatic lesions may gain the greatest benefit from radical nephrectomy, metastasectomy, and adjuvant immunotherapy.

Suggested Readings

Quek ML, Stein JP, Skinner DG. Surgical approaches to venous tumor thrombus. *Semin Urol Oncol* 2001;19:88–97.

Skinner DG, Pfister RF, Colvin R. Extension of renal cell carcinoma into the vena cava: the rationale for aggressive surgical management. *J Urol* 1972;107:711–716.

Skinner DG, Pritchett TR, Lieskovsky G, et al. Vena caval involvement by renal cell carcinoma: surgical resection provides meaningful long-term survival. *Ann Surg* 1989;210:387–393.

Vaidya A, Ciancio G, Soloway M. Surgical techniques for treating a renal neoplasm invading the inferior vena cava. *J Urol* 2003;169:435–444.

case 86

Presentation

A 63-year-old woman is referred for further evaluation of a 3-week history of urinary frequency and intermittent gross hematuria. She is a 30-pack-year smoker and has no significant past medical or surgical history. Physical examination is unremarkable. Serum creatinine is 0.7 mg/dL, hematocrit 35%, and alkaline phosphatase and liver enzymes are within the normal range. Urinalysis and culture are significant only for hematuria at this time. An abdominal and pelvic computed tomography (CT) scan is performed.

CT Scan

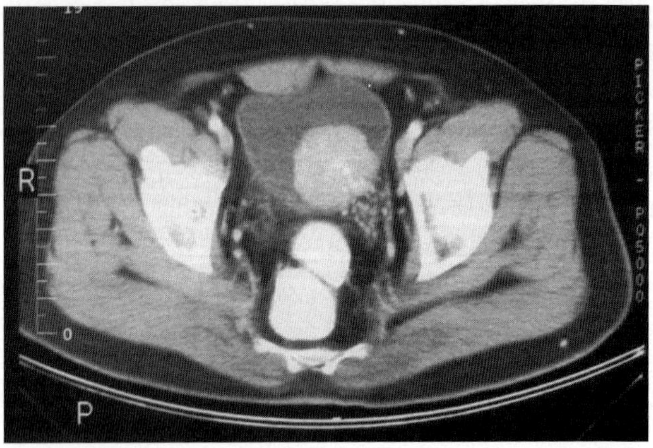

Figure 86.1

CT Scan Report

Filling defect within urinary bladder. There is no hydronephrosis or pelvic/retroperitoneal adenopathy. No urinary calculi are visualized.

Differential Diagnosis

The differential diagnosis for hematuria can be quite extensive. Associated symptoms may aid in distinguishing the etiology, such as flank pain for nephrolithiasis and frequency or dysuria for cystitis. Painless gross hematuria is the classic symptom for bladder cancer, although irritative voiding symptoms are not uncommon especially when carcinoma in situ is present. Hematuria, either gross or microscopic, is noted in over 60% of bladder cancer cases, and therefore, upper tract imaging (intravenous pyelography, CT scan, and ultrasound) and lower urinary tract inspection via cystourethroscopy are essential to rule out malignancy.

Discussion

Transitional cell carcinoma (TCC) of the bladder is the second most common malignancy of the genitourinary tract and the second most common cause of death among genitourinary tumors. Although more common in men (ratio of 2.7:1), it remains a considerable source of morbidity and mortality in women. Approximately 80% of patients with primary TCC will display a relatively indolent, low-grade tumor confined to the superficial mucosa. Most of these patients are managed with transurethral resection and selective administration of intravesical chemotherapy or immunotherapy. Despite the relatively "benign" nature of superficial TCC, the recurrence rate can be as high as 70%, thus necessitating frequent costly long-term follow-up. In addition, up to one third of recurrent superficial tumors may eventually progress to a higher grade and/or stage. Muscle-invasive tumors are diagnosed de novo in 15% to 30% of all bladder cancer patients. Unlike superficial disease, invasive TCC typically displays a highly aggressive behavior, as exemplified by the fact that nearly 50% of patients undergoing definitive local therapy for invasive tumors relapse with distant metastases within 2 years of treatment. Clearly, TCC represents a heterogeneous entity with significant malignant potential.

The gold standard for diagnosis of bladder cancer is cystoscopy with transurethral resection of the bladder tumor (TURBT). This allows histopathologic sampling of the tumor and can also be therapeutic for small superficial lesions. Further therapy depends on the histologic cell type, tumor grade, and pathologic stage, which are determined from the transurethral resection.

Recommendation

Cystoscopy and possible transurethral resection of bladder tumor.

Cystoscopic Image

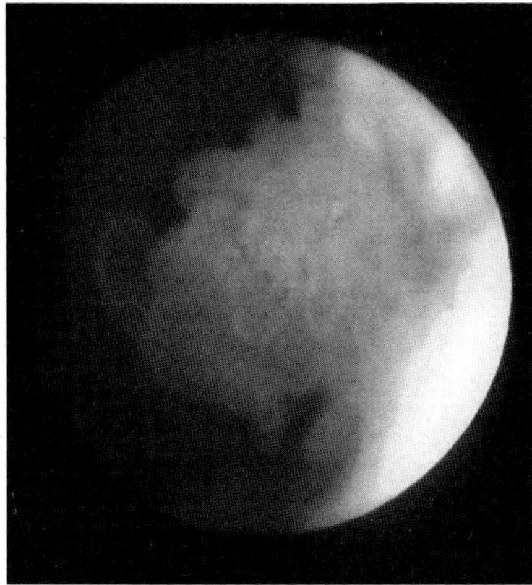

Figure 86.2

Cystoscopy Report

Cystoscopy is performed and a large sessile bladder tumor is found at the left lateral wall.

Case Continued

Transurethral resection of the tumor reveals a grade 4/4 TCC with invasion into the muscularis propria (pT2). Further staging workup, including chest x-ray, is negative.

Approach

Radical cystectomy with pelvic iliac lymphadenectomy represents the standard therapy for invasive bladder cancer. In women, this implies the en bloc removal of the anterior pelvic organs (anterior exenteration), including the bladder, urachus, ovaries, fallopian tubes, uterus, cervix, vaginal cuff, and anterior pelvic peritoneum. Improvements in surgical and perioperative care have significantly decreased the morbidity and mortality associated with radical cystectomy, with most contemporary series reporting a <10% complication rate and 2% mortality rate. Exen-

terative surgery represents the optimal local control of the tumor, with pelvic recurrence rates of <10% for lymph node-negative bladder tumors.

Urinary diversion following radical cystectomy has evolved significantly over the last 50 years from incontinent cutaneous urinary stomas to orthotopic intestinal neobladders. Although it was previously felt that orthotopic lower urinary tract reconstruction could only be performed in males, improved neuroanatomical understanding of the female urethral continence mechanism has now allowed appropriately selected women to be candidates for orthotopic neobladder formation and thus volitional voiding through the intact native urethra. Risk factors for tumor at the urethra in women include bladder neck or anterior vaginal wall involvement. Intraoperative frozen section analysis of the proximal urethral margin provides a reliable means to determine candidacy for orthotopic diversion.

Surgical Approach

The patient is admitted the day before surgery for a mechanical and antibiotic bowel preparation, intravenous hydration, and evaluation by an enterostomal therapist. She is placed in the hyperextended supine position with legs in a frog-leg position to allow access to the vagina. A vertical midline incision from pubis to epigastrium is made and the peritoneum is entered. The urachal remnant is identified, transected, and removed en bloc with the cystectomy specimen. A careful systematic intra-abdominal exploration is performed to exclude distant metastases and to determine local extent of the disease. The bowel is mobilized upon its mesenteric pedicle, thereby exposing the retroperitoneum. Both ureters are clipped and divided near the bladder and sent for frozen section analysis to ensure a tumor-free margin. An extended pelvic iliac lymphadenectomy extending from above the aortic bifurcation to Cooper's ligament and extending laterally to the genitofemoral nerve is performed. The lateral and posterior vascular pedicle to the bladder is isolated, and branches off the hypogastric artery are individually clipped and divided. The vagina is resected just distal to the cervix and the bladder, uterus, and adnexa are removed en bloc. For deeply invasive posterior bladder tumors, the anterior vaginal wall may be removed to ensure adequate surgical margins. The urethral margin is sent for frozen-section analysis to determine whether orthotopic urinary diversion is appropriate. The vaginal stump is closed and an omental pedicle graft is developed based on the left gastroepiploic artery to allow interposition of the omentum between the vaginal stump and neobladder, thereby preventing pouch-vaginal fistulization. After confirmation of a negative urethral margin, an intestinal neobladder is constructed using any number of techniques. Ileal-based neobladders are most commonly utilized consisting of an afferent limb for ureteroileal anastomosis, a detubularized spherical reservoir, and an anastomosis to the native urethra. The use of various techniques for reflux prevention is advocated, though these remain a subject of controversy. Large-bore catheter drainage is maintained with frequent postoperative irrigation to prevent mucus plugging.

Case Continued

After adequate preoperative bowel preparation and counseling, the patient is brought to the operating room for anterior exenteration, pelvic iliac lymphadenectomy, and orthotopic ileal neobladder reconstruction. Intra-abdominal exploration reveals no obvious hepatic or retroperitoneal metastases. The anterior pelvic organs are resected en bloc. Both ureteral and urethral frozen section margins are negative. An omental pedicle is developed and interposed between the vagina and neobladder. An ileal neobladder utilizing an isoperistaltic afferent limb is created and anastomosed to the urethra. A 24F catheter is left indwelling along with a pelvic drain. The patient has an essentially uneventful postoperative course with gradual advancement of oral intake. The catheter and drain are removed 3 weeks postoperatively.

Pathologic analysis of the cystectomy specimen reveals high-grade TCC with focal squamous differentiation penetrating into the deep muscularis layers and involving 7 of 78 lymph nodes (pT2b N2 M0).

Recommendation

Lymph node-positive bladder cancer portends a poor prognosis. Although recent attention has been directed toward the use of chemotherapy in the neoadjuvant setting, most would agree that adjuvant chemotherapy for node-positive TCC is indicated. The standard regimen of methotrexate, vinblastine, doxorubicin, and cisplatin (MVAC) and the newer, less toxic regimen of gemcitabine and cisplatin have shown efficacy for this indication with apparently comparable results.

Case Continued

The patient is referred to the medical oncologist for MVAC chemotherapy.

Suggested Readings

Quek ML, Stein JP, Skinner DG. Current strategies for managing locally advanced bladder cancer. *Contemp Urol* 2004;16:44–55.

Stein JP, Skinner DG. Orthotopic urinary diversion. In Walsh PC, Retik AB, Vaughan ED, Wein AJ, eds. *Campbell's urology.* 8th ed. Philadelphia, PA: WB Saunders; 2002:3835–3867.

Stein JP, Skinner DG. Radical cystectomy in women. *Atlas Urol Clin North Am* 1997;5:37–64.

Stein JP, Lieskovsky G, Cote R, et al. Radical cystectomy in the treatment of invasive bladder cancer: long-term results in 1,054 patients. *J Clin Oncol* 2001;19:666–675.

Presentation

A 63-year-old man presents with a serum prostate-specific antigen (PSA) level of 5.2 ng/mL (upper limit of normal 4.0 ng/mL). Prior PSA 1 year previously was 2.1 ng/mL. A repeat PSA with a free and total fraction is performed; this demonstrates a PSA of 5.3 ng/mL with a free-to-total fraction of 9% (more than 15% suggests benign disease). The patient otherwise is in good health. He has no smoking history, and no family history of prostate malignancy. No abnormal findings were noted on physical examination. The prostate is symmetrical, not enlarged, and free of nodules or induration.

Differential Diagnosis

The main concern in a patient with an elevation of PSA relates to the possible presence of adenocarcinoma of the prostate. Elevation in PSA can be secondary to benign prostatic hyperplasia or prostatitis. Other factors such as sexual activity, exercise, and digital rectal examination typically do not have a significant impact on PSA levels.

Prostate biopsy is the only means of establishing the diagnosis of adenocarcinoma of the prostate. A normal ultrasound does not exclude the presence of carcinoma, and the study should only be used to assist in biopsy, not to determine if a biopsy should be performed. This decision is based on the presence of an elevated PSA and/or the presence of a prostate nodule. Of 12 cores obtained (6 on each side), three were positive on the right for Gleason 6 (3+3) adenocarcinoma of the prostate.

Sagittal Ultrasonogram

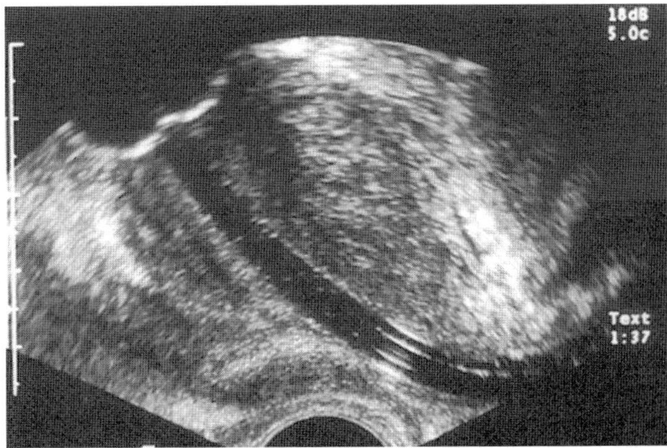

Figure 87.1

Sagittal Ultrasonography Report

Ultrasonogram is used to assist in biopsy.

Histopathologic Slide

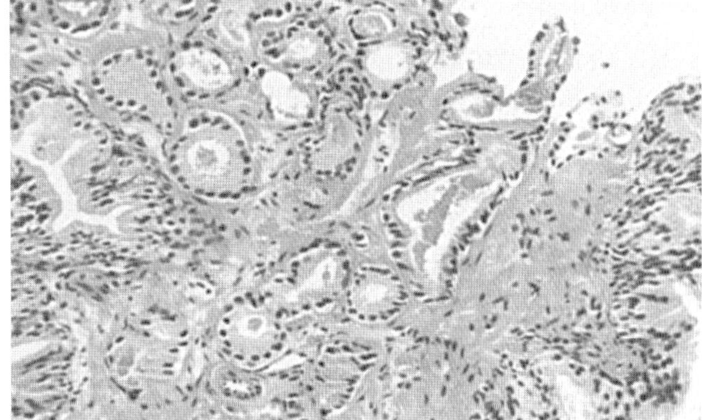

Figure 87.2

Histopathology Report

Histology demonstrates Gleason 6 (3+3) adenocarcinoma of the prostate.

Discussion

This patient with a Gleason 6 adenocarcinoma of the prostate, which is unilateral on biopsy, and a PSA <10.0 ng/mL has a high likelihood of having disease confined to the prostate. The likelihood of lymph node metastases is unlikely. It is unusual for bone metastasis to be present in patients with PSA levels <10, and therefore this study is not indicated. Additionally, because of the low likelihood of lymph node metastases, computed tomography (CT) scan and magnetic resonance imaging (MRI) are not indicated either. There is mixed evidence for the role of ultrasonography and endorectal MRI in determining the presence of extraprostatic disease; however, these studies have not been generally accepted for making this determination.

Approach

Treatment options vary and include observation, external-beam radiation therapy, brachytherapy, radical prostatectomy, and cryotherapy.

Observation with these findings would be considered in a patient with limited life expectancy, typically due to age or the existence of comorbid disease. Generally, if the patient has a life expectancy of >10 years, experience indicates that he would benefit from surgery or radiation therapy with the anticipation that his life would be extended.

Radiation therapy can be performed either with external beam or brachytherapy. Brachytherapy offers the advantage of being an outpatient procedure with no need for catherization and also avoids the need for repeated visits to the radiation therapy facility. It also appears that the side effects, particularly rectal irritation, are less than with external beam.

External-beam radiation therapy offers the advantage of being able to treat a wider field than is possible with brachytherapy, and it is typically utilized in patients requiring treatment of extraprostatic tissue. Some radiation therapists are combining brachytherapy and external beam to obtain the benefits of brachytherapy on delivering a high dose to the prostate and external beam to treat broader areas including the periprostatic tissue and possibly regional lymph nodes.

Radical prostatectomy is the other form of therapy used to cure these patients. The procedure can be performed either laparoscopically, retropubically, or by a perineal approach. All these approaches offer advantages and disadvantages; however, the goal is for the patient to have undergone complete prostate removal with maintenance of potency and continence. These statistics are impacted by patient age. Patients who are in their 50s have a 70% to 80% chance of maintaining potency; however, this falls significantly if the patient is older than 65 years of age. Incontinence rates are low; however, incontinence is severe in 1% to 2% of men and stress-related incontinence occurs in about 5% to 10%.

Cryotherapy is a relatively new therapy that continues to evolve technologically. Earlier reports were unsatisfactory due to associated high complication rates. Complications have been reduced with technological advances, but further follow-up is needed to assess the efficacy of this treatment when compared with the other standard treatment approaches.

Recommendation

Patients need to understand the pros and cons of the various treatment modalities. Most urologists favor radical prostatectomy because of the reduced local recurrence rate and the general well being of the patient.

Surgical Approach

The patient is placed in a modified lithotomy position. A 22F Foley catheter is placed. A lower midline incision is made. Modified bilateral pelvic lymph node metastases dissection is performed. If these lymph nodes show no evidence of metastatic disease, then radical prostatectomy is performed. Dissection proceeds in the space of Retzius. The puboprostatic ligaments, dorsal venous complex, and urethra are divided. With the prostate rotated up out of the pelvis, the vascular pedicle of the prostate is divided while preserving the neurovascular bundle. The bladder is entered, and after identifying the ureteric orifices, the prostate is resected. The bladder neck is reconstructed to create a stoma, following which a vesicourethral anastomosis is performed over an 18F Foley catheter.

Case Continued

The patient undergoes a radical prostatectomy. Pathologic analysis reveals a positive margin along the left lateral border of the prostate. Additionally, Gleason 7 (4+3) disease is noted to be present bilaterally. The patient undergoes follow-up examinations at 6-month intervals. At the first follow-up examination, his PSA level is in the undetectable range. However, by 1 year postoperatively, his PSA has risen to 0.3 ng/mL, and at 18 months is 0.6 ng/mL.

Approach

Various approaches exist for the individual who has developed recurrent disease. First, it is imperative that metastatic disease be differentiated from local recurrence. Of the various methods available to make this differentiation, the monoclonal antibody scanning technique known as ProstaScint (Cytogen Corporation, Princeton, NJ) has been useful, although positive and negative predictive values are problematic. The study is helpful if lymph nodes are negative, particularly if uptake is in the prostatic bed. Bone scans remain important in excluding bony metastases, in addition to laboratory studies such as PSA and alkaline phosphatase.

The differential diagnosis is differentiating local recurrence from distant metastatic disease, as both can result in an elevated PSA.

ProstaScint

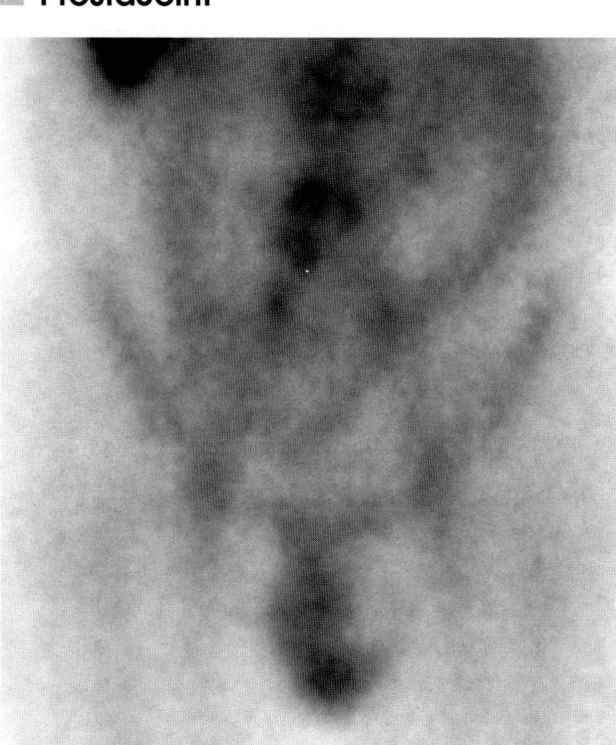

Figure 87.3

ProstaScint Report

Increased uptake in the prostatic bed with evidence of involvement of the pelvic lymph nodes. No evidence of metastatic disease to regional lymph nodes.

Case Continued

In view of the prior pathologic finding of the radical prostatectomy specimen, the prolonged period of an undetectable PSA following radical prostatectomy, and the slow rate of increase, the patient is believed to have localized disease. He receives radiation therapy to the prostatic bed.

The patient is administered 72 Gy and tolerates the treatment well. He has rectal and urinary irritability during therapy; however, 6 months after completion, he has had neither voiding nor rectal difficulties. Additionally, by 6 months, his PSA level returns to the undetectable range.

The patient is followed for another 2 years and remains disease free, until his PSA again begins to rise (0.8 ng/mL). Continued follow-up reveals a gradual rise in PSA so that by 3 years after radiation therapy, his PSA is 3.0 ng/mL.

Bone Scan

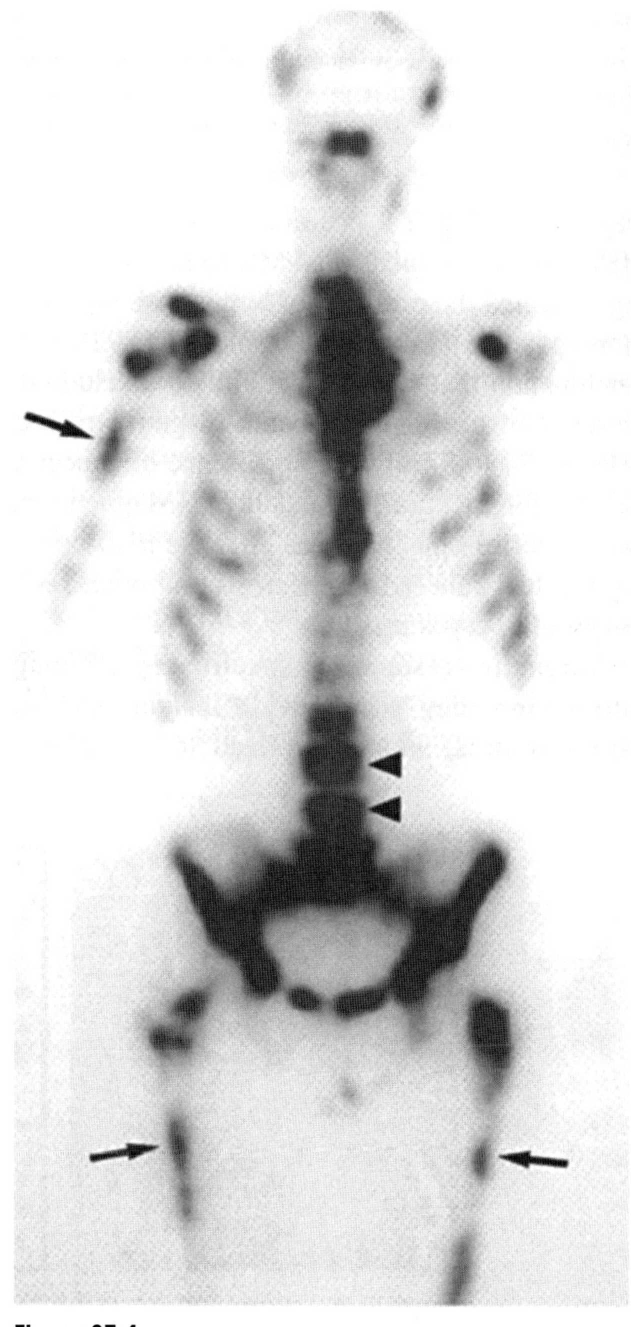

Figure 87.4

Bone Scan Report

Bone scan was normal, showing no evidence of metastatic disease.

Recommendation

The patient has recurrent disease that has not responded to radiation therapy. Multiple treatment options are available; however, the patient was followed with the anticipation that he would be placed on androgen-ablative therapy should his PSA increase consistently or be determined to have a short doubling time (e.g., <6 months).

Suggested Readings

Diblasio CJ, Kattan MW. Use of nomograms to predict the risk of disease recurrence after definitive local therapy for prostate cancer. *Urology* 2003;62(suppl 1):9–18.

Febbo PG, Sellers WR. Use of expression analysis to predict outcome after radical prostatectomy. *J Urol* 2003;170:S11–S19; discussion S19–S20.

Hu JC, Elkin EP, Pasta DJ, et al. Predicting quality of life after radical prostatectomy; results from CaPSURE. *J Urol* 2004;171:703–707, discussion 707–708.

Khan MA, Partin AW. Partin tables: past and present. *BJU Intl* 2003;92:7–11.

Khan MA, Partin AW, Mangold LA, et al. Probability of biochemical recurrence by analysis of pathologic stage, Gleason score, and margin status for localized prostate cancer. *Urology* 2003;62:866–871.

Naya Y, Slaton JW, Troncoso P, et al. Tumor length and location of cancer on biopsy predict for side specific extraprostatic cancer extension. *J Urol* 2004;171:1093–1097.

Singh H, Canto EI, Shariat SF, et al. Six additional systematic lateral cores enhance sextant biopsy prediction of pathological features at radical prostatectomy. *J Urol* 2004;171:204–209.

Stephenson AJ, Shariat SF, Zelefsky MJ, et al. Salvage radiotherapy for recurrent prostate cancer after radical prostatectomy. *JAMA* 2004;291:1325–1332.

Van Andel G, Visser AP, Zwinderman AH, et al. A prospective longitudinal study comparing the impact of external radiation therapy with radical prostatectomy on health related quality of life (HRQOL) in prostate cancer patients. *Prostate* 2004;58:354–365.

Presentation

A 53-year-old woman presents complaining of a 3-month history of fatigue, abdominal bloating, and persistent abdominal swelling such that she notes that her clothes do not fit. She has had a modest weight gain of about 10 pounds. She has noted some constipation but no pencil stools or melena. She has noted some mild nausea and decrease in appetite along with early satiety, but she denies emesis. Her family history is significant for a sister with breast carcinoma, diagnosed at the age of 47. A paternal aunt also has had breast cancer, at unknown age at diagnosis.

The abdominal examination shows moderate abdominal distension, with no enlarged liver or spleen, but there is a suspicion of a mass in the mid-epigastrium and there is a fluid wave. Pelvic examination shows normal external genitalia, bladder, urethra, and vagina. The cervix is grossly normal, and a Papanicolaou test is collected. On bimanual examination, there is a firm mass filling the cul-de-sac, not freely moveable, measuring about 15 cm in diameter. Rectovaginal examination shows the rectum to be deviated toward the right and densely adherent to this mass. Results of fecal occult blood tests (stool guaiac) are negative.

Differential Diagnosis

The differential diagnosis must include an adnexal neoplasm (benign, borderline, malignant, or metastatic), infectious causes such as tubo-ovarian abscess, appendiceal abscess, or diverticular abscess, uterine fibroid, or advanced bladder or colon neoplasm.

Discussion

Some relevant clues are revealed during this patient's history. Ovarian cancer does not have a pathognomic set of symptoms, but there are quantitative differences between the symptoms of healthy women attending a primary care clinic and women found to have ovarian carcinoma.

Ovarian cancer has often been called the "silent killer" because pathognomic symptoms are not recognized until late in the course of the disease. Recent data suggest that there are symptoms that antedate, often by several months, the diagnosis of ovarian cancer. These symptoms are not limited to women with advanced-stage ovarian cancer, thus offering some hope that early identification of telltale symptoms may help diagnose this lethal disease at an earlier, more treatable stage. The most common symptoms of ovarian cancer include bloating, increasing abdominal girth, abdominal pain, urinary urgency, and pelvic pain. The combination of bloating, increased abdominal size, and urinary urgency occurs in about half of ovarian cancer patients but in < 10% of patients attending primary care clinics. The symptoms are noted to be more severe and of shorter duration among women with ovarian cancer.

The family history in this patient is also worthy of further notice. Her sister and paternal aunt both suffered from breast cancer, and the sister was diagnosed at an early age. This family history is associated with an increased risk of carrying a BRCA1 or BRCA2 mutation within the family. This risk is substantially increased if ovarian cancer is also present within the family. Based upon her family history, the patient should be offered genetic counseling and testing for mutations in BRCA1 and BRCA2 if appropriate.

Her physical examination documents a palpable adnexal mass along with ascites and, possibly, a mass in the omentum. These findings mandate further evaluation. Testing for the CA 125 tumor marker should be ordered and an imaging study should be obtained. In cases in which the clinical suspicion of ovarian cancer is high, a computed tomography (CT) scan of the abdomen and pelvis is superior to an ultrasound. The CT scan allows evaluation of the retroperitoneal nodes, omentum, pancreas, liver, spleen, kidneys, and adrenals. Additionally, neoplasms of the stomach or colon are occasionally identified through critical evaluation of the CT images. Conversely, where the clinical suspicion of ovarian carcinoma is low, an ultrasound provides an inexpensive, low-risk method of characterizing an adnexal mass.

Case Continued

CA 125 level is elevated at 792.

■ CT Scans

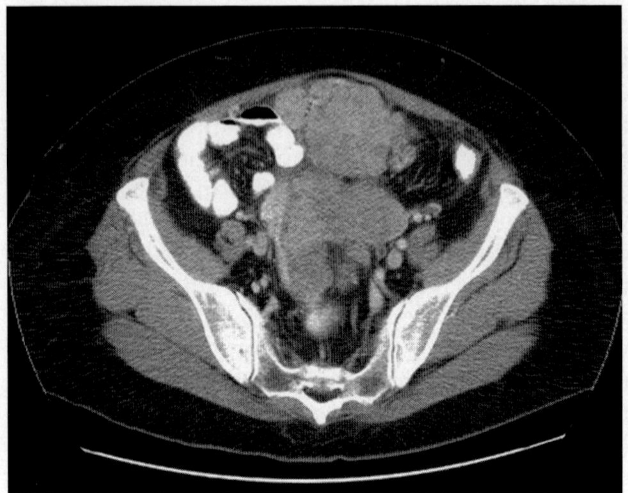

Figure 88.1A

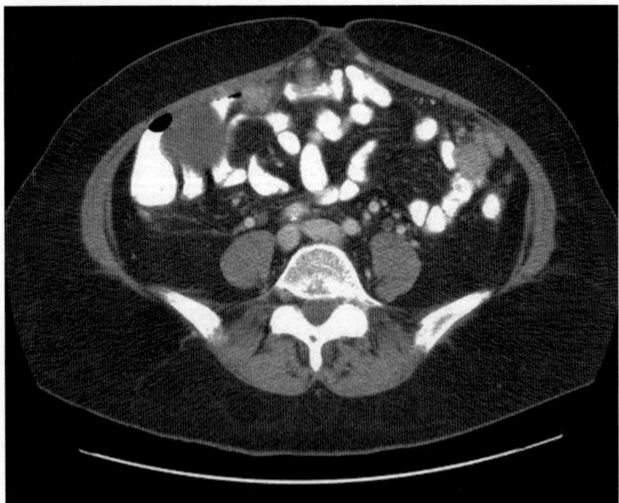

Figure 88.1B

CT Scan Report

Large pelvic mass associated with omental cake and extensive peritoneal and mesenteric metastatic implants. Distribution of disease is typical of ovarian carcinoma.

Diagnosis and Recommendation

The diagnosis appears to be ovarian cancer. The patient was offered exploratory laparotomy with total abdominal hysterectomy, bilateral salpingo-oophorectomy, omentectomy, and aggressive tumor debulking, possibly including a bowel resection or lymphadenectomy. The goals of the surgery are to confirm the diagnosis pathologically and debulk the tumor aggressively to minimal residual volume. Following recovery from surgery, the patient will need chemotherapy to treat residual disease.

■ Surgical Approach

A preoperative mechanical and antibiotic bowel preparation is ordered to allow resection of the distal colon if this proves to be necessary. The patient's abdomen is surgically explored through an adequate midline incision, taking care to rule out other primary disease such as pancreatic, gastric, or colorectal cancer. An overall assessment of the feasibility of resection is then performed. Because survival is inversely proportional to the quantity of residual disease, great effort is extended to resect as much as feasible. Typically, a total abdominal hysterectomy, bilateral salpingo-oophorectomy, and omentectomy are performed along with lymph node sampling and bowel resection where needed to provide complete debulking. At times, the argon-beam coagulator or cavitary ultrasonic surgical aspirator is helpful in ablating tumor that is coating peritoneal surfaces. In circumstances in which the upper abdomen is free of visible tumor, biopsies of multiple peritoneal surfaces, omentectomy, and lymph node sampling are performed to rule out occult metastasis. Because 30% of apparently early-stage ovarian cancers are metastatic to lymph nodes, pelvic and para-aortic lymph node sampling is a mandatory part of the evaluation of apparently early-stage ovarian cancer.

Discussion

Germ-cell ovarian tumors provide an exception to these rules. Most germ-cell tumors are unilateral, are highly responsive to chemotherapy, and typically occur in the second or third decade of life, when preservation of fertility is often strongly desired. Most ovarian germ-cell tumors should be treated by unilateral salpingo-oophorectomy with lymph node sampling, omentectomy, and tumor debulking, thus leaving the uterus and opposite adnexa in place for future fertility. Similarly, ovarian tumors of low malignant potential tend to occur among younger women, but in contrast to ovarian germ-cell tumors, they are not responsive to chemotherapy. Women with ovarian tumors of low malignant potential who desire to preserve fertility may have a procedure that conserves the uterus and the opposite adnexa; however, this approach is associated with a greater risk of recurrence.

Case Continued

The patient undergoes a total abdominal hysterectomy, bilateral salpingo-oophorectomy, omentectomy, and tumor debulking. A bowel resection is not deemed necessary and no enlarged lymph nodes are resected. The argon-beam coagulator is employed to ablate tumor implants on the bowel serosa, mesentery, and pelvic peritoneal surfaces. Residual implants under the right hemidiaphragm, measuring <1 cm in greatest diameter, are left in place. The patient is prepared for chemotherapy.

Approach

Combination chemotherapy is required in all cases of invasive epithelial ovarian cancer where residual disease is demonstrated or likely. This includes all advanced-stage cases. Early-stage ovarian cancer may be treated by surgery alone when the tumor is proven by an adequate staging operation to be limited to the ovaries, well differentiated, without large-volume ascites, and without dense adhesions requiring sharp dissection. Advanced-stage tumors and early-stage tumors not fitting these criteria are given platinum-based combination chemotherapy. Typically, six cycles are administered, once every 3 weeks, using an organic platinum derivative (either cisplatin or carboplatin) together with a taxane (paclitaxel or docetaxel). The most common side effects include nausea, alopecia, fatigue, myalgias, neutropenia, thrombocytopenia, and, over multiple cycles, peripheral neuropathy. Because epithelial ovarian tumors of low malignant potential do not respond to chemotherapy, these patients are not given chemotherapy, even when diagnosed at an advanced stage, unless metastasis with invasive implants is present. High-risk ovarian germ cell tumors are treated with four cycles of bleomycin, etoposide, and cisplatin (BEP) combination chemotherapy. Conversely, dysgerminomas or well-differentiated immature teratomas, when limited to the ovary, may be adequately treated with surgery alone, reserving chemotherapy for recurrent disease.

Discussion

Unfortunately, despite aggressive surgery and appropriate chemotherapy, the majority of patients with advanced-stage ovarian cancer experience recurrence and eventually die of their disease. In spite of this rather grim prognosis, appropriate management can prolong life and enhance quality of life. For women who present with advanced-stage epithelial ovarian cancer, the extent of primary debulking is the most important predictor of prolonged survival. Patients whose disease is rendered optimally debulked (defined as largest focus of residual disease no greater than 1 cm in diameter) enjoy a median survival time of 42 months, compared with those who had suboptimal debulking in whom the median survival time was only 18 months.

Another important predictor of long-term survival is a prompt and durable response to platinum-based chemotherapy. Approximately 10% of patients with advanced-stage ovarian carcinoma have disease that does not respond to primary chemotherapy and is unlikely to respond to any chemotherapy regimen. The prognosis for these patients is poor. Approximately 20% of patients have disease that responds to initial chemotherapy, only to return within a short follow-up interval of <6 months, implying resistance to platinum-based chemotherapy. These patients also have a poor prognosis, but may respond to a non-cross-resistant regimen. Drugs with activity in this population include liposomal doxorubicin, etoposide, topotecan, and gemcitabine. Patients who enjoyed a prolonged response to initial platinum-based therapy are likely to respond again to the same agents, particularly if the initial response lasted more than 24 months. These patients should receive a platinum/taxane combination.

Ovarian cancer remains the most lethal gynecologic malignancy among women in the industrialized world. The presenting symptoms are easily mistaken for common benign gastrointestinal or urologic conditions. Approximately 70% of cases present at an advanced stage. The diagnosis is usually suggested on examination and imaging, and confirmed at laparotomy. An aggressive initial debulking surgery followed by combination chemotherapy is essential to provide the best possible outcome for women with advanced-stage disease. This approach leads to a complete clinical response in about 70% of patients. Despite this, the majority of women with advanced-stage disease will experience recurrence and eventually die of their disease, with a median survival of about 4 years in women who receive optimal debulking at diagnosis.

Suggested Readings

Barnes-Kedar IM, Plon SE. Counseling the at risk patient in the BRCA1 and BRCA2 era. *Obstet Gynecol Clin North Am* 2002;29:341–366, vii.

Bristow RE, Tomacruz RS, Armstrong DK, et al. Survival effect of maximal cytoreductive surgery for advanced ovarian carcinoma during the platinum era: a meta-analysis. *J Clin Oncol* 2002;20:1248–1259.

Goff BA, Mandel LS, Melancon CH, et al. Frequency of symptoms of ovarian cancer in women presenting to primary care clinics. *JAMA* 2004;291:2705–2712.

Jeong YY, Outwater EK, Kang HK. Imaging evaluation of ovarian masses. *Radiographics* 2000;20:1445–1470.

Low JJ, Perrin LC, Crandon AJ, et al. Conservative surgery to preserve ovarian function in patients with malignant ovarian germ cell tumors. A review of 74 cases. *Cancer* 2000;89:391–398.

Morice P, Camatte S, El Hassan J, et al. Clinical outcomes and fertility after conservative treatment of ovarian borderline tumors. *Fertil Steril* 2001;75:92–96.

Ozols RF, Bundy BN, Greer BE, et al. Phase III trial of carboplatin and paclitaxel compared with cisplatin and paclitaxel in patients with optimally resected stage III ovarian cancer: a Gynecologic Oncology Group study. *J Clin Oncol* 2003; 21:3194–3200.

Williams S, Blessing JA, Liao SY, et al. Adjuvant therapy of ovarian germ cell tumors with cisplatin, etoposide, and bleomycin: a trial of the Gynecologic Oncology Group. *J Clin Oncol* 1994;12:701–706.

Presentation

The patient is a 22-year-old nulligravid woman who presents to the emergency room with a sudden onset of right lower quadrant pain. Her urinary pregnancy test is negative; however, she has an elevated white blood cell (WBC) count, right lower quadrant pain with guarding, rebound, and a low-grade fever to 38.2°C. She is admitted to the general surgery service where she is observed to rule out appendicitis. Her abdominal examination becomes more tender, with guarding and rebound tenderness, and she is taken to surgery for a laparotomy, during which an inflamed appendix is identified and resected. A 4-cm right ovarian cyst is identified. An intraoperative consultation is requested of the gynecology service.

◼ Intraoperative Image

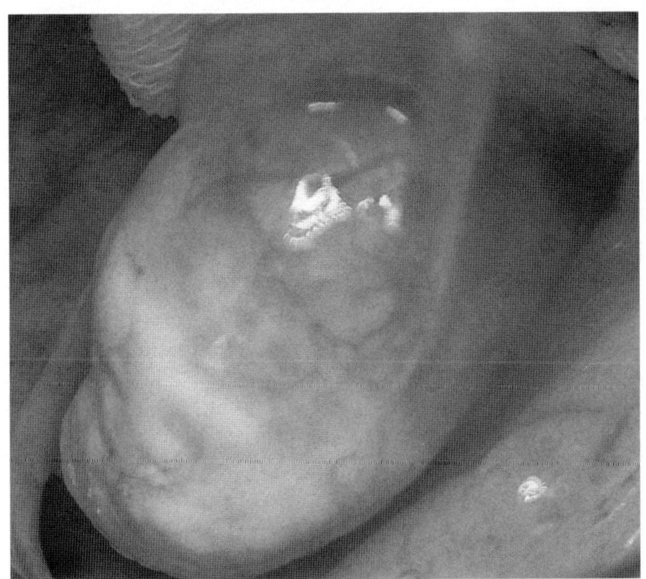

Figure 89.1

Intraoperative Report

The gynecologic consultant carefully inspects and transilluminates the ovarian mass. It is small and appears to be a simple cystic mass without solid elements.

Differential Diagnosis

The differential diagnosis of an adnexal mass is quite extensive (Table 89.1); however, a simple cystic ovarian mass is most commonly a functional cyst or, less likely, a benign cystadenoma. Small, cystic adnexal masses that do not contain any solid elements are unlikely to be malignancies. Functional cysts typically are smaller than 5 cm in diameter and invariably resolve spontaneously with observation, usually within 1 or 2 menstrual cycles. Benign cystadenomas may be small or large, but do not spontaneously resolve. These lesions will eventually require surgical resection because they may grow or cause torsion of the adnexa. For the patient in this case, surgical resection was not indicated due to the absence of a definite diagnosis and the patient's informed consent.

Discussion

Gynecologists occasionally are asked to consult intraoperatively when an unexpected adnexal mass is discovered. The absence of a preoperative evaluation and physician-patient relationship creates a dilemma for the consultant, particularly if the patient is of reproductive age. On the one hand, the patient may have a disease process that is best treated by surgical resection. On the other hand, surgical resection can compromise fertility. When an adnexal mass is unexpectedly discovered, the patient has no opportunity to be offered an informed consent, and yet deferring treatment until a later time causes even greater morbidity. For these reasons, it is

Table 89.1: Differential Diagnosis of an Incidental Adnexal Mass

Category	Condition
Pregnancy related	Ectopic pregnancy
	Abdominal pregnancy
	Theca-lutein cysts
Infectious	Pelvic inflammatory disease
Tubo-ovarian abscess	
	Tuberculous abscess
	Actinomyces (typically associated with intrauterine device or foreign body)
	Gastrointestinal: appendiceal abscess, diverticulitis
	Parasitic: hydatid cysts
Inflammatory	Endometriosis
	Hydrosalpinx
	Peritoneal pseudocyst
	Inflammatory bowel disease
	Autoimmune
Functional	Corpus luteum cyst, hemorrhagic
	Ovarian hyperstimulation
	Massive ovarian edema
	Hydronephrosis
	Transplant kidney
Postsurgical	Postsurgical abscess
	Urinoma
	Lymphocyst
	Retained foreign body (surgical sponge)
Developmental	Bicornuate uterus with obstructed outflow tract
	Transverse vaginal septum with obstructed outflow tract
	Pelvic kidney
	Gartner's duct cyst
	Vascular: arteriovenous malformation, aneurysm
Neoplastic: benign	Germ cell: teratoma
	Epithelial: serous, mucinous, endometrioid, clear-cell, Brenner
	Stromal: fibroma/thecoma
	Uterine fibroids: uterine, broad ligament, parasitic
	Paratubal cysts
	Neurofibromatosis
Neoplastic: low malignant potential	Epithelial: serous, mucinous, endometrioid
	Stromal: granulosa cell
Neoplastic: Malignant	Ovarian epithelial
	Ovarian germ cell
	Ovarian stromal
	Uterine, ovarian, or soft-tissue sarcoma
	Metastatic: other reproductive, gastrointestinal, breast, melanoma, gestational trophoblastic disease
	Primary gastrointestinal: appendix, colorectal, small bowel (gastrointestinal stromal tumor)
	Lymphoma
	Primary bladder neoplasm

important to avoid, as much as possible, the situation where an adnexal mass is found incidentally, particularly in fertile, premenopausal women. Despite everyone's best efforts, the clinician must be prepared to care for patients with adnexal masses discovered incidentally at laparotomy.

Recommendation

Evaluate the urgency of the patient's clinical condition first to determine if surgical resection is necessary. In the absence of an emergent situation, thorough exploration of the peritoneal cavity and pelvis should be performed to exclude the presence of metastatic disease. The ovarian mass is evaluated to determine the presence of any malignant features.

Approach

The approach to the management of an incidentally discovered adnexal mass can be simplified if the patient can be assigned into one of the following categories. (a) Postmenopausal women, or women who have irreversibly completed their childbearing, are less likely to desire fertility preservation. These women should have their medical condition treated without limitation based upon fertility concerns. (b) Acutely life-threatening events and severe illnesses that cause great pain or carry substantial risk of progression to an acutely life-threatening event need to be treated, even if fertility is compromised. (c) Malignant neoplasms or neoplasms of low malignant potential need adequate diagnosis and staging, but because of the absence of informed consent, every effort should be made to preserve fertility. (d) Benign conditions that are not expected to resolve spontaneously should be treated when treatment only minimally affects fertility or when the diagnosis of a malignancy is seriously entertained and cannot be resolved without surgical resection. (e) Prophylactic resection of healthy organs should not be performed without a prospectively obtained patient's informed consent.

Discussion

The most urgent indication for adnexal surgery is treatment of shock caused by an adnexal source. This situation is only rarely encountered incidentally. The typical adnexal causes of shock include hemorrhagic shock from a ruptured ectopic pregnancy or septic shock from a ruptured tubo-ovarian abscess. Treatment of shock associated with a ruptured ectopic pregnancy requires resection of the

ectopic pregnancy to control hemorrhage, along with replacement of blood and clotting factors. Similarly, septic shock from a ruptured tubo-ovarian abscess should be treated by urgent salpingo-oophorectomy and, where necessary, further resection of involved structures. In the absence of shock, there is less urgency regarding treatment and a more conservative approach is safe and warranted, such as draining the abscess cavity with decortication of the abscess wall.

The second most urgent indication for adnexal surgery is treatment of severe but not acutely life-threatening processes associated with severe pain, which risk progression to a life-threatening process or where surgical treatment improves the outcome. Examples include adnexal torsion, unruptured ectopic pregnancy, or tubo-ovarian abscess. In general, the gynecologist should manage women who have completed childbearing or who are post-menopausal without regard for preservation of fertility, whereas women likely to desire preservation of fertility should have the minimal resection adequate to correct the lesion. For women anxious to preserve fertility, tubo-ovarian abscess may be safely treated by abscess drainage or unilateral salpingo-oophorectomy if the patient is clinically stable. Unruptured ectopic pregnancy may be treated by segmental resection or salpingostomy. Alternatively, if the diagnosis of ectopic pregnancy is unclear, the adnexa should be left untreated, as medical treatment is possible with methotrexate. Adnexal torsion may be treated by untwisting the affected adnexa and performing a cystectomy of the ipsilateral adnexal cyst; salpingo-oophorectomy is necessary only for women who have suffered necrosis of the twisted adnexa.

A common reason for intraoperative consultation for an incidental adnexal mass is the concern for a malignant neoplasm. It is worth noting that the incidence of epithelial ovarian cancer is low in women of reproductive age, and most of these tumors are of low malignant potential. In a review of the Swedish tumor registry of over 10,000 women who underwent surgery for adnexal masses, only 1.4% of women aged 15 to 40 had malignant ovarian tumors while 38% had functional cysts or paratubal cysts. The incidence rate of ovarian cancer in this age group was calculated at 3.2 of 100,000 women-years of observation. Clearly, many women in this cohort were subjected to surgery for lesions with a very low risk of cancer. In the absence of informed consent, a more compelling risk of cancer should be present before fertility-compromising adnexal surgery is performed.

The intraoperative assessment of an incidentally discovered adnexal mass should include an assessment of the malignant potential of the lesion. Generally, a malignant ovarian tumor is both solid and cystic. Although this may be appreciated by palpation or transillumination, the accuracy of intraoperative evaluation for malignancy remains poor. Occasionally, malignant tumors have dense adhesions, ascites, or surface excrescences. However, ovarian fibromas are benign solid tumors with a complex surface that is easily confused with surface excrescences. The presence of metastasis to abdominal peritoneal surfaces, retroperitoneal nodes, or the omentum confirms a frankly malignant neoplasm or a neoplasm of low malignant potential. Pathologic confirmation of the gross appearance by frozen section is recommended prior to definitive surgical treatment. Although little published data exist, intraoperative ultrasound may prove useful for urgent evaluation of the malignant potential of an incidentally discovered adnexal mass.

For women beyond reproductive age, appropriate treatment of a malignant epithelial ovarian tumor requires total abdominal hysterectomy, bilateral salpingo-oophorectomy, omentectomy, and tumor debulking with the goal of maximal resection of tumor. If the patient has palpably enlarged lymph nodes, or if peritoneal metastases are absent or smaller than 2 cm in diameter, the patient should also have a pelvic and para-aortic lymph node dissection performed for debulking and staging purposes. Women who wish to preserve fertility may be treated by resecting the involved adnexa and debulking the remaining tumor while leaving the opposite adnexa and/or uterus intact. This approach preserves fertility while awaiting a final pathologic diagnosis and is particularly appropriate for tumors of low malignant potential or of low grade and early stage.

Germ-cell neoplasms of the ovary occur almost exclusively in young women who have not yet completed childbearing. Grossly they are solid ovarian tumors and, with the exception of dysgerminomas, they are typically unilateral. These neoplasms are highly sensitive to multiagent chemotherapy. The intraoperative finding of a solid unilateral adnexal mass in a young woman should be treated by ovarian resection and frozen section. Most often, these lesions will be a benign stromal neoplasm such as a fibroma. If an ovarian germ-cell malignancy is identified, the uterus and opposite adnexa should be left in place but a retroperitoneal lymph node dissection, omentectomy, and staging biopsy should be performed. In those rare cases when bilateral dysgerminomas are identified incidentally and the patient's wishes regarding fertility cannot be obtained, the larger lesion should be resected and the smaller ovarian mass should be left in place and treated with chemotherapy.

Endometriosis is a common nonmalignant cause of severe pelvic pain and a pelvic mass. Because endometriosis has a variety of management strategies, ranging from hormonal suppression to complete extirpation of reproductive organs, the surgeon discovering endometriosis incidentally should be conservative. Treatment should range from biopsy alone, simply to prove the diagnosis, to ovarian cystectomy with excision of involved lesions.

Most incidental adnexal masses are benign asymptomatic lesions. The most common lesions include benign serous cystadenomas, mature cystic teratomas, paratubal cysts, and functional ovarian cysts. In women of reproductive age, it can be very difficult to grossly differentiate between a functional ovarian cyst and a benign serious cystadenoma. In premenopausal women in whom the lesion is <5 cm in diameter, observation is appropriate because many lesions are functional cysts that resolve spontaneously. Fertility following ovarian cystectomy can be reduced due to postsurgical adhesions to the ovary or ipsilateral fallopian tube. These adhesions can be minimized with bioresorbable membranes. A cystectomy or oophorectomy is warranted for ovarian cysts larger than 5 cm in size, with solid elements, or in postmenopausal women.

Surgical Approach

If the decision is made to proceed with an ovarian cystectomy, this involves careful dissection in the plane between the ovary and the incidentally discovered mass, which is then sent for frozen section. Alternatively, if a unilateral oophorectomy is to be performed, the broad ligament is opened in the region of the ovarian vessels, which can be transected between clamps and ligated or secured with a linear stapling device. The ovary along with the mass is resected en bloc and sent for frozen section. Further surgical resection will depend on the results of the frozen section.

Case Continued

The gynecologic consultant chose not to resect the adnexal mass, but asked the patient to have a followup pelvic ultrasound and physical examination in 2 months. At that time, the mass had spontaneously resolved, as confirmed on examination and ultrasound. No further management was recommended.

Discussion

Discovery of an incidental adnexal mass poses ethical and medical challenges for the consulting gynecologist. For women desiring future pregnancies, it is important to establish a diagnosis and treat the abnormality with as little impact on fertility as possible. Although postmenopausal women are often less concerned about fertility, they may be reluctant to have their reproductive organs removed. The consultant must carefully balance the certainty of benefit with the loss of autonomy the patient must suffer when surgical treatment is performed in the emergency setting without an informed consent. When it is impossible to obtain an informed consent from the patient, the gynecologic surgeon should seek the consent of a surrogate decision maker, if possible. Even with the consent of a surrogate decision maker, in the absence of the patient's informed consent, surgery on the reproductive tract should be limited to the mini-mum resection necessary in order to minimize risk and consequences to fertility.

Suggested Readings

Dietrich M, Osmers RG, Grobe G, et al. Limitations of the evaluation of adnexal masses by its macroscopic aspects, cytology and biopsy. *Eur J Obstet Gynecol Reprod Biol* 1999;82:57–62.

Gillon R. Medical ethics: four principles plus attention to scope. *BMJ* 1994;309:184–188.

Low JJ, Perrin LC, Crandon AJ, et al. Conservative surgery to preserve ovarian function in patients with malignant ovarian germ cell tumors. A review of 74 cases. *Cancer* 2000;89:391–398.

Nelson L, Ekbom A, Gerdin E. Ovarian cancer in young women in Sweden, 1989-1991. *Gynecol Oncol* 1999;74:472–476.

Oelsner G, Cohen SB, Soriano D, et al. Minimal surgery for the twisted ischemic adnexa can preserve ovarian function. *Hum Reprod* 2003;18:2599–2602.

case 90

The patient is a 76-year old man who is referred by a medical oncologist for possible splenectomy. He presents with vague abdominal discomfort and thrombocytopenia. The patient denies weight loss, fever, or night sweats. Past medical history is significant for hypertension, coronary artery disease, and gastroesophageal reflux. Physical examination reveals no lymphadenopathy. The spleen is enlarged and easily palpated. It is nontender. The patient has had a complete blood cell (CBC) count, bone marrow evaluation, a computed tomography (CT) scan, and magnetic resonance imaging (MRI) of the abdomen.

CBC revealed hemoglobin of 12.7, white count of 7.3, and platelets of 65,000.

Peripheral smear is significant for normochromic normocytic red cells and absence of schistocytes, spherocytes, or poikilocytes. There is no evidence of lymphocytosis or atypical lymphocytes, monocytosis, or overt dysplastic changes. Absolute lymphocyte count is 2,000; moderate thrombocytopenia with normal size platelets is noted without platelet aggregates. Bone marrow biopsy was noncontributory to the diagnosis.

CT Scan

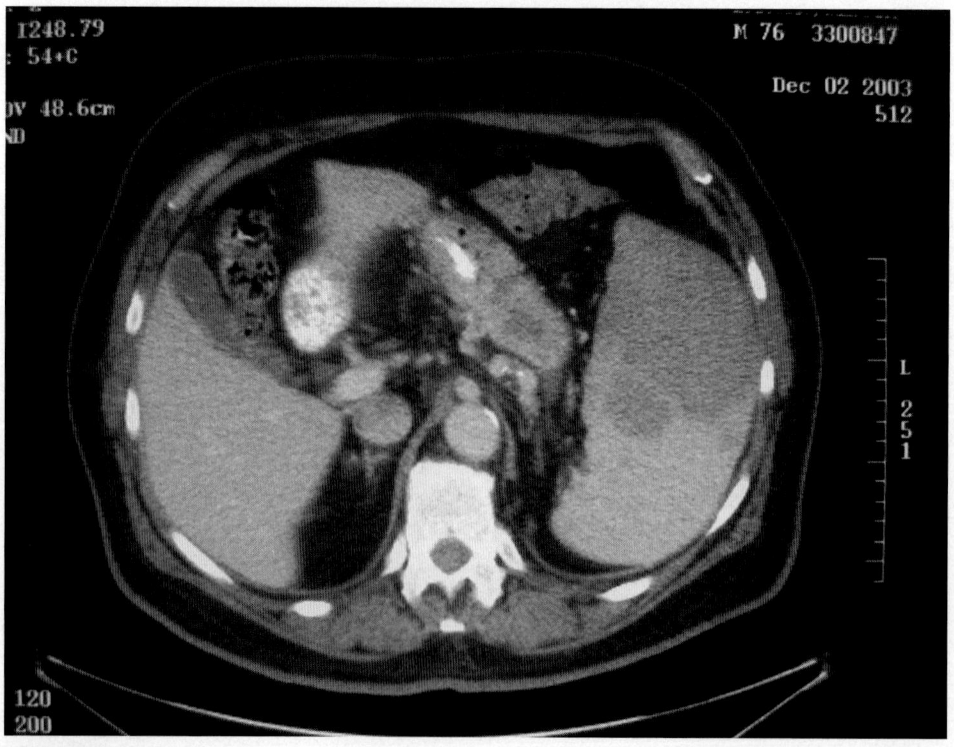

Figure 90.1A

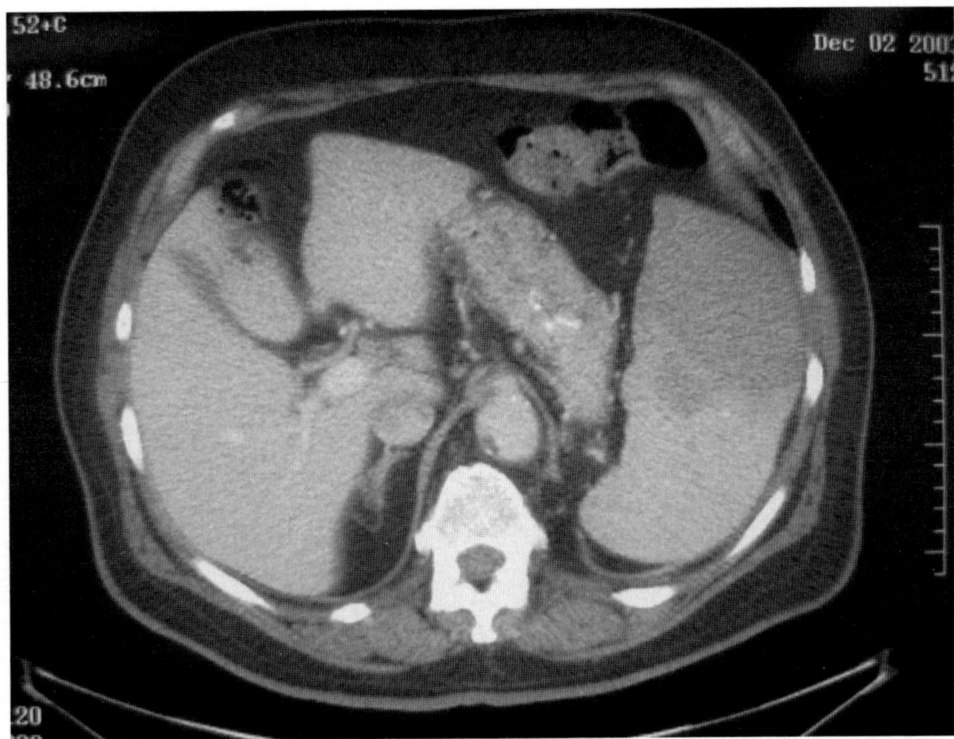

Figure 90.1B

CT Scan Report

The CT scan shows an enlarged and heterogeneous spleen. No evidence of lymphadenopathy is seen within the chest, abdomen, or pelvis. Minimal bilateral pleural effusions are shown.

▨ MRI

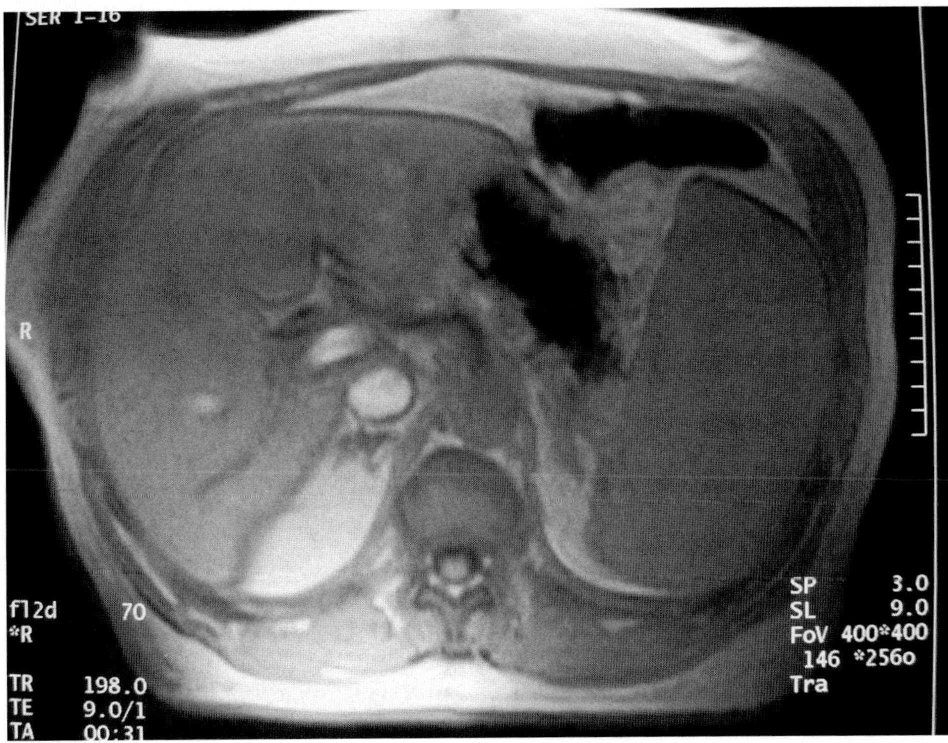

Figure 90.2A

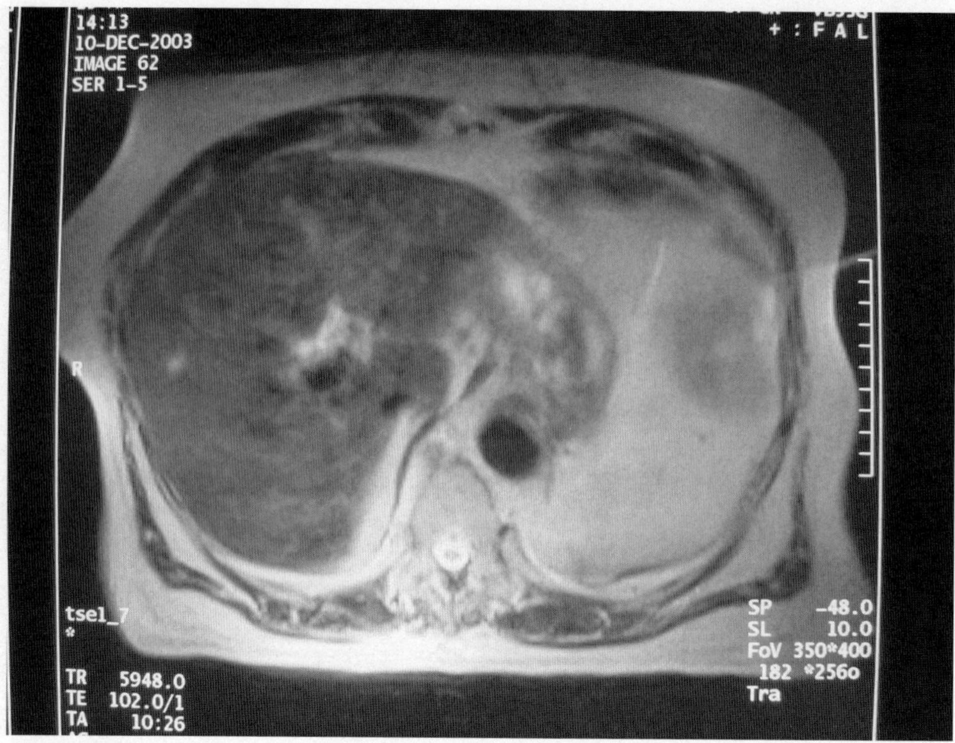

Figure 90.2B

MRI Report

MRI shows an enlarged spleen measuring 17 cm in maximum anterior-posterior (AP) diameter. On T2-weighted images, there is a 10-cm area of hypointense signal suggestive of an infiltrative mass.

Differential Diagnosis

The differential diagnosis for splenomegaly, within the context of the CT and MRI findings, includes hematologic malignancy, specifically lymphoma, a splenic infiltrative or inflammatory process, and primary or metastatic splenic tumor.

Discussion

The possible etiologies of splenomegaly are extensive and can include infectious causes (viral, bacterial, parasitic), and congestive (heart failure, cirrhosis, portal or splenic venous thrombosis), malignant (lymphomas, leukemias, polycythemia vera, multiple myeloma, agnogenic myeloid metaplasia, primary and metastatic tumors), inflammatory (sarcoid, systemic lupus erythematosus, Felty syndrome), infiltrative (amyloid, Gaucher disease, Niemann-Pick disease, glycogen storage disease), and hypersplenic states (hemolytic anemias, sickle cell diseases)

Because the spleen normally participates in the filtering of senescent red blood cells (RBCs), bacteria, and debris, as well as sequestration of the normal circulating pool of platelets (up to one third), any increase in function (hypersplenism) may be manifested by varying degrees of anemia, thrombocytopenia, or pancytopenia.

This patient presents with clinical, laboratory, and imaging data that suggest a disease process attributed to the spleen, with secondary thrombocytopenia as a result of splenomegaly. The heterogeneous attenuation suggests differential splenic perfusion, which could be due to ischemia, an infarct, or a space-occupying lesion in the spleen. Lack of systemic complaints makes an infectious etiology less likely. There is no clinical evidence of cirrhosis or congestive heart failure. A hematologic malignancy must be suspected.

Recommendation

Indications for splenectomy can be characterized as diagnostic, therapeutic, or both. Therapeutic splenectomy is performed for refractory cytopenias or to relieve bulk symptoms from the enlarged spleen. The latter include abdominal pain and early satiety. The primary indication for splenectomy in this patient is diagnostic, with a suspicion of hematologic malignancy. Secondary benefits are likely to include relief of the abdominal discomfort and resolution of the thrombocytopenia. The patient was advised to undergo splenectomy via a left subcostal incision. Procedure-specific risks were discussed, including postoperative hemorrhage, pancreatic or gastric injury, subphrenic abscess, and wound infection. Also discussed was the increased susceptibility to certain bacterial infections in the asplenic state and the use of prophylactic vaccinations.

Surgical Approach

An open approach to splenectomy was undertaken due to splenic size and the potential malignant process. A left subcostal incision was created and abdominal exploration revealed bulky splenomegaly with enlarged pathologic hilar lymph nodes. A mass was palpable within the spleen and corresponded to the abnormality noted on MRI. The lesser sac was entered below the gastroepiploic arcade to expose the pancreatic body. The splenic artery was identified at the superior border of the pancreas, encircled, and ligated without division. The gastrosplenic ligament was divided up to the short gastric vessels. The spleen and pancreas were then fully mobilized to the midline. The short gastric vessels were divided. The splenic hilar vessels were then clamped and divided, with care to avoid injury to the tail of the pancreas. After specimen removal, the operative field was carefully inspected for hemostasis.

Case Continued

The patient tolerated the procedure well, was transferred to the floor postoperatively, and discharged in stable condition on postoperative day 4. Outpatient follow-up was scheduled with the hematology/oncology service. The pathology report returned as non-Hodgkin B-cell lymphoma, follicular small cleaved cell type (grade 1) involving spleen and splenic hilar lymph nodes.

Discussion

There are many types of non-Hodgkin lymphoma with numerous clinical presentations. Indolent lymphomas may not require treatment. Localized disease is sometimes treated with radiation alone. However, most lymphomas are systemic and require chemotherapy with or without radiation. Although splenomegaly is not uncommon in association with lymphoma, most patients will not require splenectomy. Candidates for splenectomy include those presenting with the spleen as the primary site of disease, refractory cytopenias, or bulk symptoms from persistent splenomegaly, and patients with splenomegaly and undiagnosed but suspected lymphoma. Splenectomy for lymphoma should be accomplished with minimal morbidity and mortality and an expected hospital stay of 3 to 4 days.

Presentation: Case 90B

The hematology service refers a 74-year-old man with polycythemia vera, to be considered for splenectomy. He is in the "burnt out" phase of his disease and has had multiple admissions for transfusion-dependent refractory anemia. Past medical history is notable for hypertension. Recently, the patient developed symptoms of early satiety, weight loss, and exertional dyspnea. Physical examination reveals no jaundice or ascites, but a markedly enlarged, nontender spleen.

Differential Diagnosis

The differential diagnosis for symptomatic massive splenomegaly and a history of polycythemia vera includes myelofibrosis with extramedullary hematopoiesis, infection, and hematologic malignancy (lymphoma/leukemia).

Discussion

This patient presents with refractory anemia and bulk symptoms related to massive splenomegaly. The latter include gastric compression with early satiety and weight loss, and diaphragm displacement with exertional dyspnea. Anemia and high-output congestive heart failure related to increased flow through the splenic artery may also contribute to respiratory compromise. With polycythemia vera, the spleen may act as a site of extramedullary hematopoiesis, resulting in progressive splenic enlargement. This is the most likely scenario in this case. Evaluation should include CBC and bone marrow biopsy. Given the history of polycythemia vera, causes of splenomegaly other than hematologic disease would be uncommon. Splenectomy should be considered to potentially decrease transfusion requirements and relieve bulk symptoms. A CT scan may be obtained for further evaluation of the spleen.

Recommendation

Bone marrow biopsy, CBC count, and CT scan of the abdomen and pelvis.

Case Continued

The CBC count revealed hemoglobin of 7.3, hematocrit of 26.3, white cell count of 8,600, and platelet count of 366,000. Bone marrow aspiration and biopsy revealed a hypercellular marrow with marked megakaryocytic and erythroid hyperplasia. Myelocyte series showed full maturation but with 10% blasts seen. Cytogenetic study showed no further abnormalities. CT scan was obtained.

CT Scan

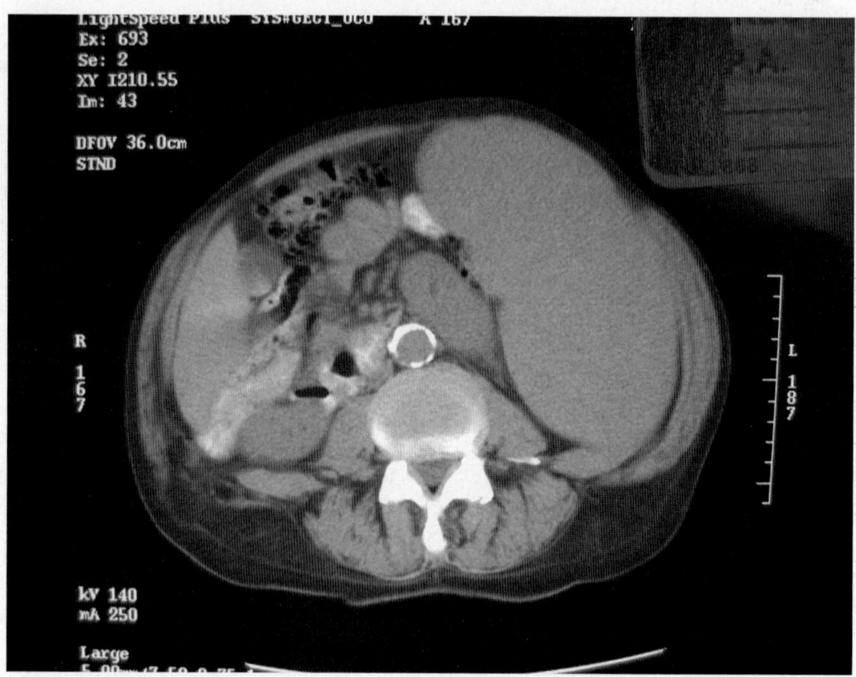

Figure 90.3A

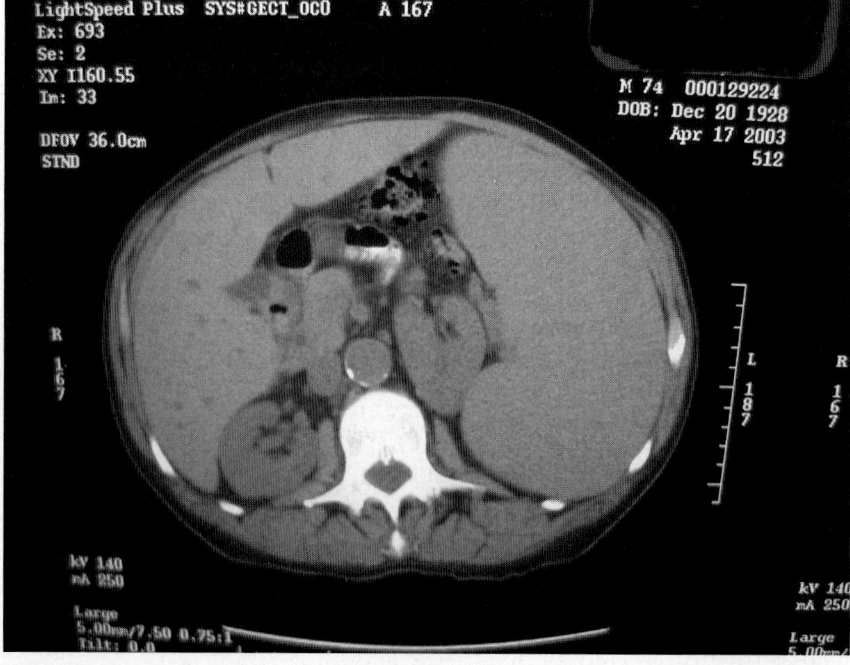

Figure 90.3B

CT Scan Report

The CT scan shows massive splenomegaly measuring 25 cm in craniocaudal dimension, with possible infarct in the periphery of the spleen and associated mass effect on adjacent intra-abdominal structures. Extensive diverticulosis is present.

Diagnosis and Recommendation

This patient has a chronic myeloproliferative disorder, polycythemia vera, with associated massive splenomegaly. In the "burned out" phase of polycythemia vera, RBC life span is markedly decreased. This, in combination with splenomegaly from extramedullary hematopoiesis, has resulted in a transfusion-dependent refractory anemia. In addition, the patient has developed significant bulk symptoms from the enlarged spleen. Splenectomy is offered to relieve symptoms and reduce the transfusion requirement. Risks of surgery include hemorrhage, infection, injury to adjacent organs, and thrombosis. The patient should receive standard splenectomy vaccines preoperatively. Antiplatelet and/or low-dose heparin therapy may be required postoperatively.

Surgical Approach

The size of the spleen necessitates open splenectomy. Standard approaches include midline or left subcostal incision. Choice of incision is related to age, body habitus, and prior abdominal surgery. Midline incisions may be more appropriate in younger patients to avoid abdominal wall weakness or numbness. The subcostal approach facilitates splenectomy in obese patients and those with a wide costal angle. After complete abdominal exploration, the lesser sac is entered below the gastroepiploic arcade to expose the pancreas. The splenic artery is encircled at the superior border of the pancreas and ligated without division. This maneuver quickly decreases the size of the spleen and reduces bleeding during mobilization. The gastrosplenic ligament is divided and the spleen and pancreas are mobilized to the midline. The short gastric vessels are controlled and divided. The vessels in the splenic hilum are then controlled and divided with removal of the specimen.

Case Continued

The patient suffered no hemorrhagic or thrombotic complications and recovered uneventfully. He is discharged on postoperative day 3 with scheduled hematology and surgery follow-up. Pathology reveals marked extramedullary hematopoiesis with fibrosis. Small infarcts were present. The spleen weighed 1,739 g and measured 25 × 15 × 7.3 cm in greatest dimension.

Discussion

Polycythemia vera is a chronic myeloproliferative disorder characterized by erythrocytosis, an elevated RBC mass, due to clonal proliferation of myeloid cells in the bone marrow. Physical examination usually reveals splenomegaly and often hepatomegaly. Characteristic laboratory findings include an elevated hematocrit, thrombocytosis, and leukocytosis. With aggressive treatment, survival often exceeds 10 years. Patients with polycythemia have a predisposition to myelofibrotic transformation over time and may develop myelofibrosis with myeloid metaplasia, or acute myeloid leukemia. Death can result from thrombotic complications, hematologic malignancy, or infection. Medical treatment may include phlebotomy, hydroxyurea, busulfan, and antiplatelet agents. With appropriate perioperative management, splenectomy can be safely performed. Attention must be given to potential thrombotic complications, as well as the risk of blast transformation or acceleration. Published series report mortality of 8% to 9% and morbidity of 31% to 40%, with hemorrhagic/thrombotic complications in about 17% of patients. When splenectomy is performed in the setting of anemia, improvement of anemia is seen in about 50% at 1 year.

This patient underwent splenectomy for polycythemia vera in "burnt out" phase with refractory anemia, massive splenomegaly secondary to extramedullary hematopoiesis, and significant compressive symptoms. In patients who are not surgical candidates, splenic irradiation may be considered.

Presentation: Case 90C

A 53-year-old woman with a history of myelofibrosis and myeloid metaplasia is referred for splenectomy. The duration of her disease is 27 years. She has had a chronically enlarged spleen and now presents with disease progression. One month prior to her visit she was seen by her hematologist with weakness and dyspnea on exertion. She was noted to have a massively enlarged spleen. Laboratory evaluation revealed hemoglobin of 7.3, white cell count of 14,000, and platelet count of 1,000,000. She was started on busulfan and received 2 units of packed RBCs. She was re-evaluated 3 days prior to this visit, at which time she continued to have massive splenomegaly with a hemoglobin of 8.6, white blood cell count of 3,020, and platelet count of 276,000. She received two more units of packed RBCs and splenectomy was recommended. At this visit, she notes left upper quadrant discomfort, abdominal distention, and dyspnea on exertion. Physical examination of the abdomen reveals a markedly enlarged spleen extending across the midline and into the pelvis. The liver is not enlarged. There were no signs of portal hypertension or ascites.

Differential Diagnosis

Massive splenomegaly is frequently associated with myelofibrosis and myeloid metaplasia secondary to extramedullary hematopoiesis. Other causes of splenomegaly in this clinical scenario would be unlikely.

Discussion

This patient presents with symptomatic massive splenomegaly due to the progression of a chronic myeloproliferative disorder. Myelofibrosis and myeloid metaplasia (MFMM) is characterized by bone marrow fibrosis and extramedullary hematopoiesis in the spleen, liver, and lymph nodes. Although absent in this patient, hepatomegaly is seen in about 50% of cases. The most common initial laboratory abnormality is anemia. The white blood cell count and platelet count may be normal, elevated, or low. Busulfan or hydroxyurea may be used in patients with marked thrombocytosis.

The course of MFMM is that of progressive splenomegaly that leads to compressive symptoms. Portal hypertension and its associated complications may develop. Acute leukemic transformation may occur as a terminal event.

Recommendation

Administer standard preoperative splenectomy vaccines and proceed with splenectomy.

Surgical Approach

An upper midline incision was utilized. The gastrosplenic ligament was divided and the splenic artery was ligated at the superior border of the pancreas prior to splenic mobilization. The remainder of the procedure was completed as previously described.

With markedly enlarged spleens, care must be taken to avoid traction injuries of the pancreas.

Case Continued

The hospital course is unremarkable and the patient is discharged on postoperative day 4. Pathology revealed an enlarged spleen measuring $28.5 \times 17 \times 8.9$ cm and weighing 2,304 g. The spleen and six hilar lymph nodes demonstrate extramedullary hematopoiesis. The patient is feeling well, with relief of symptoms 6 weeks after splenectomy. A CBC count shows a hemoglobin of 11.1, white count of 7,230, and platelet count of 357,000. She remains clinically stable 1 year after surgery. At 1 year, the hemoglobin is 11 and the platelet count is 588,000. However, the white count rose to 89,000 with 35% polymorphs, 15% lymphocytes, 7% monocytes, and 43% eosinophils. She is started on interferon.

Discussion

The role of splenectomy for MFMM remains controversial. Potential indications include refractory anemia and/or thrombocytopenia, abdominal discomfort due to massive splenomegaly or splenic infarcts, and other compressive symptoms. Indications for splenectomy in this patient included anemia and bulk symptoms. To date, her symptoms and transfusion requirements have been relieved. However, in some patients, splenectomy may be followed by progressive hepatomegaly and recurrent anemia or thrombocytopenia. There is also potential for severe thrombocytosis with resultant thrombosis or hemorrhage. Morbidity and mortality of splenectomy for MFMM can be minimized through careful patient selection, and referral to hematologists and surgeons experienced in the management of this problem. Patients who have developed portal hypertension with significant ascites and cachexia are prohibitive risks and should not undergo splenectomy.

Suggested Readings

Barosi G, Ambrosetti A, Buratti A, et al. Splenectomy for patients with myelofibrosis with myeloid metaplasia: pretreatment variables and outcome prediction. *Leukemia* 1993;7:200–206.

Ben-Ezia J. B-cell lymphoproliferative disorders. *Hematol Oncol Clin North Am* 2002;16:321–333.

Brodsky JT, Abcar A, Styler M. Splenectomy for non-Hodgkin's lymphoma. *Am J Clin Oncol* 1996;19:558–561.

Cunningham S. Splenectomy for massive splenomegaly of polycythemia vera. *Am J Surg* 2004;188;94-95.

O'Reilly RA. Splenomegaly in 2,505 patients in a large university medical center from 1913 to 1995. *West J Med* 1998;169:78–87.

Presentation

A 47-year-old menopausal woman presents to your office with dyspnea, progressive abdominal distention and discomfort, anorexia, fatigue, lower extremity swelling, and weight loss over 8 weeks. Past medical history is significant for her having had a total abdominal hysterectomy (for fibroids) and bilateral salpingo-oophorectomy several years ago. She is on no medications, has never smoked, and drinks alcohol on rare occasions. Her family history is significant for a maternal aunt with breast cancer diagnosed at age 60, and a father who died from non-small cell lung cancer at age 72. Examination is significant for cachexia and ascites, with no palpable adenopathy or masses. Breast, pelvic, and rectal examinations are unrevealing.

Complete blood cell count, comprehensive metabolic profile, and urinalysis are all normal, except for the following values: platelets 748 K/uL (normal range for institution, 150 to 375) and alkaline phosphatase 144 U/L (normal range, 38 to 126).

Chest x-ray reveals minimal to moderate bilateral pleural effusions, and several subcentimeter-sized nodules in the right lower and left upper lobes. Abdominal ultrasonography shows massive ascites, no organomegaly, and multiple hepatic lesions. Subsequent computed tomography (CT) scans of the chest, abdomen, and pelvis show pulmonary nodules as previously described, moderate bilateral pleural effusions, and no mediastinal or hilar adenopathy. The CT scans also show multiple hepatic lesions (ranging in size from 1 to 3 cm), omental thickening and nodularity, retroperitoneal adenopathy, ascites, and sclerotic lesions in the thoracic and lumbar spine on bone windows. Kidneys, adrenal glands, spleen, stomach, pancreas, and small and large bowel all appear normal.

Differential Diagnosis

In this clinical scenario, cancer should be considered as the primary diagnosis until proven otherwise. In a young, previously healthy woman with evidence of likely widespread metastases involving lung, liver, omentum, nodes, peritoneum, and bone, potential primary sites include ovarian, peritoneal, gastrointestinal (colorectal, pancreatic, gastric), renal, breast, lung, lymphoma, melanoma, and germ cell tumors, among others.

Recommendation

Open biopsy of omental, nodal, or hepatic lesion(s) with complete morphologic and immunohistochemical analysis including evaluation for estrogen and progesterone hormone receptors. Additionally, this patient should have a mammography and positron emission tomography (PET) scanning, if possible, to help rule out potential primary sites. As well, upper and lower endoscopy should be considered if feasible and if it does not delay other evaluation and treatment. Head imaging (CT or magnetic resonance imaging [MRI]) should be performed to rule out brain involvement and the need for prompt surgical and/or radiation intervention. Additional laboratory evaluation should include serum human chorionic gonadotropin (HCG) and alpha-fetoprotein (AFP) to help exclude a primary germ-cell tumor. Additional tumor markers are unlikely to be helpful in diagnosing and confirming a primary site, but may be useful as baseline values in following disease response with eventual treatment. These markers include CA 125, carcinoembryonic antigen (CEA), CA 19-9, CA 15-3 or CA 27, 29, and lactate dehydrogenase (LDH). In this patient, it may also prove useful to review the operative and pathology reports from her hysterectomy and oophorectomy from several years ago to rule out any suspicious or premalignant findings.

Case Continued

A biopsy of an omental mass is performed by laparotomy without complication. No additional information is obtained at surgery to help confirm a primary site. Additional examination yields no new suspicious findings. She reports having recently had "normal" gynecologic evaluations, mammography, esophagogastroduodenoscopy, and colonoscopy in the last 2 years.

Pathology is consistent with a poorly differentiated adenocarcinoma. Complete immunohistochemical analysis is nonspecific for a primary tumor site. Immunohistochemistry is positive for cytokeratin-7, and TTF-1 and negative for CD-20, S-100, CD-117 (or C-KIT), Mart-1, hormone receptor, and neuroendocrine markers.

HCG and AFP are within normal limits. Abnormal tumor markers otherwise include LDH of 670 U/L (reference range, 313 to 618); CEA of 68 ng/mL (reference value <2.5 for a nonsmoker); CA –125 of 687 U/mL (reference value <35); and CA 19-9 of 5,395 U/mL (reference value <37).

PET scanning shows hypermetabolic activity correlating with the lesions seen on CT in the lungs, liver, peritoneum, and bones, including uptake in the right midfemur, right humerus, and lower cervical spine. Head imaging (CT with contrast) reveals no evidence of metastases.

Diagnosis and Recommendation

The diagnosis is carcinoma of unknown primary site. Despite a thorough evaluation, no specific finding(s) definitively establish a primary diagnosis. Therapeutic paracentesis and bilateral thoracenteses should be offered for symptomatic relief (of abdominal discomfort, dyspnea). Systemic chemotherapy, ideally as part of a clinical trial, should be offered.

Approach

At this point in the evaluation, additional radiographic studies, laboratory evaluations, genetic testing, and other interventions to attempt to identify a primary source will rarely be helpful, and can add unnecessary delay in treatment and the potential hardship of additional testing for the patient. Although this situation can often be emotionally unsettling for the patient and family, moving forward

at this point with care aimed at a cancer of unknown primary site is prudent. Addressing the effusions and discomfort promptly and planning for initiation of systemic chemotherapy and supportive care (e.g., intravenous bisphosphonate treatment, nutritional support) is now appropriate.

Surgical Approach

In this patient, early surgical intervention is important in ensuring an adequate biopsy specimen is obtained. Open biopsies are always preferred when image-guided biopsies are deemed technically difficult or unsafe, or likely to yield insufficient material for complete histologic and immunhistochemical evaluation. Although center-dependent, fine-needle aspirates rarely are acceptable as the sole modality in establishing the initial pathologic diagnosis. Additional surgical intervention may be necessary from a therapeutic standpoint at some point in her care for a variety of clinical circumstances (e.g., palliative bypass surgery for bowel obstruction, placement of a portacath for chemotherapy or shunt for persistent ascites, performing pleurodesis for recurring symptomatic effusion(s), or resection of isolated brain, or otherwise symptomatic, metastases.) In rare occasions after systemic therapy, surgical resection (or radiation) of residual tumor(s) should be considered.

Discussion

Approximately 80,000 to 90,000 cases of cancer of unknown primary site are diagnosed each year in the United States. As a group, these cancers comprise various histologies and associated clinical characteristics. Most patients with unknown primary cancers will present with symptoms of advanced disease and multiorgan involvement. Establishing a diagnosis involves the exclusion of more common solid tumors through physical, laboratory, radiographic, and pathologic evidence. Many patients with cancer of unknown primary site fit into recognizable clinical and/or pathologic presentations with more established evaluations and treatments (Table 91.1). However, many patients do not readily fit a defined clinical subset, and the approach and treatment must be individualized.

Four major histologic subtypes constitute the majority of cancers of unknown primary sites: (a) poorly differentiated carcinoma/poorly differentiated adenocarcinoma (30% of the group as a whole); (b) well-differentiated and moderately differentiated adenocarcinoma (60%); (c) poorly differentiated neoplasm (5%); and (d) squamous cell carcinoma

Table 91.1: Cancer of Unknown Primary Site: Treatable Subsets

- Features of extragonadal germ-cell tumor in young men
  Treatment for germ-cell tumor

- Squamous cell carcinomas (cervical or inguinal regions)
  Treatment for locally advanced head and neck cancer, or if inguinal, local treatment only (surgery, radiation, or chemotherapy)

- Axillary nodal metastases in a woman
  Treatment for early-stage node-positive breast cancer

- Peritoneal carcinomatosis in a women
  Treatment for advanced ovarian cancer

- Blastic skeletal metastases or increased prostate-specific antigen in serum or tumor in men
  Treatment for advanced prostate cancer

- Neuroendocrine carcinoma: poorly differentiated
  Treatment for extensive-stage small cell lung cancer

- Neuroendocrine carcinoma: well differentiated
  Treatment for advanced carcinoid tumor

- Solitary metastatic site
  Consideration of local modality treatment (surgery, radiation, or chemotherapy)

(5%). Each of these major groups can be further subdivided based on specific pathologic and clinical features.

In the case presented, the patient was diagnosed with a poorly differentiated adenocarcinoma involving multiple organs. Some of these patients will have disease that is very responsive to chemotherapy and have more favorable outcomes than might be anticipated given the advanced stage. In general, patients in this group are young, and the time from symptom onset to diagnosis may be brief. Relative to well-differentiated adenocarcinomas, this subgroup has fewer primary sites discovered at autopsy.

Peritoneal carcinomatosis in women is a favorable clinical subset of unknown primary cancers. The clinical and pathologic features of this subset are similar to presentations of ovarian cancer. Ovarian or other primary gynecologic cancer in this patient seem less likely given that she has had a hysterectomy and oophorectomy and has otherwise widespread disease; however, this is not absolute. Primary peritoneal carcinoma could readily account for the pathologic and clinical findings in this presentation, although skeletal and pulmonary metastases would be less common in this setting.

Treatment of cancers of unknown primary site is predicated on identifying clinical subsets (e.g., women with axillary nodal cancer, young men with features of germ-cell tumors) in which therapies model more established treatments for known primary cancers (see Table 91.1). The majority of patients with cancer of unknown primary site do not readily fit into such recognized subsets, and should be treated empirically based on available evidence.

Platinum-based chemotherapy is a standard regimen in the treatment of some patients with poorly differentiated adenocarcinomas, as in this case. In a large prospective study, over 60% of patients with poorly differentiated carcinomas or poorly differentiated adenocarcinomas who received platinum-based chemotherapy had objective responses (26% complete responses), with 16% disease free at 5 years and a median survival time of 20 months. Several "good-risk" features associated with a more favorable prognosis have been identified subsequently from this large study and include patients with predominant retroperitoneal, mediastinal, or peripheral nodal disease (suggesting a germ-cell primary). Also, features of primary peritoneal carcinoma, poorly differentiated neuroendocrine carcinoma, or an extragonadal germ-cell syndrome are generally associated with a better prognosis.

More recently, combinations of the newer cytotoxic drugs (paclitaxel, docetaxel, gemcitabine, and irinotecan) with a platinum and/or etoposide, or with each other, have improved the overall survival of these patients, and further studies of these agents are ongoing.

Case Continued

With informed consent, this patient elected to participate in a clinical trial in which she received combination systemic chemotherapy with carboplatin, paclitaxel, and etoposide every 3 weeks, in addition to intravenous bisphosphonate therapy and subcutaneous erythropoietin. After one cycle of treatment, she noted a dramatic improvement in her symptoms. After completing six scheduled cycles without complications, she had evidence of a partial response (complete disappearance of pulmonary lesions, pleural effusions, and ascites, and approximately an 80% decrease in hepatic disease). She is entirely asymptomatic except for alopecia and mild neuropathy related to treatment. As part of the trial, she is currently receiving "maintenance" gefitinib, to remain on this as long as there is no evidence of progressive disease or undue toxicity.

Suggested Readings

Briasoulis E, Pavlidis N. Cancer of unknown primary origin. *Oncologist* 1997;2:142–152.

Greco F, Hainsworth J. Cancer of unknown primary site. In: DeVita V, Hellman S, Rosenberg S, eds. *Cancer: principles and practice of oncology.* 7th ed. Philadelphia, PA: Lippincott Williams & Wilkins; 2004.

Hainsworth JD, Greco FA. Treatment of patients with cancer of an unknown primary site. *N Engl J Med* 1993;329: 257–263.

Hainsworth J, Johnson D, Greco F. Cisplatin-based combination chemotherapy in the treatment of poorly differentiated carcinoma and poorly differentiated adenocarcinoma of unknown primary site: results of a 12-year experience. *J Clin Oncol* 1992;10:912–922.

Hainsworth J, Erland JB, Kalman LA, et al. Carcinoma of unknown primary site: treatment with 1-hour paclitaxel, carboplatin, and extended-schedule etoposide. *J Clin Oncol* 1997;15:2385–2393.

Hainsworth J, Wright EP, Johnson DH, et al. Poorly differentiated carcinoma of unknown primary site: clinical usefulness of immunoperoxidase staining. *J Clin Oncol* 1991;9:1931–1938.

Mintzer DM, Warhol M, Martin AM, et al. Cancer of unknown primary: changing approaches. A multidisciplinary case presentation from the Joan Karnell Cancer Center of Pennsylvania Hospital. *Oncologist* 2004;9:330–338.

van de Wouw AJ, Jansen RL, Speel EJ, et al. The unknown biology of the unknown primary tumor: a literature review. *Ann Oncol* 2003;14:191–196.

A

Abdominal cancer
    chordoma, 299–302
    pelvic chondrosarcoma, 279–285
    retroperitoneal sarcoma, 273–278
Actinic keratoses, 322
Adnexal masses, 397–401
Adrenal mass suspicious for malignancy, 372–376
Adrenal pheochromocytoma, 343–346, 362–364
Anal canal SCC, 165–169
Androgen ablative therapy, 392
Angiograms
    hepatocellular carcinoma, single, 180
    osteosarcoma, 288
Anorectal mucosal melanoma, 173–177
Anthracycline regimen, 234
Appendiceal cancer
    neuroendocrine tumor with carcinoid features,
        111–113
    pseudomyxoma peritonei syndrome,
        114–118
Askin's sarcoma, 60

B

Barium contrast studies
    esophageal cancer, squamous cell, 68–69
    rectal submucosal masses, 159
    small bowel adenocarcinoma, 99
Barrett's carcinoma, 77
Bevacizumab (Avastin), 134, 193
Bile duct tumors, 205
Bladder cancer, 386–388
Bone cancer
    Ewing's sarcoma. *See* Ewing's sarcoma
    osteosarcoma, shoulder, 286–292
Breast cancer, 225–226
    ductal carcinoma, invasive, 223–227
    ductal carcinoma in situ, 249–252
    inflammatory, 232–235
    lobular carcinoma in situ, 245–248
    locally advanced carcinoma, 228–231
    male, 261–264
    Paget's disease of the nipple, 253–256
    pregnancy-associated, invasive, 241–244
    primary, with metastases to the axilla,
        257–260
    recurrent breast carcinoma, 236–240

C

Capecitabine, 149
Carboplatin, 395
Carcinoids, 102
    appendiceal neuroendocrine tumor with carcinoid
        features, 111–113
    liver tumors, 194–198
    small bowel, with lymph node metastases, 101–105
Carcinoma of unknown primary site, 409–411
Cervical esophageal SCC, 63–67
Cetuximab (Erbitux), 134
Chemoradiation
    for anal canal SCC, 167
    for duodenal carcinoma, 97
    for esophageal cancer
        cervical esophageal SCC, 64–65
        squamous cell carcinoma, 64–65, 70, 73
    for gastric cancer, 82
    for lung cancer
        Pancoast tumor, non-small, 38
        small cell, 34, 35
    for oropharynx carcinoma, 6, 7
    for Pancoast tumor with Pancoast syndrome,
        38
    for rectal cancer
        distal rectal adenocarcinoma, 142
        locally advanced, 147
        rectal SCC, 171
    for squamous cell carcinoma from unknown source, 21
    for SVC syndrome, 41
Chemotherapy
    for abdominal cancer
        pelvic chondrosarcoma, 284
        retroperitoneal sarcoma, 275
    for adnexal masses, 400
    for anal canal SEC, 167
    for anorectal mucosal melanoma, 176
    for bladder cancer, 388
    for bowel obstruction, 134
    for breast cancer
        inflammatory, 234, 235
        locally advanced carcinoma, 230
        male, 264
        pregnancy-associated, invasive, 243
        primary, with metastases to the axilla, 259
        recurrent breast carcinoma, 239–240
    for carcinoma of unknown primary site, 411

Chemotherapy *(continued)*
    for central chondrosarcoma, 61
    for distal esophagus adenocarcinoma, 77
    for duodenal carcinoma, 97
    for Ewing's sarcoma, in right femur, 297
    for hematuria, 388
    for Kaposi's sarcoma, 337
    for liver cancer
        carcinoid tumors, 198
        colorectal cancer, metastatic, 190–191
        gallbladder carcinoma, 202
        hilar cholangiocarcinoma, 208
        intrahepatic cholangiocarcinoma, 213
    for lung cancer
        metastases from soft tissue sarcoma, 48
        small cell lung cancer, 34
    for Merkel cell carcinoma, 320
    for mucoepidermoid carcinoma, 27
    for obstructions
        bowel obstruction, 134
        sigmoid colon, obstructing carcinoma of, 130
    for osteosarcoma, 287–288, 289, 292
    for ovarian cancer, 395
        adnexal masses, 400
    for pelvic chondrosarcoma, 284
    for pharyngolarynx cancer, 17
    for pseudomyxoma peritonei syndrome, 116, 117–118
    for rectal cancer
        anal canal SEC, 167
        anorectal mucosal melanoma, 176
        locally advanced, 148, 149
        locally advanced, recurrent, 151, 152
    for renal cell carcinoma, 385
    for skin SCC, high-risk invasive, 326, 327, 328
    for stomach cancers
        adenocarcinoma of stomach, 82
        carcinomatosis of stomach, 85, 86
        gastric lymphoma, primary intermediate grade
            B-cell, 87, 89
    for testicular cancer, 378
        metastatic nonseminomatous, 380
Chest melanoma, 303–306
Cholangiocarcinoma tumors, 212–213
Chondroma, 59
Chondrosarcomas, 59–60, 284–285
    central chondrosarcoma, 59–62
    pelvic, 279–285
CHOP with rituximab, 88
Chordoma, 299–302
Cisplatin
    for anal canal SCC, 168, 169
    for anorectal mucosal melanoma, 176
    for esophageal cancer
        distal esophagus, adenocarcinoma of, 77
        squamous cell carcinoma, 70, 73
    for hematuria, 388
    for intrahepatic cholangiocarcinoma, 210
    for lung cell cancer, small, 34
    for mesothelioma, 53
    for osteosarcoma, 288, 289, 292
    for ovarian cancer, 395

    for rectal cancer
        anal canal SCC, 168, 169
        anorectal mucosal melanoma, 176
        squamous cell carcinoma, 172
    for testicular cancer, 371
        metastatic nonseminomatous, 380
Colon cancer
    obstructing colon carcinoma of the sigmoid colon,
        126–130
    polyps. *See* Colon polyps
Colon polyps, 119–122
    tubulovillous adenoma, adenocarcinoma within,
        123–125
Colorectal cancer
    of the liver, 188–193
    of the rectum, 136–139
Computed tomography. *See* CT scans
Concurrent chemotherapy and radiotherapy. *See*
        Chemoradiation
Cryotherapy
    liver, colorectal cancer, 190
    prostate, adenocarcinoma of, 390
CT scans
    abdominal cancer
        pelvic chondrosarcoma, 279–280
        retroperitoneal sarcoma, 274–275
    adrenal cancer
        mass suspicious for malignancy, 372, 373, 375
        pheochromocytoma, 362–363
    anal canal SCC, 166
    appendiceal neuroendocrine tumors with carcinoid
        features, 112
    bladder cancer, 386
    bowel obstruction, 132, 133, 134
    breast cancer
        inflammatory, 234
        locally advanced carcinoma, 229
        pregnancy-associated, invasive, 241
        primary, with metastases to the axilla, 258
    carcinoma of unknown primary site, 409
    central chondrosarcoma, 60
    colon
        bowel obstruction, 132, 133, 134
        polyps. Colon polyps, *below*
        sigmoid colon, obstructing carcinoma of, 128
    colon polyps, 120
        tubulovillous adenoma, adenocarcinoma within, 124
    colorectal cancer, 137–138
        liver cancer, 188–189, 190
    esophageal cancer
        cervical esophageal SCC, 64
        distal esophagus, adenocarcinoma of, 75
        squamous cell, 69–70, 71
    gallbladder carcinoma, 200, 201
    glottic carcinoma, 12, 13
    insulinoma, 351
    liver cancer
        carcinoid tumors, 194, 196, 197
        colorectal cancer, metastatic, 188–189, 190
        hepatic tumors, 184, 187
        hilar cholangiocarcinoma, 203, 204

intrahepatic cholangiocarcinoma, 209, 210, 211, 212
metastatic disease, 339, 340
single hepatocellular carcinoma, 179–180
lung cancer
adenocarcinoma, stage IA, 44, 45, 46
metastases from soft tissue sarcoma, 47, 48
non-small cell Pancoast tumor, 37, 38, 40
non-small lung cell cancer, 30
small lung cell cancer, 34
melanomas
metastatic, 312
residual, 308, 309
Merkel cell carcinoma, 342
mesothelioma, 53, 54, 56
mucoepidermoid carcinoma, 24, 25
nasopharynx carcinoma, 9
oral lesions, 2–3, 6
osteosarcoma, 286, 287
ovarian cancer, 393, 394
pancreatic cancer
carcinoma, 214, 215
cystic lesions, 217–218, 219, 220, 221
insulinoma, 351
pharyngolarynx, 15, 16
pheochromocytoma
adrenal cancer, 362–363
Merkel cell carcinoma, 342
pseudomyxona peritonei syndrome, 115
rectal cancer
colorectal cancer, 137–138
distal rectal adenocarcinoma, 140, 141–142
locally advanced, 146, 147, 149
locally advanced, recurrent, 150
neuroendocrine tumor of lower rectum, deeply
invasive, 157
rectal SCC, 173
submucosal masses, 160, 163
renal cell carcinoma, 382–383, 384, 385
retroperitoneal sarcoma, 274–275
small bowel
adenocarcinoma, 99
carcinoid with lymph node metastases, 101
gastrointestinal stromal tumors, 106, 107, 110
soft tissue sarcomas, 265, 266, 269–270
splenomegaly, 402–403, 406–407
squamous cell carcinoma from unknown source, 18,
19
stomach cancer
adenocarcinoma of stomach, 79–80
gastric lymphoma, primary intermediate grade
B-cell, 87, 88
gastrointestinal stromal tumors, 91–92, 106, 107, 110
total carcinomatosis of stomach, 84
SVC syndrome, 41
testicular cancer, 379, 380
thyroid, papillary carcinoma of, 355, 356, 358, 359
Zollinger-Ellison syndrome, 348
Cyclophosphamide
for breast cancer
inflammatory, 234
male, 264
pregnancy-associated, 243
for gastric lymphoma, 88
for liver cancer
carcinoid tumors, 198
metastatic disease, 341

D
Dacarbazin, 314
Desmoid tumor, 59
Differential diagnosis
for abdominal cancer
chordoma, 299
pelvic chondrosarcoma, 281–282
retroperitoneal sarcoma, 273
for adnexal masses, 397–398
for adrenal cancer
mass suspicious for malignancy, 372–373
pheochromocytoma, 362
for anal canal SCC, 165–166
for anal mucosa, nodular melanoma of, 173
for appendiceal neuroendocrine tumor with carcinoid
features, 111
for bladder cancer, 386–387
for breast cancer
ductal carcinoma, invasive, 224
ductal carcinoma in situ, 249–250
inflammatory, 232
lobular carcinoma in situ, 246
locally advanced carcinoma, 228
male, 261
Paget's disease of the nipple, 253–254
primary, with metastases to the axilla, 257–258
recurrent breast cancer, 237–238
for carcinoma of unknown primary site, 409–410
for central chondrosarcoma, 59–60
for colon cancer
for colon polyps, sigmoid colon, obstructing
carcinoma of, 127
for colon polyps, 119
tubulovillous adenoma, adenocarcinoma within,
123–124
for duodenal adenocarcinoma, 95, 96
for esophageal cancer
cervical esophageal SCC, 63
distal esophagus, adenocarcinoma of, 74–75
squamous cell carcinoma, 68
for Ewing's sarcoma, in right femur, 294
for gallbladder carcinoma, 200
for gastrointestinal stromal tumors, 91, 107
for glottic carcinoma, 12
for hematuria, 386–387
for insulinoma, 350
for Kaposi's sarcoma, 335–336
for liver cancer
carcinoid tumors, 194
colorectal cancer, metastatic, 188–189
hepatic tumors, 183–184
hilar cholangiocarcinoma, 203
intrahepatic cholangiocarcinoma, 209–210
metastatic disease, 339–340
single hepatocellular carcinoma, 179

Differential diagnosis *(continued)*
   for lung cancer
      adenocarcinoma, stage IA, 45
      metastases from soft tissue sarcoma, 48
      non-small cell Pancoast tumor, with Pancoast
         syndrome, 29
      non-small lung cell cancer, 29
      small cell lung cancer, 33
   for melanomas
      metastatic, 311–314
      residual, 307–308
   for mucoepidermoid carcinoma, 23
   for nasopharynx carcinoma, 8
   for osteosarcoma, 287–288
   for ovarian cancer, 393–394
      adnexal masses, 397–398
   for Paget's disease of the nipple, 253–254
   for pancreatic cancer
      carcinoma, 214–215
      cystic lesions, 218
      insulinoma, 350
   for pharyngolarynx carcinoma, 16
   for pheochromocytoma, 344
      adrenal cancer, 362
   for pseudomyxoma peritonei syndrome, 114
   for rectal cancer
      anal canal SCC, 165–166
      anal mucosa, nodular melanoma of, 173
      colorectal cancer, 136
      distal rectal adenocarcinoma, 140–144
      locally advanced, 146
      locally advanced, recurrent, 150
      neuroendocrine tumor of lower rectum, deeply
         invasive, 155
      rectal SCC, 170–172
   for retroperitoneal sarcoma, 273
   for skin cancer
      basal cell carcinoma, 330–331
      squamous cell carcinoma, high-risk invasive,
         322–323
   for small bowel cancers
      adenocarcinoma, 98
      carcinoid with lymph node metastases, 101
      gastrointestinal stromal tumors, 107
   for splenomegaly, 404, 405, 408
   for squamous cell carcinoma
      anal canal SCC, 165–166
      cervical esophageal SCC, 63
      esophageal cancer, 63, 68
      rectal SCC, 170–172
      skin cancer, 322–323
      tongue lesions, 1, 5
      from unknown source, 18
   for stomach cancer
      adenocarcinoma of stomach, 78
      gastric lymphoma, primary intermediate grade
         B-cell, 87
      gastrointestinal stromal tumors, 91
      total carcinomatosis of stomach, 83–84
   for testicular cancer, 377–378
      metastatic nonseminomatous, 379–380
   for thyroid cancer
      papillary carcinoma, 354, 357
      primary hyperparathyroidism, 365–366, 369
   for tongue lesions, 1, 5
   for tubulopapillary neoplasm, 51
   for Zollinger-Ellison syndrome, 347
Docetaxel
   for breast cancer, inflammatory, 234
   for carcinoma of unknown primary site, 411
   for ovarian cancer, 395
Doxil, 337
Doxorubicin (Adriamycin)
   for breast cancer
      male, 264
      osteosarcoma, 288, 289, 292
      pregnancy-associated, 243
   for gastric lymphoma, primary intermediate grade
      B-cell, 88
   for hematuria, 388
   for Kaposi's sarcoma, 337
   for ovarian cancer, 395
   for pulmonary metastases from soft tissue sarcoma,
      48, 49
Duodenal adenocarcinoma, 95–98
Duodenal tumors, 349
Dysphagia, 74–77

E
Endometriosis, 400
Endorectal ultrasound
   anal canal SCC, 166, 167
   distal rectal adenocarcinoma, 140, 141
   neuroendocrine tumor of lower rectum, deeply
      invasive, 157
   rectal SCC, 171
Endoscopic images
   distal esophagus, adenocarcinoma of, 74
   duodenal adenocarcinoma, 95
   gastrointestinal stromal tumors, 90, 91
   nasopharynx carcinoma, 8
   stomach
      adenocarcinoma of, 78–79
      total carcinomatosis of, 83
   tubulopapillary carcinoma, 52–53
   Zollinger-Ellison syndrome, 347
Endoscopic retrograde cholangiograms, 199–200
Endoscopic ultrasound (EUS)
   duodenum carcinoma, 95, 96
   esophageal cancer, squamous cell, 70, 71
   pancreatic cystic lesions, 218
   rectum, deeply invasive endocrine tumor of,
      157
Endoscopic ultrasound with needle aspiration (EUS-NA),
      30
Epirubicin, 77
Esophageal cancer
   cervical esophageal SCC, 63–67
   distal esophagus, adenocarcinoma of, 74–77
   pharyngo-laryno-esophagectomy, 64
   squamous cell, 68–73

Etoposide
    for esophageal cancer
        distal esophagus, adenocarcinoma of, 77
        squamous cell, 70, 73
    for lung cell cancer, small, 34
    for ovarian cancer, 395
Ewing's sarcoma, 60, 291
    in femur, 293–298

F
Fibrous dysplasia, 59
Fine-needle aspiration biopsy (FNAB)
    adrenal mass suspicious for malignancy, 373
    breast cancer, with metastases to the axilla, 237
    breast cancer
        male, 261, 262
    gastrointestinal stromal tumors, 93
    mucoepidermoid carcinoma, 24, 25
    pancreatic cystic lesions, 218–219
    pregnancy-associated, 241–242
    soft tissue sarcomas, 266
    squamous cell carcinoma from unknown source,
        19
    SVC syndrome, 42
    thyroid, papillary carcinoma of, 354, 356, 358
Fluorouracil
    for anal canal SCC, 167
    for bowel obstruction, 134
    for breast cancer, pregnancy-associated, 243
    for esophageal cancer, squamous cell, 70, 73
    for gallbladder carcinoma, 202
    for liver cancer
        carcinoid tumors, 198
        colorectal cancer, metastatic, 193
        hilar cholangiocarcinoma, 208
        intrahepatic cholangiocarcinoma, 210
    for pseudomyxoma peritonei syndrome, 116,
        117–118
    for rectal cancer
        colorectal cancer, 139
        distal rectal adenocarcinoma, 142, 145
        locally advanced, 148
        locally advanced, recurrent, 151, 152, 153
    for sigmoid colon, obstructing carcinoma of, 130
    for skin SCC, high-risk invasive, 327, 328
Focal nodular hyperplasia, 184, 185, 186
FOLFOX regimen, 148
Follicular lesions, stages of, 354
5-FU. *See* Fluorouracil

G
Gallbladder carcinoma, 199–202
Gastrectomy, 80–81
Gastric cancer. *See* Stomach cancer
Gastrinomas, 349
Gastrografin studies
    esophageal SCC, cervical, 65
    sigmoid colon, obstructing carcinoma of, 127–128
Gefitinib (Iressa), 193
Gemcitabine
    for carcinoma of unknown primary site, 411

    for hematuria, 388
    for mesothelioma, 58
    for ovarian cancer, 395
    for skin SCC, high-risk invasive, 329
Glottic carcinoma, 12–14
Gy
    for anal canal SCC, 168
    for breast cancer
        inflammatory, 234, 235
        Paget's disease of the nipple, 255
        recurrent breast carcinoma, 240
    for esophageal SCC, 70
    for lung cancer
        Pancoast tumor, non-small cell, 38
        small cell, 34
    for nasopharyngeal carcinoma, 10
    for oropharynx carcinoma, 6
    for Paget's disease of the nipple, 255
    for prostate, adenocarcinoma of, 391
    for rectal cancer
        adenocarcinoma, distal, 142
        locally advanced, recurrent, 152
        rectal SCC, 171, 172
    for squamous cell carcinoma from unknown source,
        21
    for tongue SCC, 4, 6

H
Hemangioma, 186
Hematuria, 386–388
Hepatic adenoma, 186–187
Hepatic angiograms, 180
Hepatic tumors, 183–187
Hepatocellular carcinoma, single, 178–182
Histopathology slides
    appendiceal neuroendocrine tumors with carcinoid
        features, 111
    breast cancer
        ductal carcinoma, invasive, 226–227
        Paget's disease of the nipple, 255
    colon polyps, 119, 120
    gastrointestinal stromal tumors, 92–93, 110
    mesothelioma, 53
    mucoepidermoid carcinoma, 24, 26, 27
    Paget's disease of the nipple, 255
    pancreatic cystic lesions, 219–220
    prostate, adenocarcinoma of, 389
    rectal neuroendocrine tumor, 156
    rectal submucosal masses, 160, 161
    thyroid, papillary carcinoma of, 358, 360

I
Ifosfamide, 288, 289, 292
Imatinib, 163, 164
Inflammatory breast cancer, 232–235
Insulinoma, 350–353
Interferon
    for anorectal mucosal melanoma, 176
    for Kaposi's sarcoma, 337
    for metastatic melanoma, 314–315
    for renal cell carcinoma, 385

Interleukin, 385
Intraductal carcinoma, 249–252
Irinotecan
    for bowel obstruction, 132
    for carcinoma of unknown primary site, 411
    for liver colorectal cancer, metastatic, 193
    for rectal cancer
        locally advanced, 149
        locally advanced, recurrent, 151, 152
Isolated limb infusion, 310

K

Kaposi's sarcoma, 335–338
Kidney cancer, 382–385

L

Laryngeal cancer, 12–14
"Leather bottle" stomach, 85, 86
Leucovorin
    for bowel obstruction, 132, 134
    for rectal cancer
        distal rectal adenocarcinoma, 145
        locally advanced, 148
        locally advanced, recurrent, 151, 152
    for sigmoid colon, obstructing carcinoma of, 130
Linitis plastica, 85, 86
Lipiodol CT scans, 180
Liver cancer
    carcinoid tumors, 194–198
    cholangiocarcinoma
        hiler, 203–208
        intrahepatic, 209–213
    colorectal cancer, metastatic, 188–193
    hepatic tumors, 183–187
    hepatocellular carcinoma, single, 178–182
    metastatic disease, 339–342
Lung cancer
    adenocarcinoma, Stage IA, 44–46
    metastases from soft tissue sarcoma, 47–50
    non-small lung cell, 29–31
    non-small Pancoast tumor with Pancoast syndrome,
        36–40
    small lung cell cancer, 32–35
Lymphoscintigrams
    anal mucosa, nodular melanoma of, 174
    male breast cancer, 263

M

Magnetic resonance imaging. *See* MRIs
MALT lymphoma, 89
Mammograms
    ductal carcinoma, invasive, 223–224, 225
    ductal carcinoma in situ, 250
    lobular carcinoma in situ, 245–246
    locally advanced carcinoma, 229, 230
    male breast cancer, 261–262
    Paget's disease of the nipple, 254
    recurrent breast cancer, 236
Mediastinoscopy
    for non-small lung cancer, 30
    for SVC syndrome, 43

Melanomas
    anorectal mucosal melanoma, 173–177
    chest melanoma, 303–306
    metastatic melanoma, 311–315
    residual melanoma, 307–310
Merkel cell carcinoma, 316–320
Mesothelioma, 51–58
Methotrexate
    for breast cancer, pregnancy-associated, 243
    for hematuria, 388
    for osteosarcoma, 288, 292
    for ovarian adnexal masses, 399
    for skin SCC, high-risk invasive, 327
Miltefosine, 240
Mitomycin, 167
Mohs Micrographic Surgery
    basal cell carcinoma, 331–333
    squamous cell carcinoma, 323–327
MRIs
    adrenal mass suspicious for malignancy, 373
    breast cancer
        inflammatory, 233–234
        male, 262
        Paget's disease of the nipple, 254
        pregnancy-associated, 242
        primary, with metastases to the axilla, 257
    carcinoma of unknown site, 409
    central chondrosarcoma, 61
    colorectal cancer, 137
        liver cancer, 190
    Ewing's sarcoma, in right femur, 294–295,
        296
    liver cancer
        carcinoid tumors, 195
        colorectal cancer, metastatic, 190
        hepatic tumors, 184, 187
        hilar cholangiocarcinoma, 204, 205–206
    liver metastatic disease, 339
    melanomas
        metastatic, 312
        residual, 309
    Merkel cell carcinoma, 319
    nasopharynx carcinoma, 9
    non-small cell Pancoast tumor, with Pancoast
        syndrome, 37, 38
    Paget's disease of the nipple, 254
    pancreatic cystic lesions, 219, 220
    pelvic chondrosarcoma, 281
    pheochromocytoma, 343, 345
    pulmonary metastases, 47, 48
    rectal cancer
        anal canal SCC, 167
        colorectal cancer, 137
        distal rectal adenocarcinoma, 140
        locally advanced, 148
        locally advanced, recurrent, 150, 151, 153
        neuroendocrine tumor of lower rectum, deeply
            invasive, 157
        submucosal masses, 160, 163
    renal cell carcinoma, 383
    sacral chordoma, 300

skin SCC, high-risk invasive, 322
soft tissue sarcomas, 266–267
splenomegaly, 403–404
thyroid, papillary carcinoma of, 355, 356
Zollinger-Ellison syndrome, 348
Mucoepidermoid carcinoma, 23–28
MUGA examination, 48, 49
MVAC-regimen, 388
Myeloma, 60

N
Nasopharynx carcinoma, 8–11

O
Obstruction
bowel obstruction, 131–135
sigmoid colon, obstructing carcinoma of, 126–130
Octreotide scans
liver, carcinoid tumors, 195–196
small bowel carcinoid with lymph node metastases, 103
Octreotide therapy, 104
Oral ulcers, 1–7
Oropharynx carcinoma, 5–7
Osteochondroma, 59
Ovarian cancer, 393–396
adnexal masses, 397–401
Oxaliplatin
for bowel obstruction, 134
for liver colorectal cancer, metastatic, 193
for rectal cancer
distal rectal adenocarcinoma, 145
locally advanced, 148
locally advanced, recurrent, 152
for sigmoid colon, obstructing carcinoma of, 130

P
Paclitaxel
for carcinoma of unknown primary site, 411
for ovarian cancer, 395
for skin SCC, high-risk invasive, 327
Pancoast syndrome, 36–40
Pancreatic cancer
carcinoma, 214–216
cystic lesions, 217–222
insulinoma, 350–353
Parotid masses, 23–28
Pedunculated polyps, 121
Pelvic chondrosarcoma, 279–285
PET scans
anal canal SCC, 167
bowel obstructions, 134
carcinoma of unknown primary site, 409
esophageal cancer
cervical esophageal SCC, 64
squamous cell, 69–70, 71
liver cancer
colorectal cancer, metastatic, 189
hepatic tumors, 184
hilar cholangiocarcinoma, 206

lung cancer
adenocarcinoma, stage IA, 44, 45
non-small cell lung cancer, 30
non-small cell Pancoast tumors, 37
melanomas
metastatic, 312
residual, 308, 309
Merkel cell carcinoma, 319
nasopharynx carcinoma, 9
rectal cancer
colorectal cancer, 137
locally advanced cancer, recurrent, 150
neuroendocrine tumor of lower rectum, deeply invasive, 157
submucosal masses, 163
squamous cell carcinoma from unknown source, 19, 20
thyroid, papillary carcinoma of, 356, 359
Pharyngolarynx carcinoma, 15–17
Phenoxybenzamine
for liver metastatic disease, 339, 340
for pheochromocytoma, 344
Pheochromocytoma, 343–346, 362–364
Plasmacytoma, 60
Platinum-based chemotherapy
for carcinoma of unknown primary site, 411
for ovarian cancer, 395
Prednisone, 88
Prostascints, 391
Prostate, adenocarcinoma of, 389–392
PSA tests and results, 389–392
Pseudomyxoma peritonei syndrome, 114–118
Punch biopsy, 254

R
Radiographs. *See* X-rays
Radiotherapy
for abdominal cancer
pelvic chondrosarcoma, 284
retroperitoneal sarcoma, 275
for adrenal mass suspicious for malignancy, 374
for anal canal SCC, 167, 169
for breast cancer
inflammatory, 234, 235
locally advanced carcinoma, 230
Paget's disease of the nipple, 255
primary, with metastases to the axilla, 259
recurrent breast carcinoma, 239, 240
for central chondrosarcoma, 61
for chordoma, sacral, 301
for colorectal cancer, 139
for Ewing's sarcoma, in right femur, 297, 298
for gastric lymphoma, primary intermediate grade B-cell, 88, 89
for laryngeal cancer, 13
for melanoma, metastatic, 314
for Merkel cell carcinoma, 320
for mucoepidermoid carcinoma, 27
for nasopharynx carcinoma, 10, 11
for oropharynx carcinoma, 6, 7
for Paget's disease of the nipple, 255

Radiotherapy *(continued)*
    for Pancoast tumor, non-small, 38
    for pelvic chondrosarcoma, 284
    for pharyngolarynx cancer, 17
    for prostate, adenocarcinoma of, 390, 391
    for rectal cancer
        anal SCC, 168, 169
        colorectal cancer, 139
        locally advanced, 147, 148
        locally advanced, recurrent, 151
        rectal SCC, 171
    for renal cell carcinoma, 385
    for retroperitoneal sarcoma, 275
    for skin cancer
        basal cell carcinoma, 333
        liver metastatic disease, 342
        squamous cell carcinoma, high-risk invasive, 326, 329
    for soft tissue sarcomas
        retroperitoneal sarcoma, 275
        thigh, 268
    for squamous cell carcinoma
        anal canal SCC, 167, 169
        base of tongue, 6, 7
        oral tongue, 4
        rectal SCC, 171
        skin cancer, 326, 329
        from unknown source, 20, 21
    for testicular cancer, 378
Rectal cancer
    anorectal mucosal melanoma, 173–177
    colorectal cancer, 136–139
    distal rectal adenocarcinoma, 140–145
    locally advanced, recurrent, 150–154
    neuroendocrine tumor of lower rectum, deeply invasive, 155–158
    squamous cell carcinoma, 170–172
    submucosal masses, 159–164
Renal cell carcinoma, 382–385
Residual melanoma, 307–310
Retroperitoneal sarcoma, 275
Rituximab, 88

S

Sacral chordoma, 299–302
Sagittal ultrasonography, 389
Sentinel node biopsy, 173, 174, 176
Sessile polyps, 121, 123–125
Sestamibi scans and SPECT, 366, 370
Shoulder osteosarcoma, 286–292
Sigmoid colon, obstructing carcinoma of, 126–130
Skin cancer. *See also* Melanomas
    basal cell carcinoma, 330–334
    squamous cell carcinoma, high-risk invasive, 321–329
Small bowel cancers
    adenocarcinoma, 98–100
    carcinoid with lymph node metastases, 101–105
    gastrointestinal stromal tumors, 106–110
Soft tissue sarcomas
    retroperitoneal sarcoma, 273–278
    thigh, 258, 265–272

Solitary exostosis, 59
Somatostatin, 196
Splenomegaly, 402–408
Sputum cytology
    lung cancer diagnosis, 29
Squamous cell carcinoma from unknown primary site, 18–22
Stereotactic core biopsy
    ductal carcinoma, invasive, 250
    ductal carcinoma in situ, 250
    lobular carcinoma in situ, 246
Stomach cancers. *See also* Small bowel cancers
    adenocarcinoma of stomach, 78–82
    gastric lymphoma, primary intermediate grade B-cell, 87–89
    total carcinomatosis of stomach, 83–86
Streptozocin, 198
Surgery
    for abdominal cancer
        pelvic chondrosarcoma, 282–283
        retroperitoneal sarcoma, 276–278
    for adrenal cancer
        mass suspicious for malignancy, 373–375
        pheochromocytoma, 363
    for anal canal SCC, 168
    for anal mucosa, nodular melanoma of, 173–174
    for appendiceal neuroendocrine tumors with carcinoid features, 112–113
    for bladder cancer, 387–388
    for bowel obstruction, 133, 134–135
    for breast cancer
        ductal carcinoma, invasive, 225
        ductal carcinoma in situ, 250–251
        inflammatory, 234, 235
        lobular carcinoma in situ, 247
        locally advanced carcinoma, 230–231
        male, 263–264
        Paget's disease of the nipple, 255
        pregnancy-associated, invasive, 242–243
        primary, with metastases to the axilla, 259
        recurrent breast carcinoma, 238–240
    for carcinoma of unknown primary site, 410–411
    for central chondrosarcoma, 61–62
    for chest melanoma, 303–305
    for chordoma, sacral, 300–301
    for colon cancers
        bowel obstruction, 134–135
        sigmoid colon, obstructing carcinoma of, 128–129
    for colon polyps, 120
        tubulovillous adenoma, adenocarcinoma within, 124
    for duodenal carcinoma, 96–97
    for esophageal cancer
        cervical esophageal SCC, 65, 66, 67
        distal esophagus adenocarcinoma, 76, 77
        squamous cell, 71–72
    for Ewing's sarcoma, in right shoulder, 296–297
    for gallbladder carcinoma, 200–202
    for gastrointestinal stromal tumors, 94, 107, 108–109
    for hematuria, 387–388
    for insulinoma, 352–353
    for laryngeal cancer, 13

for liver cancer
  carcinoid tumors, 197
  colorectal cancer, metastatic, 189–193
  hepatic tumors, 185–186
  hilar cholangiocarcinoma, 206, 207
  intrahepatic cholangiocarcinoma, 210–211
  metastatic disease, 340–341
  single hepatocellular carcinoma, 181–182
for lung cancer
  adenocarcinoma, stage IA, 45
  metastases from soft tissue sarcoma, 48–50
  non-small cell Pancoast tumor, with Pancoast syndrome, 38–40
  non-small lung cell cancer, 31
  small lung cell cancer, 34
for Merkel cell carcinoma, 319–320
for mesothelioma, 56
for mucoepidermoid carcinoma, 25
for nasopharynx carcinoma, 10
for oropharynx carcinoma, 7
for osteosarcoma, 288–289
for ovarian cancer, 394–395
  adnexal masses, 399–400
for Paget's disease of the nipple, 255
for pancreatic cancer
  carcinoma, 215
  cystic lesions, 219
  insulinoma, 352–353
for pelvic chondrosarcoma, 282–283
for pharyngolarynx carcinoma, 16–17
for prostate, adenocarcinoma of, 390–391
for pseudomyxoma peritonei syndrome, 116–117
for rectal cancer
  anal mucosa, nodular melanoma of, 173–174
  anal SCC, 168
  colorectal cancer, 138, 139
  distal rectal adenocarcinoma, 142–145
  locally advanced, 145, 148
  locally advanced, recurrent, 151–152
  neuroendocrine tumor of lower rectum, deeply invasive, 158
  squamous cell carcinoma, 170–171
  submucosal masses, 160–162
for retroperitoneal sarcoma, 276–278
for skin cancer
  basal cell carcinoma, 331–333
  squamous cell carcinoma, high-risk invasive, 323–327
for small bowel cancers
  adenocarcinoma of small bowel, 99
  carcinoid with lymph node metastases, 104
  gastrointestinal stromal tumors, 107, 108–109
for soft tissue sarcomas
  retroperitoneal sarcoma, 276–278
  thigh, 268–271
for splenomegaly, 404–405, 407, 408
for squamous cell carcinoma
  anal SCC, 168
  base of tongue, 7
  cervical esophageal SCC, 65, 66, 67
  esophageal cancer, 65, 66, 67, 72
  oral tongue, 3

rectal cancer, 170–171
  from unknown source, 20
for stomach cancers
  adenocarcinoma of stomach, 80–82
  small bowel cancers, *above*
  total carcinomatosis of stomach, 84–86
for SVC syndrome, 41–42
for testicular cancer, 378
  metastatic nonseminomatous, 381
for thyroid cancer
  papillary carcinoma, 355–357, 358–360
  primary hyperparathyroidism, 370–371
  primary hyperparathyroidism, secondary to inferior parathyroid adenoma, 366–367
for tongue lesions, 3–4
SVC syndrome, 41–43

T
Tamoxifen
  for lobular carcinoma in situ, 247–248
  for pregnancy-associated breast cancer, 243
Testicular cancer, 377–378
  metastatic nonseminomatous, 379–381
Thigh sarcomas, 265–272
Thoracentesis, 52
Thyroid cancer
  papillary carcinoma, 354–361
  primary hyperparathyroidism, 369–371
    secondary to inferior parathyroid adenoma, 365–368
Tongue, squamous cell carcinoma of, 1–7
Topotecan, 395
Transthoracic needle aspiration (TTNA)
  lung cancer diagnosis, 29, 30
  SVC syndrome, 42
Tubulovillous adenoma, adenocarcinoma within, 123–125

U
Ultrasonography
  breast cancer
    inflammatory, 234
    locally advanced carcinoma, 229
    male, 262
    Paget's disease of the nipple, 254
    pregnancy-associated, 241
    primary, with metastases to the axilla, 257, 258, 259
  gallbladder carcinoma, 199
  insulinoma, 352
  liver cancer
    colorectal cancer, metastatic, 191–192
    hepatic tumors, 183–187
    hilar cholangliocarcinoma, 204
    single hepatocellular carcinoma, 178–179
  Paget's disease of the nipple, 254
  primary hyperparathyroidism, 366
  prostate, adenocarcinoma of, 389
  soft tissue sarcomas, 265, 267
  testicular cancer, 377
Upper gastrointestinal imaging (UGI), 90, 91

V

Ventilation-perfusion (V/Q) scans, 55
Vinblastine, 388

X

X-rays
    bowel obstructions, 132
    breast cancer, pregnancy-associated, 242
    central chondrosarcoma, 59, 62
    Ewing's sarcoma, in right femur, 293–294, 297
    follicular lesions, stages of, 354
    lung cancer
        non-small cell, 29
        non-small Pancoast tumor, with Pancoast
            syndrome, 36, 37

    mesothelioma, 57
    osteosarcoma, 289, 290
    pancreatic carcinoma, 214
    pelvic chondrosarcoma, 280, 284
    renal cell carcinoma, 384
    sigmoid colon, obstructing carcinoma of,
        126, 127
    soft tissue sarcomas, 269–270
    thyroid, papillary carcinoma of,
        354–361
    tubulopapillary neoplasm, 51, 54

Z

Zollinger-Ellison syndrome (ZES),
    347–349